A Textbook of

PANCHAKARMA

AF520711

A Textbook of PANCHAKARMA

According to the Latest Syllabus of CCIM, New Delhi

SECOND EDITION

Anup Jain MD Panchakarma
Assistant Professor
PG Department of Panchakarma
Chaudhary Brahm Prakash Ayurved Charak Sansthan
New Delhi, India

Foreword
HM Chandola

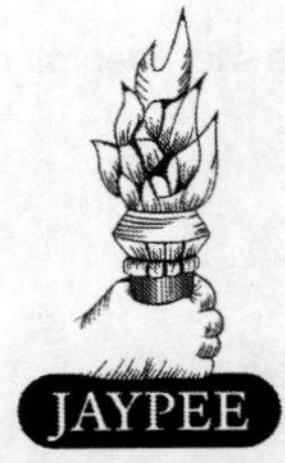

JAYPEE BROTHERS MEDICAL PUBLISHERS
The Health Sciences Publisher
New Delhi | London

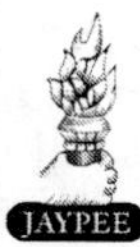

Jaypee Brothers Medical Publishers (P) Ltd

Headquarters
EMCA House
23/23-B, Ansari Road, Daryaganj
New Delhi 110 002, India
Landline: +91-11-23272143, +91-11-23272703
+91-11-23282021, +91-11-23245672
E-mail: jaypee@jaypeebrothers.com

Corporate Office
4838/24, Ansari Road, Daryaganj
New Delhi 110 002, India
Phone: +91-11-43574357
Fax: +91-11-43574314
E-mail: jaypee@jaypeebrothers.com

Overseas Office
J.P. Medical Ltd
83 Victoria Street, London
SW1H 0HW (UK)
Phone: +44 20 3170 8910
E-mail: info@jpmedpub.com

EU GPSR Authorised Representative
Logos Europe, 9 rue Nicolas Poussin
17000, La Rochelle, France
Phone: +33 (0) 6 67 93 73 78
E-mail: contact@logoseurope.eu

Website: www.jaypeebrothers.com
Website: www.jaypeedigital.com

© 2019, Jaypee Brothers Medical Publishers

The views and opinions expressed in this book are solely those of the original contributor(s)/author(s) and do not necessarily represent those of editor(s) of the book.

All rights reserved. No part of this publication may be reproduced, stored or transmitted in any form or by any means, electronic, mechanical, photocopying, recording or otherwise, without the prior permission in writing of the publishers.

All brand names and product names used in this book are trade names, service marks, trademarks or registered trademarks of their respective owners. The publisher is not associated with any product or vendor mentioned in this book.

Medical knowledge and practice change constantly. This book is designed to provide accurate, authoritative information about the subject matter in question. However, readers are advised to check the most current information available on procedures included and check information from the manufacturer of each product to be administered, to verify the recommended dose, formula, method and duration of administration, adverse effects and contraindications. It is the responsibility of the practitioner to take all appropriate safety precautions. Neither the publisher nor the author(s)/editor(s) assume any liability for any injury and/or damage to persons or property arising from or related to use of material in this book.

This book is sold on the understanding that the publisher is not engaged in providing professional medical services. If such advice or services are required, the services of a competent medical professional should be sought.

Every effort has been made where necessary to contact holders of copyright to obtain permission to reproduce copyright material. If any have been inadvertently overlooked, the publisher will be pleased to make the necessary arrangements at the first opportunity. The **CD/DVD-ROM** (if any) provided in the sealed envelope with this book is complimentary and free of cost. **Not meant for sale**.

Inquiries for bulk sales may be solicited at: jaypee@jaypeebrothers.com

A Textbook of Panchakarma

First Edition: 2016

Second Edition: **2019**

Reprint: **2026**

ISBN 978-93-5270-254-1

Printed at: Samrat Offset Pvt. Ltd.

Dedicated to

पूज्य दादाजी स्व. श्री दर्शन लाल जैन व
दादीजी स्व. श्रीमती शांति देवी जैन जी को समर्पित

My respected Grandfather Late Mr Darshan Lal Jain
and
Grandmother Late Mrs Shanti Devi Jain

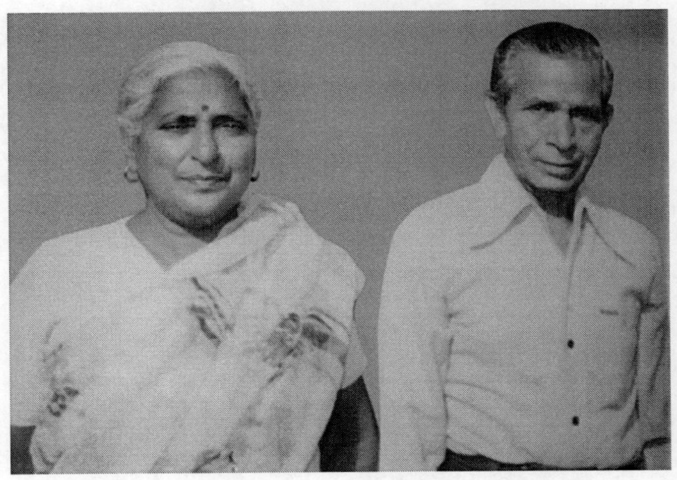

Foreword

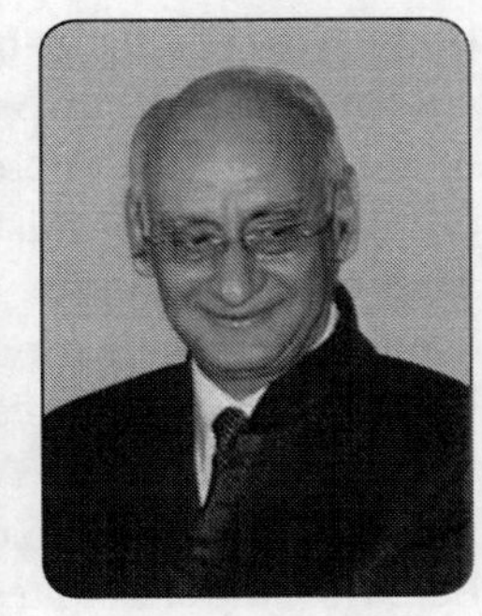

Panchakarma is a specialized branch of Ayurveda which has global acceptance by giving tremendous results through the biopurificatory and rejuvenating procedures. It is an integral part of Ayurvedic treatment to have body-mind healing experience by detoxifying the body, strengthening the immune system and restoring balance and well-being. It promotes detoxification and rejuvenation. It is recommended on a seasonal basis, as well as when an individual feels out of balance or is experiencing illness. Hence, it is beneficial not only for diseased but also for healthy individuals, as it focuses on prevention of diseases by purification therapies when Doshas are still in the stage of Sanchaya for accumulation and stagnation. It is highly individualized therapy based on the needs of the individual depending on the body constitution, doshic imbalances, age, digestive strength, immune status, etc. and disease condition. It removes the excess doshas and correct metabolic imbalances as well as eliminates the harmful Ama, the root cause for disease out of the body.

Normally, the body has the innate ability to efficiently process and remove these waste materials including vitiated doshas. However, due to dietary indiscretion, lack of physical activity, sedentary lifestyle, and genetic predisposition, the digestive enzymes, metabolic cofactors, hormones, and agnis which regulate the body's internal homeostasis become disorganized. This can lead to the accumulation and spread of toxins throughout the physiology resulting in disease. All the learned scholars of this Ancient Science of Life since beginning of the present era have highly appreciated the importance and therapeutic efficacy of *Panchakarma* speciality. The description of *Panchakarma* is found to be popular in Ayurvedic classics viz *Charak Samhita*, *Sushrut Samhita*, *Ashtang Hridayam*, *Ashtang Sangraha*, *Sharangdhara* and *Vangsena*, etc.

A Textbook of Panchakarma authored by Dr Anup Jain, Assistant Professor in *Panchakarma* at prestigious Chaudhary Brahm Prakash Ayurved Charak Sansthan—an autonomous institution under the Government of NCT of Delhi, who completed his Doctorate in Medicine with Ayurvedic *Panchakarma* specility from Bharati Vidyapeeth, Pune, is based on the latest syllabus by Central Council of Indian Medicine (CCIM). The book presents the classic description of the important aspects of the subject spread over nine different chapters dealing with Snehana, Svedana, Vamana, Virechana, Basti Karma, Nasya Karma, Raktamokshana, and Physiotherapy. The author has intensely worked for providing related textual references from Brihattrayi and Laghutrayi in running body of the book with abridged English version. All the chapters include photographs of the correct way to perform procedures and also the plants used in *Panchakarma* for ease of identification for the students. Many traditional therapies have been depicted with the help of line art and graphics so that the students can have a better idea of how the procedures should be performed.

The author has made great efforts by describing each therapy analytically and critically by using various Ayurvedic texts, contemporary theories for describing mode of action on scientific lines. It is a well-known fact that enteric nervous system (ENS) has same tissues as central nervous system (CNS) during fetal development. It has many structural and chemical similarities to the brain. Even when the vagal supply is severed, it continues to function because of its own nervous system and can operate autonomously, thus also called as Second brain. Thus, Basti does not just work at gastrointestinal tract (GIT) level but it works on the whole system of body. Now when gut-brain axis (GBA) theory is well established, mechanisms underlying GBA communications involve neuro-immuno-endocrine mediators. Gut microflora also contributes in gut-brain axis. There is a possibility of some neuro-immuno-endocrine process induced by administration of Basti and thus shows systemic therapeutic effect. Thus, it is a need of the hour to describe the valid basis for each and every indications of the each therapy through establishing their mode of action on scientific lines for their global acceptance. As such the book carries a rich reference manual on *Panchakarma*. Prima facie, it is an excellent addition to the contemporary Ayurvedic literature for English readers. In the end it includes about 250 questions in the form of MCQs, short answer questions and long answer questions, which will help the students to test their knowledge.

I hope that this textbook will serve as a ready reckoner document for undergraduates and postgraduate students, practitioners, academicians, research scholars of Ayurveda in general and *Panchakarma* in particular for precise and deeper understanding of the principles, concepts and practices of *Panchakarma* therapy.

Dr Anup Jain is an active, energetic and dynamic scholar with deep insight and vision. He possesses all qualities of a capable teacher, good researcher and skilled *Panchakarma* physician. He is known to me for several years while I rendered services at Chaudhary Brahm Prakash Ayurved Charak Sansthan as Director-Prinicipal. I appreciate his understanding of the subject and the painstaking efforts to compile this important text of Ayurveda. I congratulate the author for this brilliant scholarly work and wish that many more such useful books may come out from his talented brain and versatile pen for the benefit of Ancient Indian Wisdom-Ayurveda to make it Medicine of the Millennium.

HM Chandola
MD (Ay) PhD Dip Yoga PGDIPR (BHU)
Professor and Hospital Director
Uttaranchal Ayurvedic College, Dehradun
Formerly, Dean and HOD-IPGT and RA, Gujarat Ayurved University, Jamnagar
Ex-Director-Principal, Chaudhary Brahm Prakash Ayurved Charak Sansthan, New Delhi

Preface

Ayurveda is the oldest form of medical science and comprises of eight branches namely Kayachikitsa, Balroga, Graha, Urdhvanga or Shalakya tantra, Shalya tantra, Danshtra or Agada tantra, Jara or Rasayana, Vrishya or Vajitantra. Out of these, Kayachikitsa holds the best position as it deals with not only the treatments but also prevention of all the major ailments of a body and with promotion of health. *Panchakarma* is a specialized branch of Kayachikitsa which meets all these efficiently as it purifies the body of the doshas. As Charak says, doshas which are won over by the process of langhan pachana, etc. may get vitiated again, but when they are controlled/purified by sanshodhana, there is least chance of recurrence.

दोषाः कदाचित् कुप्यन्ति जिता लङ्घनपाचनैः। जिताः संशोधनैर्ये तु न तेषां पुनरुद्भवः॥

(Ch. Su. 16/20)

Panchakarma is a branch of Ayurveda which for long has been giving tremendous results in clinics and hospitals across the globe and is still growing strong. *Panchakarma* deals with an ailment at two levels, through sanshodhana, i.e. purification and also sanshamana, i.e. pacification. It is wrongly stated at times that *Panchakarma* is only for ailing and by purification procedures only; on the contrary, *Panchakarma* deals with not only the ailing but also serves the larger purpose of Ayurveda by establishing prevention of diseases and promotion of health. This book *A Textbook of Panchakarma* is an effort in the direction to comprise a detailed description of not only the Pradhana Karma but also the Purvakarma while keeping in mind the CCIM syllabus of Undergraduate and Postgraduate courses of *Panchakarma* in mind. The book details all the therapies along with the possible modern scientific correlation and mode of action according to Ayurveda and modern science to the best of my knowledge. It has been endeavored to keep the book in as simple language as possible and also to include all the aspects of Trividha Karma. I hope this book will benefit physicians and students alike who practice *Panchakarma* on concise theoretical as well as practical aspects of performing these procedures along with the photographs and computer line diagrams wherever necessary especially in the cases of Trayodasha Sagni Sveda which has not been tried by the authors earlier.

Sample questions in the form of MCQs, short answer questions and long answer questions have also been added to help the students prepare better for the exams and also to provide an insight into what kind of questions can be expected in not only the Undergraduate or Postgraduate examination but also in further exams. Efforts have been made to include all the aspects of each procedure in detail and to depict them with diagrams or photographs, and hope that it helps all those who read in gaining more knowledge about the subject. In the end, I would like to ask for suggestions and corrections in the book from all the readers.

Anup Jain

Acknowledgments

First and foremost, I am thankful to Lord Dhanvantari who imparted the knowledge of Ayurveda on earth and without whose blessings none of us would have been having the knowledge of this beautiful science. After Lord, teachers and gurus are the one who guide, shape and help a student to achieve the wisdom and blossom into a person they become. I desire to express my deep sense of gratitude and indebtedness to my teachers and gurus especially Vaidya Acharya Shri Tarachand Sharma, famous Ayurvedic Physician and author of many books, who has taught me over the years in the science of Ayurveda and also who keeps on inspiring me about authoring the knowledge we gain while we study and practice. Words cannot describe my gratitude towards Vaidya Shri Rasik S Pawaskar, famous Ayurvedic Physician, teacher and above all a wonderful human who took me under his wings fairly early while I was still doing my BAMS and helped me to understand the theoretical and practical aspects of Ayurveda. I express my gratitude towards my respected teachers especially Prof (Dr) SM Vedpathak, Dr Santosh Chavan, and Dr Pravin Sawant in PG Department of Panchakarma, College of Ayurved, Bharati Vidyapeeth, Pune, for all the support and knowledge I gained under their guidance.

Nothing can be achieved without the support of family and blessings of the parents, and I take this opportunity to express my deepest gratitude towards my parents Smt Sharda and Sh Rakesh Kumar Jain, who always inspire me to become better everyday and for their unconditional love. It would be pertinent to express my adoration towards my wife, Dr Namita Jain, Physiotherapist by profession and who has also helped with suggestions, especially on the parts related to Physiotherapy and Massage therapy and also for being so supportive.

Words are not sufficient to describe my gratitude towards management of my Institute, Chaudhary Brahm Prakash Ayurved Charak Sansthan, New Delhi, India. I also wish to acknowledge the contribution of my colleagues Dr Subash Sahu, HOD and Dr Monica, Assistant Professor of Dravyaguna department, CBPACS for the help provided in compiling the photographs of all the plants used in the *Panchakarma*. I am thankful to Professor Arun Gupta, HOD Panchakarma at CBPACS, New Delhi, who has always been supportive during all the works and also comes up with various ideas for the development of Panchakarma as a field. Also, this book would not be complete without thanking my postgraduate students who have helped in proofreading and corrections of the manuscript, especially Dr Pooja, Dr Vishal, Dr Pragati, Dr Divya, Dr Richa, and Dr Pankaj.

My sincere gratitude to Shri Jitendar P Vij (Group Chairman), Mr Ankit Vij (Managing Director), Mr MS Mani (Group President), Ms Ritu Sharma (Director-Content Strategy), Ms Sunita Katla (Executive Assistant to Group Chairman and Publishing Manager), Ms Pooja Bhandari (Production Head), Ms Samina Khan (Executive Assistant to Director-Content Strategy), Dr Pinky Chauhan (Development Editor), Ms Seema Dogra (Cover Visualizer), Mr Deep Kumar (DTP Operator), Ms Ritika Ahuja (Proofreader), Mr Ram Kumar (Graphic Designer), and their team members, for all their support and work on this project and make it a success. Without their cooperation, I could not have completed this project.

Contents

CHAPTER 1

Introduction

INTRODUCTION TO PANCHAKARMA

Panchakarma is a specialized branch of Ayurveda, which deals with both the aspects of ayurvedic treatment which are purification as well as pacification of the tridosha, viz. Vata, Pitta and Kapha; bringing the body to a state of Sama dosha (normal health). It is effective in physical as well as mental disorders.

Among Ashtanga Ayurveda, Kayachikitsa stands first and it has been considered the branch dealing with sarvanga sanshrita vyadhis. Also, it is convenient to say that for all Kayachikitsa sadhya conditions, Panchakarma is considered as the best method for treatment. Therefore, it is not only a part of Kayachikitsa but also can be considered as a swatantra vigyana. Panchakarma treatment not only helps in radical elimination of the disease causing factors, it also helps in achieving equilibrium of doshas. Panchakarma is not just limited to only Kayachikitsa but through its various procedures and ability to cure all types of diseases, this branch has proven that it can help in all the eight branches of Ashtanga Ayurveda. Although, Panchakarma procedures have been discussed at length in the classical texts, still it has never been defined; however, Acharya Mukundi Lal Dwivedi along with Vaidya Tarachand Sharma defined it as under:

''स्नेहस्वेदादि द्वारा शरीरस्य उत्क्लिष्ट दोषाणां यथासन्न मार्गेण बहिर् निर्हरण कर्तुत्वं संशमनं कर्तुत्वं च पञ्चकर्मत्वम्। (Ayurvediya Panchakarma Vigyan)

Panchakarma is a procedure in which utklishta doshas are expelled out through the nearest route after Snehana and Svedana. It is followed by shamana therapy.

The word Panchakarma is made up from two separate words, i. e. "Pancha" and "Karma" –

'Pancha' meaning 'Five'

'Karma' meaning work done or treatment procedures

बहु इति कर्तव्यता योगि दोष निर्हरण शक्तिर् ज्यायस्त्वम्। (Ch. Su. 2/15 Teeka)

Here Pancha is sankhya pradhana and karma refers to the procedure which has multi-dimensional therapeutic effects and having the capacity to expel the Doshas in larger quantity. So, Panchakarma in essentiality means five purification procedures namely, Vamana, Virechana, Asthapana Basti, Anuvasana Basti and Nasya (Dalhana includes Raktamokshana as the fifth Karma after merging both types of Basti as one). The word Panchakarma is mostly used by Acharya Charaka; other Acharyas like Vagbhata and Sushruta have not put much emphasis on the word Panchakarma, although the commentators on these texts have used the term to elaborate the concepts. These are the procedures capable of removing vitiated Doshas in bulk quantity, and are hence given importance as the five important modalities of treatment.

तानि उपस्थित दोषाणां स्नेह स्वेदोपपादनैः। पञ्चकर्माणि कुर्वीत मात्राकालौ विचारयन्॥ (Ch. Su. 2/15)
चक्रपाणिटीका: ''उपस्थित दोषाणाम् इति शाखां त्यक्त्वा कोष्ठ आगमनेन तथा लीनत्व परित्यागेन प्रधानावस्था प्राप्त दोषाणाम् इति।'' (Ch. Su. 2/15 teeka)

After attaining Upasthita doshavastha by Snehana and Svedana, Panchakarma should be done by considering proper Matra and Kala. Here Chakrapani says that, Upasthita Dosha means:

- The doshas which have left the Shakha and are moving towards Koshtha.
- The doshas which have lost leenatva (deep seated or sthana sanshraya).
- Pradhana avastha – Have attained the qualities to be expelled.

Concept of Chikitsa

Ayurveda emphasizes on three folds therapeutic management of the diseases, viz. Sanshodhana (purification), Sanshamana (pacification) and Nidana Parivarjana (avoiding causative factors).

संशोधन संशमन निदानस्य च वर्जनम्। एतावद्भिषजा कार्य रोगे-रोगे यथाविधि॥ (Ch.Vi.7/30)

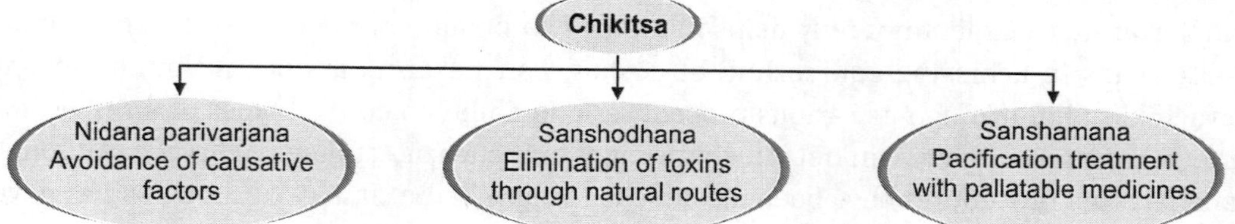

What is Sanshodhana Therapy?

यदीरयेद्बहिर्दोषान् पञ्चधा शोधनं च यत् ॥ (A. H. Su. 14/6)

Shanshodhana or shodhana therapy is the procedure or upakrama which helps in removal of the vitiated or vikara of dosha, dhatu and mala, etc. from the body. It is of five types.

Panchakarma or Sanshodhana is one of the important therapies of Ayurveda which deals mainly with elimination of the aggravated Doshas from the body. These Doshas (toxins and waste material) should be eliminated from natural as well as nearest route of the body.

This Sanshodhana therapy consists of a number of Physico-Physiologic measures advocated in the treatment of the diseases. It is divided into three major parts, viz. Purva Karma (Preparatory methods like Oleation and Fomentation), Pradhana Karma (Main Sanshodhana measures) and Pashchata Karma (Post-therapy regimen). The Pradhana Karma should always be preceded by suitable Purva Karmas in order to mobilize the Doshas from the discrete parts of the body (Shakha). It is believed that imbalanced Doshas spread from the Koshtha to the Shakha and thus are able to produce various types of diseases depending upon the Dosha Dushya-Adishthana pattern.

Now, before going in detail of subject some question related to the topic should be analyzed such as:

What is Panchakarma?
Why there is only five karmas (procedures) included not more or less than that?
What is its utility in achieving healthy life?
What is its field of action or where it is applicable?

What is Panchakarma?

Panchakarma is made of two words, i.e. Pancha + Karma.

Karma : Kri Dhatu + Manin Pratyaya + Adhadarchadi Sutra + Karma + Karya.

The work done by the subject is known as karma. Here subject refers to Physician and Karma refers to treatment procedure. The thing to be done for work is known as Karma. Its synonyms are Karma, Kriya, Yatna, Karya Samarambha. This procedure of doing work is known as "Pratikarma Samarambha". Karma and Pratikarma both denotes Chikitsa, i.e. treatment.

Acharya Sushruta uses Kriya word for Karma and divided into Chhedanadi karma and Snehanadi karma. Further Acharya Dalhana opines that this Snehanadi word comprises of following procedures namely Snehana, Svedana, Vamana, Virechana, Asthapana, Anuvasana, Dhupana, Nasya, Kavala, Gandusha and Deepana-Pachanadi Sanshamana Karma.

Thus the procedure of treatment is known as Karma. According to Ayurveda "Dhatusamaya Kriya is Chikitsa" i.e. the procedure that brings normalcy of vitiated Dhatu and prevent their further vitiation is called Chikitsa or Karma. It will be worthful to mentioned here that Dhatu in the above context refers to vitiated Doshas.

Why only Five Karma are Included in Panchakarma Not More or Less Than That?

Pancha: In Ayurveda there is numerical description of subjects such as Pancha Mahabhuta, Tridosha, Sapta Dhatu, etc. Similarly in the description of diseases also details are given with their symbolic numerical description as 8 Udara roga, 5 Shvasa roga, 4 Grahani roga, etc. There is no logic behind choosing any number and it is only the knowledge of the subject gained by the 4 Pramana (though extensive exploration of the subject by mean of different scientific tools) on the basis of which it can be said that there are Panchakarmas.

The term Panchakarma is mainly used by Acharya Charaka. Acharya Sushruta and Vagbhatta did not give much importance to the word. Although commentators like Dalhana, Arundutta and Hemadri used the word at many places in their explanation.

There are numerous references from Charaka Chikitsa Sthana for the word Panchakarma. "Karmbhivamanadibhi" is line of management for Apasmara roga. In Unmada Chikitsa also he directed the use of Vamanadi Karma and in Urustambha the use of Panchakarma is contraindicated. In Siddhi sthana the second chapter entitled as "Panchakarma Siddhi" whereas first chapter starts with the heading of "का कल्पना पच्चसु कर्मसूक्ता".

As said above that Acharya Sushruta and Vagbhata had not given much emphasis on this word and at very few places the word is used. In Madhumeha treatment Acharya Sushruta recommends the use of Sanshamana therapy in those who are not curable by Panchakarma. Dalhana while commenting on the above clarifies that word Panchakarma signifies three meaning :

1. Vamanadi Panchakarma: Including Vamana, Virechana, Basti, Nasya and Raktamokshana.
2. Using Sanshamana: Abhyanga, use of Guggulu, use of Shilajit and Sanshodhana as five karma.
3. Using the treatment for Rasagata Vyadhi, Raktagata Vyadhi, Mansagata Vyadhi, Medogata Vyadhi and Purva karma comprises five karmas.

Acharya Vagbhatta uses the word Panchakarma in chapter "Siravyadhavidhi" and while commenting Arundutta clarifies that it consists of five procedures namely—Vamana, Virechana, Niruha, Anuvasana and Nasya.

Which Karma are Included in Panchakarma

As directed by Acharya Charaka that it comprises five procedures of purification which are:

1. Vamana
2. Virechana
3. Niruha basti
4. Anuvasana basti
5. Shirovirechana/Nasya.

Acharya Sharangdhara and Bhavaprakasha have the same opinion. According to Acharya Sushruta there are three main procedures Purva karma, Pradhana karma and Pashchat karma. According to Dalhana there may be three possible way to explain this as follows :

1. Procedure from Langhana up to Virechana (Langhana, Pachana, Deepan, Snehana, Svedana, Vamana and Virechana) are included under Purva karma and Ropana, Patanadi, karma are taken under the heading of Pradhana karma whereas measures used to enhance the Bala, Varna and Agni are known as Pashchata karma.
2. At the different stages of Kriyakala (Six stages in the pathogenesis of disease). The procedure employed before Roga-utpatti, i.e. manifestation of disease is purva karma; treatment given after manifestation of diseases is Pradhana karma and treatment modality used to prevent relapses and complications are included under Pashchata karma.
3. Pachana, Snehana and Svedana used before Shodhana karma are included under Purva karma; Vamana, Virechana, Basti, Nasya and Siramokshana are Pradhana karma and using Sansarjana krama by Peya, Vilepi, Yushadi, etc. is Pashchata karma.

A point of conflict occurs when including Raktamokshana among five procedures. Acharya Charaka has not included Raktamokshana in Panchakarma whereas Acharya Dalhana and Vagbhatta included it. The reason behind this may be the difference in field of speciality. As Sushruta is Shalya pradhana tantra it focuses more on surgical procedures and that may be the reason of his acceptance Rakta as a fourth Dosha. Thus to remove vitiated Rakta by its nearest route the only way is Raktamokshana. Importance of Raktamokshana in Shalyatantra can be understood by the fact that Sushruta told Raktamokshana as "Chikitsa-ardhanga" and it enjoys the same position as by Basti in Kayachikitsa. Acharya Charaka also accepts the fact that vitiated Pitta cause vitiation of Rakta due to their dependence on each other (Ashraya-ashrayi bhava). And Vidhah cannot occur without vitiated Rakta thus to disrupt the pathogenesis the only way is to remove vitiated Rakta by its nearest route, i.e. Raktamokshana (Ch. Chi. 5/37). So it can be concluded that Raktamokshana should be included under Panchakarma.

Panchakarma according to different Acharya			
Charaka	*Sushruta*	*Dalhana*	*Sharangdhara/ Bhavaprakasha*
Vamana	Vamana	Vamana	Vamana
Virechana	Virechana	Virechana	Virechana
Asthapana	Asthapana	Basti	Asthapana
Anuvasana	Anuvasana	Shiro Virechana	Anuvasana
Shiro Virechana	Shiro Virechana	Raktamokshana	Shiro Virechana

PANCHAKARMA AND SHODHANA

Panchakarma is not only meant for shodhana, but is also a measure for Langhana, Brihana, Lekhana and Shamana. It is a Vyapaka chikitsa (pervades many areas) and is a great measure to attain all types of phala shrutis (benefits).

यद् इर्येद् बहिर् दोषान् पञ्चधा शोधनं च तत्। निरुहो वमनं कायशिरोरेको अस्रविस्रुतिः॥

(A.H.Su. 14/5)

शोधनं यत् कुपितान् दोषान् निःसार्य बहिः रोगोपशमनं करोति। (A.S.Su. 1/37 Indu teeka)

Procedure for evacuation of Prakupita Doshas (aggravated doshas) from the body for the purpose of Roga upashamana (pacifying disease) is known as Shodhana. Vagbhatta named 5 types of Shodhana popularly known as Pancha Shodhanas, viz., Vamana, Niruha, Kaya vireka, Shiro vireka, Asra visruti.

Doshanusara Shodhana

वमयेत् श्लेष्म रोगांञ्च पैत्तिकाश्च विरेचयेत्। निरूहयेद् वातरोगान् रक्तजांञ्च अवसेचयेत्॥

(Bhe.Su. 5/19)

Vamana – Shleshma Nirharanartha in Shlaishmika roga
Virechana – Pitta Nirharanartha in Paittika roga
Basti – Vata Shodhanartha in Vatika roga
Raktaavasechana – Rakta Shodhanartha in Raktaja vyadhi

IMPORTANCE OF PANCHAKARMA

The importance of Panchakarma can be studied under following headings:

1. Panchakarma in Svastha (Preventive Measure)
2. Rasayanadi Asadharana Guna Prapti (Promotive Purpose)
3. Roganusara Panchakarma. (Curative purpose)

Panchakarma in Svastha

मलापहं रोगहरं बलवर्ण प्रसादनम्। पीत्वा संशोधनं काले सम्यक् आयुषा युज्यते चिरम्॥

(Ch.Su. 15/22)

If Shodhana is administered properly, then it expels out the vitiated Doshas (toxins), pacifies the disease and increases Strength and Varna of the person.

Here Panchakarma can be performed as a Dinacharya, Ritucharya and as a treatment measure for all types of Vegavarodhajanya Vyadhis (diseases occurring due to retention of natural urges).

Panchakarma in Dinacharya

Snehana, Abhayanga, Shiro Abhyanga, Nasya, Karnapurana, Shiropichu, Udvartana, Matra Basti, etc. comes under Panchakarma and can be done daily for Swasthya Rakshanartha in Svastha (for the purpose of maintaining and promoting health).

Panchakarma in Ritucharya

Ritu	*Panchakarma indicated*
Hemanta ritu (Margashira and Pausha—November to January)	• Abhyanga, Utsadana, Murdhni taila, Jentaka sveda, Ushna sadana, Atapa Sveda
Vasanta ritu (Chaitra and Vaishakha Masa (March to May)	• As there is a kapha prakopa, Vamana in Kaphotklesha condition • Virechana in Pitta Sansrishta kapha • Nasya for Kapha jayartha • Virechana, Asthapana, Anuvasana in Vata Pitta Prakopavastha
Sharada ritu (Ashwini and Kartika Masa (September to November)	As there is Pitta Prakopa, Tikta Ghritapana, Virechana, Rakta mokshana are to be carried out during this season
Shishira ritu (Magha and Phalguna Masa (January to March)	Hemanta samana vidhi (same procedures as followed in Hemanta ritu)
Varsha ritu (Shravana and Bhadrapada Masa (July to September)	As there is a Vata Prakopa-Basti is indicated

Rasayanadi Asadharana Guna Prapti

Panchakarma has got a great importance as purva karma for Swastasya Urjaskara Chikitsa.

ना अविशुद्ध शरीरस्य युक्तो रासायनोविधिः। न भाति वाससि क्लिष्टे रंगयोग इवाहिः।। (Su.Chi.27/4)

Acharyas have highlighted that; Shodhana of Shareera is an essential pre-requisite for the administration of Rasayana therapy. Because, if Srotasa, are not clean then Rasayana effect will not be achieved to the maximum extent-just as unclean cloth does not take up the color. Hence, if Shodhana is administered before Rasayana, it will help in cleaning all the Srotasas of the body and thus this helps in getting maximum benefits from the Rasayana.

बुद्धि प्रसादं बलम् इन्द्रियाणं धातु स्थिरत्वं ज्वलनस्य दीप्तिम्।
चिरात् च पाकं वयसः करोति संशोधनं सम्यग् उपास्य मानम्।। (A.H.Su. 18/60)

Shodhana helps in the proper attainment of Rasayana effect by Srotoshodhana (cleansing the channels) and provides Buddhi and Indriya prasada (clarity of intellect and sense organs), Dhatu sthiratva (stability of body tissues), Agnidipana (increase in digestive power). This leads to Chirat vayasa paka that is, delayed process of aging.

Roganusara Panchakarma (Curative Purpose)

रोगाः सर्वेऽपि मन्देऽग्नौ.........। (A.H.Ni.12/1)

Mandagni is the cause for all disease. For correction of Agni, Panchakarma is the best treatment.

एवं विशुद्ध कोष्ठस्य कायाग्नेराभिवर्धते। व्याधयश्च उपशाम्यन्ति प्रकृतिश्च अनुवर्तते।
इन्द्रियाणि मनो बुद्धिर् वर्णश्च अस्य प्रसीदति। बलं पुष्टिर् अपत्यं च वृषताचास्य जायते।
जरां कृच्छ्रेण लभते चिरंजीवत्यनामयः। तस्मात् संशोधनं काले युक्ति युक्तं पिबेत् नरः॥

(Ch.Su. 16/17)

Acharya Charaka has highlighted the following benefits of Panchakarma in the 16th chapter of Sutrasthana, i.e., Chikitsa Prabhrutiya Adhyaya. He says that once the Koshtha of a person becomes clean after Shodhana, then the person will achieve.

- Agni vriddhi – increase in the digestive capacity
- Vyadhi upashanti – diminution in the severity of diseases
- Prakriti anuvartate – there will be normalcy in all the components of body
- Increase in the strength and sexual potency
- Delayed process of aging
- The person live a long life without any diseases.

IMPORTANCE OF PANCHAKARMA/SANSHODHANA

भगवन् पंचकर्माणि समस्तानि पृथक तथा। निर्दिष्टान्यामयानां हि सर्वेषामेव भेषजम्॥
...........अस्त्यूरुतम्भ इत्युक्ते गुरुणा तस्य कारणम्॥ (Ch.Chi.27/5-6,7)

The morbid Doshas subdued by Langhana and Pachana may sometimes be again evoked, but in the case of those which are purified by Sanshodhana, there is no possibility of such recurrences.

If the root cause of a disease is not eradicated, it reappears like the saplings reoccur if we do not cut a plant from the root completely.

To show the importance of Shodhana therapy, Charaka has mentioned in the context of Vajikarana (Ch. Chi. 2/1/50-51) that, as dirty clothes can not take up the color properly, likewise the medicines given to the body without Shodhana therapy do not serve the purpose. Therefore medicines should be given only after proper Shodhana (i.e. biopurification by Panchakarma therapy) of the body.

This Shodhana therapy also form a part in the regimen of Svasthavritta (i.e. preventive medicine) indicated as prophylactic measures in the context of epidemics and pandemics. Besides the application in the treatment of disease, they are also stated as preparatory measures before institution of Surgery and also before administration of Rasayana (Rejuvenation therapy) and Vajikarana therapy and in Kshetrikarana treatment (Before internal administration of Medicinal preparation).

In this way the Shodhana or Panchakarma therapy is not merely a therapeutic regime but also a management of the individual which improves the body resistance and thereby checks the pathogenesis of the disease confirming its promotive and preservative effects of normal health. Thus, Panchakarma therapy has a direct reference to both the healthy as well as the ailing.

Benefits of Sanshodhana

Judiciously and timely performed Sanshodhana will increase the Agni, relieaves from suffering diseases and restore the state of homeostasis. Sense, mind, intellect and complexion will be clear, increases strength, facilitates the conception, delays the aging and person will live for a longer time without diseases.

मलापहं रोगहरं बलवर्णप्रसादनम्। पीत्वा संशोधन सम्यगायुज्ञा युज्यते चिरम्।। (Ch.Su.15/22)

One acquires long life by properly performing the Bio-cleansing treatment that cleanses one from impurities, relieves from disease and restores vitality and complexion.

Charaka Explained the Benefits of Shodhana Therapy as Follows

''दोषाः कदाचित् कुप्यन्ति जिता लंघन पाचनैः। जिताः संशोधनैर्ये तु न तेषां पुनरुद्भवः।।

(Ch.Su. 16/20)

The Dosha's which are pacified by Shodhana never reoccur but those pacified by Langhana-Pachana may reoccur. By Shodhana, the dosha's will be detached from their root. By this, the chances of establishment of disease is nil.

TRIVIDHA KARMA

There are mainly 3 types of Karma's explained in the classics. These are done in order to achieve Samyaka Shodhana, and for Prakriti stapanartha (getting back to normalcy).

त्रिविधिं कर्मं पूर्वकर्मं प्रधान कर्मं पश्चात् कर्मं इति। (Su.Su.5/3)

पाचनैः दीपनेः स्नेहैः तान् स्वेदैः च परिष्कृतान्। शोधयेत् शोधनैः काले यथासन्नं यथा बलम्।।

(A.H.Su.13/30)

संशोध्यस्य पाचन स्नेहन स्वेदनानि पूर्वकर्मं, वमन विरेचन बस्ति नस्य सिरामोक्षणानि प्रधानं कर्मं, पेयादि अन्न संसर्जनं पश्चात् कर्मः। (Su.Su.5/3 Dalhana)

Purva karma	*Pradhana karma*	*Pashchat karma*
Deepana and Pachana	Vamana	Sansarjana krama
Snehana	Virechana	Tarpanadi krama
Svedana	Basti	Shamana/ Rasayan
	Nasya	
	Raktamokshana	

Purva karma

Deepana and Pachana

Deepana

दीपनः दीपनीयं वह्लेरुध् दीपनाय हितम। (Ch.Su.4. Gangadhara)

Deepana drugs are those which are capable of performing stimulation of Jatharagni.

पचेत् न आमं वह्नि कृच्च दीपनं तद् यथा मिशि। (Sha.Pu.4)

According to Sharangadhara, drugs having deepana karma do not digest the Ama but increases Agni. For example, Mishi, Deepana drugs helps in separation of dosha from dhatus. (A.H.Su 13/29 Hemadri).

Accordingly—Deepaniya drugs may also perform Pachana action sometimes. This may be the reason for not mentioning Pachaniya dashaimani in Charaka.

Drugs

1. Dipaniya gana. Ch. Su. 4/9
2. Guduchyadi gana
3. Chaturjataka, Panchakola
4. Haritakyadi gana

These drugs act better on empty stomach. It improves Abhyavaharana shakti (increases quantity of food intake).

Pachana

These are the group of drugs which undertake the digestion of Ama alone without causing Agni deepana. These are useful in conditions like Ajeerna, Grahani, Amavata, Agni mandya, etc. they increase Jarana shakti for example Mustadi gana.

Importance of Deepana and Pachana

Before expulsion of Doshas from the body, it is mandatory for the Doshas to be in a Pakva state (ripened state). This process of transformation of morbid doshas from their unripened state to ripened state is achieved by pachana chikitsa.

Snehana and Svedana

स्नेहन् अग्रे प्रयुञ्जीत ततः स्वेदम् अनन्तरम्।
स्नेह स्वेद उपपन्नस्य संशोधनम् अथेतरत्।। (Ch. Su. 13/99)

Snehana and Svedana are the major preoperative procedure to be performed before Shodhana. The entire procedure depends upon the proper mobilization of doshas from Shakha to Koshtha. This is achieved with the help of Snehana and Svedana.

Snehana

स्नेहनं स्नेह विष्यन्दं मार्दव क्लेद कारकम्। (Ch.Su.22/11)
स्नेहो अनिलं हन्ति मृदु करोति देहं मलानां विनिहन्ति सङ्गं।। (Ch.Si. 1/7)

Snehana is the procedure which imparts Snigdhata (unctuousness), causes Vishyandana of Doshas (melting of Dosha's) and imparts Mardavata (Softness) and Kledata (moisture) to the body. Snehana means oleation therapy; the therapy which provides the body with Snigdhata as well as makes the vitiated doshas easily expellable from the body.

Svedana

स्तम्भ गौरव शीतघ्नं स्वेदनं स्वेदकारकम्। (Ch.Su. 22/11)

स्निग्धस्य सुक्ष्मेषु अयनेषु लीनं स्वेदस्तु दोषं नयति द्रवत्वं। (Ch.Si.1/8)

Svedana is a procedure which relieves Stambha (stiffness), Gaurava (heaviness), Sheeta (coldness) from the body and induces sweating. Svedana means Sudation therapy, which helps to liquefy the vitiated doshas that have spread throughout the micro-channels of body.

Importance of Purva Karma

पाचनैः दीपनैः स्नेहैः तान् स्वेदैः च परिष्कृतान्। शोधयेत् शोधनैः काले यथा सन्नं यथा बलम्।।

(A.H.Su.13/29)

पाचनैः पक्वत्म्। दीपनैर् धातुभ्यः पृथक्त्वं। स्नेहैर् उत्क्लिष्टत्व। स्वेदैः कोष्ठगतत्वं।।

(A.H.Su.13/30 Hemadri teeka)

After Deepana, Pachana, Snehana and Svedana, dosha should be expelled from the nearest route at a proper time according to the strength of Roga and Rogi. Hemadri, commenting on this, says that Pachana does ripening of Ama, Deepana does the separation of dosha from dhatu, Snehana does Uthkleshana of dosha and Svedana brings the Dosha from Shakhas to Koshtha.

स्निग्ध स्विन्नस्य भैषज्यैर् दोषैर् तु उत्क्लेशितो बलात्। निलीयते न मार्गेषु स्निग्धे भाण्ड इवोदकम्।।

(Su. Chi. 33/40)

स्निग्धात् पात्राद् यथा तोयम् अयत्नेन प्रणुध्यते। कफादयः प्रणुध्यन्ते स्निग्धाद् देहात् तथा औषधैः

(Ch. Si. 6/11)

Just like in a vessel smeared with oil, water escapes without sticking to the vessel, similarly, Kapha and other morbid doshas will be expelled out easily from a body which has undergone Snehana and Svedana.

आर्द्रं काष्ठं यथा वह्निर् विष्यन्दयति सर्वतः। तथा स्निग्धस्य वै दोषान् स्वेदो विष्यन्दयेत् स्थिरान्।।

(Ch. Si. 6/12)

As fire makes the water in moist wood trickle out from each and every pore, similarly Svedana causes the adhered doshas to melt and flow out from the body in a person who has undergone Snehana priorly.

स्नेह स्वेदाव अनभ्यस्य यस्तु संशोधनं पिबेत्। दारु शुष्कमिवान् आमे देहस्तस्य विशीर्यते।।

(Su. Chi. 33/46)

If, Sanshodhana is given without undergoing Snehana and Svedana then it may destroy the body. Here Acharyas have given an example that if we try to bend a dried wood then it will break. In the same way, if Shodhana is administered without mobilization of Doshas, then the body will get destroyed.

Importance of Purva karma in Pancha Karma Therapy

Probable mechanism of Snehana and Svedana in expelling out the Doshas:

- ❑ Lipid soluble drugs diffuse by dissolving in the lipoidal matrix of the membrane, the rate of transport being proportional to lipid : water partition coefficient of the drug. A more lipid soluble drug attain higher concentration in the membrane and diffuse quickly. (K.D.T., Medical Pharmacology, 4th edition, P.N.11).

- As temperature increases, (externally by sudation) both the cell membrane and the proteins can be affected. The fatty acid tails of the phospholipid bilayer can "melt"at high temperatures meaning that they become more fluid and allow more movement. This affects the permeability of the cell which increases permeability.
- The osmotic pressure of a solution may be calculated from Van't Hoff's Law : P = iRTc

Where 'i' is the number of ions formed by dissociation, R the ideal gas constant, T the absolute temperature and c the molar concentration. Thus osmotic pressure directly depends upon temperature.

Heat is expected to enhance the body fluid circulation, blood vessel wall permeability, rate-limiting permeability, and drug solubility. According to Kligman, diffusion is a temperature-dependent process, so raising the skin temperature should add thermodynamic drive. Heat is known to increase the kinetic energy of both the drug molecules and the proteins, lipids, and carbohydrates in the cell membrane. Heating prior to or during topical application of a drug will dilate penetration pathways in the skin, increase kinetic energy and the movement of particles in the treated area, and facilitate drug absorption. Heating the skin after the topical application of a drug will increase drug absorption into the vascular network, enhancing the systemic delivery but decreasing the local delivery as the drug molecules are carried away from the local delivery site. (The journal of applied research; Wade Hill. et.al.)

Knuston et al. recently investigated the mechanisms involved in temperature-enhanced skin permeability. Results indicated that the increased skin permeability of lipophilic drugs results from temperature-induced alteration of the lipid structure, which involves the disordered arrangement of the lipid bilayer structure and its fluidization. Further studies indicate that temperature changes of approximately 5°C are necessary to cause measurable changes in cell membrane permeability.

External heating induces changes in hemodynamics, body fluid volume, and blood flow distribution, which in turn affect the pharmacokinetics or bioavailability of administered drug. The body's initial response to heat is peripheral vasodilation followed by perspiration, which results in a large fraction of the total blood volume being circulated through the skin vessels for cooling.

Diaphoresis, or sweating, is one of the Six Hygienic Purification Methods of Greek Medicine. It cleanses the blood by releasing toxins via the sweat.

Thus Snehana and Svedana helps in mobilizing the toxin from cell into circulation and then into GI tract for their easy expulsion. Therefore appropriate Purva karma in the form of Snehana and Svedana is always done before Pradhana karma.

Pradhana Karma

Pradhana karma includes Vamana, Virechana, Asthapana basti, Anuvasana basti and Nasya. After proper Purva karma is performed dosha's will be brought from Shakha to Koshtha so that they may be easily expelled from the nearest route.

Vamana

Vamana is defined as "A process by which malas (Dosha) are eliminated through the upper chanels, i.e. mouth". Chakrapani mentions that the Urdhvabhaga should be considered as Urdhvamukha. Vamana karma, the first measure amongst Panchakarma, has been considered as the best line of treatment for Kaphaja disorders.

Virechana

Virechana is the procedure by which the orally administered drug acts on internally situated doshas, specifically on pitta dosha and expels them out of the body through anal route (Adhobhaga). Virechana is the prime modality of treatment for pitta dosha nirharana. Amashaya is considered as Samanya sthana for Pitta and Kapha doshas, Virechana holds good for both.

Basti

Vata is responsible for the dislodgement or combination of Vit, Mutra, Pitta and Kapha. Hence any malfunction in the body is caused by vata dosha and Basti is the prime line of treatment for vata dosha. None of the treatment modalities are as effective as Basti chikitsa for mitigation of vata dosha. Hence, it is considered as Ardha chikitsa.

Nasya

Nasya karma which is one among the Panchakarma has got an important role in the management of 'Urdhva Jatrugata Vikaras'. Medicine administered through the nose spreads throughout the Shiras and helps in the evacuation of Dosha and thereby pacifying the diseases.

Raktamokshana

Removing vitiated blood from body (blood letting) is known as Raktamokshana. It is of six types :

1. Shringa
2. Alabu
3. Sirahmokshana
4. Jalaukavacharana
5. Pracchana
6. Ghatiyantra

It helpes in raktaja and pitta pradhan roga.

Pashchata Karma

Pashchata karmas are the procedures and set of rules and regulations which are to be carried out after performing Shodhana. These play a very important role in protecting and increasing Agni gradually. Thereby these procedures aid in bringing back body to normalcy. This mainly includes Sansarjana krama.

Peyadi Sansarjana Krama

वमितश्च विरिक्तश्च मन्दाग्निश्च विलङ्घितः। अग्नि प्राण विवृद्ध्यर्थं क्रमं पेयादिकं भजेत्॥

(Ch.Si. 6/57)

Peyadi Sansarjana krama is advised to those who have undergone Vamana, Virechana, Mandagni purusha and Vilanghitha for Agni sandhukshana. (Increasing the agni)

अग्नि संधुक्षणार्थं तु पूर्वं पेयादिना भिषक्। रसोत्तरेण उपचरेत् क्रमेण क्रमकोविदः॥ (Ch.Si.12/6)

After Vamanadi sanshodhana karma jatharagni should be made strong by giving Peya first and Mansarasa at last.

Classification of Sansarjana Krama

- ❑ Peyadi sansarjana krama
- ❑ Tarpanadi sansarjana krama
- ❑ Rasa sansarjana krama

Order of Peyadi Sansarjana Krama

पेयां विलेपीम् अकृतं कृतं च यूषं रसं त्रिर्द्विर् अथैकशश्च।
क्रमेण सेवेत विशुद्ध कायः प्रधान मध्य अवर शुद्धि शुद्धः॥ (Ch.Si. 1/11)

Acharya Charaka has advised duration of Sansarjana krama based on the number of vegas. Sansarjana krama starts with Peya followed by Vilepi, Akrita yusha, Krita yusha, Akrita rasa, Krita rasa and normal food at last. The duration of Sansarjana krama depends on the level of Shuddhi achieved. According to Ayurveda, there are 2 annakala's in a day.

According to Shuddhi

Type of shuddhi	*Anna kala (1 anna kala-meal time)*	*Duration*
Pradhana shuddhi	3	7 days
Madhyama shuddhi	2	5 days
Avara shuddhi	1	3 days

According to the Quantity of Eliminated Dosha

Acharya Sushruta have advised the duration of Sansarjana krama based on the quantity of Hritadosha (eliminated Dosha).

- ❑ One prastha (avara)- 1 annakala each of Peya, Manda, Vilepi, Odana, Mansarasa.
- ❑ Half adhaka (madhyama)- 2 annakala each of Peya, Manda, Vilepi, Odana, Mansarasa.
- ❑ One adhaka (uttama)- 3 annakala each of Peya, Manda, Vilepi, Odana, Mansarasa (Su. Chi. 39/6-7)

Sushruta has also considered other factors such as vaya, bala and agni for advising Sansarjana krama. There are basically 3 types of Bala.

According to Bala

Pravara	–	1 Annakala
Madhyama	–	2 Annakala
Avara	–	3 Annakala (Su.Chi. 39/17-18)

Peya

Rice is cooked by adding fourteen times of water and boiled till rice is almost dissolved to become liquid and that is known as Peya.

पेया सिक्थ युता सिद्धा चतुर्दश गुणे अम्भसि। (Kai. De. Ni. Kritannavarga 44)

Properties of Shali

Rasa	–	Madhura
Guna	–	Snigdha
Veerya	–	Sheeta
Paka	–	Laghu
Doshaghnata	–	Pittaghna

Peya Guna

पेया लघ्वी हिता ग्लानि पिपासा क्षुत् श्रम प्रणुत्। स्तम्भ अतिसार दौर्बल्य कुक्षिरोग ज्वरापहा।।
दीपनी पाचनी दोष मल स्वेद अनुलोमनी। (Kai. De. Ni. Kritannavarga 45)

Peya is Laghu, good for health, removes tiredness, Pipasa (Thirst), Kshut (Hunger), Shrama (tiredness) and stiffness.

It is good in conditions like Atisara (Diarrhea), Daurbalya (weakness), Kukshi -roga (disease of GI-tract), and Jvara (Fever).

It is Deepana (increases digestive power), Pachana (digests toxins) and Anulomaka (helps in downward movement of Vata).

Vilepi

Rice is cooked by adding four times of water till it becomes semi-liquid. This is termed as Vilepi.

विलेपी घन सिक्था स्यात् सिद्ध तोये चतुर्गुणे। (Kai. De. Ni. Kritannavarga)

Vilepi Guna

विलेपी दीपनी हृद्या ग्राहिणी क्षुत् तृषापहा। लघ्वी स्वादुरसा नित्यं स्नेहनाय उपयोगिनी।।
बल्या संतर्पणी पथ्या व्रण शुक्र अक्षि रोगिणे। (Kai.De.Ni. Kritannavarga.43)

Vilepi is Agni deepaka (increases digestive capacity), Hridya (good for heart) and Grahi. It removes Kshut (Hunger) and Trishna (thrist). It is Laghu (light in digestion), Madhura (sweet in taste), good during Snehana, Balya (strengthening) and Santarpana (nourishing) in nature.

Yusha

Eighteen times of water is added to any one of the pulses (shimbi dhanya) and is cooked properly so that it contains more liquid and less of solid. When it is taken as such without adding anything, it is termed as Akrita Yusha, but when added with Saindhava Lavana, Shunti, Pippali, etc. Katu dravyas along with Sneha then it is named as Krita Yusha.

Types : There are two types of yusha:

1. Akrita yusha
2. Krita yusha

अष्टादश गुणे तोये श्रृतो यूषस्तु शिम्बिजैः। सः स्यात् कृताख्यो लवण कटु स्नेहादि संयुतः॥
अकृताख्य स्तद् रहितः क्रमाद् गुरुलघु मतौ। (Kai. De. Ni. Kritannavarga 62-63)

Properties of Mudga

Rasa	–	Madhura
Guna	–	Laghu, Ruksha
Veerya	–	Sheeta
Doshaghnata	–	Kapha-Pitta hara
Other karma	–	Jvaraghna, Chakshushya

Yusha Guna (Mudga Yusha)

मुद्गानाम् उत्तमो यूषो दीपनः शीतलो लघु। व्रणो उर्ध्वजत्रु रुक् दाह कफ पित ज्वर अस्रजित्।
(Kai. De. Ni. Kritannavarga 64)

Mudga Yusha is Uttama (best) among Yusha preparations. It is Deepana (increases digestive capacity), Sheetala (cold), Laghu (easily digestible), good in Vrama (would), Juara dehn Urdhva jatru vikaras (diseases occurring above sternoclavicular joint), Kapha Pitta and rakh vitiated conditions.

Mansa Rasa

Cleaned meat is cut into small pieces and a soup is prepared by adding water and cooking it properly. When it is taken as such, without adding anything. It is termed as Akrita Mansa Rasa. But, preparing the same by adding Saindhava, Shunti, Pippali, etc. Katu dravya along with Sneha dravyas- is known as Krita Mansa rasa.

रसे साध्यं जलं देयं मांस सिध्यति यावत्। पलाष्टकम् जले प्रस्थे घनेऽथ मध्यमेतुषट्॥
मांसस्यवंटनं कुर्यात् कूडवं तनुके रसे। (Dra. Gu. Vi)

Types

Two types :

1. Akrita Mansa rasa
2. Krita Mansa rasa

Properties of Aja Mansa

त्रिदोषघ्नं गुरु पीनस नाशनं। लघुपाकं नाति शीतं नाति स्निग्धं अदाहिच॥
शरीर धातु सामान्याद् अनभिष्यन्दि बृंहणम्। (Kai. De. Ni. Kritannavarga)

Tridoshaghna (mitigates all the 3 dosha's), Guru, Peenasa nashana (helps in curing running nose), easily digestible, not too Sheeta (cold) in Veerya, not too Snigdha (Unctous), does not cause Daha (burning sensation), good for Dhatus (body tissues), not Abhishyandi (does not increase secretions in body), Brihana (increases bulk of body).

Tarpanadi Sansarjana Krama

कफ पित्ताधिकान् मद्यनित्यान् हीन विशोधितान्। पेय अभिष्यन्दयेत् तेषां तर्पणादि क्रमो हितः॥

(Su.Chi. 39/13)

Tarpanadi Krama is advised in the following conditions :

- In heena vishodhitha (not undergone proper purification)
- Kapha pitta predominance
- Madya nitya (cosumption of alcohol daily)

कफपित्ते विशुद्धेऽल्पं मद्यपे वात पैत्तिके। तर्पणादि क्रमं कुर्यात् पेया अभिष्यन्दयेद्धितान्॥

(Ch.Si.6/25)

Tarpanadi krama is indicated if Kapha and Pitta are partially expelled due to Ayoga of Shodhana karma, in Madyapa (one who consumes alcohol daily) and Vata pitta predominant conditions. Peya due to its Abhishyandi guna (increasing secretion in body) will cause Srothorodha (obstruction to body channels).

In the above conditions, instead of Peya-Svachcha Tarpana (light) and instead of Vilepi-Ghana Tarpana (thick) are advised. This is followed by Yusha-Akrita and Krita and Mansa rasa-Akrita and Krita.

Svaccha Tarpana Preparation: 1 part of Laja (parched rice) cooked in 14 parts of water.
Ghana tarpana: 1 part of Laja (parched rice) cooked in 4 parts of water.

Properties of Laja

Rasa—Kashaya, Madhura, Guna—Laghu, Veerya—Sheeta

Rasa Sansarjana krama

संसर्गेण विवृद्धे अग्नौ दोषकोप भयाद् भजेत्। (Su.Chi. 39/19)

After Sansarjana Krama, Agni is to be increased. To avoid dosha kopa due to increased agni, Rasa Sansarjana krama is to be followed.

Order of Rasa Sansarjana

स्निग्धाम्ल स्वादु हृद्यानि ततो अम्ल लवणौ रसौ। स्वादु तिक्तौ ततो भूयः कषाय कटुकौ ततः॥
अन्योन्य प्रत्यनीकानां रसानां स्निग्ध रूक्षयोः। व्यत्यासाद् उपयोगेन प्रकृतिं गमयेद् भिषक्॥

(Ch.Si.12/7-8)

Rasa Used	*Action*
Snigdha (Unctuous), Amla (Sour), Madhura (Sweet) and Hridya (good to heart)	To alleviate Vata
Amla and lavana	Agni sandhukshanartha
Madhura and tikta	To alleviate Pitta
Kashaya and katu	To alleviate Kapha

Rasa	Example of food items
Madhura	Guda, Sita, Ripened fruits, etc.
Amla	Dadima, Chincha, etc.
Lavana	Saindava lavana, etc.
Katu	Maricha, Shunthi, etc.
Tikta	Nimba, Methika, etc.
Kashaya	Hareetaki, Vibhitaki, etc.

Complications if Sansarjana krama is not followed :
Agni mandya, Ama, Ajeerna, Dhatukshaya and Durbalta are the conesquences as complications if correct Sansarjana krama is not followed. Sansarjana is very important for the gradual increment of Agni (Digestive activity).

Benefits of Sansarjana Krama

यथा अणुर् अग्निस्तृण गोमयाद्यैः संधुक्ष्यमाणो भवति क्रमेण।
महान् स्थिरः सर्व पचस् तथैव शुद्धस्य पेयादिभिर् अन्तरग्निः॥ (Ch.Si.1/12)

Following are the benefits which can be achieved through proper Sansarjana krama:

Just as small flame of fire gets ignited by addition of Trina (dry grass), Gomaya (Dry cow dung), etc., in the same way Agni which has become Manda due to Shodhana will get increased by Sansarjana krama. Agni of a person after Sansarjana krama will achieve the following qualities :

Agni becomes	
Mahan	Strong
Sthira	Stable
Sarva pachati	Capacity to digest any kind of food

Diet Regimen Based on Shuddhi

Meal time	Hina Shuddhi	Madhya Shuddhi	Pravara Shuddhi
1st	Peya	Peya	Peya
2nd	Vilepi	Peya	Peya
3rd	Krita Yusha	Vilepi	Peya
4th	Krita Mansa Rasa	Vilepi	Vilepi
5th	Routine diet	Akrita Yusha	Vilepi
6th	—	Krita Yusha	Vilepi
7th	—	Akrita Mansa Rasa	Akrita Yusha
8th	—	Krita Mansa Rasa	Krita Yusha
9th	—	Routine diet	Krita Yusha
10th	—	—	Akrita Mansa Rasa
11th	—	—	Krita Mansa Rasa
12th	—	—	Krita Mansa Rasa
13th	—	—	Routine diet

Also, it is seen these days that sometimes patients complain about having a feeling of hunger before the next annakala and paricharaka and vaidya often get in a fix over what to do in this condition. It is advisable to repeat the same diet of Sansarjana krama prescribed in that annakala, e.g. if a patient is advised to take Peya in 1st annakala of second day after uttama shuddhi and is complaining of hunger before evening, they shall be given Peya again.

Similarly, another doubt arises for the patients who are vegetarians and are not giving consent for intake of Mansa rasa, in those cases yusha can be extended as Akrita - 3 annakala and Krita - 3 annakala if required in Pradhana shuddhi, or Krishra (with higher water content) can be used instead of Mansarasa.

It is also said that after completion of the Sansarjana krama a wise vaidya should advise the patient for rasabhyasa krama under which initially hridya, snigdha dravya which are madhur and amla in rasa shall be given followed by madhur and tikta rasa shall be given and in the end Kashaya and katu rasa shall be given. This helps in the patient to get accustomed to his usual diet.

1. **Shamana chikitsa after Shodhana:** Only after completion of sansarjana krama, shamana aushada can be planned.
2. **Rasyanadi karma:** When Shodhana is used as Purva karma for Rasyana then after Pradhana karma, Rasyana drug should be given.
3. **Shamana yoga:** When Shodhana Chikitsa is used as a part of treatment for a particular disease then the specific medicine for it should be given.

INDICATORS OF SHODHANA

1. Before administration of Rasayana and Vajeekarana Aushadha yoga.
2. बहु दोषाणां पुनर्दोष अवसेचनम् एव कार्यं। अविपाको अरुचिः स्थौल्य पाण्डुता गौरवं क्लमः॥
   पिडका कोठ कण्डूनां संभवो अरतिरेव च। आलस्य श्रम दौर्बल्यं दौर्गन्ध्यं अवसादकः॥
   श्लेष्म पित्त समुत्क्लेषो निद्रानाशो अतिनिद्रता। तन्द्रा क्लैब्य अबुद्धित्वम् अशस्तस्वप्नदर्शनं॥
   बलवर्ण प्रणाशश्च तृप्यतो बृंहणैरपि। बहुदोषस्य लिङ्गानि तस्मै संशोधनं हितं॥
   ऊर्ध्वं च एव अनुलोमं च यथा दोषं यथा बलम्॥ (Ch.Su.16/13-16)

   Shodhana is indicated in Bahudoshavastha. Bahudoshavastha is characterized by symptoms such as Avipaka (improper digestion), Aruchi (Tastelessness), Sthaulya (Obesity), Panduta (Anemia), Gaurava (Heaviness), Klama (tiredness without doing any work), Pidaka (various skin eruptions), Kandu (itching), etc.
3. Before administration of Rasa Aushadhi, Shamana yoga, Surgery (e.g. Ashmari).
4. क्रमाद् अपाम् अपि मणौ पङ्को अवश्यं भवति। उत्तिष्ठेत यथाकालं मलानां शोधनं प्रति॥

   (A.S.Su. 5/22)

   Vaghbhatta has advised Shodhana for prevention of seasonal diseases. He gives an example that even though a Mani (gem) stays in clean water, after sometime there will be gradual deposition of Panka (sediment) over it. In the same way even though person stays healthy, there is a seasonal deposition of some amount of Dosha's which may lead to diseases in future. To prevent these diseases, it is very important to undergo Shodhana according to the seasons.

5. तत्र चयपूर्वकं कोपम् आगताः संशोधन विधानेन् एव शमयितव्या। (Su.Chi.33/3.Dalhana)

   Dalhana said that Shodhana should be performed in Chayapurva-Prakopa Avastha. This means that there is a gradual deposition of Doshas.

6. तत्र संशोधनैः स्थौल्य बल पित्त कफ अधिकान्। आम दोष ज्वर च्छर्दि अतीसार हृदामयैः।
   विबन्ध गौरव उद्गार हृल्लास आदिभिर् आतुरान्॥ (A.H.Su.14/12-13)

   According to Vagbhatta, Shodhana is indicated in Sthaulya, aggravated Pitta and Kapha conditions, Ama dosha, Jvara, Cchardi, Atisara, Hridroga, Vibhandha, Gourava, Udgara and Hrillasa.

Shodhana According to Ritu

Ritu	*Shodhana indicated*
Vasanta	Vamana
Varsha	Basti
Sharad	Virechana, Raktamokshana

GENERAL PRINCIPLES OF DOSHAGATI

There are mainly 2 types of doshagatis which are important in the context of Shodhana. They are:

1. Movement of doshas from Koshtha to Shakha
2. Movement of doshas from Shakha to Koshtha.

Movement of Doshas From Koshtha to Shakha

व्यायामाद् ऊष्मात् तैक्ष्ण्यात् हितस्य अनावचारणात्। कोष्ठात् शाखा मलायान्ति द्रुतत्वान्मारुतस्य च॥
(Ch.Su.28/31-32)

Vyayama (exercise), Ushma (heat) and Teekshna (penetrating) dravya sevana, Ahita or Atimatra sevana (consumption of unhealthy articles in excessive quantity), Maruta Drutatva (Vitiation of Vata) are the causes for movement of Dosha from Koshtha to Shakha.

- ❑ While describing the concept of movement of dosha's from Koshtha to Shakha; Chakrapani comments that:
- ❑ Vyayama causes Kshobha to mala/ morbid dosha's accumulated in koshtha which forces them to move out towards shakha
- ❑ Ushma and Tikshna guna help in making Agni to become tikshna, which in turn causes vilayana of koshthashrita dosha and they move out towards shakha
- ❑ Hitasya anavcharnata means following ahita, ahara and vihara. This leads to aggravation of Dosha's in large quantities, which leads them to move out from there sthana and achieve prasaravastha (moving out from there sthana to shakha).
- ❑ Drutatvat marutasya cha means, aggravation of Vata due to its causative factors and the morbid dosha's are then thrown out of koshtha to shakha by this aggravated Vata.

Movement of Doshas From Shakha to Koshtha

वृद्ध्यात् विष्यन्दनात् पाकात् स्रोतोमुख विशोधनात्। शाखा मुक्त्वा मलाः कोष्ठं यान्ति वायोश्च निग्रहात्।। (Ch.Su.28/33)

Vriddhi (excessive increase of dosha), Vishyanadana (Liquification of dosha), Paka (Digestion of dosha), Srotomukha vishodhana (Cleaning of openings of Channels), Vayu nigrahat (Controlling of vayu) are the factors responsible for movement of dosha from Shakha to Koshtha which will be carried out by Purva karma of Shodhana.

While describing the concept of movement of dosha's from Shakha to Koshtha; Chakrapani comments that:

- Vriddhi means increase in volume of dosha in shakha; which results in them getting detached, which in turn initiates the movement of dosha's to koshtha
- Vishyandan means vilayan or liquification of dosha's, these liquefied dosha then naturally move towards Koshtha which is Nimna (at lower level of gravity)
- Pakat means the Dosha which were initially sama in nature, achieve niramavastha and leads to Abaddhata or dislodgement of Dosha from Shakha and these dosha then naturally move towards Koshtha which is Nimna
- Srotomukha vishodhana means removal of Margavrodha and Vayur nigrahana means pacification of aggravated vata which initially pushed the morbid doshas out of the koshtha, which in turn facilitates the natural return of the doshas to the Koshtha.

Actions	*Achieved by*
Vriddhi and Vishyandana	Snehana and Svedana
Paka	Pachana and Svedana
Srotomukha Vishodhana	Svedana
Vayoshcha nigrahat	Snehana and Svedana

GENERAL PRECAUTIONS DURING PANCHAKARMA (PARIHARYA VISHAYAS)

Dietetic and behavioral restrictions which are to be observed before, during and after the course of Panchakarma therapy are together called as Pariharya Vishaya.

Precautions During Snehapana

द्रवम् उष्णं अनभिष्यन्दि भोज्यम् अन्नं प्रमाणतः। नातिस्निग्धं असंकिर्णं श्वः स्नेह पातुमिच्छता।। (Ch.Su.13/60)

Before Snehapana, use of Drava (liquid articles), Ushna (hot articles), Anabhisyandi (does not increasing secretions), not Atisnigdha (which is not too unctuous), Asankeerna (not veerya virudda, not opposite in nature), Agnivardhaka Ahara (that which increase digestive activity) is advised. Also, it is advised that the Ahara shall be in right quantity.

उष्णोदक उपचारि स्यात् ब्रह्मचारी क्षपाशयः। शकृत् मूत्र अनिल उद्गार अनुदीर्णाश्च न धारयेत्॥
व्यायाम् उच्चैर् वचनं क्रोध शोकौ हिमातपौ। वर्जयेद् अप्रवातं च सेवेत शयनासनं॥
स्नेहं पीत्वा नरः स्नेहं प्रतिभुञ्जान् एव च। स्नेह मिथ्योपचाराद्धि जायन्ते दारुणा गदाः॥

(Ch.Su.13/62-64)

After administration of Snehapana, Ushnodakpana (consumption of hot water) is advised as it helps in the digestion of Sneha. After the sneha is digested Ushna Yavagu, Sugandhi Sneharahit Yusha, Mansarasa or Alpa Ghritayukta Vilepi should be taken as pathya; as it helps to avoid the various complications that might arise in Snehapana such as Bhrama, Trishna, Alasya, etc.

Brahmacharya (observing celibacy), Kshapashaya (sleeping only during night) and Shayanasana in Apravata Sthana (staying inside non-ventilated room) are the pathya viharas to be followed in Snehapana as it helps in the maintenance of balance of the Tridoshas.

Vegadharana and Vegodeerana, Vyayama, Uchchairvachana, Hima Atapa, Krodha and Shoka should be avoided as they are the prominent causes of complications in Snehapana.

Precautions During Svedana

स्निग्धः स्वदैर् उपक्रम्य स्विन्नः पथ्याशनो भवेत्। तदहः स्विन्नगात्रस्तु व्यायामं वर्जयेत् नरः॥

(Ch.Su. 14/67)

During Svedana, Anabhisyandi Ahara should be consumed. In addition to the said Pathyas, Shanai Shanai Mardana (repeated pressing of muscular parts), Ushna Jala Snana, covering the body with clothes and stay in Nivata Sthana is advised as Pathya Vihara; as it helps in controlling Vata which, in long run prevents complications due to Svedana. Similarly Vyayama should be avoided during Svedana.

Regimens to be Followed During Pradhana Karma

Vamana

Before Vamana, Kaphotkleshakara Ahara such as Mansa or Mansarasa of Gramya, Anupa or Audaka Pashu, Pakshi, along with Ksheera, Dadhi, Masha and Tila is to be taken for proper Utkleshana of Kapha dosha.

In Vihara, Bahya Snehana and Svedana karma is to be done for proper movement of the doshas from Shakha to Koshtha. After the completion of Vamana, Sansarjana krama is an important aspect to be followed which is dependent on the level of Shuddhi attained.

Virechana

For proper Virechana, Laghu Bhojana, Amla Phala Rasa, Snigdha, Drava, Ushma ahara and Jangala Mansarasa is advised to be taken as Pathya. Laghu Bhojana, Amla phala Rasa, Ushna Udaka will help to alleviate Pitta Dosha and will help in Kapha avajayartha, further in the Vishramakala, Bahya Snehana and Svedana should be done for proper mobilization of Doshas from Shakha to Koshtha. After Virechana Sansarjana krama is advised as Pathya for achieving results from Virechana and is dependent on the level of shuddhi attained.

Basti

In Basti, Mansa Rasa is preferably used as Pathya in Vata based disorders whereas use of Ksheera in Pitta based disorders is found to be beneficial. Further, Yusha is pathya in Kapha based disorders. Before the administration of Anuvasana basti, Laghu ahara should be taken according to dosha.

Nasya

Mainly Ushna ahara and vihara are advised during Nasya karma. Ushna Ahara and Vihara will help to check both Vata and Kapha. Since, Nasya is the preferred modality of treatment for Urdhavajatrugata Vikaras and Urdhava jatru is the seat of Kapha, both Kapha and Vata should be equally tackled. Ushna upachara will help to balance the same. Shira snana (head bath) is to be avoided.

Raktamokshana

After bloodletting, intake of foods and drinks which are neither too hot or too cold, light and stimulants of digestion are recommended. Exercise, sexual intercourse, cold bath, day sleep, exposure to breeze, food having Kshara, Amla, Katu Rasa and Shoka should be avoided till the body gets normal strength.

Ashta Mahadoshakara Bhava

उच्चैर् भाष्यं रथक्षोभम् अतिचन्क्रमण आसने। अजीर्ण अहित भोज्ये च दिवास्वप्नं समैथुनम्॥

(Ch.Si.12/11)

The Ashta Mahadoshakara bhavas are the eight factors which are apathya (to be avoided) during any process of Shodhana. These factors are Uchchabhashana (speaking loudly), Rathakshobha (excessive travelling), Atichankramana (excessive walking), Atyasana (prolonged sitting), Ajeerna (indigestion) or Adhyashana (consumption of food prior to digestion of previous meals), Divaswapna (Day sleep), Ahitabhojana (eating unhealthy food) and Maithuna (Coitus).

Uchcha Bhashya

Speaking loudly leads to Shirastapa (raise of temperature in head region), Shankha Karna Nistoda (pain in temples and ears), Srotorodha (blocking of channels), Mukha, Talu and Kantha Shosha (dryness of mouth, tongue and throat), Timira (eye disease), Pipasa (excessive thirst), Jvara (fever), Tamaka (Asthma), Hanugraha (stiffness of temperomandibular joint), Manyastambha (stiffness in cervical region), Nishtheevana (excessive spitting), Ura Parshwa Shula (pain in head and flanks), Swara Bheda (hoarseness of voice), Hikka (hiccup) and Shvasa (dyspnea).

Chikitsa

Administration of Abhyanga, Svedana, Upanaha, Dhuma, Nasya, Snehapana (Snehapana after food), Mansa Rasa, Ksheera, and other Vatahara Chikitsa.

Ratha Kshobha

Excessive traveling leads to Sandhi Parshwa Shaithilya (loosening of joints and flanks), Hanu, Nasika Karna, Shira, Shula and Toda (pain and pricking sensation in maxillary joint, nose, ears and head region) Kukshi Kshobha (difficulty in abdominal region), Atopa (increased bowel sounds), Antra Kujana, Aadhmana (distension of abdomen), Hridayendriyoparodha, (blocking in hridya and indriya), Vedana in Sphik, Parshwa, Vankshana, Vrishana, Kati and Prishtha, Daurbalya in Sandhi, skandha and greeva, Anga Abhitapa, Pada Shopha and Harshana.

Ati Chankramana

May lead to Shula (pain) in Paada, Jangha, Uru, Janu, Vankshana, Shroni, Prishtha, Sakthi, Pindikodweshtana, Anga Marda, Anga Abhitapa, Sira Dhamani Harsha, Shvasa, Kasa.

Atyasana

Leads to Vedana in Sphik, Parshwa, Vankshana, Vrishana, Kati Prishtha.

Chikitsa

Snehana, Svedadi Vatahara Karma, Nidana Varjana.

Ajeerna and Adhyashana

Mukha Shosha, Adhmana, Shula, Nistoda, Pipasa, Gatra Sada, Cchardi, Atisara, Murccha, Jvara Pravahana, Amavisha.

Chikitsa

Niravashesha, Cchardana, Ruksha Svedana, Langhaniya, Pachaniya and Deepaniya Aushadhavacharana.

Vishama and Ahita Bhojana

Leads to Anannabhilasha, Daurbalya, Vaivarnya, Gatrasada, Grahani and Arsha due to Vatadi Dosha Prakopa.

Chikitsa

Dosha Pratyanika Chikitsa.

Divaswapna

Leads to Arochaka, Avipaka, Agnimandya, Staimitya, Kandu, Pama, Daha, Cchardi, Angamarda, Hritstambha, Jadya, Tandra, Atinidra, Granthi, Daurbalya, Talu Lepa.

Chikitsa

Dhumpana, Langhana, Vamana, Shirovirechana, Vyayama, Ruksha Ahara, Arishta, Deepaniya Aushadha Pragharshana, Unmardana, Parishechana and Shlesmahara Chikitsa.

Maithuna

Leads to Aashubalanasha, Shula in Shira, Basti, Guda, Medhra, Vankshana, Uru, Janu, Jangha, Pada Hridaya Spandana, Netra Peeda, Shukra Marga Shonita Gamana, Kasa, Shvasa, Shonita Shtheevana.

Chikitsa

Jeevaniya Siddha Ksheera, Sarpi, Vatahara Sveda and Abhyanga, Upanaha, Vrishya Ahara, Vatahara Snehapana, Yapana and Anuvasana Basti.

SPECIFICATIONS OF PANCHAKARMA THEATER AND NECESSARY EQUIPMENT

Panchakarma Setup

स उदपान उदूखल मुसल वर्चः स्थान स्नानभूमि महानसन्। (Ch.Su. 15/6)

The setup should contain a water tank, kitchen, grinder, pestle, attached bathroom and toilet, and separate rooms for ladies and gents. The measurement of each therapy room should be minimum of 10×10 ft.

वास्तुविद्याकुशलः प्रशस्तं गृहमेव तावत् पूर्वम् उपकल्पयेत्। (Ch.Su. 15/6)

An expert architect should design a good as well as a strong building.

Location

अनुपत्यकं धूम आतप जल रजसाम् अमन अभिगमनीयम्। (Ch.Su. 15/6)

The building should be built in such a place which is away from mountains, it should be big and devoid of dust, smoke, sun and water.

Space

सुखविचारम्।

The room should be spacious so that one can carry out all activities comfortably.

Ventilation

निवातम् और प्रवातैकदेशम्

The room should have enough air ventilation but devoid of pravata and proper light.

Wall and Floor

Anti-skid floor with tiles having grip, light colored walls preferably tiled up to 7 ft. height, water outlet facility, exhaust fan and chimney.

Water supply: Hot and cold separately.

Sound: Calm atmosphere.

Interior decoration: Simple paintings on the roof, in-built cupboards, room fragrance, rubber/ cotton mat on the floor etc.

Waste disposal: Separate waste disposal system for solids and liquids preferably following the BMW guidelines.

Specifications of a Panchakarma Center

Infrastructure of Panchakarma Theater Room (Fig. 1.1)

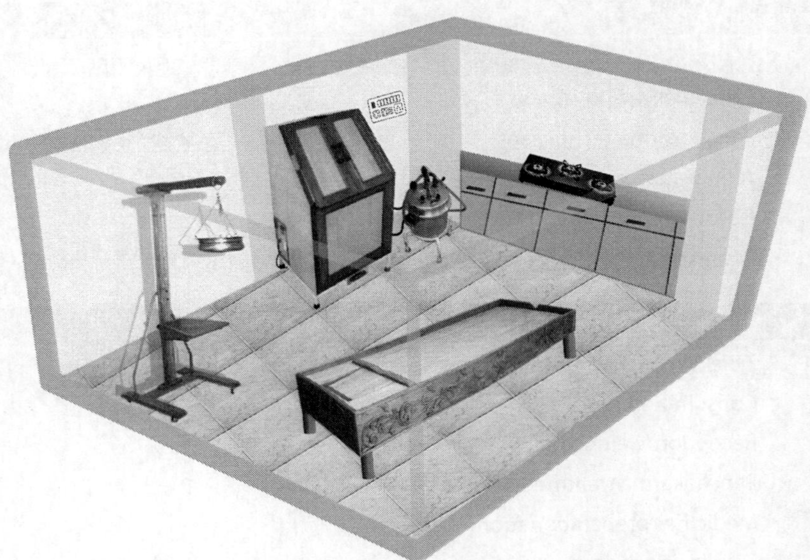

Fig. 1.1: Panchakarma theater

Ancient View

In Charaka Samhita Sutrasthana 15th chapter Upakalpaniyadhayaya there is an explanation of setup of a hospital.

- First of all an expert architect should design good building.
- The building should be strong and it should not be exposed to direct wind.
- It should be constructed so as to allow wind only through the passage.
- It should provide comfortable moving place.
- The building should not be situated in a mountain place nor should it be located near a big building.
- Besides, the building should not be exposed to smoke, sun, water, dust or undesirable noise nor it should have undesirable contacts, taste, sight or smell.
- The building should be well equipped with a water reservoir or water pot, mortar, pestle, latrine, bathroom and kitchen.
- The requirements enumerated above are meant for both the therapy and any complication in the course of the administration of the therapy as well as management of the patients afterwards.

Various Requirements of Panchakarma Speciality Center

Guidelines for establishing standard Panchakarma center with minimum requirements.

Man power requirement		
S. No.	*Man power*	*Requirement*
1.	Panchakarma physician	2
2.	Panchakarma technicians	4
3.	Admin staff	1
4.	House keeping staff	2
5.	Pharmacist	1

Infrastructure requirements		
S. No.	*Type of rooms*	*Requirement*
1.	Consultation room	1
2.	Reception/waiting hall	1
3.	Panchakarma treatment rooms	2
4.	Medicines preparation room	1
5.	Dispensing room	1
6.	Store room	1
7.	Bath room	2
8.	After panchakarma rest room	1

- ❑ At least one treatment room should be attached with bathroom which are well furnished.
- ❑ One room should be with multipurpose treatment tables for the administration or abhyanga, pinda sveda, nadi sveda, basti karma, etc.

Miscellaneous Requirements

- ❑ Daily supply of fresh medicinal leaves for treatment or as the requirements patras like eranda, nirgundi, arka, dhatura, karanja, nimba, etc.
- ❑ Office stationary, computer, racks, tables, chairs, stool, telephone, posters, etc.
- ❑ Essential furniture in all rooms
- ❑ Double top stools 2′ × 2′ × 3′
- ❑ Cot with bed in rest room
- ❑ Floor should be non-slippery
- ❑ Apart from general equipment and tools required in an ayurvedic setup the therapy section of the center should have following equipment:
  - Face steamer
  - Rubber catheter
  - Uterine cannula

- IV drip set
- Electric heating apparatus or other heating device

- Medicines used in the center should be of good quality and from reputed firms and duly labelled.

Qualities of Panchakarma Technician

- Qualified
- Dedicated
- Honest
- Well dressed
- Apron
- Well behaved
- Hygiene

Essential Equipment

Snehana

Various types of Panchakarma tables are available namely abhyang table, shirodhara table, droni, multipurpose Panchakarma table (Figs 1.2A to D). They are made of various materials as under:

- Fiber glass/wooden
- Movable/fixed
- Single piece/double piece
- Medicinal wood (kupeelu) with brass support
- Droni stand: Tilting type steel table – with lever or handle wheel, height of the stand may be adjustable.

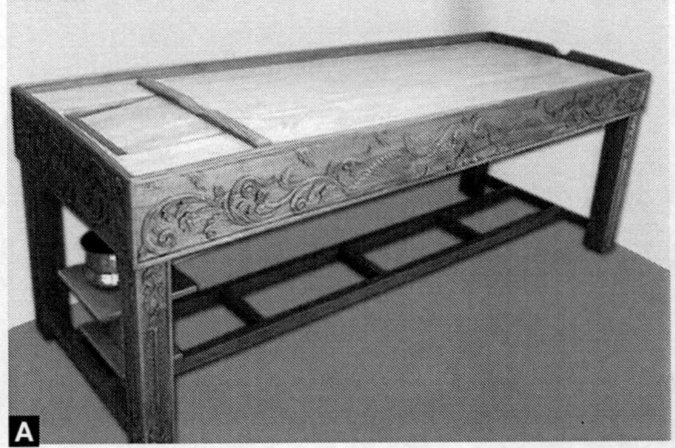

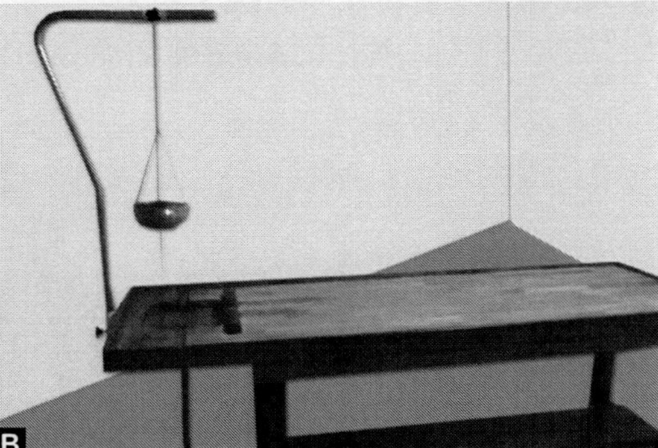

Figs 1.2A and B

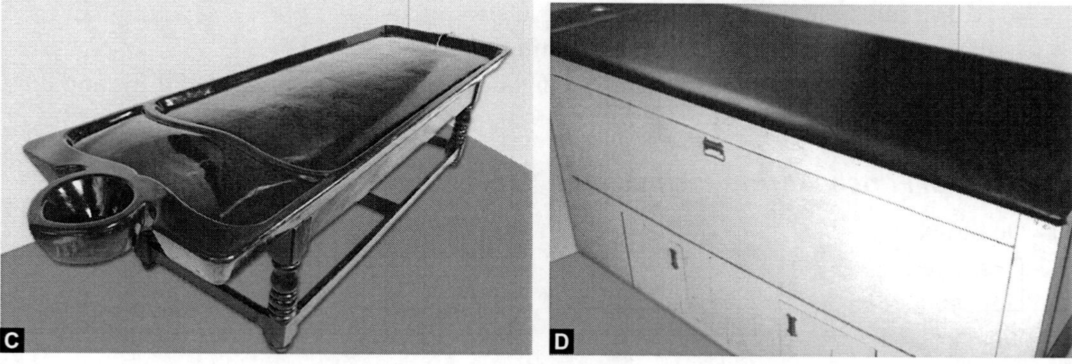

Figs 1.2C and D

Figs 1.2A to D: Various types of Panchakarma tables

Svedana Karma (Figs 1.3 to 1.5)

- Steam chamber : Sitting – 6 feet × 3 feet × 2.5 feet
  Lying – 7 feet × 3 feet
- Pressure cooker and flexible tube, Dhara sveda, bath tub for Avagaha Sveda, Kindhi.

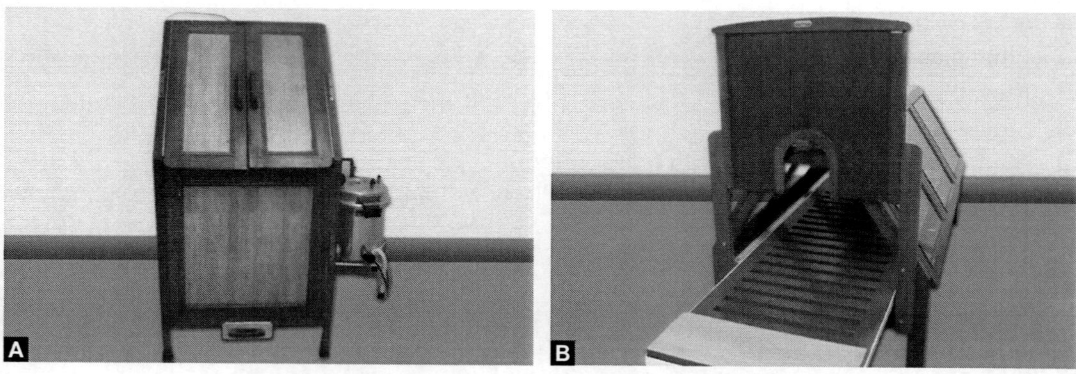

Figs 1.3A and B: Sitting and laying down types of Svedana box

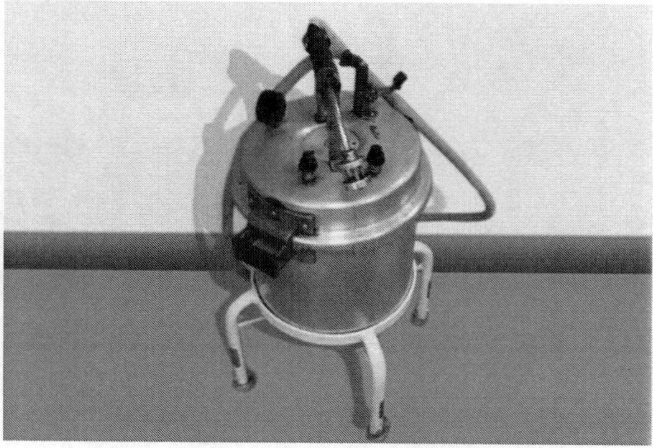

Fig. 1.4: Nadi Svedana yantra

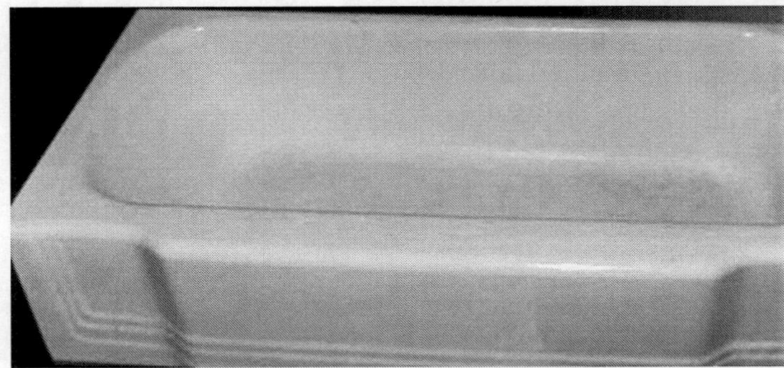

Fig. 1.5: Avgaha Svedana yantra

Vamana Karma (Fig. 1.6)

Comfortable knee high chair for relaxing with hand support, vomiting tray and stand with measuring vessel.

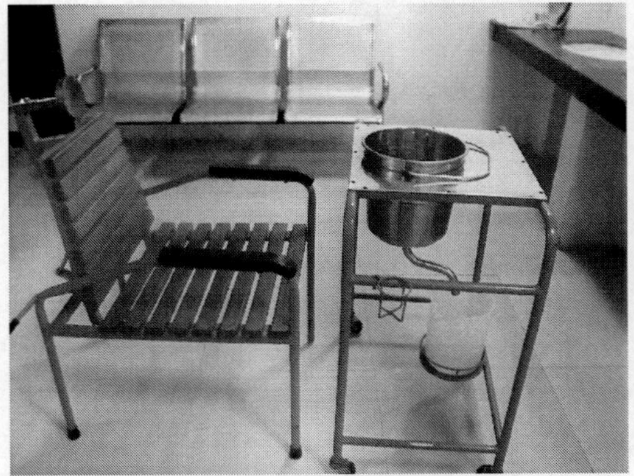

Fig. 1.6: Vamana chair

Virechana Karma

Virechana seat with collecting calibrated vessel.

Basti Karma (Figs 1.7A and B)

Basti netra, Enema pot.

Nasya Karma (Figs 1.8A and B)

Gokarna, sputum cup, cotton, dwimukha nadi.

Raktamokshana

- Jalauka—with a well maintained tank
- Pracchana—Shephalika patra, insulin needle, etc.
- Siravedha—Venesection scalpel
- Alabu
- Shringa
- Sterilizing facility
- Flat twain
- Kidney tray
- Gloves
- Rakta pravartaka dravyas and sthambhaka dravyas

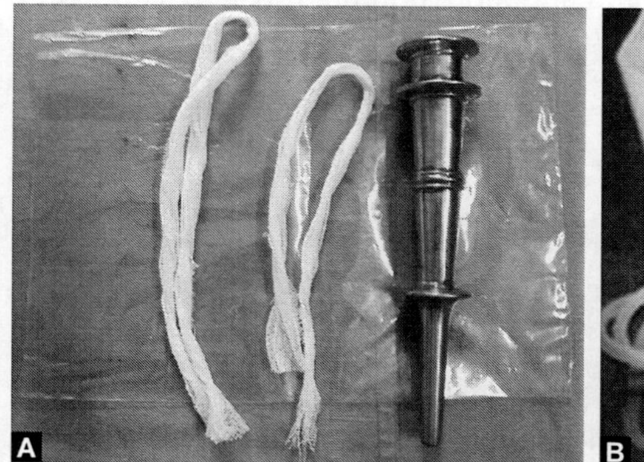
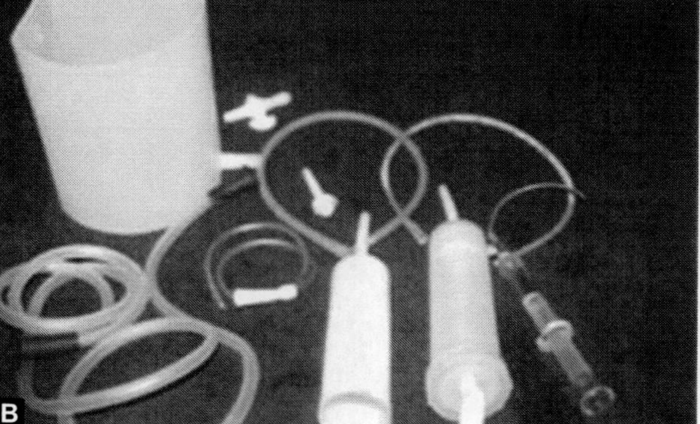

Figs 1.7A and B: Basti karma yantra

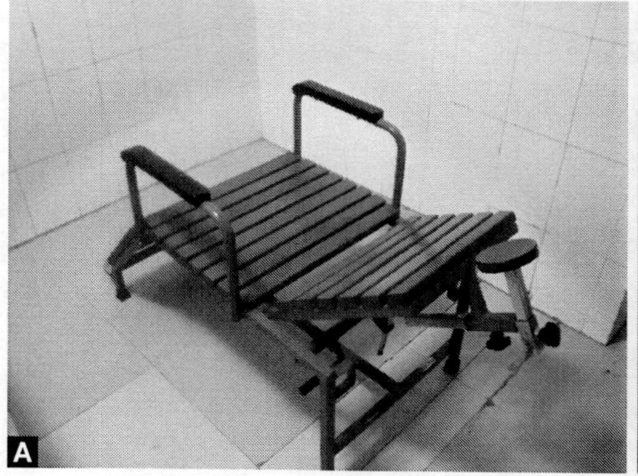
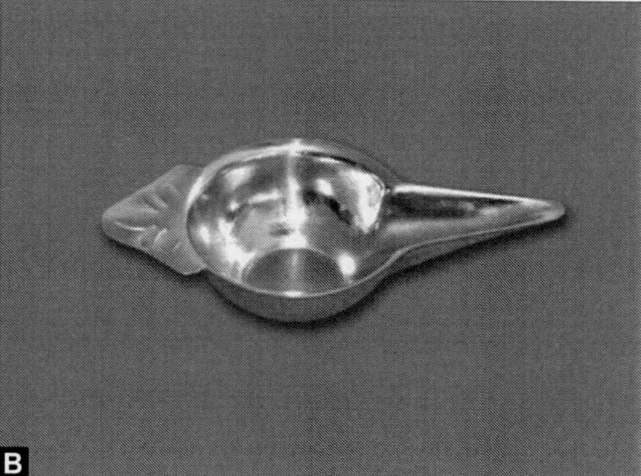

Figs 1.8A and B: (A) Nasya karma peetha (B) Gokarna yantra

Other Equipment

- ❑ Shirodhara pot (Fig. 1.9)
- ❑ Shirobasti yantra (Fig. 1.10)
- ❑ LPG cylinder and double burner stove
- ❑ Stainless steel utensils
- ❑ BP apparatus, torch
- ❑ Stethoscope
- ❑ Wash basin

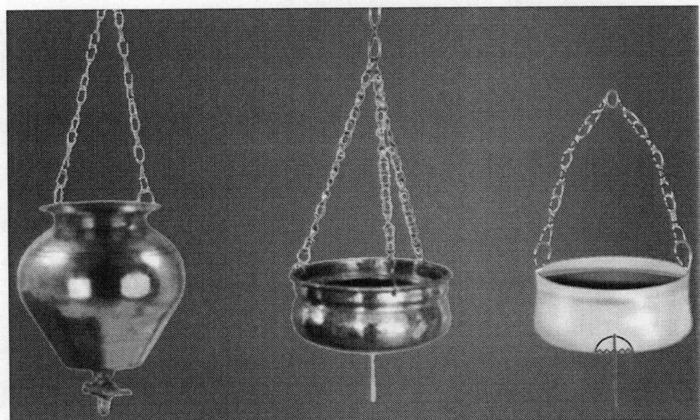

Fig. 1.9: Various types of Shirodhara pot

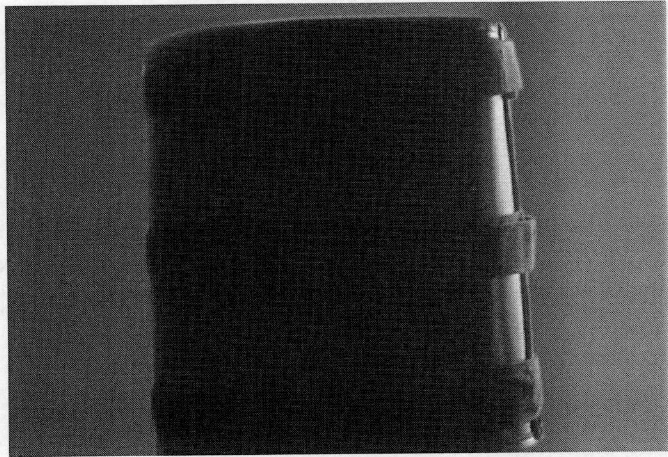

Fig. 1.10: Shirobasti yantra

IMPORTANCE OF KOSHTHA AND AGNI PARIKSHAN

Agni Pariksha

There are 13 types of Agni mentioned in classics, 5 Bhutagni, 7 Dhatvagni and 1 Jatharagni.

सर्वाग्निषु जाठराग्नेः प्राधान्यम्। (च.पा.)

Among all 13 types of Agni, Jatharagni has a prime importance.

- According to Charaka, Agni assessment is based on two components, viz. Abhyavarana shakti and Jarana shakti
- If the digestion process (Abhyavarana shakti) is proper then at the end of digestion Jeerna ahara lakshanas are produced like Utsaha, Laghuta, Udagara shuddhi, Kshudha pravritti and proper malotsarga.

Koshtha Pariksha

The word koshtha and its clinical considerations have different meanings. These are:

- Koshtha may be considered as the Thoraco abdominal region anatomically and surgically.
- Koshtha may be considered as many of the system on the basis of physiology.
- Koshtha may be considered as the gastrointestinal system on the basis of treatment.

  ग्रहणी कोष्ठस्थ अग्निधिष्ठान भूठा नाडी। (Ch.Su.13/69.Chakrapani)

  Koshtha is the Agni adhistana.

  तत्र मृदुः क्रूरो मध्यम इति त्रिविधः कोष्ठोभवति। (Su.Chi.33/21)

  3 types of koshtha, Mridu, Madhyama and Krura Koshtha.

- Koshtha is assessed based on two factor, i.e. Agni and Bowel habit.

  बहु पित्तो मृदुः कोष्ठः क्षीणेणापि विरेच्यते। (A.H.Su.18/34)

  In Mridhu koshtha person pitta is predominant; he will pass the loose stool even by taking Ksheera.

  प्रभूतमारुतः क्रूरः कृच्छ्राच्छयामादिकैरपि।। (A.H.Su.18/34)

  In Krura koshtha person Vata is dominant and person will not pass stool regularly or has Kathina or Shushka mala pravritti. Requires drastic purgatives to pass stool (e.g. Nilini, Trivrit, etc.)

  बहुश्लेष्मा समदोषश्च मध्यः स साधारणः।। (A.H.Su.18/34)

  In Madhyama koshtha person bahu shelshma and dosha are in the sama avastha, he will pass formed stool daily once. Requires medium dose of purgatives and does not purgates on minor laxatives or milk etc.

Importance of Agni and Koshtha Pariksha

- To decide द्रव्य प्रमाण/औषध मात्रा
- To decide स्नेहपान मात्रा
- अज्ञात (If Koshtha is not known): ह्रसीयसी मात्रा (A.H. 16/17-18)
- To assess duration of Snehapana karma
  - For Mridu koshtha person—3 days of snehapana
  - Madhyama koshtha person—4 to 6 days
  - Krura koshtha person—Upto 7 days

- In Vamana to decide dosage of medicine

	मृदु	मध्यम	क्रूर
वाग्भट्ट	अल्प	मध्यम	उत्तम
शार्ङ्गधर Kvatha	9 prastha	6 prastha	3 prastha
शार्ङ्गधर Kalka, Avaleha and Churna	3 pala	2 pala	1 pala

- In Virechana to decide dosage of medicine

	मृदु	मध्यम	क्रूर
शार्ङ्गधर Kvatha	½ pala	1 pala	2 pala
Kalka, Avaleha and Churna	1 karsha	2 karsha	1 pala
वंगसेन	1 karsha	½ pala	1 pala
Churna	½ karsha	½ pala	1 pala
Swarasa	Half of Kvatha		

- Dose of Anupana
  Ushna jala as anupana matra is explained according to koshtha by Vangasena; for Mridu koshtha (1 pala), Madhyama koshtha (2 pala), Krura koshtha (3 pala)
- Selection of Aushadha
- To avoid complications
- Planning of Sansarjana krama.

INTRODUCTION TO KERALIYA PANCHAKARMA

Various modified forms of traditional Panchakarma therapies are practiced in Southern India especially in Kerala which are now very famous across the globe as Keraliya Panchakarma. Following are some of the famous and practiced in abundance procedures amongst Keraliya Panchakarma therapies:-

1. Dhara Kalpa
2. Pinda Sveda (Navrakizhi, Elakizhi, Poddikizhi etc.)
3. Kaya Seka (Pizzichil)
4. Anna lepana
5. Mastikshya or Talapottichil

Dhara Kalpa

In this procedure medicated oils, Kvatha, milk, etc. are poured slowly on head through special pot known as Dhara Pot or Dhara Patra hanged on specific height, it is also called Shirodhara.

Pinda Sveda

In this a bolus made up of different materials, e.g. Payasa of Shashtika Shali cooked in milk and Bala Kvatha in case of Shashtika shali pinda sveda also known as Navrakizhi, or of leaves in case of Patrapinda sveda also called as Elakizhi, is used for fomentation on the body. Abhyanga is done before the procedure of Snigdha pinda sveda. In case of Ruksha pinda sveda, e.g. by dry bolus made of powders of various herbs in case of Churna pinda sveda also called as Poddikizhi in not preceded by abhyanga. It is used in various types of musculoskeletal disorders.

Kaya Seka

In this procedure medicated oil, decoction, etc. are poured on whole body from appropriate height (12 angula). Light massage is also carried out simultaneously in this procedure. It is useful in various neuromuscular and musculoskeletal diseases.

Anna Lepa

In this procedure Anna is prepared by using medicines or herbs as part of cooking medium and the Payasa thus prepared in used for massage on body. Anna is directly used for massage without making a bolus unlike in Shashtika shali pinda sveda. It is brihana in nature and useful in motor neuron and musculoskeletal disorders.

Thalapothichil

In this procedure, paste of boiled amlaki is smeared over the forehead leaving the anterior fontanel open, which is filled with medicated oil and then covered with leaves. It is useful in psychological and brain disorders.

Correlation of Keraliya Panchakarma with Shastriya Panchakarma

The procedures of Keraliya Panchakarma are famous as different form of Pancha karma, but essentially they are not different but a modified and more evolved form of various purva karma (Snehana and Svedana) already mentioned is Shastriya Panchakarma.

S. No.	*Keraliya Panchakarma*		*Comparative Shastriya Panchakarma*
1.	Dhara kalpa		Murdhni taila and seka or shirahseka
2.	Pinda sveda	Navrakizhi	Snigdha Sankara sveda
		Elakizhi	Snigdha – ruksha sankara sveda
		Poddikizhi	Ruksha sankara sveda
3.	Kayaseka		Parisheka
4.	Annalepa		Snigdha sankara sveda
5.	Thalapottichil		Mastishkya

ADHARABHUTA SIDDHANTA OF PANCHAKARMA

Basic concepts of Panchakarma have been taken from shad vidha upakram mentioned in Charaka Samhita which are included in the dividha upakrama mentioned by Vagbhatta which are:

लंघनं बृहणं काले रूक्षणं स्नेहनं तथा।
स्वेदनं स्तंभनं चैव जानीते यः स वै भिषग्।। (C. Su. 22/4)

A proper bhishak or vaidya is one who knows the detailed concept of Langhana, Brihana, Rukshana, Snehana, Svedana and Stambhana.

Inclusion of Shadvidha upkrama in Divividha upkrama

S. No.	*Shadvidha upkrama*	*Divividha upkrama*
1.	Langhana	Langhana or Apatarpana
2.	Rukshana	
3.	Svedana	
4.	Brihana	Brihana or Santarpana
5.	Snehana	
6.	Stambhana	

All the panchakarma and associated purva and pashchata karma get included in the above said upkramas.

S. No.	*Shadvidha upkrama*	*Examples of Panchakarma (trividha karma) included*
1.	Langhana	Deepana, Pachana, Vyayama, Kshudha, Vamana, Virechana, Asthapana basti, Lekhana basti, Vaitrana basti, kshara basti, Raktamokshana, Peya, vilepi, yusha, etc.
2.	Rukshana	Maruta sevana, Udvartana, Valuka sveda, Churna pinda sveda, Pradhamana Nasya
3.	Svedana	13 types of Agni sveda, 10 types of Niragni sveda
4.	Brihana	Snehapana, bahya snehana, Shashtika shali pinda sveda, annalepana, mashapinda sveda, Kukkutanda pinda sveda, Anuvasana basti, Matra basti, Ksheera basti, Yapana basti, brihana nasya Marsha and Pratimarsha nasya, Snehana nasya Tarpanadi krama, etc.
5.	Snehana	Abhyantara and bahya snehana, Anuvasana basti, Matra basti, Ksheera basti, Yapana basti, Brihana nasya Marsha and Pratimarsha nasya, Snehana nasya, etc.
6.	Stambhana	Avapida nasya, piccha basti, etc.

Thus, it is clear that various forms of purva, pradhana and pashchat karma are essentially fine parts of Shadvidha upkrama. And within these Shadvidha upkrama lies the basic concepts or siddhanta of Panchakarma.

CHAPTER 2

Snehana

INTRODUCTION

Sneha means Snigdhata (lubrication). Snehana or oleation therapy means the process which provides lubrication to the body. It is a treatment which brings viscosity, softness, solubility and kleda in body. Acharya Charaka has defined Snehana as the treatment, which produces viscosity, softness, solubility and kleda in the body (Ch.Su.22/10). It is one among the Shadvidhopakramas.

The therapy which provides the body with Snigdhata as well as it makes the vitiated Doshas easily extractable. It is a process of administering Sneha dravya to achieve the desired effect in precise duration prior to Vamana and Virechana Karma, not merely, simple administration of Sneha irrespective of dose, time, duration, etc.

Snehana is of two types, i.e. the Abhyantara and Bahya Snehana both are related with the Purva karma of Shodhana Chikitsa. The aim of Shodhana therapy is to prepare the body for Shodhana karma, i.e. to bring the Doshas situated in Shakha to the Koshtha so that they can be easily expelled out. (Su.Chi. 33/47) (Bhe. Su. 14/11).

Importance of Snehana-Svedana before Shodhana is quoted in Samhita that, if without these, Shodhana is induced; the body will break like a dry wood (Su.Chi. 33/46). Sneha helps in loosening the Doshas which are adherent to the wall of minute channels. According to Charaka, Kaphadi Doshas are easily expelled out from the snigdha body as from a smooth container; contents easily separate without any effort. (Ch. Si. 6/11).

As Kutshita (dirt) Mala of any cloth is easily washed by water, if it is loosen from its site in the similar way- Mala are easily expelled out by Shodhana if they are Utklishta by Purva karma, i.e. Snehana and Svedana. (Ch. Si. 6/13). Snehana is amongst the two major preparatory procedures to be performed before Shodhana.

The entire Shodhana procedure depends upon the proper mobilization of doshas from the shakha towards koshtha which can only be achieved with the help of proper Snehana and Svedana. Due to above mentioned reasons; Snehana should be thoroughly understood as told by Chakrapani:

वमनादिप्रवृत्तौ स्नेहस्यैव प्रथमं विधीयमानतया तथा दोष प्रधानस्य वातस्य प्रधानभेषजत्वाच्च।

(Chakrapani on Ch.Su. 13/2)

Two main reasons for Snehana are:

1. As a Purva karma of Vamanadi Shodhana karma.
2. As Pradhana karma for various Vataja disorders.

ETYMOLOGY AND DEFINITION OF SNEHA AND SNEHANA

Sneha word is derived by adding ल्युट् प्रत्यय to स्निह् धातु (वाचस्पत्य) and is नपुंसक लिंग.
The meaning of word Sneha is Snigdha (unctuous). A substance which induces Snigdhata (unctuousness) is Sneha
The word Sneh (स्नेह) has two meanings:

1. स्निह् – प्रितौ means to render affection and
2. स्नेह् – स्नेहने means to render lubrication.

The meaning of the term Sneha means, a substance that brings oilyness or unctuousness. Sneha literally means oiliness, unctuousness, fattiness, greasiness, lubricity, viscidity, affection, love, kindness and tenderness. (Monier Williams - Sanskrit-English dictionary)

Definition

स्नेहनं स्नेहविष्यन्दम् मार्दवक्लेदकारकम्। (Ch.Su. 22/11)

The procedure by which body achieves Sneha (snigdhata), vishyandam (vilayana or dissolution of dosha), mardavata (softness) and kledana (increase in "apa" content) is known as Snehana.

SNEHA YONI/SNEHA ASHAYA

Sneha Dravyas are Obtained from its Two Natural Sources Namely

Sthavara sneha: Plant source
Jangama sneha: Animal source

स्नेहानां द्विविधः सौम्य योनिः स्थावरजङ्गमाः।

Sthavara Sneha (Plant Source)

तिलः प्रियालाभिषुकौ बिभीतकश्चित्राभयैरण्डमधूकसर्षपाः।
कुसुम्भबिल्वारुकमूलकातसीनिकोचक्षोडकरञ्जशिग्रुकाः॥
स्नेहाशयाः स्थावरसंज्ञिता.................................... (Ch.Su. 13/10)

The oil extracted from the seeds of certain plants is used for Snehana :

- ❑ Tila (*Sesamum indicum*) (Fig. 2.1A)
- ❑ Priyala (*Buchanania lanzan*) (Fig. 2.1B)
- ❑ Bilwa (*Aegle marmelos*) (Fig. 2.1C)
- ❑ Aaruka (*Prunus persica*) (Fig. 2.1D)
- ❑ Abhishuka (*Pistacia vera*) (Fig. 2.1E)
- ❑ Moolaka (Raphanus sativa) (Fig. 2.1F)
- ❑ Bibhitaka bellirica (*Terminalia belerica*) (Fig. 2.1G)
- ❑ Atasi (*Linum usitatissimum*) (Fig. 2.1H)
- ❑ Chitra (*Baliospermum montanum*) (Fig. 2.1I)
- ❑ Nikochaka (*Artocarpus lakoocha*) (Fig. 2.1J)
- ❑ Abhaya (*Terminalia chebula*) (Fig. 2.1K)
- ❑ Akshoda (*Juglans regia*) (Fig. 2.1L)
- ❑ Eranda (*Ricinus communis*) (Fig. 2.1M)
- ❑ Karanja (*Pongamia pinnata*) (Fig. 2.1N)
- ❑ Madhuka (*Madhuca indica*) (Fig. 2.1O)
- ❑ Shigru (*Moringa oleifera*) (Fig. 2.1P)
- ❑ Sarshapa (*Brassica campestris*) (Fig. 2.1Q)
- ❑ Kusumbha (*Carthamus tinctorius*) (Fig. 2.1R)

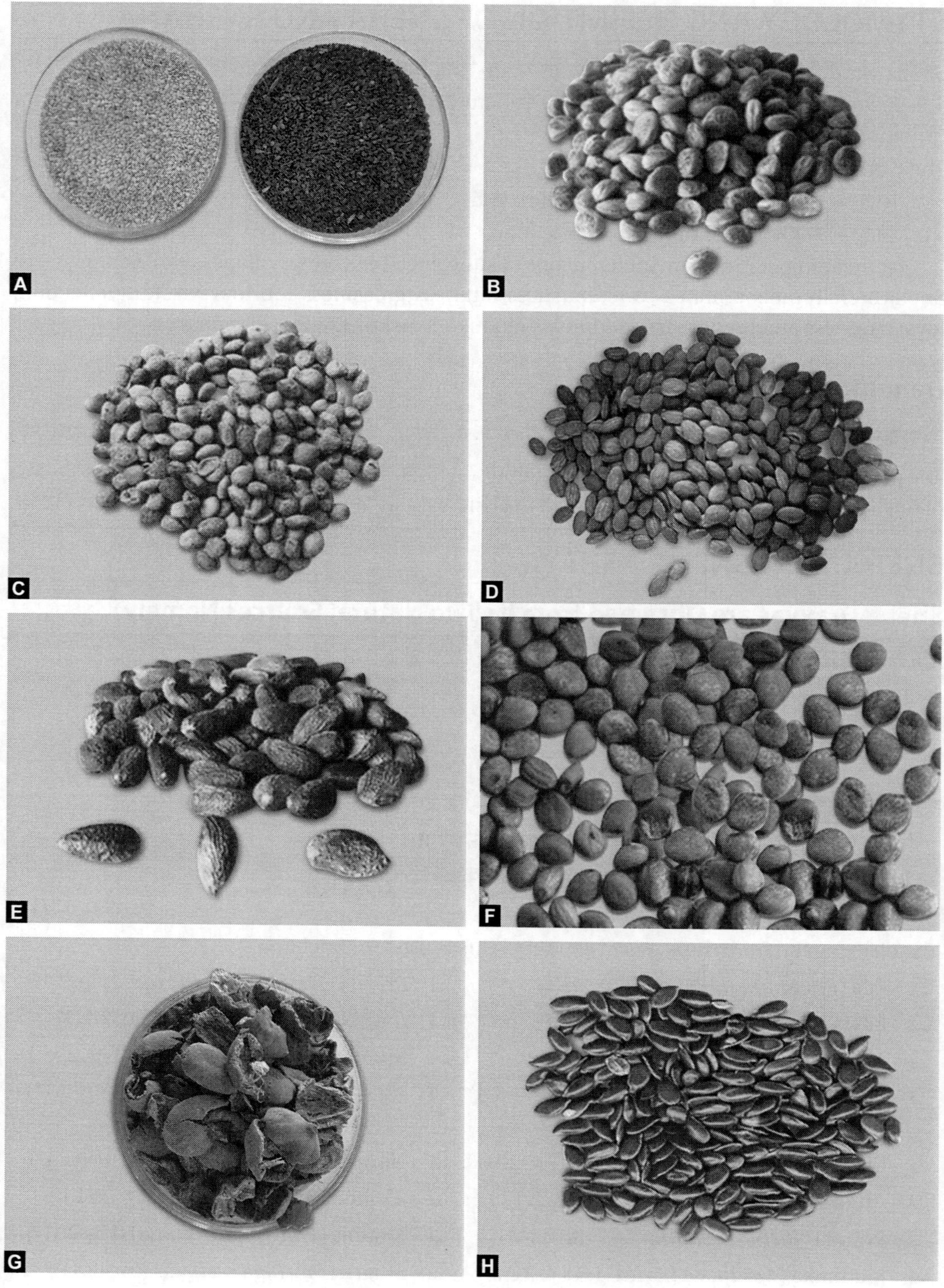

Figs 2.1A to H: Various sneha dravya

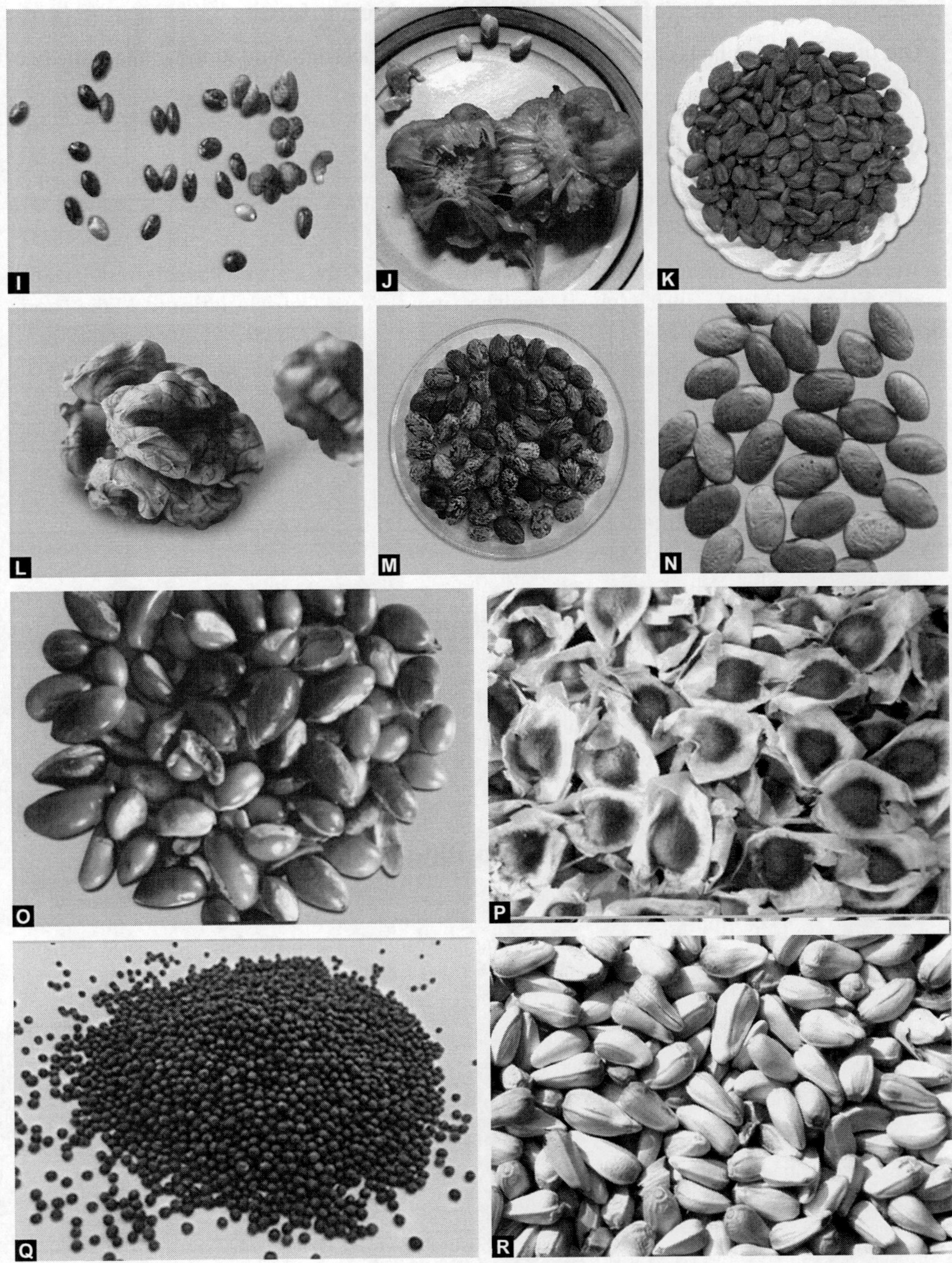

Figs 2.1 I to R: Various sneha dravya

सर्वेषां तैलजातानां तिलतैलं विशिष्यते। बलार्थे स्नेहने चाग्र्यमैरण्डं तु विरेचने।। (Ch.Su. 13/12)

Out of these, Tila taila is considered best for imparting strength and Eranda taila is the best of purgatives.

Jangama Sneha (Animal Source)

.... जङ्गमा मत्स्यमृगाः स पक्षिणः। तेषां दधिक्षीरघृतामिषं वसा स्नेहेषु मज्जा च तथोपदिश्यते।। (Ch.Su. 13/11)

The sources of Jangama Sneha are Matsya (fish), Mriga (Animals) and Pakshi (Birds). Dadhi (curd), Ksheera (Milk), Ghrita (ghee), Amisha (meat), Vasa (muscle fat) and Majja (bone marrow).

तत्र द्वियोनि श्वतुर्विकल्पोऽभिहितः स्नेहः स्नेहगुणाश्च।
तत्र जङ्गमेभ्यो गव्यं घृतं प्रधानं स्थावरेभ्यस्तिलतैलं प्रधानमिति।। (Su.Chi. 31/4)

According to Sushruta

The source of Sneha are two and it has four Vikalpa
Source: Sthavara and Jangama
Vikalpa: Sarpi, Taila, Vasa and Majja

सर्पिस्तैल वसा मज्जा स्नेह उदिष्टश्चतुर्विधः। (Ch.Su.1/86)
सर्पिस्तैलं वसा मज्जा सर्वस्नेहोत्तमा मताः। एषु चैवोत्तमं सर्पिः संस्कारस्यानुवर्तनात्।। (Ch.Su. 13/13)

Sarpi (Ghee), Taila (oil), Vasa (Muscle fat) and Majja (Bone marrow) are the four main types of Sneha. Further, out of all the four main types of Sneha, Ghrita, particularly Goghrita is considered best. It is best because when it is processed with drugs having other properties, it takes up their properties, without loosing its own property. This property is known as Sanskarasya Anuvartanam.

Classification of Sthavara Snehas according to Sushrutacharya

S.No.	*Karma*	*Dravya*
1.	Virechanopyogi	Lodhra, Eranda, Koshamra, Danti, Dravanti, Saptala, Shankhini, Vishanika, Gavakshi, Kampilaka
2.	Vamanopyogi	Jimutaka, Kutaja, Kritavedhana, Madana
3.	Shiro Virechanopyogi	Vidanga, Pilu, Jyotishmati, Kharamanjiri, Madhushigru, Siddhartaka, Jyotishmati
4.	Dushtavranopyogi	Karanja, Putika, Kritamala, Ingudi, Kirattikta
5.	Mahavyadhi upyogi	Tuvaraka, Kapittha, Kampillaka, Bhallataka, Patola
6.	Mutrasanga upyogi	Trapusa, Ervaruka, Tumbi
7.	Sharkara, Ashmari upyogi	Kapotvanga, Avalguja, Haritaki
8.	Prameha upayogi	Sarshapa, Kusumbh, Aatasi, Pichumarda
9.	Pittasansrishta vayu upayogi	Narikela, Panasa, Mocha, Priyala, Bilva, Madhuka, Shleshmataka

S.No.	Karma	Dravya
10.	Krishnikarana upayogi	Bibhitaka, Bhallataka, Madana
11.	Pandukaran upayogi	Ingudi, Priyangu, Shyonyaka
12.	Dadru, kushtha, kitibha upayogi	Sarala, Aguru, Pitadaru, Simshapa

Classification of Sneha According to their Paka

When Sneha is to be prepared using both Kvatha, i.e. decoction and Kalka, i.e. paste, proper care should be taken. Many Acharyas classify these types depending upon Agni given and quantity of water kept remaining.

Dagdha paka: First mentioned by Sushruta
Ama paka: First mentioned by Sharangdhara
Chikkana paka: Word used for Madhyama paka by Vagbhatta.

Classification of Sneha According to their Mode of Administration

स्नेहो हि पानानुवासनमस्तिष्क्य शिरोबस्त्युत्तरबस्ति नस्यकर्णपूरण गात्राभ्यङ्ग भोजनेषूपयोज्यः।

(Su.Chi. 31/3)

As mentioned above on the basis of mode of administration snehana is classified into:

- Abhyantara: Pana, Anuvasana, Uttarabasti, Bhojana.
- Bahya: Abhyanga, Shirobasti, Gandusha, Karnapurana, Mastishkya, Lepa, etc.

This type is either of pouring retaining or applying.

Classification of Sneha According to their Dose

अहोरात्रमहः कृत्सनमर्धांह च प्रतीक्षते। प्रधाना मध्यमा ह्रस्वा स्नेहमात्रा जरां प्रति॥ (Ch. Su. 13/29)

Charakacharya has classified Snehana into three groups as per the time required for their digestion (Ch. Su. 13/30-40)

1. **Uttama matra**: The matra that can be digested or assimilated within 24 hours, e.g. patients with very good digestive power, Gulma, Visarpa, Mutrakricchra.
2. **Madhyama matra**: The matra that can be digested or assimilated within 12 hours, e.g. Sphota, Vatarakta, Kushtha, etc.
3. **Hrasva matra**: The matra that can be digested or assimilated within 6 hours, e.g. Vridhha, Bala, Mandagni, Jvara, Kasa, Atisara, etc.

   Besides these, Sushruta has mentioned two more types with no indication of name

   (Su.Chi.31/28-29)

4. The matra which gets digested with in 18 hours, e.g. Bahudosha.
5. The matra which gets digested within 3 hours, e.g. Alpadosha. Here, Vagbhattacharya adds one more type. (A.H.Su. 16/18)
6. **Hrasiyasi matra**: Which digests within 3 hours. It is advised to use in those patients whose koshtha is unknown. In such condition Sneha should be administered cautiously as excess amount may lead to severe Vyapada and may lead to death too.

अज्ञातकोष्ठे हि बहुः कुर्याज्जीवितसंशयम्। (A.S. Su. 25/23)

Classification of Sneha According to their Combination

द्वाभ्यां त्रिभिश्चतुर्भिर्यमकः त्रिवृतो महान्। (A.H.Su. 16/2)

According to their uses of 2, 3 or 4 Snehas at a time it is classified as,

1. **Yamaka**: Combination of any two Snehas, e.g. Sarpi + Vasa or Sarpi + Taila
2. **Trivrita**: Combination of any three Snehas, e.g. Taila + Vasa + Sarpi
3. **Mahan**: Combination of all four Snehas. This can be used both internally and externally as per dosha vitiation, e.g. in Vatavyadhi (Ch.Chi.28/104)

Classification of Sneha According to their Preparation (Prayogika Bheda)

अच्छः केवलो यः स्नेह पीयते सा विचारणा न भवति। मूर्द्धादितर्पणादिना तु केवलस्य स्नेहस्य य उपयोगः सा च विचारणेति। (Arundutta on A.H.Su. 16/16)

Depending upon the use of Sneha alone or in combination of other substances, it is classified into two groups.

1. **Accha sneha**: The sneha which is not mixed with any other substance, i.e. sneha given alone with low or high dose (pratham kalpika). It is considered as best Sneha. (Ch.Su. 13/26)
2. **Vicharana** – Use of Sneha after mixing it with other substances, e.g. with rice, yusha, in basti, gandusha, etc. (Ch.Su. 13/23-25)

Here the basic difference, according to Chakrapani is that 'Vicharana does not come in direct contact with Jatharagni while in case of Accha Sneha digestion is compulsory'. As per Dalhana, Accha-Sneha may be medicated or non-medicated.

Classification of Sneha According to their Action on the Body

Whenever Sneha enters the body, it either pacifies the doshas or expels them out or helps in Brihana of the body. Depending on this. It is further subdivided as :

1. **Shamana snehana**: When Sneha is administered with an intention to normalize the aggravated doshas without expelling them out or disturbing the normal one. It has been explained by Hemadri that if shamana sneha is administered after the digestion of previous diet (Jirnaahare), due to vitiated Kaphadi doshas present in the srotasas, sneha will not spread in the whole body and its function to pacify doshas will not occur.
   Matra: Uttama (Charaka) or Madhyama (A.H.).
   Kala: During meal time or when one feels hungry without taking meals.
   According to Arundatta, kshudha occurs within 1 yama –

   पिबेत् सशंमनं स्नेहमन्नकाले प्रकांक्षितः। (Ch. Su. 13/61)

2. **Brihana snehana**: When sneha is administered for nourishment in the form of mixture with Mansarasa, Madya or Kshira.
   Matra: Alpa / Hrasiyasi.
   Kala: Any time with the food.
   The relation with food is beautifully described by Vagbhattacharya as-

   प्राङ्मध्योतरभक्तोऽवसावधोमध्योर्ध्वदेहजान्। व्याधीञ्जयेद्बल कुर्यादङ्गानां च यथाक्रम्॥

   (A.H.Su. 16/21)

Before food: Gives strength to Adhobhaga, e.g. uru, jangha, kati and helps in Vatanulomana process.

With food: Gives strength to Madhyama bhaga, e.g. trunk, in the diseases like Pakshaghata, Hridroga, etc. to increase Agni-bala.

After food: Gives strength and stability to sense organs in the head and cures diseases related to it.

3. **Shodhana snehana** – The sneha is to be given when the diet of previous night is completely digested in order to expel out the doshas.

   शुद्ध्यर्थं पुनराहारे नैशे जीर्णे पिबेन्नरः। (Ch. Su. 13/61)

   Matra – Madhyama

   Kala – Jirna-ahare

   It has been indicated to administered shodhanarth Sneha when previous diet taken is completely digested. If it is given at the time of hunger it will get digested by the Jatharagni and its function to expel out dosha will not take place.

According to Sub-types of Bahya Sneha

Abhyang, Lepa, Udvartana, Mardana, Parishek, etc. are the sub-types.

1. **Abhyanga**: Snehana in the direction of Loma, i.e. away from heart in downward direction. It is said to be jara-shram-vata har, drishthi, prasadak, pushtikar, cause sound sleep and nourishes the skin.
2. **Lepa**: It is less effective than Abhyanga. Pralep, pradeha and aalepa are its varieties. It may be cold or hot with difference in the thickness.
3. **Udvartana**: It is either ruksha or snigdha. Here the medicine is in the form of dry powder or sneha kalka which is massaged vigourously, opposite to the direction of Loma, i.e. towards the Heart.
4. **Mardana**: Massage with more pressure using oil.
5. **Padaghat**: It is described by Vagbhatta. Initially oil is applied all over the body and then the body is pressurized in fixed direction with the sole.
6. **Samvahana**: It means gentle application of oil without any pressure.

Miscellaneous Classification of Sneha

Sadhya Snehana

The procedure of administration of sneha to achieve snigdha lakshanas immediately or within a short duration is called Sadhya Snehana. It is a variety of Vicharana Sneha. Dalhana, Adhamalla, Chakrapani describe that it brings snigdha lakshanas quickly on administration. But both Chakrapani and adhamalla explained that it may take three days to produce 'Sadhyosnehana.' (Sadhyo-snehana <3 days).

Examples of Sadhya Snehana :

- ❑ Pancha prasritika peya
- ❑ Snigdha yavagu fried in Mansarasa
- ❑ Pippali + saindhava + four snehas + dadhi mastu
- ❑ Phanita with snehyukta tila churna

Avaritta Sneha

The Sneha prepared by repeated boiling of Sneha for 100 or 1000 times with drugs methodically is called Avaritta sneha. It is more concentrated and effective. For example, Shatapaki bala taila (Ch.Chi. 29/120) in the treatment of Vata Rakta.

Auttarbhauktika Sneha

The Sneha which is given after meal. It is indicated in Urdhva-jatrugata Vikaras.

Avapidaka Sneha

The sneha which is given in the middle of the meal. As it is churned along with food in the intenstine, it is called as Avapidika sneha.

PROPERTIES OF SNEHA DRAVYA

To understand the action of Snehana dravyas or for selection of a specific Sneha for a particular disease, proper knowledge of its properties is very important. These are described as :

द्रवं सूक्ष्मं सरं स्निग्धं पिच्छिलं गुरु शीतलम्। प्रायो मन्दं मृदु च यद्द्रव्यं तत्स्नेहनं मतम्॥

(Ch.Su. 22/15)

गुरु शीत सर स्निग्ध मन्द सूक्ष्म मृदु द्रवम्। औषधं स्नेहनं प्रायो..............................॥

(A.H.Su. 16/1)

Drava

यस्य विलोडने शक्तिः स द्रवः (Hemadri)

It liquifies doshas and helps in diffusion of Sneha throughout the body.

Sukshma

यस्य विवरणे शक्तिः स सूक्ष्मः (Hemadri)

To reach into micro-channels of body.

Sara

यस्य प्रेरणे शक्तिः स सरः (Hemadri)

To increase gati/velocity of doshas (especially Sthira Kapha).

Snigdha

यस्य क्लेदने शक्तिः स स्निगधः (Hemadri)

Bring unctuousness.

Picchila

यस्य लेपने शक्तिः स पिच्छिलः (Hemadri)

Forms a coat over doshas and keeps them in that state for longer time.

Guru

यस्य द्रव्यस्य बृहणे शक्तिः स गुरु (Hemadri)

For dosha vriddhi.

Shital

स्तम्भने हिमः (Hemadri)

Controls the movement of doshas along with increase of kapha with similar properties (Vriddhi samnaih sarvesham).

Mridu

यस्य द्रव्यस्य श्लथने शक्तिः स मृदुः (Hemadri)

Increases shaithilya in morbid doshas.

S.No.	Property	Charaka	Vagbhatta
1.	Drava (Liquid)	+	+
2.	Sukshma (Subtle)	+	+
3.	Sara (Tendency of flow)	+	+
4.	Snigdha (Unctuous)	+	+
5.	Picchila (Slimy)	+	–
6.	Guru (Heavy)	+	+
7.	Sheeta (Cold)	+	+
8.	Manda (Sluggish)	+	+
9.	Mridu (Soft)	+	+

Snehopaga Dravya

स्नेहोपगानीति स्नेहस्य सर्पिरादेः स्नेहक्रियायां सहायत्वेनोपगच्छन्तीति स्नेहोपगानि..........

(Ch.Su.4/8 Chakrapani)

The drugs which enhances the action of Sneha when administered with Sarpi, etc. is called Snehopaga.

मृद्वीका मधुक मधुपर्णी मेदा विदारी काकोली क्षीरकाकोली जीवक जीवन्ती शालपर्ण्य इति दशेमानि स्नेहोपगानि भवन्ति॥ (Ch. Su. 4/13)

S.No.	Drug	Botanical Name
1.	Mridvika	*Vitis vinifera*
2.	Madhuka	*Glycyrrhiza glabra*
3.	Madhuparni	*Tinospora cordifolia (willd) Miers*
4.	Meda	*Polygonatum verticillatum*
5.	Vidari	*Pueraria tuberosa*
6.	Kakoli	*Roscoea procera*
7.	Ksheerakakoli	*Roscoea procera*
8.	Jeevaka	*Microstylis wallichi*
9.	Jeevanti	*Leptadenia reticulate*
10.	Shalaparni	*Desmodium gangeticum*

GENERAL KNOWLEDGE OF GHRITA, TAILA, VASA AND MAJJA

Properties of Mahasneha

सर्पिमज्जा वसा तैलं स्नेहेषु प्रवरं मतम्। तत्रापि चोत्तमं सर्पि संस्कारस्य अनुवर्तनात्।
माधुर्याद् अविदाहित्वद् आजन्माद् एव च शीलनात्।। (A.H.Su.16/2)

Sarpi, Taila, Vasa and Majja are considered best among all the Snehas. Among the four, Sarpi is considered best because of its 'Sanskarasya-anuvartana' property (i.e., by proper processing qualities will get increased without losing its own properties) and also due to its Madhurya (Sweetness), Avidaha property (not causing burning sensation) and Satmya since birth.

Ghrita (Ghee)

Ghrita is one among the Jangama Sneha and it is best among all the Sneha because of its 'Sanskarsya Anuvartanat' property.

Classification

घृतमपि द्विविधं क्षीरोत्थं, दध्युत्थं। (Su.Chi. 31/4.Dalhana)

Ghrita is of two types:

1. **Ksheerottha**

   क्षीरोत्थः क्षीरमथनात् समुद्धूतनवनीतोत्थितं घृतं क्षीरघृतम्। (Su.Su.45/105 Dalhana)

   Ghrita prepared from Navaneeta (butter) obtained from churning milk.

   क्षीरघृतं पुनः संग्राहि रक्तपित्तभ्रममूर्च्छाप्रशमनं नेत्ररोगहितं च।। (Su.Su.45/105)

   It is Sangrahi, Rakta-pitta prashamaka, useful in Bhrama, Murccha and Netra roga.

2. **Dadhyottha**

   Ghrita prepared from Navaneeta (butter) obtained by churing curd.

घृतं तु मधुर सौम्यं मृदु शीतवीर्यमनभिष्यन्दि स्नेहनमुदावर्तोन्मादापस्मारशूलज्वर।
नाहवातपित्तप्रशनम् अग्निदीपनं स्मृतिमतिमेधाकान्तिस्वरलावण्यसौकुमार्योजं
बलकरमायुष्यं वृष्यं मेध्यं वयः स्थापनं गुरु चक्षुष्यं श्लेष्माभिवर्धनं पाप्मालक्ष्मीप्रशमन
विषहरं रक्षोघ्नं च।। (Su.Su.45/96)

स्मृतिबुद्ध्याग्निशुक्रौजः कफमेदोविवर्धनम्। वातपित्तविषोन्मादशोषालक्ष्मीज्वरापहम्।।
सर्वस्नेहोत्तमं शीतं मधुरं रसपाकयोः। सहस्रवीर्यं विधिभिर्घृतं कर्मसहस्रकृत्।। (Ch.Su. 27/231-32)

Rasa	*Madhura*
Guna	Saumya, Mridu, Guru, Anabhishyandi
Veerya	Sheeta
Vipaka	Madhura
Doshaghnata	Vata-Pitta Prashamana, Kaphavardhaka
Karma	Snehana, Agni deepana, Balakara, Ayushya Vrishya, Medhya, Vayasthapana, Chakshushya
Upayoga	Udavarta, Unmada, Apasmara, Shula, Jvara, Anaha
Seasonal indication	Sharada ritu

Guna (Properties)

घृतं पित्तानिलहरं रसशुक्रौजसां हितम्। निर्वापणं मृदुकरं स्वरवर्णप्रसादनम्॥ (Ch.Su. 13/14)

Mitigates Pitta-Vata, good for Rasa dhatu, Shukra dhatu and Ojas, Nirvapana (Daha prashamaka), increases softness, and nourishes voice and complexion.

Indications

वातपित्तप्रकृतयो वातपित्तविकारिणः। चक्षुः कामाः क्षताः क्षीणा वृद्धा बालास्तथाऽबलाः॥
आयुः प्रकर्षकामाश्च बलवर्णस्वरार्थिनः। पुष्टिकामाः प्रजाकामाः सौकुमार्यार्थिनश्च ये॥
दीप्त्योजः स्मृतिमेधाग्निबुद्धीन्द्रियबलार्थिनः। पिबेयुः सर्पिरार्ताश्च दाहशस्त्रविषाग्निभिः॥
(Ch.Su. 13/41-43)

तत्र धीस्मृतिमेधादिकाङ्क्षिणां शस्यते घृतम्। (A.H.Su. 16/8)

Persons of Vata-Pitta prakriti, diseases due to Vata-Pitta, those who are keen on preserving their eye-sight, injured, emaciated, old, young or weak, who are desirous of longevity, improvement in strength, complexion, voice, plumpness, progeny, youthfulness and increase of lustre, memory, talent, knowledge, power of the senses, those afflicted with heat and those who are injured by weapons, poison and fire.

Purana Ghrita

	Su.	*YR*	*BP*	*CD*	*Arunadatta*	*Ch.*
पुराणघृत	10 years	10 years	1 year		15 years	10 years
कौम्भसर्पि	11–100 years	100 years		10 years		प्रपुराणघृत
महाघृत	>100 years	10–100 years				

सर्पिः पुराणं सरं कटुविपाकं त्रिदोषहरं मूर्च्छोन्मादोदर ज्वर गर शोषापस्मार योनि श्रोत्राभि शिर शूलघ्नं दीपनं बस्ति नस्य पूरणेषूपदिश्यते। (Su.Su. 45/107)

पुराणं तिमिर श्वास पीनस ज्वर कासनुत्। मूर्च्छा कुष्ठ विषोन्माद ग्रहापस्मार नाशनम्॥
एकादशशतं चैव वत्सरानुषितं घृतम्॥ रक्षौघ्नं कुम्भसर्पिः स्यात् परतस्तु महाघृतम्।
पेयं महाघृतं भूतैः कफघ्नं पवनाधिकैः॥ बल्यं पवित्रं मेध्यं च विशेषात्तिमिरापहम्॥
सर्वभूतहरं चैव घृतमेतत् प्रशस्यते॥ (Su.Su. 45/108-111)

Guna	Sara
Vipaka	Katu
Doshaghanata	Tridoshahara
Karma	Deepana, Grahanashaka
Upayoga	Murccha, Unmada, Udara, Jvara, Gara, Shosha, Apasmara, Yoni, Shrotra, Akshi, Shira Shulaghna

Nutritional Value of Ghee

Ghee nutritional value per 100 g (3.5 oz)	
Carbohydrates	0 g
Protein	0 g
Vitamins Vitamin A Vitamin E	 3069 IU (105%) 15.7 mg
Other constituents Cholesterol	 256 mg

Fats and fatty acids	*Amounts per 100 g of ghee*
Total fat	99.5 g (153% DV)
Saturated fat	61.9 g (310% DV)
Monounsaturated fat	28.7 g
Polyunsaturated fat	3.7 g
Trans fats	4 g
Omega-3 fatty acids	1447 mg
Omega-6 fatty acids	2247 mg

Taila (Oil)

It is one among the Chatursneha and best Vatahara sneha among them.

Guna Karma

तैलं स्वयोनिवत्तत्र मुख्यं तीक्ष्णं व्यवायि च। त्वग्दोषकृ द्चक्षुष्यं सूक्ष्मोणं कफकृन्न च॥
कृशानां बृहणायालं स्थूलानां कर्शनाय च। बद्धविट्कं कृमिघ्नं च संस्कारात्सर्वरोगजित्॥

(A.H.Su.5/55-56)

मारुतघ्नं न च श्लेष्मवर्धनं बलवर्धनं। त्वच्यमुष्णं स्थिरकरं तैलं योनिविशोधनम्॥ (Ch.Su. 13/15)

Rasa	Madhura, Tikta, Kashaya anurasa
Guna	Tikshna, Guru, Snigdha, Vikasi, Sara
Veerya	Ushma
Vipaka	Madhura
Doshaghnata	Vatahara, not increases Kapha
Karma	Krimighna, Sthirakara, Tvachya, Balakara, Yoni Vishodhaka
Upayoga	Specially for Krishanam Brimhanartham and Sthulanam Karshanartham
Seasonal indication	Pravrit and Sheeta Kala (Ashadha and shravana masa)

Indications

प्रवृद्ध श्लेष्म मेदास्काश्चलस्थूलगलोदराः। वातव्याधिभिराविष्टा वातप्रकृतयश्च ये।।
बलं तनुत्वं लघुतां दृढतां स्थिरगात्रताम्। स्निग्धश्लक्ष्णतनुत्वक्तां ये च काङ्क्षन्ति देहिनः।।
कृमिकोष्ठाः क्रूरकोष्ठास्तथा नाडीभिरर्दिताः। पिबेयुः शीतले काले तैलं तैलोचिताश्च ये।।
(Ch.Su. 13/44-46)

ग्रन्थिनाडीकृमिश्लेष्ममेदोमारुतरोगेषु। तैलं लाघवदार्ढ्यार्थिक्रूरकोष्ठेषु देहिषु।। (A.H.Su. 16/9)

Those who have Kapha and Meda in excess, who have pendulous, fatty neck and belly, who are suffering from Vata disorders and who are of Vata prakriti. Person who are desirous to have strength, leanness, lightness, firmness, stability of limbs and elastic, smooth and thin skin, who are infected with intestinal worms, who are hard-bowelled, suffering from sinuses or fistula and accustomed to oil and in the cold season. For these persons taila is best.

Vasa

शुद्धमांसस्नेहो वसा। (Su.Chi.34/4.Dalhana)
वसा मांसस्नेहः। (Cha.Pa)

Fat which is extracted from muscle is known as Vasa.

Indications

विद्धभग्नाहत भ्रष्टयोनिकर्णशिरोरुजि। पौरुषोपचये स्नेहे व्यायामे चेष्यते वसा।। (Ch.Su. 13/16)
वात आतपसहा ये च रूक्षा भाराध्वकर्शिताः। संशुष्करेतोरुधिरानिष्पीतकफमेदसः।।
अस्थिसन्धिसिरास्नायुमर्मकोष्ठमहारुजः। बलवान्मारुतो येषां खानि चावृत्य तिष्ठति।।
महच्चाग्निबलं येषां वसासात्म्याश्च ये नराः। तेषां स्नेहयितव्यानां वसापानं विधीयते।।
(Ch.Su. 13/47-49)

वसा तु सन्ध्यस्थिमर्मकोष्ठरुजासु च। तथा दग्धाहतभ्रष्टयोनिकर्णशिरोरुजि।। (A.H.Su. 16/11)

Animal muscle fat is indicated in wounds, fractures, trauma, and prolapse of uterus, ear-ache and headache, for increasing virility, also in oleation procedures and after exercise.

Those who are exposed to severe wind and sun and who are dry, emaciated by carrying heavy weight and whose semen, blood, kapha and fat have decreased, who have severe pain in the bones, joints, vessels, muscles, vital parts and alimentary tract and in whom the highly provoked vata, becomes localized, has obstructed the various orifices of the body; those whose digestive power is very great and to whom animal fat is habituated in all these cases where oleation is indicated Vasa is prescribed.

Properties – These are similar with the Mansa of animals from which they are obtained.
Seasonal indication – Madhava kala.

Majja (Bone Marrow)

अस्थ्याश्रया मज्जा।
अस्थ्नः शुद्धस्नेहभागः। (A.Ko)

Indications

बलशुक्ररसश्लेष्ममेदोमज्जविवर्धनः। मज्जा विशेषतोऽस्थ्नां च बलकृत् स्नेहने हितः॥ (Ch.Su. 13/17)
दीप्ताग्नयः क्लेशसहा घस्मराः स्नेहसेविनः। वातार्ताः क्रूरकोष्ठाश्च स्नेह्या मज्जानमाप्नुयुः।
येभ्यो येभ्यो हितो यो यः स्नेहः स परिकीर्तितः॥ (Ch.Su. 13/50)
वातातपाध्वभारस्त्रीव्यायामक्षीणधातुषु। रुक्षक्लेशक्षमात्याग्निवातावृतपथेषु च॥ (A.H.Su. 16/10)

Properties – Based on the source of Majja.

Seasonal indication – Madhava Ritu.

Indications–Marrow increases strength, semen, Kapha, fat and marrow. It is especially good in increasing the strength of bones and good for oleation.

Those whose digestive fire is very active, can withstand hardships, who are ferocious eater, habitual takers of Sneha, afflicted with Vata, hard bowelled and who need oleation should use marrow for oleation.

METABOLISM OF FAT

There are three main macronutrients which are fat, carbohydrates and protein. Fats are a wide group of compounds whose base is in long-chain organic acids, called fatty acids.

The word oil, fat and lipid are often used interchangeably. Oil is the term usually used for fats that are liquids at normal room temperature, while fat is usually used for fats that are solids at normal room temperature.

Lipid constitutes a heterogenous group of compounds which are relatively insoluble in water but freely soluble in non-polar organic solvents like benzene, chloroform, ether, acetone, etc.

They are of great importance to the body as the chief concentrated storage forms of energy, besides their role in cellular structure and various other biochemical functions.

Lipids are mostly consumed in the form of neutral fats, which are also known as triglycerides. These are made of a glycerol nucleus and free fatty acids. Triglycerides are more in animal origin fat and less in food of plant origin.

Dietary Fats are Classified

1. Saturated fats
2. Unsaturated fats

Saturated Fats

The fatty acids having the maximum amount of hydrogen ions without any double bonds between carbon atoms are called saturated fatty acids.

Unsaturated Fats

These are the fatty acids formed by the dehydrogenation of saturated fatty acids.
Unsaturated fatty acids are classified into 3 types: :

1. Monounsaturated fatty acids
2. Polyunsaturated fatty acids
3. Trans-fatty acids
   1. Monounsaturated fatty acids which contain one double bond between the carbon atoms are called monounsaturated fats.
   2. Polyunsaturated fatty acids contain more than one double bond between carbon atoms. It belongs to the family of essential fatty acids (fatty acids required in diet). Omega-3 fatty acids are polyunsaturated fatty acids with a double bond (C=C) at the third carbon atom from the end of the carbon chain.
      Omega-6 fatty acids are polyunsaturated fatty acids with a double bond (C=C) at the sixth carbon atom from the end of the carbon chain.
   3. Trans-fatty acids contain a molecule with trans (across or opposite) double bonds between carbon atoms.

Type of fatty acids	*Source*	*Function*
Saturated fatty acids	Milk, cheese, butter, biscuits, fried fast food, coconut oil, palm oil, fatty meat.	• Increases blood cholesterol • Increases atherosclerosis • Increases coronary heart diseases
Monounsaturated	Oils (olive, pea, nut) Nuts (Cashew, almonds) ·	Decreases blood circulation
Polyunsaturated	Fruits, vegetables, sunflower, soya oil, flax seeds, lean meat, fish, egg	Decreases triglycerides, blood cholesterol, obesity and inflammation
Trans-fatty acids	Milk, lamb, beef, cheese	Increases low density lipo-proteins

Digestion of lipids: The enzymes involved in the digestion of lipids are called lipolytic enzymes.

In Mouth and Stomach

The lingual lipase from the mouth enters, the stomach along with the food. It has an optimum pH of 2.5–5. The enzymes, therefore, continues to be active in the stomach. It acts on short chain triglycerides present in milk, butter and ghee.

Gastric lipase is acid stable, with an optimum pH around 5.4. It is secreted by chief cells; the secretion is stimulated by gastrin. It is weak.

The lingual lipase converts triglycerides into fatty acids and 1, 2-diacylglycerols.

In Small Intestine

Role of bile salts:

Emulsification is a prerequisite for digestion of lipids. The lipids are dispersed into smaller droplets; surface tension is reduced; surface area of droplets is increased. This process is favored by:

1. Bile salts (detergent action)
2. Peristalsis (mechanical mixing)
3. Phospholipids

The bile salts cause the formation of aggregation of lipid molecules in the form of micelles. The micelles contain cholesterol, monoglycerides and fatty acids.

Role of Pancreatic Lipolytic Enzymes

Pancreatic lipase can digest only the emulsified fat molecules. Pancreatic lipase converts most of the triglycerides into free fatty acids and monoglycerides and a very small portion remains as diglycerides.

Other lipolytic enzymes of pancreatic juice are:

- ❑ Cholesterol ester hydrolase—Hydrolyses cholesterol ester into free cholesterol and fatty acid.
- ❑ Phospholipase A—Hydrolyses phospholipids into lysophospholipids.
- ❑ Phospholipase B—Converts the lysophospholipids into phosphorylcholine and free fatty acids.

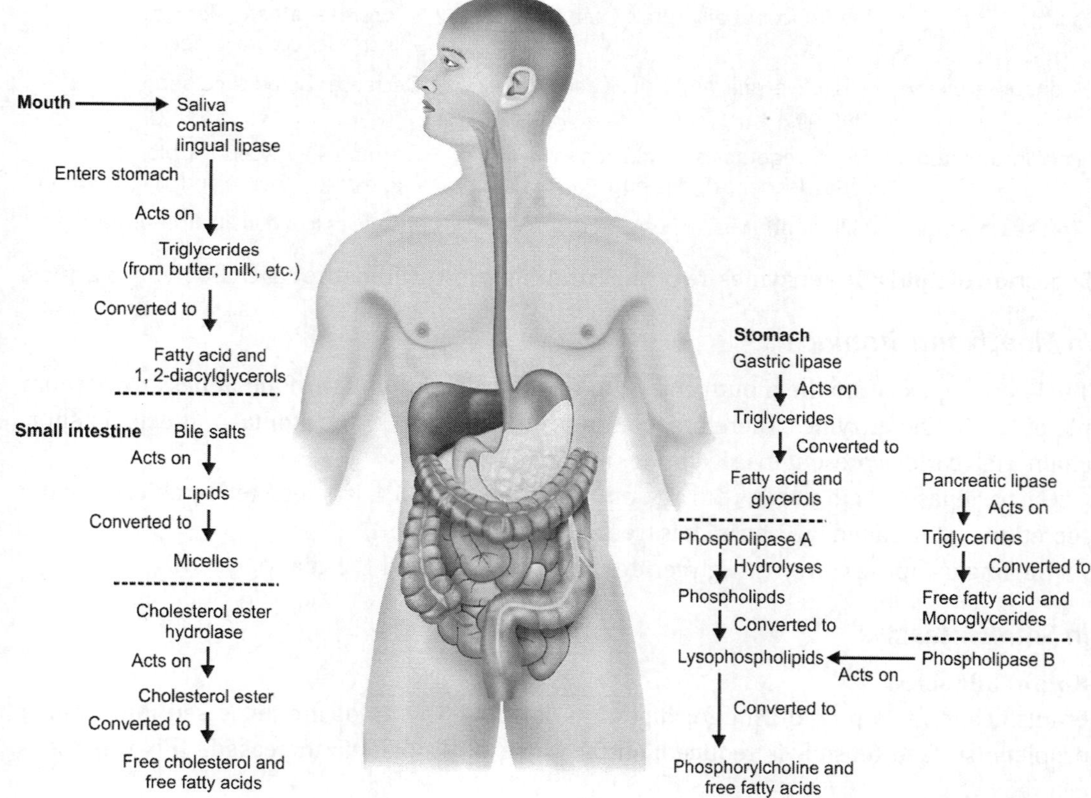

Fig. 2.2: Pictorial presentation of metabolism of fat

Absorption of Lipids

- ❑ From the micelle, fatty acids, cholesterol and monoglycerides diffuse into the epithelial cells in the mucosa of small intestine.
- ❑ The fatty acids less than 12 carbon atoms diffuse directly into the blood, which transports through portal vein to live as unesterified fatty acids.
- ❑ The fatty acids having more than 12 carbon atoms and some of the cholesterol molecules are converted into triglycerides by re- esterification.
- ❑ Lipids remaining in the intestine are aggregated into chylomicrons by the activity of endoplasmic reticulum of the epithelial cells in the intestinal mucosa.
- ❑ Chylomicrons cannot pass through the membrane of the blood capillaries because of the larger size. So these lipid materials enter the lymph vessels; and then are transferred into blood from lymph.

Importance of Lipoproteins

High density lipoproteins referred to as "good cholesterol" because they carry cholesterol and phospholipids from tissues and organs back to the liver for degradation and elimination. They prevent the deposition of cholesterol on the walls of arteries by carrying cholesterol away from arteries to liver.

Low density lipoproteins are considered as 'bad cholesterol" because they carriy cholesterol and phospholipids from the liver to different areas of the body, viz. muscles, other tissues and organs such as the heart. It is responsible for deposition of cholesterol on the walls of arteries causing atherosclerosis.

Very low density lipoproteins carry cholesterol from the liver to organs and tissues in the body. These are also associated with atherosclerosis and heart disease.

ACCHAPANA AND PRAVICHARANA OF SNEHA

Acchapana

Administration of any sneha as such without mixing with any food article is termed as Acchapeya (Acchapana).

अच्छ पेयस्तु यः स्नेहो न तमाहुर्विचारणाम्।
स्नेहस्य स भिषग्द्रष्टः कल्पः प्राथमकल्पिकः॥ (Ch.Su.13/26)

Accha Sneha means intake of large quantity of Sneha, without mixing with any other articles. Physicians emphasise regarding the intake of Accha Sneha as the best Snehana therapy. (Ch.Su.13/26).

Dalhana opines that, 'Kevala Sneha' is the synonym of Accha Sneha, which means administration of processed (or) unprocessed Sneha alone, without mixing with other liquids. (Dalhana on Su.Chi.31/19, 21)

So for defining 'Accha Peya' following criteria are considered:

- ❑ The quantity of Sneha should be comparatively more than Vicharana Sneha.
- ❑ Oral administration of pure Sneha not mixed with admixtures. However suitable Anupana as said in the classics can be used (Ch.Su.13/22).

Indications of Accha Sneha

स्नेहसात्म्यः क्लेशसहः काले नात्युष्णशीतले। अच्छमेव पिबेत् स्नेहमच्छपानं हि पूजितम्॥

(Su.Chi.31/21)

- ❑ Sneha Satmya—who have the habit of fat food consumption
- ❑ Klesha Saha—who can tolerate stress
- ❑ Naati—Sheeta/Ushna Kala-in moderate weather.

Pravicharana Sneha

प्रविचार्यते अवचार्यतेऽनुकल्पेनुपयुज्यतेऽनयेति प्राविचारणा ओदनादयः। (Cha.Pa)

The methodical administration of Sneha along with various preparations like Odana, Vilepi, etc., is known as Pravicharana Sneha. This includes even external administration of Snehas without admixture.

Different techniques are available to bring the Snehana effect. Accha Snehana is a superior method to achieve this effect. As an alternate technique to Accha Snehana, Pravicharana Snehana can be practiced.

According to Vagbhatta (A.H.Su. 16/6) Sneha which is administered for drinking is Accha Sneha and the Sneha used for Murdhadi and Tarpanadi karma is Vicharana.

In some persons, it is very difficult to consume it in the pure form due to dislike and in that case it may be administered by mixing it with some diet articles or by making it as some palatable preparations and then it is known as Pravicharana.

For instance, ghee taken by mixing with milk, curd, rice, gruel, meat soup, etc. is considered as Pravicharana.

रसैश्चोपहितः स्नेहः समासव्यासयोगिभिः। षड्भिस्त्रिषटिधा संख्यां प्राप्नोत्येकश्च केवलः॥
एवमेताश्चतुः षष्टिः स्नेहानां प्रविचारणा। ओकर्तुव्याधिपुरुषान् प्रयोज्ना जानता भवेत्॥

(Ch.Su.13/27-28)

Pravicharana can be administered in the form of Odanadi (24 in number) or Rasa Pravicharana (63 + 1 number). This should be administered considering Oka, Ritu, Vyadhi and Purusha.

Rasa Pravicharana

1. Ekarasa	-	06
2. Dvirasa	-	15
3. Trirasa	-	20
4. Chaturrasa	-	15
5. Pancharasa	-	06
6. Shadarasa	-	01
Total	-	63 + 1 Accha = 64

Varieties of Pravicharana

ओदनश्च विलेपी च रसो मांसं पयो दधि। यवागूः सूपशाकौ च यूषः काम्बलिकः खडः॥
सक्तवस्तिलपिष्टं च मद्यं लेहास्तथैव च। भक्ष्यमभ्यञ्जनं बस्तिस्तथा चोत्तरबस्तयः॥
गण्डूषः कर्णतैलं च नस्तः कर्णाक्षितर्पणम्। चतुर्विंशतिरित्येताः स्नेहस्य प्रविचारणाः॥

(Ch.Su. 13/23-25)

S.No.	Name	S.No.	Name	S.No.	Name	S.No.	Name
1.	ओदन	2.	विलेपी	3.	रस	4.	मांस
5.	पय	6.	दधि	7.	यवागु	8.	सूप
9.	शाक	10.	यूष	11.	काम्बलिक	12.	खड
13.	सक्तु	14.	तिलपिष्ट	15.	मद्य	16.	लेह्य
17.	भक्ष्य	18.	अभ्यञ्जन	19.	बस्ति	20.	उत्तरबस्ति
21.	गण्डूष	22.	कर्णतैल	23.	नस्य	24.	अक्षितर्पण

1. **Odana**: 1 part of rice boiled with 5 parts of water and then the excessive of water is strained off to get the odana. The boiled rice is added with some amount of ghrita and is then served for the purpose of vicharana sneha.
2. **Vilepi**: Vilepi is the food preparation obtained by adding 1 part of rice with 4 parts of water and boiling the mixture to make it thick. This vilepi is mixed with certain amount of ghee.
3. **Rasa**: Rasa means meat soup. Thick, average and thin soup may be prepared for the oral consumption. Thick meat soup is prepared by boiling 320 g of meat in 620 mL of water.
4. **Mansa**: Different dishes of the meat is added with extra amount of edible fat and then served in the meals as vicharana sneha.
5. **Dugdha**: Milk is to be added with certain amount of ghee before consumption to get the effect of vicharana sneha.
6. **Dadhi**: Curd consisting of sneha is mixed with specific amount of sneha before oral intake.
7. **Yavagu**: The mixture of 1 part of cereal in 6 parts of water is boiled properly till the liquid portion is barely left to get the yavagu. Before serving in the meals, this yavagu is mixed with certain amount of Sneha depending upon the plan of vicharana sneha.
8. **Soup**: The soup prepared by one part of pulse mixed with 14 part of water and the mixture is boiled to reduce it to ¼th. Thus, prepared soup is added with ghrita or taila and then given orally as vicharana sneha.
9. **Shaka**: A food preparation with different vegetables are boiled and treated with seasoning is known as shaka. In vicharana sneha this shaka is mixed with adequate amount of sneha before oral consumption.
10. **Yusha**: The liquid food prepared by 1 part of pulse added with 14 parts of water and then boiled to reduce the mixture to half is known by the name yusha. This yusha is mixed with certain amount of sneha and given orally as vicharana sneha.

11. **Kambalika**: During the preparation of yusha with one part of pulse mixed with 14 parts of water this combination is further mixed with curd, salts, amla, edible fat, tila, and masha. This mixture is boiled properly to get the kambalika to use this in vicharana sneha, kambalika is added with extra amount of edible fat.
12. **Khada**: The combination of one part of pulse and 14 of water is added with specific amount of takra, kapittha, changeri, maricha, and chitraka. This mixture is properly boiled to get the khada yusha. This khada yusha is mixed with Sneha for the vicharana sneha.
13. **Saktu**: The flour of cereal and pulse is moistened with adequate amount of fat and then given orally in the form of vicharana sneha.
14. **Tilapishta**: The cakes of tila is moistened with certain amount of ghee or oil and then eaten. This will be a form of vicharana sneha.
15. **Madya**: Different alcoholic beverages are mixed with desired amount of sneha and taken internally to get the effect of vicharana sneha.
16. **Leha**: Soft and thick confectionary, kind of sweet dish prepared with sugar and pulses like black gram is called leha. For the purpose of vicharana sneha this leha is mixed with Sneha and then consumed.
17. **Bhakshyanna**: Varities of tasty dishes are known by the name bhakshyanna. The sweet dishes are added with Sneha before consumption to get the effect of vicharana sneha.
18. **Abhyanga**: The therapeutic massage by specific maneuvers.
19. **Basti**: Administration of different medicaments in the form of enema.
20. **Uttara basti**: Administration of medicaments through the urethral route.
21. **Gandusha**: Holding the liquid medicines mixed with fat substances in the mouth.
22. **Karna poorana**: Filling of medicated oil into the ears.
23. **Nasa poorana**: Administration of oil into the nostrils.
24. **Akshi tarpana**: Administration of sneha into the eyes.

To understand Pravicharana Snehana the entire matter may be classified in the following manner:

Kevala Sneha Prayoga: Nasya, Karna - Akshi Tarpana, Gandusha, Abhyanga, and Basti.
Along with preparations: Odana, Vilepi, Yavagu, Rasa, Mansa, etc.

- **Based on route of administration–**

– **Bahya** –	Oral route	-	Gandusha
	Skin	-	Abhyanga
	Eye	-	Akshi tarpana
	Ear	-	Karna poorana
– **Abhyantara** –	Oral route	-	Along with odana, etc.
	Nasal route	-	Nasya
	Genital/Urethral	-	Uttara basti
	Rectal route	-	Basti

- **Based on action** –
  Shodhana Pravicharana
  Shamana Pravicharana
  Brihana Pravicharana

- **Based on time required for bringing Snehana effect.**
  Sadyo Snehana Pravicharana and Chira Kalina Pravicharana. So by giving due importance to Satmya, Roga, Ritu, likings (Ch. Su. 13/27) etc. the Pravicharana Sneha can be administered.

Indications of Pravicharana

स्नेहद्विषः स्नेहनित्या मृदुकोष्ठाश्च ये नराः। क्लेशासहा मद्यनित्यास्तेषामिष्टा विचारणा॥

(Ch. Su. 13/82)

1. Sukumara
2. Vriddha
3. Sneha Dvesha
4. Sneha Nitya
5. Klesha Asaha
6. Ushna Kala
7. Krisha
8. Shishu
9. Madya Nitya
10. Mridu Koshtha
11. Trishnarta

SNEHAPAKA

Ch.Ka. 12/102-104, Su.Chi.31/11, Sha.Ma. 9/17-19, A.H.Ka.6/21

स्नेहपाकस्त्रिधा ज्ञेयो मृदुर्मध्यः खरस्तथा।
तुल्ये कल्केन निर्यासे भेषजानां मृदुः स्मृतः॥ (Ch.Ka. 12/102-104)

Snehapaka is of 3 types:

1. **Mridu**: When the solution of the drugs attains the consistency of the paste added to it is known as Mridu.
2. **Madhyama**: When the solution acquires jelly consistency and can be poured out easily with spoon.
3. **Khara**: When the solution becomes so thickened that it snaps, can be rolled between the fingers.

Opinion of different authors regarding varieties of Sneha Paka and its indications are mentioned as follows:

Snehana	*Charaka*	*Sushruta*	*Vagbhatta*	*Sharangdhara*
Abhyanga	Khara	Madhyama	Khara	Madhyama
Pana	Madhyama	Mridu	Chikkana	Madhyama
Nasya	Mridu	Madhyama	Mridu	Mridu
Basti	Madhyama	Khara	Chikkana	Madhyama
Karnapurana	–	Khara		Madhyama

Opinion of different authors regarding Usage of particular Paka or Sneha for Snehana is summarized as follows:

- ❑ Abhyanga and Basti : Madhyama to Khara paka.
- ❑ Pana and Nasya : Mridu to Madhyama paka
- ❑ Karnapurana : Madhyama to Khara paka

Except for Nasya, in all other procedure Madhyama Paka Sneha, can be used.

The process by which snigdhata, vishyandata, mardavata and kledana are achieved is known as Snehana.

This has great importance regarding 'Shodhanarth Abhyantar Snehapana.'

1. **Sneha**: Snigdhata
2. **Vishyandata:** Vilayana, i.e. dissolution or diffusion which causes excretion and overflowing of doshas.
3. **Mardava**: Softness
4. **Kledana**: Increase of Apya guna (water content) in the body or Utkleshavastha.

TYPES OF SNEHANA

Sneha is broadly classified into two types:

1. Bahya Snehana
2. Abhyantara Snehana

Bahya Snehana

Application of Sneha externally for the purpose of Snehana is known as Bahya Snehana. It is practiced as a part or Dinarcharya and Ritucharya in healthy person. In diseased it is used for Shamana Chikitsa also as a part of Purva karma before the administration of Shodhana.

Bahya Snehana can be Sthanika (local application) Sarvadehika (complete body)

Various types of Bahya Snehana are as follows :

अभ्यङ्गोद्वर्तनं लेपः मर्दनोन्मर्दनं तथा। पादाघातं परिषेकं त्वचि संवाहनं तथा।।
गण्डूषो मूर्धतैलानि कर्णनासाक्षितर्पणम्। मस्तिष्क्यमवगाहं च बाह्यस्नेहे प्रयुज्यते।।

(Pan. Sam. 3/82-83)

1.	Abhyanga	2.	Udvartana	3.	Lepa	4.	Mardana
5.	Unmardana	6.	Padaghata	7.	Parisheka	8.	Samvahana
9.	Gandusha	10.	Murdha taila	11.	Karna tarpana	12.	Nasa tarpana
13.	Akshi Tarpana	14.	Mastishkya	15.	Avagaha		

Abhyanga

Abhyanga has been considered as important part of the external Snehana. Our skin is the largest organ of our body. It is also the most important and rich source of healing substances. It is very sensitive to the touch therapy, particularly to the Abhyanga with powder, oil, aromas or just to the gentle touch.

Abhyanga is one type of external oleation therapy. The word Abhyanga derived from the "Ang" Dhatu, which is used for the meaning of motion and "Abhi" Upasarga in it. Its literary meaning is to produce some motions. Rubbing or stroking after applying Ghirta, Taila, etc. on the skin, helps in their absorption.

Importance

A person should resort to Abhyanga every day if he wants to keep himself healty. In classics, Abhyanga has been mentioned as the part of Dinacharya, i.e. daily routine. (Ch. Su. 5/89, A.H. Su 2/8).

It is very useful before performing physical exercise.

The importance of Abhyanga has been shown by the way of different metaphoric illustrations. As a pitcher or a dry leather or an axis of a wheel become strong and resistant to wear and tear by the application of oil. Similarly by the Abhyanga of oil, human body, becomes strong and smooth - skinned; it becomes unsusceptible to the disease of Vata and resistant to exhaustions and exertions (Ch. Su.5/85,86).

स्नेहाभ्यङ्गाद्यथा कुम्भश्चर्म स्नेहविमर्दनात्। भवत्युपाङ्गादक्षश्च दृढः क्लेशसहो यथा॥
तथा शरीरमभ्यङ्गादृढं सुत्वक् च जायते। प्रशान्तमारुताबाधं क्लेशव्यायामसंसहम्॥

The body is compared to the tree. If the root of tree is given water regularly, then it lives for a long time. Similarly, on the above anology, if the body of an individual is oleated properly through Abhyanga, then he lives for a long time, without any decay or disease.

Type of Tailapaka

The oils used should be prepared in the form of Madhyama or Khara paka

Indication of Abhyanga

- Taila Abhyanga is indicated in Bala, Vriddha, Krisha and Rogi.
- All types of Vata Roga, Vishama Jvara and all Tvak Vikara

Contraindication of Abhyanga

- Person suffering from Kaphaja Roga
- Person suffering from Ajeerna, Nava or Taruna Jvara are contraindicated for Abhyanga.
- High fever—increased body temperature—increases metabolism - Liston (1995)
- After Sanshodhana, i.e. immediately after Vamana, Virechana and Niruha Basti, Abhyanga is contraindicated as it causes Agnimandya
- After Tarpana Kriya
- Person suffering from Netra roga, Karna roga, Atisara, Adhmana; Peenasa, Agnimandya and other Ama dosha condition
- Santarpanottha roga—diseases gets further aggravated
- Immediately after consumption of the food
- Person accustomed to Ruksha and Abhishyandhi Ahara.
- After Snana, Vyayama, Divasvapna, Vegadharana, Prajagarana, Sheta Vayu Sevana.

Local Contraindication

- Acute inflammation
- Oozing skin disease

- Fractures
- Severe varicose vein
- Thrombosis and arteriosclerosis
- Malignancy
- Open wound

Purpose of Abhyanga Therapy

Abhyanga can be done to a person for two different purposes.

1. It can be done regularly to a person for the prevention of several diseases and for the maintenance as well as promotion of positive health.
2. It can also be done as a special therapy for a limited period. This special massage therapy is generally carried out for the purposes of,
   a. Rejuvenating the body to prevent and arrest the aging process; and
   b. Curing several obstinate and otherwise incurable diseases.

Apart from the above mentioned purposes, Abhyanga therapy along with fomentation is also given before administering several categories of elimination therapies like Vamana, Virecchana, Basti and Nasya.

Method of Abhyanga

Abhyanga should be done with luke-warm medicated oil or ghee, prepared with aromatic and Doshaghna drugs suitable to the season, Prakriti, disease, Dosha, etc. It should be applied slowly, gently and in the direction of hair. Abhyanga is done particularly on head, leg and ear daily (**शिरःश्रवण पादेषु तं विशेषेण शीलयेत्**) (A.H. Su. 2/9). For Abhyanga on the head, cold or luke-warm oil may be used, because head is the place of all senses and it is considered as the most vital part, hence, it should be protected from heat. Abhyanga on limbs should be applied with warm oil. In this way Abhyanga may be administered with warm oil in cold season and with cold oil in hot season. Abhyanga may be applied in the direction of hair on relatively broad and large organs. It should be done in circular pattern on joints like elbow, shoulder, knee, ankle and lumbar joints.

The Abhyanga should be done in the following seven positions :

1. Sitting position (Figs 2.3A and B)
2. Supine position–lying on back (Fig. 2.4)
3. Left lateral lying position (Fig. 2.5A)
4. Prone position (Fig. 2.5B)
5. Right lateral lying position (Fig. 2.5C)
6. Supine position
7. Sitting position

Effect of Abhyanga on Sapta Dhatu

Dalhana the commentator of Sushruta has described the effect of Abhyanga according to the duration for which it is done, the oil used in Abhyanga reaches to the root of hair of the skin if

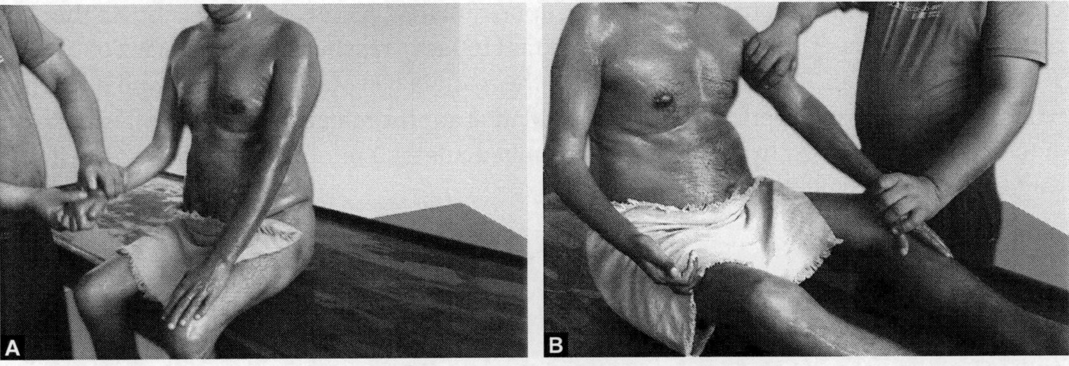

Figs 2.3A and B: Abhyanga sitting position

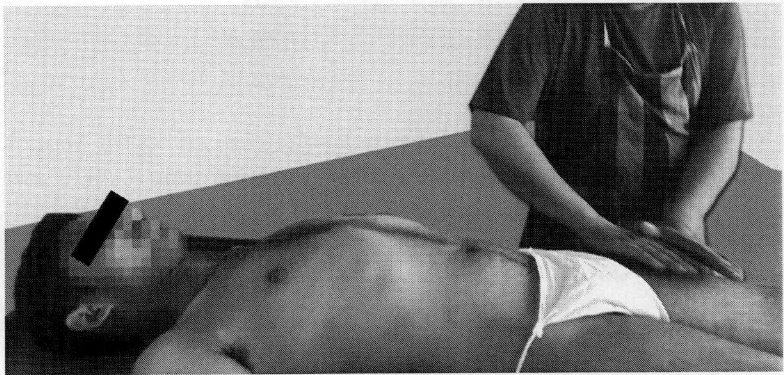

Fig. 2.4: Abhyanga supine position

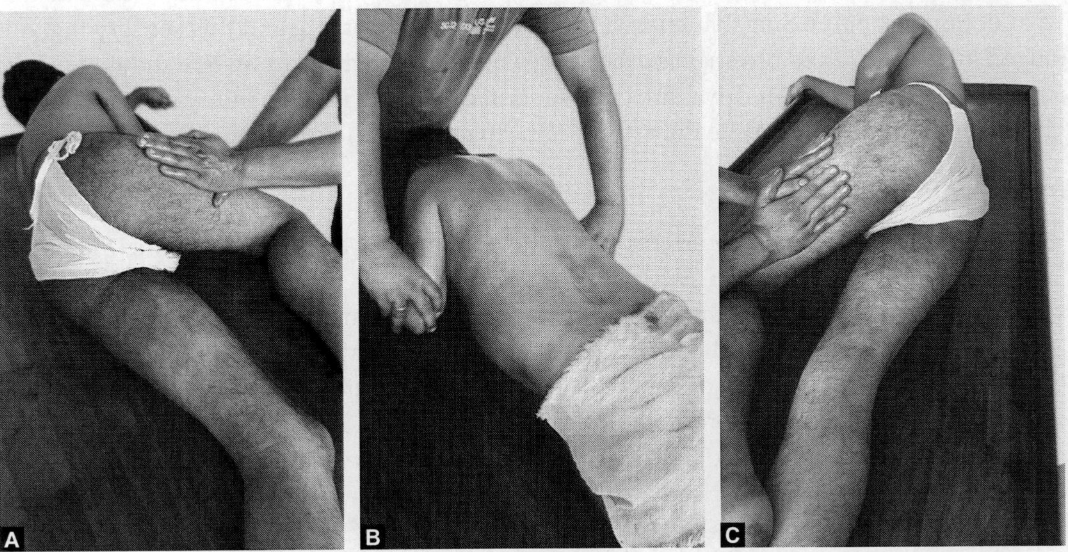

Figs 2.5A to C: (A) Abhyanga Left lateral (B) Prone (C) Right lateral position

Abhyanga is performed up to 300 Matras, i.e. approximately, 65 seconds. It reaches in the skin in 400 Matras (133 sec), in the Rakta in 500 Matras (160 sec), reaches up to Mansa in 600 Matras (190 sec.), in Meda in 700 Matras (228 sec), in the Asthi in 800 Matras (240 sec) and it reaches to the Majja if Abhyanga performed up to 900 Matras approximately 285 seconds (Dalhana on Su.S. Ci. 24/ 30). Thus Abhyanga should be applied atleast 5 minutes in each position if one wants to get its effect in deeper tissues like Majja.

S. No.	*Time taken (in Matra)*	*Dhatu reached*
1.	300	Romanta
2.	400	Tvacha
3.	500	Rakta
4.	600	Mansa
5.	700	Meda
6.	800	Till Asthi
7.	900	In Asthi

According to Sahasra Yoga, Abhyanga done to the Shareera enters the Sapta Kala in 7 days and requires 6 days to enter Raktadi Dhatu and at the same time it takes away the Dosha present in the body through Sira, Dhamani, etc.

Mode of Action of Abhyanga

Dalhana has explained in detail about the absorption of Sneha used in Abhyanga procedure, accordingly the oil used in Abhyanga can reaches up to the different Dhatus if it is applied for the sufficient time. Hence, it is clear that the drug used in the Abhyanga gets absorbed by the skin. Dalhana also mentions that when Snehana drug reaches to the particular Dhatu it subsides or cures the diseases of that particular Dhatu. Charaka has also described that Vayu dominates in the Sparshanendriya, i.e. tactile sensory organ, and this sensory organ is lodged in the skin. The Abhyanga is exceedingly beneficial to the skin, so one should practice it regularly (Ch.Su. 5/87). Indriyas are in close contact of mind, hence if indriya remain healthy mind automatically remains healthy. Thus, Abhyanga keeps body and mind healthy.

Benefits of Abhyanga

1. **Jarahara:** It prevents and corrects aging process. The Abhyanga nourishes the Dhatus and increases their strength.
2. **Shramahara:** It helps a person to overcome fatigue, because of routine hard work.
3. **Vatahara**: It prevents and corrects disorders caused by affliction of the Vata. Abhyanga helps in the promotion and regulation of the proper function of Vata.
4. **Drishti prasadakara:** It promotes eyesight. The diseases of the eye like Timira and other diseases, which are caused due to aging could be prevented and cured by Abhyanga.
5. **Pushtikara**: It helps in nourishment of the body. It nourishes all the seven Dhauts of the body.
6. **Ayushyakara**: It promotes longevity of an individual. The functions of the vital organs and tissues are improved and life span is promoted through Abhyanga therapy.

7. **Svapanakara**: It helps the individual to get sleep. The Abhyanga is very useful to overcome sleeplessness and other mental ailments.
8. **Tvak Dardhyakara**: It promotes sturdiness of an individual. Abhyanga provides a passive form of exercise even for those who cannot perform active physical exercise because of debility and old age. Even for a normal healthy person, Abhyanga provides sturdiness of the body, which keeps him healthy and happy.
9. **Klesha Sahatva**: By the sturdiness due to Abhyanga, body becomes capable to tolerate the stress and strains of life.
10. **Abhighat Sahatva**: In the persons who always undergo Abhyanga therapy, trauma cannot cause as much trouble as in other individuals.
11. **Kapha Vata Nirodhana**: According to Sushruta Abhyanga prevents both Vata and Kapha. (Su.S. Ci. 24/30)

When it comes to massage, the character of technique is more important. The classification based on the character of techniques goes as follows:

1. Stroking manipulations—superficial, deep (effleurage)
2. Pressure manipulations—kneading, petrissage, friction
3. Tapotement/percussion manipulations
4. Vibratory manipulations

General Classification of Massage

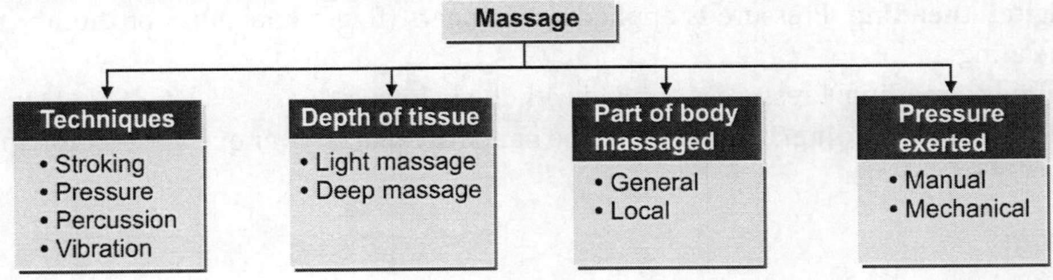

Classification of Massage Based on Techniques

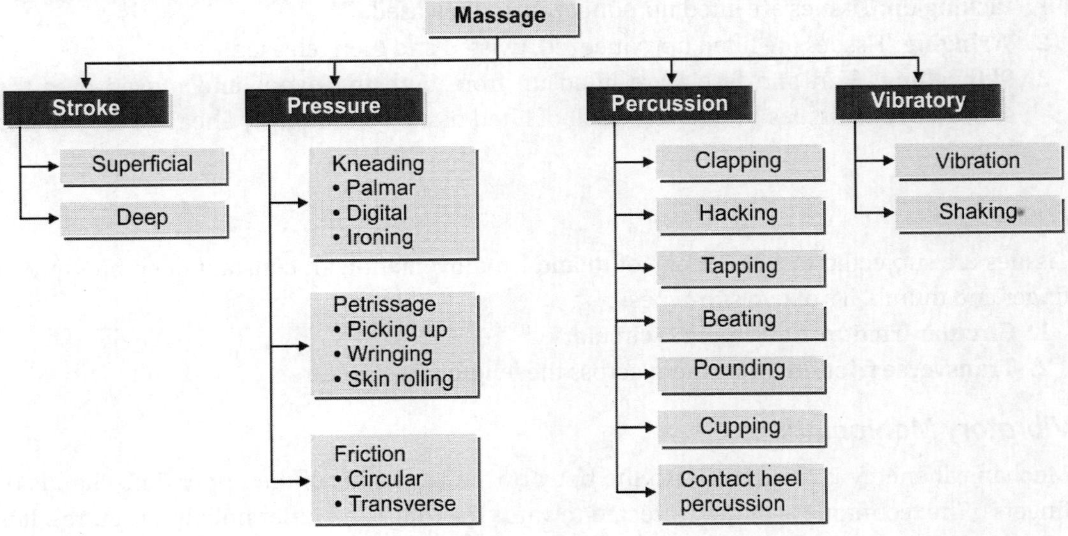

Stroking Manipulations

A linear movement of relaxed hand along the whole length of a segment is known as 'stroke'. Based on the amount of pressure applied, it is of two types:

Superficial Stroking

It is rhythmical linear movement of hand over the skin without any pressure.

Effleurage Stroking (Deep Massage)

It is a linear movement of hand, over the external surface of the body, with moderate pressure.

Pressure Manipulations

A deep localized pressure is applied to the body where, the hand of the therapist and the skin of the patient move together.
Based on the type and the direction of pressure applied, it is of three major types:
1. Kneading, 2. Petrissage, and 3. Friction

Kneading

The tissues are pressed down to the underlying firm- structure and intermittent pressure is applied in circular direction, parallel to the long axis of a bone. It is of three sub-types

1. **Digital kneading**: Pressure is applied with fingers (finger kneading) or thumb (thumb kneading)
2. **Palmar kneading**: Pressure is applied with the palm
3. **Reinforced kneading/ironing**: Both the hands are placed over one another for applying pressure.

Petrissage

The tissues are grasped and lifted away from the underlying structure with the pressure applied perpendicular to the long axis of the bone. It's of three sub types-

1. **Picking up**: Tissues are lifted up, squeezed and released.
2. **Wringing**: Tissues are lifted up, squeezed, twisted and then released.
3. **Skinrolling**: Skin and fascia are lifted up from both the hands and moved over the subcutaneous tissues by keeping a roll of lifted tissue continuously ahead of the moving thumb.

Friction

Tissues are subjected to small range of to and fro movement with constant deep pressure of finger and thumb. It's of two sub-types:

1. **Circular friction:** Movement is circular
2. **Transverse friction:** Movement across the length of a structure

Vibratory Manipulations

Mechanical energy is transmitted to the body by the vibrations of the upper limb (hands or fingers). The technique is mainly directed towards the lungs and other hollow structures. It is of two sub-types.

Vibration

Fine vibrations produced in upward and downward direction.

Shaking

Coarse vibrations produced in side way direction.

Percussion/Tapotement Manipulations

A succession of soft, gentle blows applied over the body with production of a characteristic sound in which the striking hands are not in constant touch with the skin. It is of various types :

- **Clapping**: Applied with a flat palm
- **Hacking**: Applied with the ulnar borders of 5th, 4th and 3rd digits
- **Beating**: Applied with anterior aspect of the clenched fist
- **Cupping**: Applied with a cupped palm
- **Tapping**: Applied with the pulp of the fingers
- **Pounding**: Applied with the medial aspect of the clenched fist
- **Contact heel percussion**: Applied with the heels of both the hands.

Features of Massage Technique

- Technique should apply mechanical force to soft tissue of the body.
- The force should not produce any change in the position of the joint or any change in the normal anatomical shape of the site.
- The technique must evoke some physiological or psychological effect which serve to achieve the therapeutic, restorative and the preventive goal.

Physiological Effects

- Effects on the circulatory system: On the venous and lymphatic flow and the arterial flow
- Effects on the blood
- Effects on metabolism
- Effects on nervous system
- Effects on the mobility of the soft tissue
- Effects on the respiratory system
- Effects on the skin
- Effects on the adipose tissue
- Psychological effects

Abhyanga is done in a ventilated room but direct air entry should not be there. It is advisable to perform massage in the morning after attending the natural urges in empty stomach.

After care: After completion of Abhyanga patient should rest in waiting room having no access to direct air for about 15 minute. Thereafter the oil should be sponged with a thick cloth or towel and patient is allowed to take meal after hot water bath.

Mode of Action

Massage can increase the fresh oxygenated blood supply to the muscles and organs and aid the drainage of venous blood, promoting the removal of waste products from the body. By increasing the flow of lymphatic material, waste removal is also aided and white blood cell production is increased, boosting one's natural immunity. Massage influences the equilibrium in the nervous system.

There are few newly developed scientific concepts regarding mode of action of massage:

Pain Modulation

The precise mechanism of action in massage therapy is not known. It has been proposed that increased parasympathetic activity and a slowed-down physiological state may strengthen the behavioral and physiological processes associated with massage. As discussed by Wright and Sluka, massage is thought to induce a variety of positive physiological effects that may contribute to tissue repair, pain modulation, relaxation, and improved mood. For example, these authors point to research showing that massage has beneficial effects on arterial and venous blood flow and edema. In addition, they note that vigorous massage has been shown to increase local blood flow and cardiac stroke volume, as well as improve lymphatic drainage; massage also appears to have an anticoagulant effect. Finally, Wright and Sluka maintain that massage may activate segmental inhibitory mechanisms to suppress pain and that some techniques may activate descending pain inhibitory systems, as suggested by gate theory.

The main theories regarding the analgesic effects of massage include gate theory.

Pain Gate Control Theory

The Pain Gate Control Theory was initially proposed in 1965 by Melzack and Wall based on the fact that small diameter nerve fibers carry pain stimuli through a 'gate mechanism' but larger diameter nerve fibers going through the same gate can inhibit the transmission of the smaller nerves carrying the pain signal. Chemicals released as a response to the pain stimuli also influence whether the gate is open or closed for the brain to receive the pain signal. This lead to the theory that the pain signals can be interfered with by stimulating the periphery of the pain site, the appropriate signal- carrying nerves at the spinal cord, or particular corresponding areas in the brain stem or cerebral cortex.

It is generally seen that the 'Pain gate' can be shut by stimulating nerves responsible for carrying the touch signal (mechanoreceptors) which enables the relief of pain through massage techniques, rubbing, and also the application of hot packs. The Gate can also be shut by stimulating the release of endogenous opioids which are opioid (pain relieving) type chemicals released by the body in response to pain stimuli.

Serotonin Hypothesis

The serotonin hypothesis maintains that massage increases levels of serotonin, a neurotransmitter that modulates the pain control system.

Tactile Kinesthetic Stimulation

Abhayanga and strokes of heated pack produces tactile kinesthetic stimulation. Studies have shown that such tactile kinesthetic stimulation works by Limbic system and exerts positive physiological and therapeutic action through hypothalamus by neurohormonal and neuro-psychological pathways. By this mechanism it may help to produce neuromuscular and neurobehavior development.

Myofascial Release Theory

Myofascial release therapy is an extremely effective hands-on technique that works by applying gentle, sustained pressure to eliminate pain and restore flexibility and motion to the fascia (connective tissue). The science behind myofascial release states that fascia is a densely woven sheath that interpenetrates and "houses" every muscle, bone, vein, nerve and all of our internal organs including the spinal cord. A good visualization is a spider web that in effect holds everything together in a neat package connecting every part of the body to every other part of the body.

In its natural healthy state, the fascia is relaxed and has the flexibility to stretch and move without undue restriction. If however, there has been physical trauma to the body or scarring, the normally liable fascia becomes tight and restricted, causing tension throughout the rest of the body. In such pathological conditions, myofacial release techniques like gentle massage, deep pressure, tactile stimulation; etc. restores the normal status of fascia and hence removes the facial pain syndrome.

Massage and Sensory Integration

Sensory integration is the neurological process by which we take in sensory information, make sense of it, and respond to it. An appropriate response to sensory information allows us to interact with the world and go about our daily routines with ease. The theory of sensory integration was developed by Dr A Jean Ayres, occupational therapist and graduate of the University of Southern California. Her theory of sensory integration is based on extensive research in the area of proprioception. A certain amount of sensory input is required in order for our neurological threshold to be met so that this sensory input can be perceived. Regular fluctuation in a neurological threshold through out ones day, some people have unusually high neurological thresholds while others have unusually low neurological thresholds. These people will continue to have fluctuations in their neurological threshold; however, their neurological thresholds will stay around the high or low end of the spectrum. In general those with high neurological thresholds require a lot of sensory input to reach their neurological threshold and perceive this sensory input, while those with low neurological thresholds only needs a little sensory input to reach their neurological threshold and perceive this sensory input.

Lepa

The word Lepa is derived from the root "Lip". This mainly denotes to smear. By adding "Ghan" Pratyaya to root Lip, the word Lepa is derived, which means to smear or to plaster (Sha. Ka. D)

लिप्यते अनेन इति लेपः। (Sha. Ka. D)

The act of smearing or anointing.

Synonyms: आलेपस्य च नामानि लिप्तो लेपश्च लेपनम्। (Sha. Ut. 11/1)

The synonyms of lepa are Alepa, Lipta, Lepa, Lepana, Pralep and Pradeha.

Definition: Smearing of the medicated oil or application of paste of medicinal plants mixing with oil on the body is known as Lepa. Application of Lepa is not followed by any type of manipulation or massage.

Types of Lepa

According to Sharangadhara. Ut. 11/1 : 3 types of Lepa

दोषघ्न	1/4th Angula
विषाह	1/3rd Angula
वर्ण्य – also called Mukhalepa	1/2 Angula

According to Sushruta. Su. 18/6 : 3 types

प्रलेप	शीत, तनु, अविशोषि/विशोषि	वातश्लेष्मप्रशमन, क्षताक्षत
प्रदेह	उष्ण या शीत, बहल, अबहु, अविशोषि	वातश्लेष्मप्रशमन, शोधन, रोपण, शोफवेदनापह
आलेप	मध्यम	रक्तपित्तप्रसादकृत्

According to Vagbhatta: 10 Types of Lepa

दशविधश्च समासादालेपः। स्नैहिक निर्वापणः प्रसादनः स्तम्भनो विलायनः पाचनः पीडनः शोधनो रोपणः सवर्णीकरणश्च॥ (A.S.Ut. 30/8)

Quantity of Sneha in Alepa

Vata	:	1/4th
Pitta	:	1/6th
Kapha	:	1/8th

Thickness of Lepa

According to Sushruta : महिषार्द्रचर्मोत्सेध – Thickness of fresh/moist skin of buffalo (around 3–5 mm) (Su.Su. 18/11)

According to Charaka : त्रिभागाङ्गुष्ठमात्र 1/3rd of Angushtha

According to Vagbhatta: अर्धाङ्गुष्ठभागमेव 1/2 of Angushtha

Preparation of Lepa

Lepa is prepared by grinding or crushing the fresh herbs together into a fine paste form. If the drugs are in the dried form then they are made into fine paste by triturating with water, milk, ghee or oil.

नातिस्निग्धो न रूक्षश्च न पिण्डो न द्रवः समः। (Ch.Chi.21/101)

Prepared Lepa should not be too oily, dry, thick or watery.

Lepa Vidhi

प्रतिलोममेव चानुलिम्पेन्नानुलोमम्। तथा ह्यौषधं सम्यगवतिष्ठते।
अनुप्रविशति च रोमकूपान्। न तु शुष्यदुपेक्षितव्यमन्यत्र पीडयितव्यात्।
शुष्कं हि दाहोषारागश्यावत्वशूलानि वर्धयति॥ (A.S.Ut.30/6)

Lepa should be applied in the upward/opposite direction of hair follicle. By this it will stick properly and enters into hair follicles. One should not wait till the Lepa gets dried off completely. If done, it will lead to inflammation and aggravation of pain.

न च पर्युषितं लेपं कदाचिदवचारयेत्॥
न च तेनैव लेपनं पुनर्जातु प्रलेपयेत्। (Ch.Chi.21/101-102)

Once used Lepa should not be reused again. Every time freshly prepared Lepa should be used.

Mardana and Unmardana

मर्दन – अङ्गमर्दनम्। (अ.म.को.)
उन्मर्दन – हस्ततलेन मर्दनम्। (अ.म.को.)
मर्दनं चानुलोमेन विरुद्धोन्मर्दनम् तथा। तैलादिकेन हस्ताभ्यां समुखं परिपीडनम्॥ (Pan.Sam.3/107)
मर्दनं तु गाढ़ं पादाभ्यामारभ्य कटिपर्यन्तं। (Su.Chi.24/83.Dalhana)

Performing pressure massage in downward direction after the application of oil to palm is called Mardana opposite to this is Unmardana, i.e, in upward direction.

Indications

Mardana is indicated in both in healthy and diseased persons. Mardana is indicated in various categories of disorders.

स्नेहाभ्यंगोपनाहाश्च मर्दनालेपनानि च। त्वक्मांसासृक् शिरा प्राप्ते..................॥ (Su.Chi.4/6)
स्नेहोपनाहाग्निकर्म बन्धनोन्मर्दनानि च। स्नायु संध्यास्थि संप्राप्ते कुर्यात्..........॥ (Su.Chi.4/8)

1. Sarvanga Mardana after Vyayama (Vagbhatta)
2. Hemanta ritu (Vagbhatta)
3. Twakgata vata—skin disorders due to imbalance of vata
4. Raktagata vata—disorders of blood
5. Mansagata vata—disorders of muscle tissue
6. Snayugata vata—disorders of ligaments/nerves
7. Sandhigata vata—disorders of joints
8. Asthigata vata—disorders of bone.

Bheda

According to Vatsyayanana kamasutra

Abhyanga	–	Massage with oils
Samvahana	–	Whole body massage
Keshamardana	–	Head massage
Udvartana	–	Massage with churna
Utsadana	–	Massage with kalka/with feet
Udgharshana	–	Reinforced massage with churna

According to Tiruka

- Shushkanga mardana
- Tailanga mardana
- Ksheeranga mardana
- Svayamanga mardana
- Yamalanga mardana

Padaghata (Massage with Feet) (Fig. 2.6)

पादाघात – पादाभ्यां मर्दनम्

Padaghata is a type of Bahya Snehana karma in which the therapist uses his feet to apply required pressure for massage after anointing patients body with oil.

दक्षेन मृदुभिः पद्भ्यां पादाघातं प्रकुर्वतः। व्याधयो नोपसर्पन्ति कृतव्यायमदेहिनः।। (Pan.Sam.3/109)
व्यायामस्विन्नगात्रस्या पद्भ्यमुद्वर्तितस्य च। व्याधयो नोपसर्पन्ति सिंह क्षुद्रमृगा इव।। (Su.Chi.24/43)

One should undergo Padaghata after performing sufficient exercise. If one undergoes padaghata, body will become stable, stroke and diseases run away from the body just like the small animals after seeing the lion.

Oil which alleviates Vata should be used for Padaghata.

Procedure

1. A rope is tied to the ceiling for support.
2. With minimum cloth patient is advised to lie in supine position the mat placed on the ground.
3. Oil is taken in a plate and placed beside the patient.
4. Therapist should stand on the side of the patient and should hold the rope firmly.
5. Therapist should dip his feet in the oil containing plate and apply the oil with deep pressure over chest, abdomen, upper and lower limbs.
6. After completing the massage in supine position procedure done in prone position.
7. After the completion of the procedure patient is made to take rest for an hour and is advised to take hot water bath.

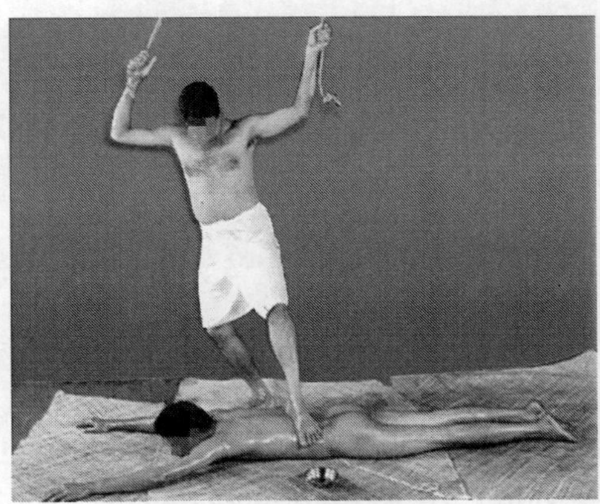

Figs 2.6: Padaghata

Precautions

- Therapist should have moderate built, i.e. neither obese nor lean.
- Therapist should have uncracked foot and trimmed nails.
- Therapist should have good control in applying pressure.

Samvahana

संवाहन सुखकरस्पर्शः। (Su.Chi.24/83. Dalhana)
हस्ताभ्यां शनैः शनैराहननमिति वदति॥ (अमितप्रभ टीकाकार)
संवाहन पाणिना पादादिप्रदेशे सुखमभिहननमुन्मर्दनं च। (Ch.Su. 7/23. Chakrapani)

After the application of oil, the hands are gently and repeatedly moved over the body of the person or mild massage or stroking with hand.

संवाहनं मृदुः स्पर्शो न किञ्चितदपि पीडनम् ।
स्नेहेन वा विना स्नेहें स्त्रीमित्रं कुरुते यदि॥ (Pan.Sam.3/125)

Samvahana is a pleasurable touch without pressure or very little pressure. It can be performed with or without Sneha. This is preferably performed by friends and females.

Benefits

प्रीतिनिद्राकरं वृष्यं कफवातश्रमापहम्। संवाहनं मांसरक्तत्वक्प्रसादकरं सुखम्॥ (Su.Chi. 24/83)
तत्तु शूलहरं हर्षं चित्ते शान्तिं ददाति च। रसायनं हितं वृष्यं मनोद्वेगहरं शिवम्॥ (Pan. Sam. 3/126)

Preetikara – Generates pleasure
Nidrakara – Induces sleep
Vrishya – Improves sexual vigour
Shramahara – Relieves fatigue
Sukhakara – Gives happiness

Nourishes Mansa, Rakta and Twak

Sukha – Pleasure
Shulahara – Reduces pain
Chitta Shanti – Generates calmness

Rasayana – Rejuvenation
Manodvegahara – Reduces exertion
Indications: Vatarakta (Su.chi 4/16) Nidravegavarodhajanya Vyadhi (Ch. Su.7/23)

Karnapurana

The procedure of filling oil/ medicated liquid into ears for a prescribed time is known as Karnapurana.

Vidhi

स्वेदयेत् कर्णदेशं तु किञ्चिन्नुः पार्श्वशायिनः। मूत्रैः स्नेहै रसैह् कोष्णैस्ततः श्रोत्रं प्रपूरयेत्॥
कर्णं च पूरितं रक्षेच्छतं पञ्च शतानि वा। सहस्त्रं वापि मात्राणां श्रोत्रकण्ठशिरोगदे॥

(Sha.Ut. 1/128-129)

धारयेत्पूरणं कर्णे कर्णमूलं विमर्दयेत्। रुजः स्यान्मार्दवं यावन्मात्राशतमवेदने॥ (A.H.Su. 22/32)

Purva Karma

- ❑ Proper examination of ear.
- ❑ Ear should be cleaned with ear buds, if there is any discharge or wax accumulation.
- ❑ Proper Abhyanga and Svedana should be given for ear and neck.

Pradhana Karma

- ❑ Patient is asked to lie in lateral position. For Karnapurana of left ear patient is should to lie in right lateral position with right hand beneath the head vice versa for rishteas.
- ❑ Luke warm medicated oil/liquid is filled into ear with the help of Gokarna yantra or dropper.
- ❑ Patient is advised not to move till the completion of the treatment.

Duration :

Karna roga	:	100 Matra
Kantha roga	:	500 Matra
Shiro roga	:	1000 Matra
Svastha	:	100 Matra

Pashchat Karma

- ❑ Filled medicated oil should be taken out with the help of a vessel by slowly turning to opposite side.
- ❑ Ear cavity should be cleaned with tissue paper or cotton.
- ❑ Ear plug should be kept in the ears.

Time of Administration

रसाधैः पूरणं कर्णे भोजनात् प्राक् प्रशस्यते।
तैलाद् यैः पूरणं भास्करेडस्नमुपागने॥ (Sha.Ut. 11/130)

If the medicated liquid is Rasadi it should be done in the morning hours before food.
If Taila is used then procedure should be done in the evening.

Yogas	*Indication*
Deepika taila	Karna shula
Shyonaka taila	Tridoshaja Karna Shula
Suajika taila	Karnanada, Shula, Badhiryr, Srava
Apamarga kahora taila	Baadhirya, Karnanada
Shambuka taila	Karna nada

Benefits

हनुमन्याशिरः कर्णशूलघ्नं कर्णपूरणम्। (Su.Chi.24/22)
न कर्णरोगा वातोत्था न मन्याहनुसंग्रहः। नोच्चैः श्रुतिर्न बाधिर्यं स्यान्नित्यं कर्णतर्पणात्॥
(Ch.Su. 5/84)

One who practices Karnapurana daily will not suffer from ear disease of Vata type, stiffness of the neck and jaws, difficulty in hearing loud sounds and deafness.

Akshi Tarpana

The literary meaning of the word 'Tarpana' is "to nourish". Akshi Tarpana is the procedure for the nourishment of eyes.

Akshi Tarpana is one of the Netra Kriyakalpa; it gives nourishment to the eyes and cures the eye diseases due to Vata and Pitta. In this process the eyes are filled upon with medicated oil or ghee for a certain period.

Indication of Akshi Tarpana

नयने ताम्यति स्तब्धे शुष्के रूक्षेऽभिघातिते। वातपित्तातुरे जिह्मे शीर्णपक्ष्माविलेक्षणे॥
कच्छ्रोन्मीलशिराहर्षशिरोत्पाततमोऽर्जुनै। स्यन्दमन्थान्यतोवातवातपर्यायशुक्रकैः॥ (A.H.Su.24/1-3)

Darkness before eyes, stiffness, dryness, trauma in eyes, Vata and Pitta disorders of eyes, squint, falling of eyelashes, blurring of the vision, paralysis of eyeball, loss of eye lashes, difficulty in opening and closing of eyes, congestion, glaucoma, nerve disorders of eyes, corneal opacity.

आतुरे शान्तरागाश्रुशूलंसंरम्भदूषिके। निवाते तर्पणं योज्यं......................॥

Contraindications

दुर्दिनात्युष्णशीतेषु चिन्तायासभ्रमेषु च। अशान्तोपद्रवे चाक्ष्णि तर्पणं न प्रशस्यते। (Su. Ut. 18/18)

Cloudy day, hot or cold seasons, worried, tiredness, giddiness, when person is having increased pain.

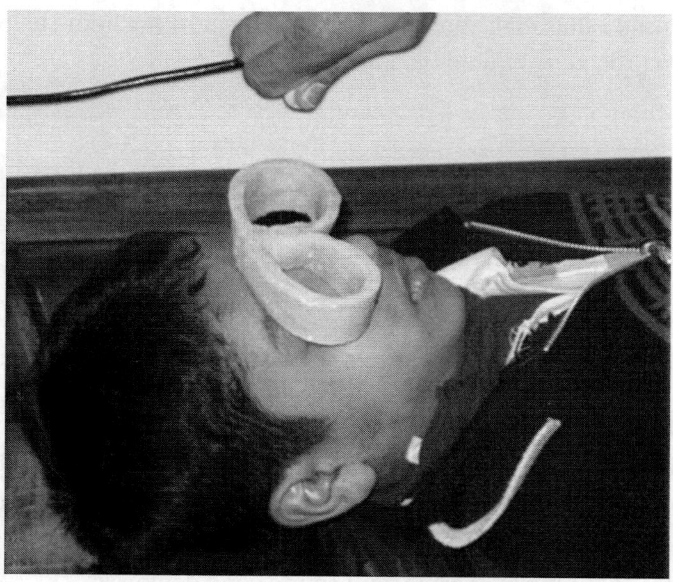

Fig. 2.7: Akshi tarpana

Akshi Tarpana Vidhi (Fig. 2.7)

I. **Purva karma:** Kaya and Shiro Shodhana

II. **Pradhana karma:**

Should be performed in Sadharana Kala either morning or evening in Nivatasthana, after digestion of previous food.

Patient should be asked to lie down comfortably in supine position.

With the paste of Yava or Masha, Masha pali is prepared and should applied eyes in 2 Angula height which should be stiff enough to prevent leaking of medicines.

Patient is asked to close his/her eyes and prescribed medicated oil is filled in the cavity up to the level of eye lashes. (आपक्ष्मग्रात्)

If ghrita is used then it has to be melted by putting the vessel on hot water.

Patient is advised to open and close his eye lids frequently up to specific time according to vitiation of doshas.

III. **Pashchat karma**

- After attaining proper symptoms of administration or specific time, medicine should be removed by making perforation in mashapali at outer canthus.
- Eyes should be cleaned after removing masha Pishti.
- Prakshalana should be done with lukewarm water.
- Vairechanika dhuma should be given.
- Advice the patient not to make effort for seeing the distant and bright things.

In case of night blindness, Vatika Timira and ptosis instead of ghee, animal fat (Vasa) is used. Commonly, Triphala ghrita is used for this process.

Duration

Disease	Duration
Sandhigata roga	300 Matra kala
Vartmagata roga	100 Matra kala
Shuklagata roga	500 Matra kala
Krishnagata roga	700 Matra kala
Drishtigata roga	800 or 1000 Matra kala
Sarva roga	1000 Matra kala
Vataja-daily	1000 Matra kala
Pittaja—once in 3 days	600 Matra kala 800 (Sushruta)
Kaphaja—once in 5 days	500 Matra kala 600 (Sushruta)
Svastha—once in 2 days	500 Matra kala

Samyak yoga

सुखस्वप्रावबोधत्वं वैशदयं वर्णपाटवम्। निर्वृतिर्व्याधिध्वंसः क्रियालाघवमेव॥ (Su. Ut. 18/13)

Induces good sleep, easy awakening at proper time, clarity of vision, ability to clearly appreciate the colours subsides, illness, no discomfort in performing movements of eyes.

Ati Yoga

गुर्वाविलमतिस्निग्धमश्रुकण्डूपदेहवत्।
ज्ञेयं दोषसमुत्क्लिष्टं नेत्रमत्यर्थतर्पितम्॥ (Su. Ut. 18/14)

Heaviness, blurness of vision, excessive oiliness, lacrimation, itching and stickiness in the eyes are the symptoms of excessive Akshi Tarpana.

Ayoga

रूक्षमाविलमस्त्राढयमसहं रूपदर्शने।
व्याधिवृद्धिश्च तज्ज्ञेयं हीनतर्पितमक्षि च॥ (Su. Ut. 18/15)

Dryness, blurness of vision, lacrimation and discharge, intolerance to the light, and aggravation of the disease are the symptoms of Ayoga of Akshi tarpana.

Talam/Mastishkya (Figs 2.8A to C)

"Thala" in Malayalam vocabulary refers to Shiras and "Pothichil" refers to Lepana. So Thala Pothichil refers to Shiro Lepana itself.

It has similar Gunas to that of Takra Dhara.

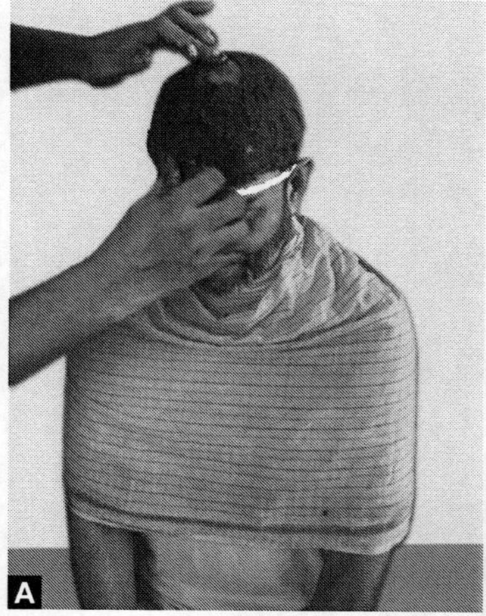

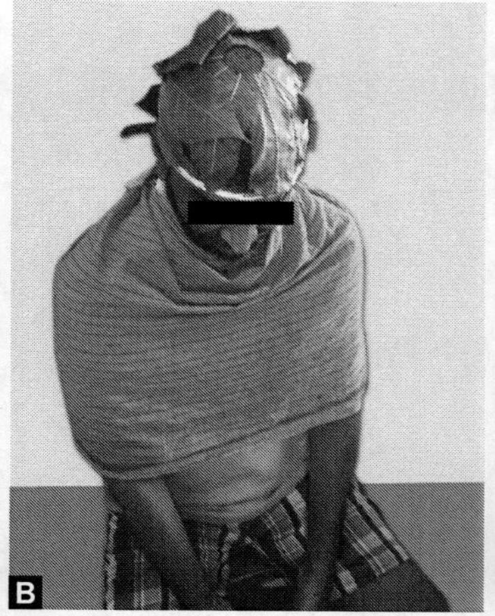

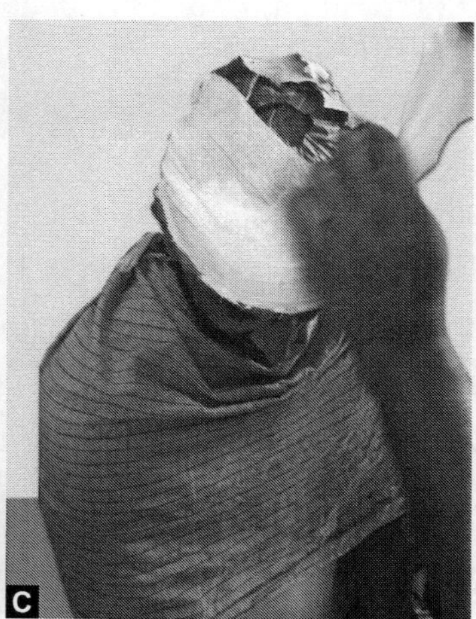

Figs 2.8A to C: Procedure of talam

Preparation

Two methods of preparation have been explained in text of Shirasekadi Vidhi by different authors

1. Boiling the drugs
2. Triturating the dry medicinal powders in butter milk

Method 1

- 1 Kudava (192 g) of dry, deseeded fruits of Amalaki are boiled with 2 Kudava (384 mL) of buttermilk mixed with an equal quantity (384 ml) of water.
- When the water gets evaporated, the vessel is removed from the fire and the contents are ground to smooth paste.

Method 2

तक्रधाराविधानेन सिद्धे प्रस्थार्धसंयुते। तक्रे चतुष्पलमितम् शुष्कधात्रीफलत्वचम्॥
मृत्पात्रे वासितम् रात्रौ पिष्ट्वा च अथ परेहनि। निरंबुचघनम् सम्यक् द्रवस्यन्द्यपि नैव वा॥

(Keraliya Panchakarma/ Shirolepa 1-2)

- Half prastha (384 mL) of butter milk (prepared as in Takra Dhaara) is taken. In this 4 Pala (192 g) of dry, pericarp of Amalaki is soaked overnight preferably in a clay pot.
- The next morning the mixture is well triturated till a fine smooth paste is obtained, which is neither too liquid nor too solid.
- If it is too liquid, it will easily ooze down the head.

Application

The method of application can be divided into three steps :

1. Purva karma
2. Pradhana karma
3. Pashchat karma

Purva Karma

अभ्यज्य मूर्धनि सुदिने कालेप्यावेष्टय वाससा। (Keraliya Panchakarma/ Shirolepa - 3)

- ❑ Abhyanga of head is done prior to the procedure.
- ❑ A strap of cloth is tied all around the forehead to prevent leakage of the substance downwards.
- ❑ Patient is asked to sit on a stool.

Pradhana Karma

पिष्ट्वादल्पम् चोन्चभागे सिरशस्तु पुरस्ततः। भागे तु दक्षिणे मृष्ठे वामे च पुनरूच्यके।
एवम् क्रमात् शिरस्सम्यगासमन्तात् समाव्रतम्।। धात्रीकल्केन लेपस्स्यान्नोनांगुल घनस्ततः।
म्लानेन रम्भापत्रेण पद्मपत्रेण वा क्वचित्।। कर्णपालि सरण्याथ सादम् सम्वेष्टय युक्तितः।
वध्नियादूर्ध्वतस्सम्यक् पत्रमौलि यथातुरः। अभ्यन्जयेद्वा सर्वान्गमासीनस्य यथा सुखम्।।
(Keraliya Panchakarma/ Shirolepa - 3-6)

- ❑ The medicinal paste is applied first at the center of the head, then on the front, right side, back and finally in the left side in the respective order. In this manner, the paste is applied over the whole scalp.
- ❑ The thickness of the paste should be about 1 Angula.
- ❑ The head is then covered with a plaintain leaf which is made flexible by heating. A lotus leaf or other suitable leaves can also be used for this purpose.
- ❑ An opening is made at the center, and the patient is made to sit unmoved for the period of half Yama (1.5 hours) or for 1 Muhurta.
- ❑ There is also a custom of placing Taila at the center of the opening while doing this procedure.

Pashchat Karma

- ❑ At the end of the procedure, the medicinal paste is wiped off.
- ❑ Abhyanga is done on the head.

Benefits

तक्रधाराफलम् चास्मदेकदेशम् समाप्नुयात्। (Keraliya Panchakarma/ Shirolepa - 10)

- ❑ It cures diseases like Klama, Apachi, etc., imparts strength to sight, and induces sleep.
- ❑ It has similar effects to that of Takra Dhaara.

Contraindication

It should never be performed in Vata predominant disorders.

Other Drugs

बलामूलं च मुस्ताम् वा यष्टयाह्वम् त्रिफलामपि।। पन्चगन्धम् तुगाक्षीरीम् दशमूलमथापि वा।
तक्रेण वापि क्षीरेण श्रृतशीत जलेन वा।। पिष्ट्वा तेन शिरोलेपम् यथावस्थम् प्रयोजयेत्।
भेषजस्य गुणे भेदात् यथेच्छम् लभते फलम्।। (Keraliya Panchakarma/ Shirolepa - 10-12)

Balamoola, Yashtimadhu, Panchagandha Churna, Tugakshiri or Dashamoola which is triturated either in milk, buttermilk or cold water as per the need of the condition may also be used.

Murdhni Taila

Head has a special importance amongst the body parts as it is considered as Uttamanga. So the oleation of the head has been separately described under the heading of Murdhni Taila.

Murdhni Taila consists of four different procedures which are as follows.

अभ्यङ्गसेकपिचवो बस्तिश्चेति चतुर्विधम्। मूर्धतैलं बहुगुणं तद्विध्यादुत्तरोत्तरम्।। (A.H.Su.22/23)

1. Shiro-Abhyanga
2. Shiro-Seka
3. Shiro-Pichu, and
4. Shiro-Basti

Successive procedures are considered as the best, i.e Seka is better than Abhyanga, Pichu is better than Seka and Basti is better than Pichu.

Shiro-Abhyanga

Introduction

- ❑ Application of oil on head followed by massage is popularly known as Shiroabhyanga.
- ❑ Usually Shiroabhyanga is performed as a part of sharirabhyanga.
- ❑ Shiroabhyanga is an important route of drug administration in patients suffering from disease of head.
- ❑ Shiroabhyanga is one among dinacharya.

अभ्यङ्गमाचरेन्नित्यं स जराश्रमवातहा। दृष्टिप्रसादपुष्टयायुः स्वप्रसुत्वक्तवदाढर्यकृत्।।
शिरः श्रवणपादेषु तं विशेषेण शीलयेत्।। (A.H.Su.2/8-9)

Materials Required

Oil/Medicated oil	50 mL
Vessel	100 mL capacity
Tissue paper/soft towel	Q.S.
Green gram powder/Snana churna	Q.S.
Masseur	One

Purva karma

- ❑ Oil in kharapaka or madhyamapaka should be selected according to climate, prakriti and disease condition of the patient.
- ❑ The oil is heated between 38°C–44°C. For shiroabhyanga, lukewarm oil is selected.

Pradhana Karma

- ❑ Patient should be seated on the droni/table, in comfortable position. The oil with optimum temperature should be applied to head, first in the anterior fontanellae and then the whole scalp.
- ❑ Then Karnaabhyanga should be done prior to the main process.
- ❑ Start massaging scalp, head and move down to neck, upper back, shoulders.

It includes total 9 steps as follows on vertex, occipital and temporal region.

1. Smearing of the oil
   - Oil is heated approximately 40°C.
   - Oil is then poured over head and is smeared over the head by dividing the hairs with the help of fingers or by using cotton dipped in oil.
2. Gharshana Hasta: Then massage the whole head, moving the palmar surface of the hand from before backwards. Complete area of scalp is massaged for a desired period.
3. Mridvanguli Tadana: Fingers of the both hands are moved as if picking up tuft of hairs.
4. Dvihasta Tadana: Gentle strokes are placed with the palmar surface on the scalp by both hands simultaneously and alternatively.
5. Taranga Hasta: Gentle strokes are placed on the Patients head by rapid rocking movement of both the palms simultaneously.
6. Anguli Kridana Hasta: Rocking movement on the head with the palmar aspect of the little finger and thumb will touch the scalp.
7. Mridu Mushti Tadana: In this maneuver gentle strokes are placed on all areas of the head with the closed fist through the ulnar border. First simultaneously then alternatively.
8. Shabdanguli Kreedana: Both the hands are clasped together with little finger folded. Stroking is done with loose hands by the other fingers producing a bubbling sound.
9. Ghatita Hasta
   - Flat of the palm is placed on the patients head and is moulded in the shape of the scalp.
   - Followed by exerting gentle and firm pressure on the head.

At the end of the procedure the medicine on the face should be wiped off with tissue paper/ towels.

Pashchat Karma

- ❑ Patient should take complete rest for 15 minutes in comfortable position.
- ❑ Patient can take bath in lukewarm water with suitable medicate soap or snana churna.
- ❑ Rasnadi churna should be applied on head after snana.

Duration : 25–35 minutes

Indications

तत्राभ्यङ्गः प्रयोक्तव्यो रौक्ष्यकण्डूमलादिषु। (A.H.Su.22/24)

Abhyanga is advised in people suffering from dryness of scalp, itching, and excessive scaling in scalp.

Contraindications

वर्ज्योऽभ्यङ्गः कफग्रस्तकृतसंशशुद्ध्यजीर्णिभिः। (A.H.Su.2/9)

Abhyanga is contraindicated in people suffering from disorders of Kapha, who have undergone sanshodhana and suffering from Ajirna.

Shirodhara (Fig. 2.9)

Continuous pouring of medicated liquid in a systematic manner on the forehead or scalp using Dhara Yantra is known as Shiro-dhara.

Synonyms

Dhara, Seka, Parisheka, Avaseka, Sechan, Prasechana
Based on the liquid used for the dhara, dhara is off many types.

- Taila-dhara
- Takra-dhara
- Kashaya-dhara
- Ksheera-dhara
- Ksheera-paka dhara
- Jala-dhara

Equipment for Dhara

Selection of Dravya for Taila-dhara

In shuddha vata	–	Mahasneha / Tila taila
In Pitta and Rakta	–	Ghrita

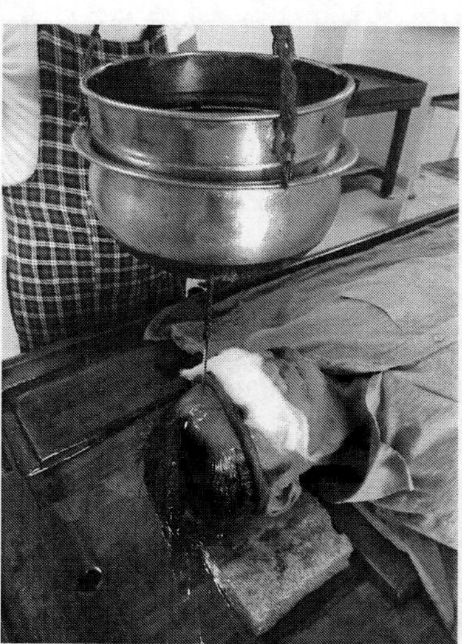

Fig. 2.9: Shiro-dhara

In kapha	–	Tila Taila
Rakta Pitta mishrita Vata	–	Equal quantity of Taila and Ghrita
Kaphaadhika vata	–	Ghrita half the quantity of Taila

Materials Required

Shiro-dhara Patra	–	1
Droni	–	1
Varti	–	1
Suitable oil	–	1 liter
Gauze	–	1
Cotton earplugs	–	2
Soft pillow covered with rexin	–	1
Rasnadi churna	–	5 gm

Specification of Dhara Patra and Varti

स्वर्णाद्यौत्तमलोहजस्तु करको मृत्संभवो वाऽत्र तन्नालाग्रं तु कनिष्ठिकाङ्गुलि परिणाहोन्मित रोगिणः।
द्विप्रस्थप्रमितो विधेय इति वा मध्यस्थरन्ध्रात् अधोगच्छाद्वर्तिरथोर्ध्वलम्ब्यपि घटः कार्यः शिरस्सेचने॥

(Sahasrayoga.Dha.Ka)

Dhara Patra

- Made up of Sphatika Gold good metal, Plakshaadi tree or mud, having 5–6 inches depth with wide open mouth, round at the bottom.
- Capacity of holding 2 prastha (approx 1.5-2 liters)
- There should be a hole in the center of the bottom measuring the size of the little finger.
- There should be three holes with equal distance to the ridges of the patra, to tie up three strings for the purpose of hanging over the stand.

Dhara Varti

- It is a wick or a string of loose cotton threads with a free end of about 4 inches coming out through the hole of dhara vessel.
- The threads of the wick should be placed firmly as not to slip from the hole, but loose enough to permit a continuous and uniform flow of the liquid poured into the Dhara patra.

Purva Karma

- Abhyanga should be done over the face, neck, shoulder and chest (Whole body abhyanga can also be done).
- Gauze is tied around the head just above the eyebrows of the patient.
- Eyes should be closed by tying the eye pad.
- Ear plug should be placed in ears.

Pradhana Karma

- Patient should lie in a supine position on the droni with a small pillow under the neck and the Shiro-dhara device should be placed near his head.
- Its height should be fixed such that oil should fall from a height of 4–5 inches in a continuous stream of little finger thickness. Serrated coconut shell should be placed inside the apparatus to maintain uniform dhara.
- Oil should be heated just above body temperature (38–40°C) and poured into the Dhara patra. A continuous stream of oil should be allowed to fall on the entire forehead, while oscillating the Dhar apatra to cover the entire head.
- Dhara oscillations should not be done too' fast or too slow uniform oscillation is required for uniform dhara. Simultaneous massage with other hand can also be done.
- The oil should be recollected from the droni, reheated and poured back into the dhara patra.

Pashchat Karma

- Gauze and earplugs should be removed.
- Head must be wiped off with the clean towel.
- Head bath should be done with lukewarm water after 45 mins.
- Rasnadi chuorna should be applied over the head after the bath.

Duration

45 minutes for the required number of days.

Precautions

- Refilling of oil should be done from side to avoid spilling of the oil into the eyes.
- Patient should not sleep during the procedure.
- Moderate height, speed, thickness and uniform flow of the fluid should be maintained.
- Hair of the patient may be shaved or cut short as much as possible.

Benefits of Taila-dhara

स्थैर्य वाङ्मनसो शरीरबलम्प्याहारकांक्षाधृतिर्माधुर्य। वचस्यत्वचोऽपि मृदुता नेत्रे प्रकाशो अगदः॥
शुक्रासृक् परिपोषणं रतरतिर्दीर्घाल्पोंष्णता। दुस्वप्नं घृततैलसेचनगुणेनाऽस्तीति जाग्रत्सुखम्॥

(Sahasrayoga. Dha. Ka)

Increases stability in speech and mind, increases strength, increases relishness towards food, increases sweetness in voice, smoothness of skin, improves eyesight and prevents eye disorders, nourishes Shukra and Rakta, increases desire, longevity and prevents disturbed sleep.

Complications and its Management

Fainting, headache, rhinitis, coldness of foot, apply rasna churna over anterior fontenelle and do ushna upachara.

Takradhara

Takradhara is a variety of Shiro-dhara, in which medicated Takra is poured in a continuous stream over the forehead, in a specified manner.

Materials Required

Shiro-dhara patra	–	1
Droni	–	1
Cotton pad	–	1
Amalaki chuorna	–	200 g
Milk	–	600 mL
Musta	–	75 g
Oil for talam	–	10 mL
Rasnadi Churna	–	5 g
Attendants	–	2
Water	–	5400 mL

Preparation of the Medicine

धारायास्त्वेक वर्षातपहिमपरिशेषातिशुद्धप्रकीर्णम्। धात्रीप्रस्थं सपादं भिषगथ पटुधीः संत्यजेत् बीजप्रस्था।। उत्क्वाथोऽष्टादशाख्यामितकुडुवजले षष्टभाहावशिष्टम्। तत्तुल्यं चाऽम्लतकं विधिरिति मुनिभिः प्रोक्त आत्रेय मुख्यैः।।

(Sahasrayoga.Dha.Ka)

- ❑ Amalaki, one year old which is dried in sunlight and kept in mist during night should be taken in the quantity of 1 prastha.
- ❑ 1/6th Kashaya is prepared by adding 18 Kudava of water.
- ❑ Equal quantity of sour butter milk should be added to the prepared kashaya and used for the treatment.

Preparation of Takra

- ❑ 600 mL of milk diluted with 2400 mL water is boiled with 75 g of Musta tied in a muslin bag, and is reduced to 600 mL. The bag of medicament is taken out and squeezed well. When cooled, this prepared milk is fermented by the addition of a little sour curd over night.
- ❑ Next morning the fermented medicated curd is churned by adding 750 mL of Amalaki Kvatha. The butter is removed completely and this mixture is used for dhara after filtering

Indications

केशादिनां च शौकल्यं क्लममपि तनुतां दोषकोपं शिरोरुक्। अबाधामोजः क्षयं तत्करचरणपरिस्तोदनं मूत्रदोषं।। संधीनां विश्लथत्वं हृदयरुगगरुचीर्जाठराग्नेश्च मांद्यं। धात्री तक्रोत्थ धारा हरति शिरसि व कर्णनेत्रामयौधम्।।

(Sahasrayoga.Dha.Ka)

Dhara prepared from Amalaki and Takra is useful in early greying of hair, dullness and thinning of hair, aggravation of Tridosha headache, Ojokshaya, numbness in palm and sole, urinary tract disorders, joint disorders, heart diseases, tastelessness, reduced digestive fire and in disorders of head, eyes and ears. It is also found to be useful in

- In diabetic mellitus
- Psoriasis
- Hypertension
- Loss of memory
- Neurological disorders like headache, neuropathy
- In psychosomatic disorders such as IBS

Purva Karma

- Make the patient to lie on Droni in comfortable position in a well room devoid of any disturbance.
- Brief regarding the procedure and benefits out of it.
- Then eyes should be covered with eye pads and gauze should be tied around the head just above the eyebrows to prevent the entry of medicine into eyes.

Pradhana Karma

- The dhara pot should be kept in such a way as to allow steady flow of the liquid, poured into it, over the forehead of the patient.
- The tip of dharavarti should be 4–5 cm above the forehead of the patient.
- Takra falling should be poured again into the vessel after collecting it from the Droni.
- The vessel should be oscillated continously so that the takra will fall into the patient's entire forehead without interruption.
- In short all the procedures are same as shiro-dhara, but takra should not be heated or reused next day.

Duration

The process should be done daily for a period of 7 to 14 days. The duration of treatment as well as the time period is according to the nature of the disease and the physical condition of the patient. It is done usually for a fixed time (45 minutes to 1 hour).

Pashchat Karma

The head should be wiped with towel and rasnadi churna is applied. Patient is advised to take rest for a period same as the period of the procedure, then asked to take bath.

Complications and Management

Shivering is observed in some patients due to excess sheeta. In such case the procedure is stopped immediately and the patient is managed with ushnopachara.

Shiropichu

A small cotton piece or swab is dipped in the medicated oil and kept on the anterior fontanelle is known as Shiro-pichu. **पिचुः केशशातस्फुटन धूपने नेत्रस्तम्भे च।** (A.H.Su.22)

It is indicated for the local scalp disorders like; hair fall, splitting of hair and loss of movement of eyeball.

Shirobasti

One of the meanings of Basti is filling and as in this process oil is kept, on the head with the help of a cap, therefore it is known, as Shirobasti.

Vidhi

विधिस्तस्य निषण्णस्य पीठे जानुसमे मृदौ । शुद्धरक्तस्विन्नदेहस्य दिनान्ते गव्यमाहिषम्॥
द्वादशाङ्गुमविस्तीर्णं चर्मपट्टं शिरः समम् । आकर्णबन्धनस्थानं ललाटे वस्त्रवेष्टिते॥
चैलवेणिकया बद्ध्वा माषकल्केन लेपयेत् । ऊर्ध्वं केशभुवो यावदङ्गुलम्। (A.H.Su.22/27-29)

For this purpose a special cap opened at both ends is prepared from thick and firm leather or rexine, having height of about 9 inches (12 Angula) and the circumference nearly equal to the circumference of the head of the patient.

Shirobasti is done on empty stomach preferably in the evening or at night. For sealing the cap dough is prepared from the flour of black gram (Masha). After whole body massage the patient is asked to sit comfortably on the knee high chair. At first a Shirobasti Patta is prepared by using the black gram paste and smearing it on a bandage (Fig. 2.10). This prepared patta is then fixed around the forehead of the patient to help fix the shirobasti cap (Figs 2.11A and B). The cap is put on the head so that it reaches up to the level of behind and above the ear lobe. Then the cap is sealed from inside and outside with the dough of black gram so that no oil leaks from the head. Thereafter a bandage is tied outside the cap at its lower end. Then the oil having about 37°C temperature is slowly poured in the cap from the side of the cap (Figs 2.12A to C).

The level of the oil in the cap should be up to 4 inches (2 Angula) above the skin of scalp. The patient is asked to sit calm in upright position without moving head for the specified period or till the symptoms of proper performance appear, which ever is earlier. The relief in the symptoms and increase in the mouth and nose secretions are the symptoms of proper performance of Shirobasti.

Duration

Vata	–	10,000 Matra (52 minutes)
Pitta	–	8,000 Matra (42 minutes) and for
Kapha	–	6,000 Matra (32 minutes)
Svastha	–	1000 Matra

Pashchat Karma

स्कन्धादि मर्दयेत्।

Thereafter the oil is taken out of the cap with the help of a spoon and the remaining oil is removed by tilting the head.

The cap is removed and the extra oil is wiped with a towel.

Then back of neck, shoulder and forehead are gently massaged.

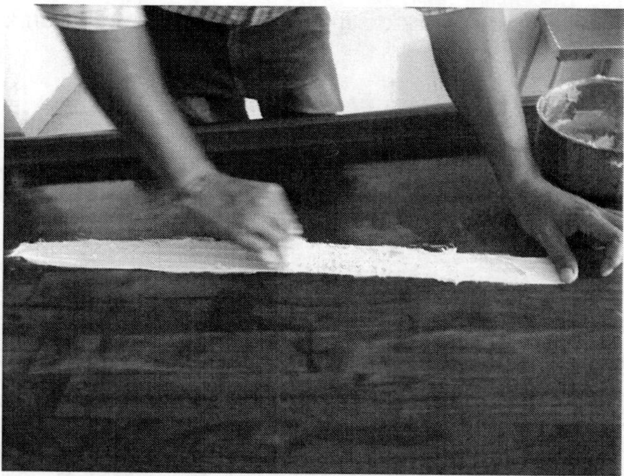

Fig. 2.10: Preparing shirobasti patti

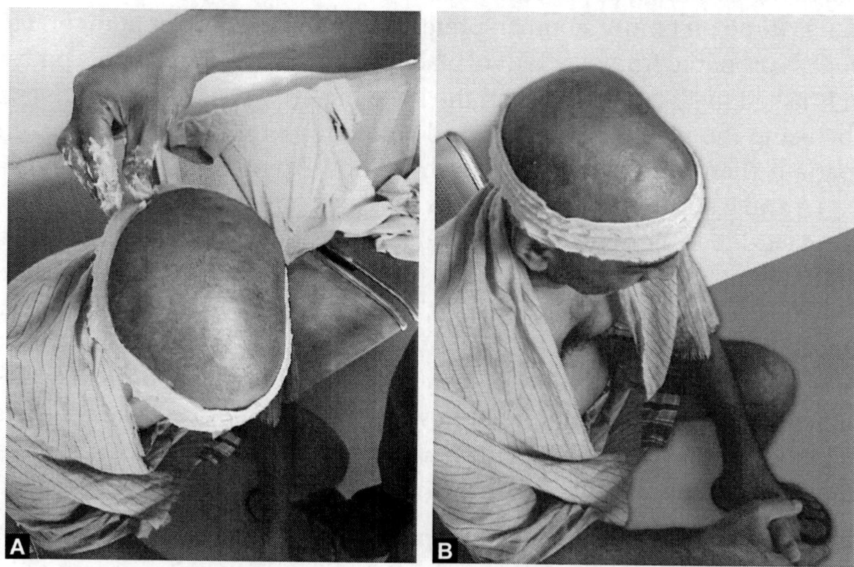

Figs 2.11A and B: Fixing shirobasti patti

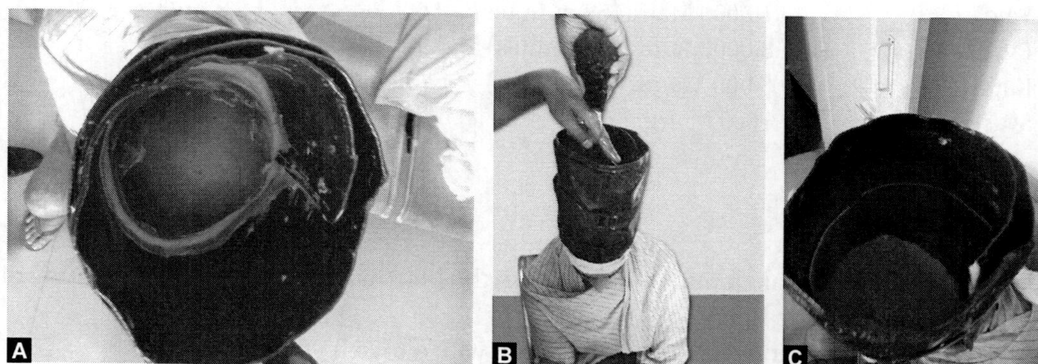

Figs 2.12A to C: (A) Fixed shirobasti cap; (B) Pouring sneha; (C) Filled shirobasti

After taking some rest in waiting room, the patient is allowed to take hot water bath and consume light diet.

Shirobasti is done daily for 3, 5 or 7 days, depending upon the response of the patient.

Indications

.... बस्तिस्तु प्रस्पुप्त्यर्दितजागरे। नासास्यशोषे तिमिरे शिरोरोगे च दारुणे॥ (A.H.Su. 22/26)

Shirobasti is indicated in facial paralysis, insomnia, headache particularly migraine, dandruff, timira, dryness of nose and mouth and loss of sensation. Shirobasti is considered better than Shiro dhara.

Abhyantara Snehana

The administration of Sneha internally through oral route for the purpose of Snehana. Based on the action Abhyantara Snehapana is of three types :

1. Shodhananga Snehapana
2. Shamananga Snehapana and
3. Brihananga Snehapana.

Shodhananga Snehapana

ह्यस्नने जीर्णरावान्ने स्नेहोऽरहाः शुद्धये बहुः। (A.H.Su. 16/9)

Shodhananga Snehapana is one of the essential Purva karma for Sanshodhana. Hence in almost all the Shodhana Arha conditions Shodhananga Snehapana is advised. In the Utklishta Avastha of the Dosha Shodhana can be administered without Snehanadi Purva karma. If necessary, Sadyo sneha can be given.

Shamananga Snehapanna

Administration of snehapana to pacify the morbid Dosha is known as Shamananga Snehana. This can be administered in the morning at the time of breakfast around 9 am.

न शोधयति यद्दोषान् समान्नोदीरयत्यपि।
समीकरोति क्रुद्धांश्च तत् संशमनमुच्यते॥ (Su.Su. 1. Dalhana teeka)

That which do not expel out Dosha, nor aggravates normal Dosha and mitigates the aggravated Dosha is called Shamana.

शमनो—य रोगस्य शमनायापयुज्यते स्नेह॥ (A.H.Su. 16/19. Hemadri)

Hemadri defines Shamana Snehana as, administration of Sneha in different disorders with an intention to normalize the aggravated Doshas without expelling them and disturbing the normal Doshas.

पिबेत् संशमनं स्नेहमन्नकाले प्रकीक्षितः। (Ch.Su.13/60)
शमनः क्षुद्वतोऽनन्नो मध्यमात्र शस्यते। (A.H.Su.16/19)

Vagbhatta opines that, Shamana Snehana is a procedure of administration of Madhyama Matra of Accha Sneha during mealtime or Annakala when one feels hungry.

शमनो हि स्नेहो यत्रतत्रस्थं दोषं कुपितं।
सर्वशरीर व्यापित्वा च्छमनरूपत्वात् शमयति। (A.H.Su.16/19.Hemadri)

Shamana Sneha is administered when one feels hungry spreads throughout the body and mitigates the aggravated Dosha in its own site.

During Shamana Snehana, Pathya and Apathya prescribed in connection with the Virechana are to be followed. (Cha.Su.13/81)

Indication

स्नेहो हितो दुर्बलवह्निदेहसन्धुक्षणे व्याधि निपीडितस्य। (Su.Chi.31/57)

Sushruta says that Sneha is beneficial for people suffering from diseases as it imparts strength to the durbala jatharagni and once the agni is stabilized, diseases start to pacify.

Brihananga Snehapana

बृंहणो रसमद्याद्यैः सभक्तोऽल्पः। (A.H.Su.16/20)

The administration of Sneha along with Mansa Rasa, Madya, Kshira, etc., are known as Brihana Snehana. The dose of Sneha should be Alpa (or even less than quantity of Hrasiyasi Matra).

Indications

बाल वृद्ध पिपासार्त स्नेहविध्वेशि मध्यशीलिषु । स्त्री स्नेहनित्य मन्दाग्नि सुखित क्लेश भीरुषु।
मृदुकोष्ट अल्पदोषेषु काले चोष्णे कृशेषु च॥ (A.H.Su.16/21)

Brihana Snehana is indicated for Bala, Vriddha, Pipasarta, Snehadveshi, Madhyashila, Stree - Sneha nitya, Mandagni, Sutika, Krisha, Bhiru, Mridu Koshtha, Alpa Dosha and Ushnakala.

Relation between Brihana Snehapana time and Food

Administration

स्नेहः प्राग्भोजनात् कुर्यादूरुजङ्घाकटीबलम् । वेगानुलोम्यमारोग्यमधः कायगदक्षयम्॥
मद्ये बृहत्वाग्निबलस्थिरताकुक्षिरुक्शमान्। इन्द्रियस्थिरतामूर्ध्वमूर्ध्वजत्रुगदक्षयम्॥ (A.S.Su.25/24)

Before food	Gives strength to Uru, Jangha and Kati. Vega Anulomana, Cures diseases of lower limb.
With food	Enhances Agnibala Gives strength and stability Reduces Kukshi Shula.
After food	Enhances stability of sense organs Cures disorders of head and neck

Time and Regimen of administering particular Sneha:

यथादोषं यथाकालं यथाव्याधियर्थाबलम्। स्नेहं पक्वमपक्वं वा पाययित्वा चिकित्सकः।

(Vangasena Snehapanadhikara)

Sneha phala shruti depends upon proper time of administering Sneha, strength of patient, doshas vitiated and disease. Wrong time of administration can induce many diseases.

Dosha	Charaka	Sushruta	Vagbhatta
Vata-Kapha	Mid-day	Day	Day
Vata, Vata-Pitta	Evening	Night	Night

As per regimen

1. Ghrita – Sharada
2. Vasa-Majja – Madhav
3. Taila – Pravrita
4. Any Sneha – Sadharana ritu and Prashast day.

These time periods seemed to be for Shamana Sneha.

INDICATIONS OF SNEHANA

स्वेद्याः शोधयितव्याश्च रूक्षा वातविकारिणः।
व्यायाममद्यस्त्रीनित्याः स्नेह्याः स्युर्ये च चिन्तकाः।। (Ch.Su.13/52)
स्वेद्यसंशोद्यमद्यस्त्रीव्यायामासक्तचिन्तकाः। वृद्धबालाबलकृशा रूक्षाः क्षीणास्त्रेरेतसः।।
वातार्तस्यन्दतिमिरदारुणप्रतिबोधिनः। (A.S.Su. 25/9)

Snehana is indicated in those who are undergoing Svedana (sudation), Shodhana (purification procedures), Rukshana (dryness), Suffering from vata disorders, one who regularly indulges in exercise, alcohol and women and also who constantly indulges in thinking.

Also indications mentioned in Shamananga and Brihananga Snehana.

Yogya	Ch.	A.H.	A.S.	B.P.	K.S.
Svedya	+	+	+	+	-
Shodhayitvya	+	+	+	+	-
Ruksha	+	+	+	+	-
Vata-vikar	+	+	+	+	-
Vyayama nitya	+	+	+	+	+
Madya nitya	+	+	+	+	+
Stri nitya	+	+	+	+	+
Chintaka	+	+	+	+	+

CONTRAINDICATION OF SNEHAPANA

विवर्जयेत् स्नेहपानमजीर्णी तरुणज्वरी। दुर्बलोऽरोचकी स्थूलो मूर्च्छार्तो मदपीड़ितः।।
छर्द्यर्दितः पिपासार्तः श्रान्तः पानक्लमान्वित। दत्तबस्तिर्विरिक्तश्च वान्तो यश्चापि मानवः।।
अकाले दुर्दिने चैव न च स्नेहं पिबेन्नरः। अकाले च प्रसूता स्त्री स्नेहपानं विवर्जयेत्।।
संशोधनाहृते येषां रूक्षणं संप्रवक्ष्यते। न तेषां स्नेहं शस्तमुत्सन्नकफमेदसाम्।।
अभिष्यण्णाननगुदा नित्यमन्दाग्नयश्च ये। तृष्णामूर्च्छापरीताश्च गर्भिण्यस्तालुशोषिणः।।
अन्नद्विषश्छर्दयन्तो जठरामगरार्दिताः। दुर्बलताश्च प्रतान्ताश्च स्नेहग्लाना मदातुराः।।
न स्नेह्या वर्तमानेषु न नस्तोबस्तिकर्मसु। स्नेहपानात् प्रजायन्ते तेषां रोगाः सुदारुणाः।। (Ch.Su. 13/53-56)

- ❑ Those who have been administered Rukshana without Shodhana
- ❑ Those in whom Kapha and Meda have increased
- ❑ Who have profuse discharge of mucous from mouth and rectum
- ❑ Who have low digestive fire constantly
- ❑ Who are suffering from thirst and fainting
- ❑ For women pregnant
- ❑ Dryness of palate
- ❑ Who have aversion towards food
- ❑ Suffering from vomiting
- ❑ Who are afflicted with diseases of stomach
- ❑ Digestive disorder and chronic poisoning (Gara Visha)
- ❑ Those who are weak and excessively attenuated
- ❑ Aversion towards oil
- ❑ Chronic alcoholic
- ❑ Who are undergoing procedure of Nasya or Basti.

Contraindications of Snehapana: In below indicated diseases, Snehapana is contraindicated If used it will cause complications.

Ayogya	*Ch.*	*Su.*	*A.H.*	*A.S.*	*Ka.*	*Sha.*	*B.P.*
Vriddha	-	+	+	+	-	-	-
Bala	-	+	+	+	-	-	-
Abala	-	+	+	+	-	-	-
Kshina	-	+	+	+	-	-	-
Asraretasa	-	+	+	+	-	-	-
Abhishyandana	-	+	+	+	-	-	-
Timira	-	+	+	+	-	-	-
Darun pratibodhaka	-	+	+	+	-	-	-
Adhva krisha	-	-	-	-	+	+	+
Bala-kal-vaya-agni atmya	-	-	-	-	+	+	+
Atimandagni	+	-	+	+	-	-	-
Atitikshnagni	-	-	+	+	-	-	-
Atisthula	-	+	+	+	-	-	-
Durbala	+	+	+	+	-	-	-
Urusthambha	-	-	+	+	-	-	-
Atisara	-	-	+	+	-	-	-
Galaroga	-	-	+	+	+	+	+
Garadita	+	-	+	+	-	-	-
Udara roga	+	-	+	+	-	-	-
Murccha	+	+	+	+	-	-	-
Cchardi	+	+	+	+	+	+	+

Ayogya	Ch.	Su.	A.H.	A.S.	Ka.	Sha.	B.P.
Aruchi	-	+	+	+	+	+	+
Trishna pidita	+	+	+	+	-	-	-
Madya pidita	+	+	+	+	-	-	-
Apa prasuta	-	+	+	+	-	-	-
Datta nasya	+	-	+	+	+	+	+
Datta basti	+	+	+	+	+	+	+
Datta virechana	-	+	+	+	-	-	-
Rukshnarha	+	-	-	-	-	-	-
Uttasnna kapha	+	-	-	-	-	-	-
Uttasnna meda	+	-	-	-	-	-	-
Abhishanna anana	+	-	-	-	-	-	-
Abhishanna guda	+	-	-	-	-	-	-
Garbhini	+	-	-	-	+	+	+
Talu shoshini	+	-	-	-	-	+	+
Anna dveshi	+	-	-	-	-	-	-
Pratanta	+	-	-	-	-	-	-
Sneha glani	+	-	-	-	-	-	-
Ajirna	+	-	-	-	+	+	+
Tarun jvari	-	+	-	-	+	+	+
Shranta	-	+	-	-	-	-	-
Klama	-	+	-	-	-	-	-
Vanta	-	+	-	-	-	-	-
Akale, durdina	-	+	-	-	-	-	-
Kapha prakopa	-	-	-	-	+	+	+
Dagdha	-	-	-	-	+	+	+
Kshirapa, jadya	-	-	-	-	+	+	+
Glani	-	-	-	-	+	+	+
Shramanvita	-	-	-	-	-	-	-

SHODANARTHA SNEHANA

Importance of Deepana-Pachana

Achieving normal status of Agni is important before the administration of Snehapana. If Agni is not in normal condition Sneha will not undergo digestion properly inturn leading to complication. So Acharya Vagbhatta has mentioned.

स्नेहस्य पानात् पूर्वञ्च दातव्यं मृदु भेषजम्। उत्तेजनं हुताशस्य कोष्ठलाघवकारि च। (A.S.Su.25/32)

Before the administration of Sneha one has to administer mild medicines which increases the Agni and brings the laghuta in the Koshtha.

Rukshana in Shodanartha Snehana

Rukshana is the Vishishta Purva karrna before the administration of Shodhananga Sneha in specific conditions like :

मांसला मेदुरा भूरिश्लेष्माणो विषमाग्नयः। स्नेहोचिताश्च ये स्नेह्यतान् पूर्व रूक्षयेत्ततः।। (A.H.Su.16/37)

Mansala (Upachita Mansa)
Medura (Medasvina)
Bhurishleshma (Excess of kapha)
Vishamagni (Altered state of digestive strength)

Rukshana should be done before the administration of sneha except Vishamagni. If it is not performed then it results in Snehavyapad. In Sneha Satmya condition if Snehapana is administered then there will be Anuthkleshana of Dosha. Here Pachana is indicated, i.e. nothing but Rukshana.

Properties of Rukshana Dravya

रूक्षं लघु खरं तीक्ष्णमुष्णं स्थिरमपिच्छिलम्। प्रायशः कठिनं चैव यद्द्रव्यं तद्धि रूक्षणम्।।

(Ch.Su.22/14)

Rukshana is mainly achieved by Sneha Abhava. It is Ruksha guna pradhana karma and dravya karya is very important here.

Ruksha	Dry
Laghu	Light
Khara	Rough
Tikshna	Penetrative
Ushna	Hot
Sthira	Stable
Apicchila	Non viscous
Kathina	Hard

While explaining Rukshana Guna Vagbhatta says Vipareeta Gunas of Snehana should be considered. Arundatta explains Laghu, Ushna, Sthira, Ruksha, Tikshna, Sthula, Kathina, Sandra are the Gunas of Rukshana. He also explains opposite qualities of these can also have Rukshana property like Yava is having Guru, Sheeta, Sara Guna, etc. but it is a Rukshana drug, i.e Katu, Tikta, Kashaya Rasa Pradhana Dravya.

Indications of Rukshana

अभिष्यण्णा महादोषा मर्मस्था व्याधयश्च ये। ऊरुस्तम्भ प्रभृतयो रूक्षणीया निदर्शिताः।।

(Ch.Su.22/30)

- ❑ Abhishanna- Drava Pradhana Shleshma Vikara like Prameha.
- ❑ Mahadosha- Kapha Vriddha state of Bahudosha like Prameha, Udara, etc.
- ❑ Marmastha Vyadhi like Hridroga.
- ❑ Urusthamba.

Samyak Rukshana Lakshana

वातमूत्रपुरीषाणां विसर्गेगात्र लाघवे। हृदयोद्गारकण्ठास्यशुद्धौ तन्द्राक्लमे गते॥
स्वेदे जाते रुचौ चैव क्षुत्पिपासासहोदये। कृतं लङ्घनमादेश्यं निर्व्यथे चान्तरात्मनि। (Ch.Su.22/34-35)

Samyak Vata, Mutra, Mala Pravritti
Udgara Shuddhi
Asya Shuddhi
Tandra Nasha
Sveda
Kshuta Pipasa Sahodaya
Utsaha
Gatra Laghuta
Hridaya Shuddhi
Kantha Shuddhi
Indriya Prasannata
Klama Nasha
Ruchi
Vyadhi Mardava
Nirvyathe Antaratma

Rukshana Atiyoga Lakshana

पर्वभेदोऽङ्गमर्दश्च कासः शोषो मुखस्य च। क्षुत्प्रणाशोऽरुचिस्तृष्णा दौर्बल्यं श्रोत्रनेत्रयोः॥
मनसः संभ्रमोऽभीक्ष्णमूर्ध्ववातस्तमो हृदि। देहाग्निबलनाशश्च लङ्घनेऽतिकृते भवेत्॥ (Ch.Su.22/36-37)

Parvabedha : Pain in joints
Angamarda : Bodyache
Kasa : Cough
Mukha Shosha : Mouth dryness
Kshuta pranasha : Absence of hunger
Aruchi : Lack of taste
Trishna : Thrist
Shrotra netra daurbalya : Impairment of hearing and vision
Mana Sambrama (Mana Asthirata) : Altered state of mind
Urdhva vata : Upward movement of vata
Tamo hrudi : Discomfort in the chest
Deha bala nasha : Loss of weight and strength
Agni bala nasha : Loss of digestive strenth

Consideration of Agni and Koshtha in Snehana

Koshtha

मृदुकोष्ठस्त्रिरात्रेण स्निह्यत्यच्छोपसेवया। स्निह्यति क्रूरकोष्ठस्तु सप्तरात्रेण मानवः॥
गुडमिक्षुरसं मस्तु क्षीरमुल्लोडितं दधि। पायसं कृशरां सर्पिः काश्मर्यत्रिफलारसम्॥
द्राक्षारसं पीलुरसं जलमुष्णमथापि वा। मद्यं वा तरुणं पीत्वा मृदुकोष्ठो विरिच्यते॥
विरेचयन्ति नैतानि क्रूरकोष्ठं कदाचन। भवति क्रूरकोष्ठस्य ग्रहण्यत्युल्बणानिला॥
उदीर्णपित्ताऽल्पकफा ग्रहणी मन्दमारुता। मृदुकोष्ठ तस्मात् स सुविरेच्यो नरः स्मृतः॥ (Ch.Su.l3/65-69)

Person having Mridu Koshtha (soft bowel) gets oleated in three days while a Krura Koshtha (hard bowel) person takes seven days to get oleated.

Soft bowelled person gets virechana by the intake of jaggery, sugarcane juice, milk, churned curds, ghee, juice of Kashmarya, Triphala, grape juice, Peelu rasa, warm water or fresh wine.

The hard bowelled person fail to virechana by intake of these as Vata will be predominant in the Grahani.

The soft bowelled person is said to easily purgates as Grahani consists predominant Pitta, Alpa Kapha and Manda Vata.

Indication of Different Matra

Achieving Snigdha lakshana with in the required number of days depends on the proper dose of Shodhana. If the Sneha is administered in less than the required quantity it will fail to produce Snigdha Lakshana and if the excessive quantity is administered it is likely to produce Atisnigdha lakshana.

Fixing the dosage of Sneha in numerical value is not possible with the reason that, dose will vary from person to person based on Doshadi factors. Hence with this idea, dosage of the Sneha is explained based on the time required for the digestion of Sneha viz.

Vagbhatta	*Charaka*	*Sushruta based on digestion time*
Hrasiyasi Matra	Hrasva Matra	3 hours
Hrasva Matra	Madhyama Matra	6 hours
Madhyama Matra	Uttama Matra	9 hours
Uttama Matra		12 hours
		24 hours

Authors like Bhavamishra, Sharangdhara have mentioned Sneha Matra in the numerical value as mentioned in below table :

Author	*Hrasiyasi Matra*	*Hrasva Matra*	*Madhyama Matra*	*Uttama Matra*
Arunadatta	1 Pala	2 Pala	4 Pala	6 Pala
Sharangdhara	-	2 Tola	3 Tola	4 Tola
Bhavamishra		2 Tola	3 Tola	4 Tola
Chakradatta		1/2 Pala	3 Parsha	1 Pala

From the table it seems that those dosage schedule given by the authors are only for the daily use of Sneha along with other food stuffs. When person is subjected for Shodhanapurva Snehapana then these dosages may hold good only for the starting day. Therefore, dose fixation should be done based on Agni factor.

Sneha Matra According to Sushruta

या मात्रा परिजीर्येत चतुर्भाग गतेऽहनि। सा मात्रा दीपयत्यग्निमल्पदोषे च पूजिता॥
या मात्रा परिजीर्येत तथाऽर्धदिवसे गते। सा वृष्या बृंहणीया च मध्यदोषे च पूजिता॥
या मात्रा परिजीर्येत चतुर्भागावशेषिते। स्नेहनीया च सा मात्रा बहुदोषे च पूजिता।
य मात्रा परिजीर्येत्तु तथा परिणतेऽहनि। ग्लानिमूर्च्छामदान् हित्वा सा मात्रा पूजिता॥
अहोरात्रादसंदुष्टा या मात्रा परिजीर्यति। स तु कुष्ठविषोन्मादग्रहापस्मारनाशिनी॥ (Su.Chi.31/25-30)

Dose	Time required for digestion	Action	Indication
Prathama Matra	3 Hrs	Agnidipti	Alpa Dosha
Dvitiya Matra	6 Hrs	Vrishya, Brihana	Madhyama Dosha
Tritiya Matra	9 Hrs	Snehaniya	Bahu Dosha
Chaturtha Matra	12 Hrs	Pujaniya	Glani, Murccha, Mada Kushtha, Visha, Unmada, Graha, Apasmara
Panchama Matra	24 Hrs		

Indications of Sneha Matra

Dose	Criteria for selection		Action
	Individual	Disease	
Uttama Matra (24 hours)	• Prabhuta Sneha nitya • Kshut-Pipasa Saha • Uttama-Agnibala • Sharira Bala • Manasa Bala	• Gulma Sarpa-danshtra • Visarpa Unmatta • Mutrakrcchra • Gadha Varcha	• Shighravikāra Shamana • Soshanukarshini • Pervades through all Marga • Balya • Rejuvenates-body, sense organs and mind
Madhyama Matra (12 hours)	• Madhyama- Sharira bala • Manasa bala • Agnibala • Mridu Koshtha	• Arushka • Sphota • Pidaka • Kandu • Pama • Kushta	• No much complication • Does not effect strength much • Brings Snehana comfortably • Used as Shodhanartha Snehana
Hrasva Matra (6 hours)	• Vriddha • Bala • Sukumara/Sukhochita • Mandagni • Durbala/Avara bala • Person not able to withstand hunger	• Chronic condition of disease like-Jvara • Atisara • Kasa	• Brihaniya • Snehaniya • Vrishya • Balya • Long lasting benefits • Does not cause complications

Hrasiyasi Matra is a trial dose, which is administered on the first day of the Snehapana.

One of the actions of Uttama Matra Snehapana is explained to Vikara Shamana and that of Hrasva Matra as Brihana in the table. Chakrapani mentions that Uttama Matra should be used for Shamana and not for Shodhana Purva Snehana.

But Dalhana commenting on Su. Chi. 31/14 clears this mentioning that, the Uttama, Madhyama and Hrasva Matra, can used as Shodhana Snehapana Matra in appropriate condition.

Arohana Snehapana

The word Arohana means the act of rising, ascending. [Monier Williams 1899].

Arohana Snehapana can be defined as an oral administration of Sneha in the increment dosage.

The clear-cut reference of Arohana Snehapana is available in Kalyanakaraka (6th AD), where it is quoted that the individual whom posted for Snehapana should drink Ghrita or Taila in the incrpermentKrama Vardhitam Pibet Dosage for 3, 5 or 7 days.

स्वयं नरस्नेहतत्पतरो घृतं तिलोद्भवं वा क्रमवर्द्धितं पिबेत्।
त्रिपंचसप्ताहमिह प्रयत्नतः ततस्तु सात्म्यं प्रभवोन्निषेवितम्॥ (Kalyanakaraka.22)

Then Vangasena [9th AD] described the method of Arohana Snehapana.
Opinion of Vangasena regarding dosage of Arohana Snehapana :

त्रिकर्षादर्धकर्षेण वृद्धिः सार्धपलं तथा। ततः कर्षाभिवृद्धिश्च भवेद्यवत्पलत्रयम्॥
ततोऽपि च पलार्धेन वृद्धिर्यावच्च षट्पलम्। मात्रेयं स्नेहपानस्य जघन्यमध्यमोत्त्माः॥
एकाहमुत्तमा पेया त्र्यद्धमेव तु मध्यमा। स्नेहमात्रा यथायोगं सप्ताहन्तु कनीयसी॥ (Vangasena. Snehadikara)

Dosage			*Day*				
Matra	1	2	3	4	5	6	7
Uttama	12 Karsha	14 Karsha	16 Karsha	18 Karsha	20 Karsha	22 Karsha	24 Karsha
Madh yama	6 Karsha	7 Karsha	8 Karsha	9 Karsha	10 Karsha	11 Karsha	12 Karsha
Hrasva	3 Karsha	3½ Karsha	4 Karsha	4½ Karsha	5 Karsha	5½ Karsha	6 Karsha

By going through all the opinions mentioned in table it seems that the Arohana krama Snehapana is advised to achieve Snigdha lakshana within 7 days. But, the method of Arohana Krama Snehapana is left to the discretion of the physician.

Method of Shodhanartha Snehapana

The administration of Shodhannanga Snehapana for the sake of convenience is undertaken in three different stages such as Purva karma, Pradhana karma and Pashchat karma.

Purva Karma

Purva karma is of 2 types: Samanya and Vishishta

A. Samanya Purva karma includes:
- Atura Pariksha
- Atura Siddhata
- Sambhara Sangraha

I. Atura Pariksha—Dasha vidha, Pariksha bhava, Koshtha pariksha

Atura pariksha is necessary for deciding the Bala of Rogi and Roga which inturn helps in the selection of appropriate Sneha and fixation of dosage and Anupana.

II. Atura Siddhata
- Pachana-Deepana
- Diet regimen
- Manasopachara

Pachana: Deepana should be administered till the attainment of Nirama Lakshana. The diet regimen before and during Snehapana should be explained. Proper counselling should be done to gain the confidence of the patient.

III. Sambhara Sangraha — Required Sneha in sufficient amount
Medicaments to treat Vyapad if any

Atura Pariksha

दोषकाल वयोवह्निबलान्यालोक्य योजयेत्। (Bh. P. Snehadhikara 6-7)

The first step of Snehana is to decide the suitability of the patient which has been termed as Arhata or Anarhata. The Dosholbanata is also studied which helps to decide a particular type of Sneha and matra of the same. Charakacharya has described Dashavidha Pariksha for it.

Prakriti: It plays a vital role. Ghrita is used for Vata-Pitta type while Taila is used for Vata-Kapha type. According to Charaka, Vata-Pitta, Kapha prakriti patients should be given Sneha for 7, 5, 3, days respectively.

Vikriti: The study of dosha, dushya plays a very important role. Which dosha is involved? It is in sama or nirama avastha? Location of vitiated doshas ? All this has to consider while deciding Sneha, For example:

- ❑ In Vata pradhana vyadhi, taila is administered.
- ❑ In Rakta-pradoshaja vyadhi, ghrita is more helpful.
- ❑ In ati-medovridhhi, Snehapana is contraindicated.
- ❑ In Samavastha, Snehapana worsens the condition.

Sara, Samhanana, Pramana, Satva, Bala, Vyayama, shakti: This enables us to decide bala of the patient which helps in deciding the Sneha matra. A patient with Avara satva can't tolerate high dose of Sneha.

Ahara shakti: Assessment of Agni helps to fix initial dose and Vardhamana dose in later stage.

Satmya: As per some Acharyas, habituated Sneha should be preferred.

Vaya: Kaphadhikya in children reduces their requirement of Sneha dravya while good digestion power in yuvaavastha increase the amount of Sneha dravya required.

Desha: As Vata is more prominent in Jangala pradesha, Sneha treatment is more effective.

Indication of Snehapana: Indications and contraindications of Snehana are described as carlier. Before the administration of Sneha Dashvidha pariksha should be carried.

स्नेहादिषूपयोगाय तत् व्यापच्छमनाय च। कुर्यात्प्रागेव तद्योगिद्रव्यसम्भारसङ्ग्रहम्॥ (A.S.Su. 25/2)

Pradhana Karma

Includes following steps, viz,

1. Administration of Sneha and Anupana
2. Observation of
   a. Sneha jeeryamana Lakshana
   b. Sneha jeerna Lakshana
   c. Snigdha, Atisnigdha and Asnigdha Lakshan

Administration of Sneha

अथ खलु लघुकोष्ठायातुराय कृतमङ्गमस्वस्तिवाचनाय उदयगिरिशिखरसंस्ति।
प्रतप्तकनकनिकरपीतलोहिते सवितरि यथाबलं तैलस्य घृतस्य वा मात्रां प्रयच्छेत्।। (Su.Chi.31/14)

Early morning when\ the sun rises and attains golden yellow color those individuals exhibiting Jeerna Ahara Lakshana except Kshudha (Hunger), after performing auspicious rituals, the appropriate quantity of Sneha should be given to drink.

Anupana of Snehana

Anupana should be given along with the Sneha. It helps in breakdown, softening, digesting, proper assimilation and in diffusion of the Sneha taken. Specific Anupana for Sneha are:

जलमुष्णं घृते पेयं यूषस्तैलेऽनुशस्यते।
वसामज्जोस्तु मण्डः स्यात् सर्वेषूष्णमथाम्बु वा।। (Ch.Su.13/22)

1. Ushnodaka: For all the Snehas, except Tuvaraka and Bhallatak Taila
2. Yusha: For Taila
3. Manda: For Vasa and Majja
4. Shita Jala: For Bhallataka and Tuvaraka

The dosage of the Anupana may be decided on the basis of nondigestion capacity and also the traditional practice.

Jeerna and Jeeryamana Lakshana

स्नेह जीर्यमान लक्षणः शिरोरुग्भ्रमनिष्ठीवमूर्च्छासादारतिक्लमैः।
जानीयाद् भेषजं जीर्यत्।.....................।। (A.S.Su.25/28)

Jeeryamana lakshana	*Jeerna lakshana*
Shiroruk	Shamana of jeeryamana lakshana
Bhrama	Leghava
Nishtheeva	Vatanulomana
Murccha	Swasthya
Sada	Kshut
Arati	Trishna
Klama	Udgara Shuddhi

Samyak Yoga, Ayoga and Atiyoga of Snehana, Vyapat and Their Management

Samyak Snigdha Lakshana

वातानुलोम्यं दीप्तोऽग्निर्वर्चः स्निग्धमसंहतम् । मार्दवं स्निग्धता चाङ्गे स्निग्धानामुपजायते।।
(Ch.Su.13/58)

सुस्निग्धा त्वग्विट्शैथिल्यं दीप्तोऽग्निर्मृदुगात्रता। ग्लानिर्लाघवमङ्गानां अधस्तात् स्नेहदर्शन।।
सम्यक् स्निग्धस्य लिङ्गानिस्नेहोद्वेगस्तथैव च।। (Su.Chi.31/53)

Symptoms of proper oleation are regulation of flatus, improvement in digestion, unctuous and loose stool, unctuousness and softness of the body.

Asnigdha Lakshana

पुरीषं ग्रथितं रूक्षं वायुरप्रगुणो मृदुः। पक्ता खरत्वं रौक्ष्यं च गात्रस्यास्निग्धलक्षणम्॥ (Ch.Su.13/57)
पुरीषं ग्रथितं रूक्षं कृच्छ्रादन्नं विपच्यते। उरो विदहते वायुः कोष्ठादुपरि धावति॥
दुर्वर्णो दुर्बलश्चैव रूक्षो भवति मानवः॥ (Su.Chi.31/51-52)

Symptoms of under oleation are dry and hard stool, nonregulation of Vata, poor digestion and persisting of roughness and dryness of the body.

Atisnigdha Lakshana

पाण्डुता गौरवं जाडय पुरीषस्याविपक्वता। तन्द्रीररुचिरुत्क्लेशः स्यादितस्निग्धलक्षणम्॥ (Ch.Su.13/59)
भक्तद्वेषो मुखस्रावो गुददाहः प्रवाहिका। पुरीषातिप्रवृत्तिश्च भृशस्निग्धस्य लक्षणम्॥ (Su.Chi. 31/54)

Symptoms of excessive oleation are heaviness, dullness, anorexia, nausea, unformed stools, pallor and drowsiness.

Special Considerations During Snehapana

केवलं पैत्तिके सर्पिर्वातिके लवणान्वितम्। देयं बहुकफे चापि व्योषक्षारसमायुतम्॥ (Su.Chi.31/19)

Pitta	–	Kevala Sarpi
Vata	–	Lavana with Sneha
Kapha	–	Vyosha, Kshara with Sneha

विसर्पपिडकाशोफकामलापाण्डुरोगिणः। अभिघातविषार्ताश्च नातिस्निग्धान् विरेचयेत्॥ (Cha.Si.6/8)

In those suffering from Visarpa, Pidaka, Shopha, Kamala, Pandu, Abhighata and Visha, Shodhananga Snehapana should be stopped after observing Snigdha lakshana and alter on Shodhana should be carried out.

Those suffering from Kushtha, Shopha and Prameha should not use Gramya-Anupa-Oudaka mansa, Guda, Dadhi, Kshira, Tila for Snehana.

Pashchat Karma

For easy understanding purpose Pashchat karma is categorized as:

- ❑ **On the days of Snehapana :**

ततो गुरुप्रावरणो निवातशयनस्थितः।
जरणान्तं प्रतीक्षेत तृष्यन्नुष्णाल्पवारिपः॥ (A.S.Su.25/26)

Guru Pravarana (covering body with thick cloth), nivata shayana sthitaha (residing in a room devoid of breeze), Jarananta, pratiksheta (awaiting of digestion), drinking little quantity of Ushna jala or any other specified Anupana if thirsty.

परिषिच्याद्भिरुष्णांभिर्जीर्णस्नेहं ततो नरम्।
यवागुं पाययेच्चोष्णां कामं क्लिन्नाल पतण्डुलाम्॥ (Su.Chi.31/34)

When Sneha gets digested, taking hot water bath and consume Yavagu, etc., food.

❑ Diet During Snehana

Pathyaapathya

उष्णोदकोपचारी स्याद्ब्रह्मचारी क्षपाशयः। शकृन्मूत्रानिलोद्गारानुदीर्णाश्च न धारयेत्।।
व्यायाममुच्चैर्वचनं क्रोधशोकौ हिमातपौ। वर्जयेदप्रवातं च सेवेत शयनासनम्।। (Ch.Su.13/62-63)

Ushnodaka upachara (should take hot water), Brahmacharya (should maintain celibacy), Kshapashaya (Should sleep during night time only).

Should not do Dharana nor induce Mala, Mutra and Anila vega, Vyayama (exercise), Uchha vachana (loud speech), Krodha (anger), Shoka (depression), Hima (mist), Atapa (sunlight) and Pravata (open breeze).

द्रवोष्णमनभिष्यन्दि भोज्यमन्नं प्रमाणतः। नातिस्निग्धसंकीर्णं श्वः स्नेहं पातुमिच्छता।। (Ch.Su.13/60)

A. Before, during and after taking the Sneha, the patient is allowed to take proper quantity of simple hot and liquid diet containing only little fat and not obstructing the channels. (Anabhishyandi).

B. After attaining Samyak Snigdha Lakshana : When the individual attains Samyak Snigdha Lakshana. Shodananga Snehapana is stopped and they are posted for further process like Sarvanga Abhyanga, Svedana and Shodhana.

Post Snehana Therapies

Gap days, the period between completion of Shodhananga Snehapana to the day of Vamana or Virechana are known as Vishrama Dina. During this period the individual will be subjected for Sarvanga Abhyanga, Svedana and provided with appropriate diet.

The following table illustrates Vishrama Dina for Vamana and Virechana.

Shodhana	*Vishrama Dina*	*Diet advised*
Vamana	1 day	Kaphotkleshakara Ahara with Mansarasa, Dadhi, Masha, Tila
Virechana	3 days	Laghu-drava, Bhuyista Ushna Ahara (Charaka) Laghu Ahara, Ushnodaka, Amalphala (Sushruta)

Sneha Vyapat (Complications)

तन्द्रा सोत्क्लेश आनाहो ज्वरः स्तम्भो विसंज्ञता। कुष्ठानि कण्डुः पाण्डुत्वं शोफार्शांस्यरुचिस्तृषा।
जठरं ग्रहणीदोषाः स्तैमित्यं वाक्यनिग्रहः। शूलमामप्रदोषाश्च जायन्ते स्नेहविभ्रमात्।।

(Ch.Su.13/75-76)

The complications of Snehapa can be divided under two headings, i.e. Immediate complications and late complications

Immediate Complications

1. Ajeerna
2. Jvara
3. Trishna
4. Anaha
5. Tandra
6. Shula
7. Aruchi
8. Sangya nasha

Late Complications

1. Kushtha
2. Pandu
3. Udara
4. Arsha
5. Kandu
6. Shotha
7. Grahani

Vyapat Chikitsa

तत्राप्युल्लेखनं शस्तं स्वेदः कालप्रतीक्षणम्। प्रति प्रति व्याधिबलं बुद्ध्वा स्रंसनमेव च॥
तक्रारिष्टप्रयोगश्च रूक्षपानान्नसेवनम्। मूत्राणां त्रिफलायाश्च स्नेहव्यापत्तिभेषजम्॥ (Ch.Su.13/77-78)

Principles of management include Pathya sevana, Pachana, deepana, Rukshana and Doshavasechana.

- ❑ Upavasa/Trishna: Beneficial in alpa Dosha avastha and enhances Agni Bala.
- ❑ Ullekhana: In Utklishta Dosha Avastha Sadyo Vamana is beneficial and is also advised in conditions like Snehajirna, Utklesha, Snehajanya trishna.
- ❑ Svedana: In conditions such as Sthambha, Svedana is beneficial.
- ❑ Rukshana: Rukshana therapy is highly beneficial in Sneha Atiyogajanya Vyapat. Rukshana Dravya can be administered in the form of Pana, Anna and Bheshja.
- ❑ Trisha: cold water sprinkling, Ruksha anna + Sheeta jala followed by Vamana. Ushnajala vamana if there is vitiation of tridoshas.

Management

Takrarishta prayoga
Mutra prayoga
Pachana dravya
Panchakola pana
Ruksha annapana sevana
Triphala prayoga
Shankha vati
Shunthi jalapana etc.

Snehana Prakarsha Kala (Duration of Shodhanartha Snehana)

Shodhananga Snehapana is the process of administering Sneha to achieve the desired Doshotkleshana within a specific number of days.

स्नेहस्य प्रकर्षौ तु सप्तरात्रत्रिरात्रकौ। (Ch.Su.13/51)
मृदुकोष्ठस्त्रिरात्रेण स्निह्यत्यच्छोपसेवया।
स्निह्यति क्रूरकोष्ठस्तु सप्तरात्रेण मानवः॥ (Ch.Su.13/65)

The minimum and maximum number of days for Shodhananga Snehapana is 3 and 7 days respectively, i.e. the person with Mridu Koshtha for 3 days, in Madhyama Koshtha for 5 days and Krura Koshtha for 7 days.

Based on Tara-Tama of the Koshtha Dalhana quotes as–

Koshtha	Mridu tama	–	1 day
	Mridu tara	–	2 day
	Mridu	–	3 day
	Madhyama tama	–	4 day
	Madhyama tara	–	5 day

Madhyama	–	6 day
Krura	–	7 day
Krura tara	–	8 day
Krura tama	–	9 day

त्र्यहावरं सप्तदिनं परं तु स्निग्धो नरः स्वेदयितव्य उक्तः।
नातः परं स्नेहनमादिशन्ति सात्म्यीभवेत् सप्तदिनात् परं तु॥ (Ch.Si.1/6)

The doses of Shodhanartha Sneha should be planned in such a way that the proper Snehana occurs within 3 to 7 days. Generally in Mridu Koshtha person, Snehana occurs in three days, while it may take 7 days in Krura Koshtha persons. The administration of Sneha should be continued once in a day till the symptoms of Samyak Sneha are achieved, but it should not be given beyond seven days because thereafter it become Satmya to the person. It means if it is given beyond 7 days then it start behaving as diet article and its drug value ceases.

The main therapeutic action of Shodhanartha Snehana is to excite the Dosha, so that they may be taken out by Shodhana and this therapeutic action of Sneha ceases when it becomes Satmya after 7 days.

Sadyo Snehana

Sometimes it becomes necessary to prepare a patient urgently. The administration of Sneha mixed with salt enhances the process of Snehana and is useful for instant (Sadyo) Snehana.

It is based on the principles of Pravicharana Snehana.

Sneha added with Lavana oleates an individual instantaneously (Sadyo Snehana), because salt by nature is Abhishyandi, Sukshma, Aruksha, Ushna and Vyavayi.

सद्यः स्नेहनमिति तदहरेव। (Su.Chi.31.Dalhana)

सद्यः इति तस्मिन्नेव दिवसे त्वरया स्नेहनं करोति। (Adhamalla)

सद्यः स्नेहप्रयोप्रयोगेणैकदिनेनापि स्नेहनममनुजानीत इति ब्रुवते। (Ch.Si.1.Chakrapani)

Dalhana, Adhamalla and Chakrapani commentaries give the description that; Sadyo Snehana brings Snigdha Lakshana quickly on the day of administration.

सद्यः स्नेहप्रयोगा अपि त्र्यहेणैव स्नेहयन्ति। (Ch.Su.13.Chakrapani)

Chakrapani and Adhamalla opine that the Snehana therapy which is said to produce snehana instantaneously may also take three days to bring Snigdha Lakshana. Only for praising, it is said as Sadyo Snehana.

सद्यः स्नेहनाः – त्रिचतुरैरहोभिर्विनाऽपि स्नेहनाः। (Arunadatta)

Sadyo Snehana quickly oleates within 3, 4 days.

Sadyo Snehana Yogas

Many references regarding Sadya Snehana Yogas are available in the classics but their dosage and method of administration is not clearly mentioned. While explaining Pancha Prasratika Peya dosage is mentioned in the numerical value. As an example few Sadyo Snehana Yogas are mentioned here:

- ❑ Pippali, Saindhava, four Snehas and Dadhi, Mastu taken together [Su.Chi.31/38]
- ❑ Intake of Snigdha Yavagu fried in Mansarasa, well prepared and added with plentiful soup [Su.Chi.3139]
- ❑ Intake of Sukshma Yavagu of little rice cooked in milk and added with Ghee. [Su.Chi.31/40]
- ❑ Pippali, Saindhava, Ghee, Tila Pishta, and Varaha Vasa taken together [Su.Chi.31/41]
- ❑ Milk of cow mixed into a vessel containing ghee mixed with powdered sugar. This yoga is indicated specially for Ruksha persons [Su.Chi.31/42].
- ❑ Ghee cooked with decoction of Yava, Kola and Kulattha, milk, curd and Sura added with paste of Pippali. This yoga indicated for Raja and Rajasamebhya persons [Su.Chi.31/43, 44].
- ❑ Mansa Rasa prepared by boiling large quantities of meat of animals of Jangala or Anupa region.
- ❑ Above Mansa Rasa along with Sneha Bharjita Vayagu.
- ❑ Phanita along with Snehayukta Tila Churna.
- ❑ Krishara along with Sneha and Phanita.
- ❑ Sadyo Dugdha with ghee and sugar or ghee and salt.
- ❑ Ghee processed with curd, Vyosha, juice of Amalaki and Draksha.
- ❑ Payasa prepared with addition of Masha and many kinds of fatty substances [A.S.Su.25/46 and A.H.Su. 16/40,41].

Pancha Prasritika Peya

सर्पिस्तैलवसामज्जातण्डुलप्रसृतैः शृता। पाञ्चप्रसृतिकी पेया पेया स्नेहनमिच्छता।। (Ch.Su.13/90)

Pancha Prasritika Peya is prepared with one Prastha each of Chatura Sneha and one Prasta of rice.

Sadyo Snehana Indications

बलहीनेषु वृद्धेषु मृद्वग्निस्त्रीहतात्मसु। अल्पदोषेषु योज्याः स्युर्ये योगाः सम्यगीरिताः।। (Su.Chi.31/45)
बालवृद्धादिषु स्नेहपरिहारअसहिष्णुषु। योगानिमाननुद्वेगान् सद्यः स्नेहान् प्रयोजयेत्।। (A.H.Su.16/39)

Bala	Vriddha
Sneha Parihara Asahishnushu	Balahina
Mridu Agni	Stri Hatatmasu
Alpa Dosha	Raja

Avapeedaka Snehapana

Avapeedaka Sneha is the treatment procedure administered for 'Mutra Vegarodha janya' Vikaras, Adhonabhigata vata vikaras, in which Sneha is consumed immediately before food and after digestion.

It can also be done in infertility, BPH, IBS, spastic colon, etc. Sneha is selected according to physician's Yukti.

Quantity- The quantity of medicated ghee is Uttama Matra. The measurement is variable and subjective.

Procedure

भोजनपूर्वं घृतपानं जीर्णान्तिकञ्च घृतं प्रशस्यते। जीर्णान्तिकं यद्ध्वस्तनेऽन्ने जीर्णे युज्यते, उत्तमया मात्रया अहोरात्रजरणलक्षणया इति प्राग्भक्तस्नेहयोजना जीर्णान्तिस्नेहयोजना च। उभयमवपीडकमुच्यते। (A.S.Su.5/7 Indu)

1. The procedure involves two steps of administration of sneha. One before food intake and second after the digestion of food.
2. For the Shamana purpose, on the day of Snehapana, patient should be observed for the Lakshanas of Vega Pravritti, Agnideepti and initially half portion of Sneha is given, followed by little quantity of hot water. The patient should be advised to take morning food soon after.
3. After the digestion of the food which is evidenced by clean belching, evacuation of bowels, lightness, thirst and hunger; the remaining portion of Sneha should be given.
4. Patient should drink a little quantity of hot water as necessary. He should be made to stay in a place devoid of breeze and by covering himself, awaiting the digestion of Sneha.
5. Feeling of lightness, relief from the symptoms like headache, giddiness, exhaustion, etc. and escape of flatus appearance of appetite, thirst and pure belching indicates the complete digestion of Sneha.
6. For Shodhana purpose 3/4th of full dose initially given, then food, after digestion 1/4th of total dose is given.

Indications

मूत्रजेषु तु पाने च प्राग्भक्तं शस्यते घृतम्।। जीर्णान्तिकं चोत्तमया मात्रया योजनाद्वयम्। अवपीडकमेनत् च संज्ञितं।। (A.H.Su.4/7)

Avapeedaka snehapana is indicated in diseases which appear due to Mutra vegavrodha, e.g. severe pain in body, ashmari (calculus), pain in genitourinary tract including in renal region, etc.

Avapeedaka Guna

पित्तानिलामयघ्नं बस्त्यूरुकटिदृढिकरं वृष्यम्। ऊर्जस्करं श्रमघ्नं विद्यात् स्नेहावपीडं तु।। (Ka.Su.22/47)

Pacifies diseases of Pitta and Vata, give stability to Basti, Uru and Kati, Vrishya, Urjaskara, Shramaghna.

Selection of Aushadhi (Example)

- ❑ Pranavaha Srotas
  - Kantakari Ghrita
  - Indukanta Ghrita
  - Vidaryadi Ghrita
  - Pippalyadi Ghrita
- ❑ Annavaha Srotas
  - Dadimadi Ghrita
  - Indukanta Ghrita
  - Sukumara Ghrita
- ❑ Rasavaha Srotas
  - Pippalyadi Ghrita
  - Dadimadi Ghrita

- Khadira Ghrita
- ❑ Raktavaha Srotas
  - Tiktaka Ghrita
  - Mahatiktaka Ghrita
- ❑ Mansa and Medovaha Srotas
  - Varunadi Ghrita
  - Guggulutiktaka Ghrita
- ❑ Asthi and Majjavaha Srotas
  - Phala Sarpi
  - Kalyanaka Ghrita
  - Dadimadi Ghrita
- ❑ Mutravaha Srotas
  - Vasthyamayantaka Ghrita
  - Varunadi Ghrita
  - Dhanvantara Ghrita
- ❑ Manovaha Srotas
  - Panchagavya Ghrita
  - Brahmi Ghrita
- ❑ Netra
  - Triphala Ghrita
  - Jeevantyadi Ghrita

MODE OF ACTION OF SNEHANA

Actions of Snehana

In Siddhisthana, while dealing with the Snehana Karya, Charaka very vividly explains them as:

❑ Sneho Anilam Hanti
❑ Mridu Karoti Deham
❑ Malanam Vinihanti Sangam [Ch.Si.1/7]

Chakrapani clarifies that these are functions of Shodhana Snehana; on the basis of above version actions of Shodhananga Snehana may be analyzed as follows:

- **Sneho Anilam Hanti**
  Vata Nigraha is one of the criteria mentioned by Charaka to bring Doshas back to Koshtha. As Sneha is having exactly opposite Guna to Vata Dosha, Sneha allots the proper Gati to Vata and helps to bring the Shakhagata Dosha into Koshtha. Vatashamana effect of Snehana can be known by observing Vatanulomana action.
- **Mridu Karoti Deham**
  Sneha by virtue of its Snigdha, Mridu qualities brings softness in Dosha Sanghata, Srotas and Deha, which are very important to bring Dosha to Koshtha and Utklesha stage. This Mridukarana effect of Sneha can be confirmed by observing Gatra Mardavata.
- **Malanam Vinihanti Sangam**
  Mala Sanga generally occurs due to Rukshata, Sneha overcomes this Rukshata by its Snigdha and Vishyanda properties and the Sanga sets right.
  To substantiate the importance of Shodhana Snehana and mode of action many references are available in the classics. For example, few of such references are explained below
- Snehana is required to be administered first, then Svedana; finally Shodhana is to be administered (Ch. Su. 13/99).

स्निग्धात् पात्राद् यथा तोयम् अयत्नेन प्रणुदयते। कफादयः प्रणुदयन्ते स्निग्धाद देहात् औषधैः॥
आर्द काष्ठं यथा वह्रिर् विष्यन्दयति सर्वतः। तथा स्निग्धस्थ वै दोषान् स्वेदो विष्यन्दयेत् स्थिरान्॥

(Ch. Si. 6/11-12)

As from unctuous utensil water is removed without any effect Kapha, etc. are detached from the oleated body with the help of Shodhana.

By going through this version we can understand that Snehana brings softness in the Srotas by that Dosha will come back to Koshtha from Shakha and when Shodhana is administered vitiated Dosha and expelled out without causing discomfort to the individual.

क्लिष्टं वासो यथा उत्क्लेश्य मलः संशोध्यत् अम्यसा। स्नेह स्वेदैस्तथा उत्क्लेश्य शोध्यते शोधनै मलः ॥

(Ch. Si. 6/13)

As the dirt of the cloth is washed with water after deterging (with alkali, etc.), the impurity of the body is eliminated by Shodhana measures after deterging (Utklesha) with Snehana and Svedana.

This version is of extreme importance for explaining the mode of action of Snehana and Svedana as Purva karma to Shodhana in bringing Doshotkleshana. Among these two Purva karma Snehana by virtue of its Vishyandana, Vriddhi properties aids in bringing Lina and Anutklishta Doshas to Utklishta Avastha.

Actions of Snehana can be attributed to properties present in the Sneha Dravya. In this regard it is very much necessary to discuss the actions of these properties with respect to Shodhana Snehana.

Drava

- Brings moistness in the Srotas and constituents of the body.
- Helps in diffusion of Sneha over the body.
- Helps in Dosha Vilayana process.
- Acts like a dissolving media to the Dosha.

Snigdha

- Snigdha and Drava both are complimentary to one another.
- Snigdha brings softness of Srotas and by this there is a better conveyance of Dosha, Dhatu and Mala.

Picchila

- Shleshmala property is important to bring Dosha Utklesha.
- Helps Sneha to come in contact with Doshas for longer duration.
- Picchila is having Pranadharana and Ojo Vivardhana action; hence it protects the body structures from negative onslaught of Shodhana.

Mridu

- Brings Srotomardavata.
- By generating softness, laxity, loosens the Dosha Sanghata.

Sukshma

- By virtue of Sukshma property Sneha reaches to each and every part of the body.
- Sukshma is having Sroto Vishodhana property, thus aiding in bringing the Doshas back to Koshtha.

Sara

- Sara is having 'Vyaptishilatva,' i.e. spreading nature, thus helps in spreading of Sneha all over the body.

- Prerana and Vatanulomana action of Sara Guna helps in the movement of Doshas back to Koshtha.

Though Guru, Shita and Manda are mentioned as properties of Sneha, but these have more of Shamana or Brihana value than aiding in Shodhanga Snehana action.

Human cell membrane is made up of phospholipids. Water-soluble substance cannot cross the cell membrane, while lipid and lipid soluble substance are permeable to the cell membrane. Cell membrane acts as a barrier to the passage of water soluble molecules, but provides free passage to lipids and lipid soluble substances.

From above description it can be said that Sneha, by its Sukshma Guna reaches the cellular level and it can be correlated with the "Actions of Sneha". Phospholipids which are a part of class of fat increase during Snehapana. Phospholipids function as a carrier of various cellular elements. Increase in their level may enhance this transport which must be helpful in some way in various diseases. This could also be compare with Gati of Dosha from Shakha to Koshtha.

Snehapana produces Kledana in body because one gram of fat on combustion gives 1.07 g of water as a side product, while combustion of protein produces 0.41 g of water and carbohydrate produces 0.55 g of water. This water may help in dissolution of various Dosha and this can be compared with the Kledana property described to Sneha dravya. Lipid consuming is helpful in excretion of lipid soluble substance. It suggests that Sneha liquefies the compact Dosha and destroy morbid Mala.The membrane permeability is important for functioning and it depends on its lipid components. Phospholipids composed of chains of poly-unsaturated fatty acids increases the membrane permeability by bonding some chains and double bonds prevent them from compacting themselves. By increasing cellular permeability Sneha directs the Dosha from Shakha to Koshtha.

Action of Snehana karma as Purva karma to Shodhana - Sneha acts as a solvent and it increases Apyansha of the body which ultimately leads to Klinnata or Utkleshavastha.

1. Action as a solvent: Ghee acts as good solvent for many metabolic waste products and it enters the cells easily because cell wall is made up of phospholipids. Compared to other non-oily substances, ghee, etc. fat materials stays in the body for a stipulated period without causing any harm and also possesses better permeability property. According to Sushruta, the disease occurs due to dislodgement of vitiated Doshas in the channels during their circulation in the body. Sneha administered internally reaches to Srotansi and acts as a solvent to remove the obstruction by dissolving Doshas in it, resulting in the removal of Srotorodha which is one of the important steps in the Samprapti Vighatana.
2. Increase in the Apyansha of the body: This specifies the Vriddhya, Vishyandana and Kledakaraka properties of Sneha.This particular phenomenon should be understood regarding Vriddha, i.e. increase in the Apyansha of the body which ultimately lead to Utklesha and Rasa and Kleda Vriddhi during Snehapana. Sneha has predominence of Aap Mahabhuta, which was also corroborated by the specific qualities ascribed to it by various Acharyas like Charaka and Vagbhatta and also it is hydrophilic in nature.
3. After proper Snehana all the cells of body become completely saturated with fats. Then the fat material comes out of the cell to extracellular fluid by osmosis process. So due to the aqueous properties of Sneha and liquefied Malas brought from the tissues, the levels

of fatty acids, etc. increases in the blood resulting in the high plasma volume. To keep up the equilibrium of the normal plasma level, the extra amount of liquid from it, reaches to the Koshtha for expulsion. This is called as Anupravana Bhava.

4. Later on when Virechana is administered, this increased amount of body fluids are evacuated by which the vitiated Doshas are expelled out resulting in the radical cure of disease. By the combined effect of Snehana and Svedana, excessive increase of Dosha, liquification of Dosha, digestion of Dosha, opening of Srotomukha and control of Vata occurs so that the Doshas come to the Koshtha by Anupravana Bhava, and they are expelled out through nearest route by proper Virechana Karma.

Importance of Snehana

दीप्तान्तराग्निः परिशुद्धकोष्ठः प्रत्यग्रधातुबर्लवर्णयुक्तः।
दृढेन्द्रियो मन्दजरः शतायुः स्नेहोपसेवी पुरुषः प्रदिष्टः॥ (A.H.Su.16/46)

Snehana increases the digestive power thus helping the GIT to function proper. It increases the strength of Dhatus, improves general Bala, Varna, make Indriya more efficient, reducing ageing process. Thus gives a long life to the person up to 100 years.

Mostly Snehana is used as Purva Karma for Panchakarma therapy. However it also happens to be the prime treatment for Vataja vikara attaining the significance of Pradhana Karma, too.

In balyavastha Kapha dosha is present as main dosha. Kapha itself has snigdhha guna hence children required less quantity of sneha to get oleated and can be subjected to shodhan chikitsa directly whenever necessary.

The saptadhatus present in the body are abundant in snigdha guna. This property is comparatively lower in the preceding dhatu which is gradually increased in the next dhatu. Thus shukra dhatu is a snigdha guna pradhan dhatu. Oja is the sara of all the dhatus and therefore is a sneha pradhan ghatak. Prana is assocated with para-oja.

So prana is also said to be Sneha Bhuyistha.

Sapta dhatu → Shukra dhatu (maximum Sneha) → Oja → Prana

SPECIAL PROCEDURES

Takra Dhara

Pouring of medicated liquids over the forehead is called as Shirodhara. It is one among the four types of Murdhni taila procedures. Murdnitaila means application of medicated oils over the head in different forms.

Materials Required

1. Shirodhara yantra – 1
2. Vessels – 3
3. Cotton pad : 1
4. Amalaki Churna : 190 g
5. Milk : 600 mL
6. Musta : 75 g
7. Oil or talam : 10 mL
8. Rasnadi Churna : 5 g
9. Attendents – 2
10. Water : 5,400 mL

Preparation of the medicine

a. Takra : 600 mL of milk diluted with 2400 mL water is boiled with 75 g of Musta tied in a muslin bag, and is reduced to 600 mL. The bag of medicament is taken out and squeezed well. When cooled this prepared milk is fermented by the addition of a little sour buttermilk over night. Next morning the fermented medicated curd is churned by adding 750 ml of Amalaki Kvatha. The butter is removed completely and this mixture is used for dhara of filtering.
b. Amalaki Kvatha : 1,909 of dried Amalaki fruit boiled with 3,000 mL of water and reduced to 750 mL.

Purva Karma

Make the patient to be in comfortable position in a well ventilated room devoid of any disturbance. Brief regarding the procedure and benefits out of it. Then eyes should be covered with eye pads and gauze should be tied around the head above the eyebrows with the main intention of preventing entry of medicine to eye.

Pradhana Karma

The dhara pot should be kept in such a way as to allow steady flowing of the liquid, poured into it, over the forehead of the patient. The tip of dharavarti should be 4-5 cm above the forehead of the patient. Takra falling should be poured again into the vessel after collecting from the droni. The vessel should always be kept oscillating around oscilation per minute in gentle manner so that the oushada will fall into the patient's entire forehead without interruption.

In short all the procedures are same as Shirodhara, but Takra should not be heated or reused for the next day.

Duration

The process should be done daily for a period of 7 to 14 days. The duration of treatment as well as the time period is according to the nature of the disease and the physical condition of the patient. It is done usually for a fixed time (45 minutes to 1 hour).

Pashchat Karma

The head should be wiped with towel and rasnadi churna is applied. Patient is advised to take rest for a period same as the period of the procedure, then to take bath.

Complications and Management

Shivering is observed in some patients due to excess sheeta. In such case the procedure is stopped immediately and the patient is managed with Ushnopachara.

Indications

This Shirodhara is indicated in the diseases like irritable bowel disease, anxiety, neurosis, sleeplessness, hypertension, paralysis, premature greying of hair and premature baldness, stress, diabetes mellitus, psoriasis, neurological disorders like headache, neuropathy, etc.

Udvartana

The powder of different drugs is used for massaging the body and the strokes are applied with pressure in the opposite direction of the hair. It is indicated in Vata and Kapha disorders by causing liquefaction of Kapha and Meda (fat) promotes the metabolism and complexion of the skin.

Paribhasha

उद्वर्तनं गात्र मर्दनम्। (Su.Chi.24/51 Dalhana)
ऊर्ध्वं वर्तनमुद्वर्तनम्।

Udvartana is one of the Bahirparimarjana chikitsa which is performed in Pratiloma gati means from below upwards by using required pressure on the body.

Types of Udvartana

1. Udgarshana
2. Udsadana

उद्धर्षणम् अस्नेहौषधचूर्णादिभिर्घर्षणम्।
सस्नेहकल्केनोद्धर्षणमुत्सादनम्। (Su.Chi 24/52 Dalhana)

General Procedure of Udvartana

Purva Karma

- Examination of patient and select suitable one.
- According to patient select the drugs which should be finely powdered (either paste or powder).
- Patient is advised to lie down on the table.

Pradhana Karma

Medicament is poured in very little quantity over dorsum of the foot first and rubbed in opposite direction of hair root. Simultaneously on both sides the process is continued in upward direction (Figs 2.13A and B).

Duration

No specific duration is mentioned, can be continued as in Abhyanga. (Same Matra Kala may be adopted).

Pashchat Karma

- Patient is allowed to clean the body with cloth followed by Ushna Jala Snana.
- It can be done for 7-14-21 days depending on the conditions.

Indications

It is indicated as a part of Dinacharya (A.H.Su. 2 and A.S.Su. 3)
'Indu' had highlighted the utility of Kashayarasa dravya for daily udvartana.

- ❑ Specially in Vasanta ritu, Medura person
- ❑ As Shodhana purva Rukshana.

Contraindications

- ❑ Durbala
- ❑ Ati Karshya
- ❑ Ati Ruksha persons.

Uses

उद्वर्तनं कफहरं मेदसः प्रविलायनम् । स्थिरी करणमङ्गानां त्वक्प्रसादकरं परम्॥ (A.H.Su.2.15)

Arunadatta commented

Udvartanasya kaphaharadaya schatwaro gunah

Hemadri commented

- Udvartanam kaphaharadigunam
- Atah kuryadityartha siddham
- Pravilayanam draveekarnam
- Draveekrutya medasah shoshanamityarthah.

उद्वर्तन वातहरं कफ मेदो विलापनम् स्थिरीकरणमङ्गानां त्वक्प्रसादकरंपरम्॥
सिरामुखविविक्तत्वं त्वक्स्थस्याग्रेश्च तेजनम् उद्धर्षणोत्सादनाभ्यां जायेयातामसंशयम्॥
(Su.Chi.24/51-52)

- ❑ **Dalhana commented**
  - Udvartanam gatramardanam
  - Vilayanam draveekaranam

Sthirikaran Anganam

Sthirikaranarn anganam is achieved by removing excessively deposited Kapha and Meda. This results in removing the obstruction in the channel of circulation which carry the nutrient materials to the site of organs. Thus enhance the functioning of these organs resulting into Sthirikarana.

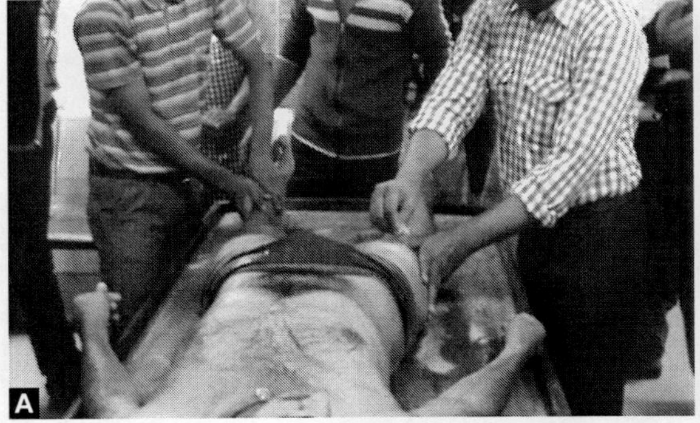

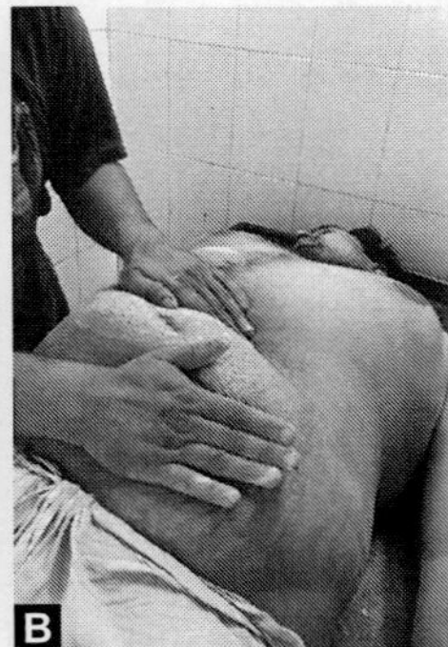

Figs 2.13A and B: Udvartana

Tvakprasadana

It increases the complexion by increasing the absorptive power of skin and also increasing the function of Bhrajakagni and Twachagni

दौर्गन्ध्यं गौरवं तन्द्रां कण्डूं मलमरोचकम्।
स्वेदबीभत्सतांहन्तिशरीरपरिमार्जनम्।। (परिमार्जनम् उद्वर्तनं) (Ch.Su.5/93)

Because of Medodhatvagni Mandya there is excessive accumulation of Medodhatu in the body. Sveda being Mala of Medodhatu, excessive sweating results into bad smell of the body.

Udvartana removes the unwanted and unpleasant toxins, bad smell produced due to Sveda.

- ❑ **Gaurava:** This lakshana is also because of vitiation of Kapha and medadhatu. Udvartana relieves this because of their opposite qualities to pathogenesis.
- ❑ **Tandra:** Ashtangasangrahakar says tandra is having predominance of vatadosha and alpa Kapha. Udvartana is having both Kapha and Vata nashana properties. It alleviates tandra resulting into Indriyarthajnana and lightness of the body.
- ❑ **Kandu:** It is a feature of kaphamedo vitiated or aggravated condition. Hence it can also be alleviated.
- ❑ **Malanashaka:** Toxins accumulated in skin are removed.
- ❑ **Arochaka:** By Udvartana, Agni present in Twacha Bhaga enters into Amapakvashayarnadhya and increases the function of antaragni and there by alleviates Arochaka.
- ❑ **Svedabibhatsata Hanti:** Udvartana helps in alleviating excessive production of sweat.

Utsadana

उत्सादनाद् भवेत् स्त्रीणां विशेषात् कान्तिमद्वपुः।
प्रहर्ष सौभाग्य मृजालाघवादिगुणान्वितम्। (Su.Chi 24/53)

The powder of herbs mixed with oil rubbed against the hair follicle is referred as utsadana, specfically indicated in females and it also imparts good skin and lightness of the body.

Udgharshana

When the dry powder of herbs is rubbed against the body it is called Udgarshana.

उद्घर्षणं तु विज्ञेयं कण्डूकोठानिलापहम्।। (Su.Chi 24/55)

Udvartana Yogas

- ❑ Kolakulatthadi churna
- ❑ Rasnadi churna
- ❑ Pichumandadi churna
- ❑ Triphala churna
- ❑ Karpoora, Shveta Chandana, Lodhra, Shireesha,Ushira, Nagakesara
- ❑ Priyangu, Lodhra, Haritaki, Chandana
- ❑ Musta, Patha, Nimba, Devadaru, etc.

In this procedure of Ruksha Udvartana mainly Katu, Tikta, Kashaya Rasa dravyas having laghu, Tikshna and Ruksha guna and Ushna veerya are used more.

The site of action also involves action of drugs on a particular stage of samprapti.

- The drugs applied and rubbed over skin get digested by Bhrajakagni or Tvachagni which is present in Avabhasini layer
- Its veerya and vipaka enter Rasadhatu which is present beneath the avabhasini. They remove the obstruction in the Rasa and Svedavaha srotas
- Veerya of the drugs resolve the Dosha dushya Sammurcchana and its gunas and vipak, veerya spreads all over the body and perform its action they produce systemic effect.

Important Qualities of Rubbing

- It gives mechanical stimulation causing contraction followed by relaxation and thus greatly influences the muscles.
- It increases the peripheral circulation and influence the venous drainage by its alternate pressure and relaxation techniques.
- It improves the nutrition of the particular area by proper circulation.
- It raises temperature locally by continuous friction.
- It increases elimination of waste products especially in the form of sweating.
- It increases secretion and absorption capacities of the skin.
- It conditions the nervous system by stimulating the cutaneous nerve endings.
- It influences the general metabolism when applied on large areas.

Physiological Effects

- As the skin covers nearly the whole body its surface is affected by massage as well as the structures which lie beneath it. It increases the cutaneous circulation, stimulates the sensory nerve ending and influences the vasoconstrictors and vasodilators in the skin.
- The pressure of deep massage exerts a simultaneous influence on all the tissue of the body. Further it accelerates the activity of the heart, helps in assimilation of food and influences general metabolism of the body.
- Influence of rubbing on the circulation of fluid including lymphatic is also of great importance.
- Rubbing stimulates both motor and sensory nerve endings. The influence of rubbing on motion of the molecules to participate in chemical activity results in the antioxidant process.

Kriya Kalpa

Need of Kriya Kalpa - When drugs are administered systemically, many of the drugs can not cross the blood aqueous, blood vitreous and blood retinal barrier.

This may be the reason for frequent usage of Kriya Kalpa in our classics.

In recent years significant advances have been made in optimizing the delivery of drugs to target tissues within the eye.

- ❑ Netra roga shamanartha
- ❑ Netra prasadanartha
- ❑ Kriya kalpas are planned as per Sama and Nirama Lakshana of netra Roga.
- ❑ Specially designed according to the site, stage and severity of the disease
- ❑ Prevention aspect.

Kriya kalpa in amavastha of netra: the common procedures which can be employed in amavasta of netra are Ashchyothana, Seka, Pinda and Bidalaka

Kriya kalpa in pakvaavastha of netra: the common procedures which can be employed in pakvavastha are anjana, tarpana and putapaka.

Putapaka

Keeping the medicaments prepared out of plant extracts, fats and certain metals and minerals for stipulated period (3-5 minutes) making concentric boundary around the orbit.

Procedure same as Tarpana

Quantity- 25 mL each eye

Snehana Putapaka - Sneha (animal fat), Jeevaniya gana etc.

Duration - 200 matra Kalas.

Lekhana Putapaka- Honey, Pippali, Maricha, Bhasma of gold, silver, loha and copper.

Duration: 100 Matra Kalas aprox. 1 minute

Ropana / Prasadana- Mansa, ghee and Madhura Dravyas and Tikta Rasa Dravyas.

Duration: 300 Matra Kalas

Course of the treatment: 1 to 3 days after Tarpana.

Putapaka Kalpas

Lekhana: Yakrit, Mansa and Tamra Bhasma

Snehana: Animal Fat, Kakolyadi Gana Dravyas, etc.

Prasadana: Ksheera, Ghee and Tikta Ropana dravya.

Leaves of Agastya, Shrigru, Punarnava

Churnas: Triphala, Yashti, Shatavari

Ashchyothana

सर्वेषामक्षिरोगाणां आदौ आचश्योतनं हितं। रुक तोद कण्डू घर्षाश्रु दाहरागनिबर्हणम्।। (A.H.Su.23/1)

- ❑ First line of treatment in occular inflammatory conditions like Ruk, Toda, Kandu, Daha, Ashru Srava, Shopha to instilled into the conjunctival sac with open eye.
- ❑ Instillation of 8-10 drops.

Drugs

Fresh leafs of Amrita, Durva, Shigru, Bhumyaamalaki, etc.

Dry Drugs

Triphala, Lodhra, Haridra, etc.

The decoction should be neither concentrated nor dilute (ideal SPH- 6.6-7.4) Temperature should not be too hot or too cold.

Lekhana	–	8 drops is Kapha doshahara.
Snehana	–	10 drops is Vata doshahara.
Ropana	–	12 drops is Pitta doshahara

Drugs for Ashchyothana

Babula
Bhumyamalaki
Vibhitaki
Daruharidra
Chaturangula
Eranda
Guduchi

Ashchyothana Kalpas

Brihatpanchamula	–	Vataja Abhishyanda
Triphala Kashaya	–	Sarva Abhishyanda
Stanya	–	Netraja Raktapitta
Drakshadi Kshirapaka	–	Pitta Raktaja Draksha, Madhuka, Manjeeshtha, Jeevaniya Dravya
Lodhra Ashchyotana	–	Raga, Shotha
Shveta Palandu Ashchyotana	–	Cataract
Dadimadi Paka	–	Conjunctivitis

Anjana

निरुक्ति''अनक्ति अनेन इति अंजनम्''।
व्यक्तरजेषु दोषेषु शुद्धकायस्य केवले। तेन एव स्थिते दोषे प्राप्तमन्जनमाचरेत्।।
लेखनं रोपणं चापि प्रसादनमथापि वा।। (Su.Ut.18)

Application of medicaments in the form of paste into the conjunctival fornices with an applicator (Shalaka). Anjana is indicated when Doshas are localized in the eye and acute inflammatory signs like congestion, redness, srava (epiphora) are subsided by Seka and Ashchyotana.

Drug used: Compound drugs prepared out of metals, minerals and herbs.

Classification of Anjana

A. According to mode of action
   1. Lekhana
   2. Ropana
   3. Prasadana
   4. Snehana

B. According to Akriti
   1. Gutika - Useful in Mahabala Roga
   2. Rasa - Useful in Madhyambala Roga
   3. Churna - Useful in Hinabala Roga
C. According to Dosha
   1. Vataghna - Amla, Lavana Rasa
   2. Pittaghna - Tikta, Kashaya Rasa
   3. Kaphaghna - Katu, Tikta Rasa
   4. Raktadoshahara - Tikta, Kashaya Rasa
   5. Sannipataghna - According to the Dominant Dosha.

Pramana

Texts have described the Pramana of Anjana to be used according to the type of Anjana Dravya as follows:

1. Tikshana Anajana - 1 Harenuka
2. Rasakriya - 1 Vidanga
3. Mridu Rasakriya - 2 Vidanga
4. Tikshna Churna - 2 Shalaka
5. Mridu Churna - 3 Shalaka

Shalaka

Snehana - Tamra
Lekhana - Kamsya
Ropana - Loha and Anguli
Prasadana - Swarna and Rajata

Anjana Kalpas

Bilwadi Gutika
Chandrodaya Varti
Jathimukuladi Varti
Samudraphenadi Varti
Darvyadi Rasakriya - once in 7 days
Guduchyadi Rasakriya
Dadimadyanjana

Rasakriya
Narikela Rasakriya Anjana

Sauviranjana

Sauvira Anjana, Triphala Kashaya, Stanya - All eye diseases
Marichadi Anjana-Maricha, Pippali, Samudraphena, Saindhaya, Saurviranjana in disease Kancha.
Shirishyadi Anjana-Shirisha Beeja, Maricha, Pippali Saindhava-Savranashrukra.
Chandanadi Anjana-Chandana, Saindhava, Pathya, Palasha-Shukra Arma.

Special Properties

- ❑ Disposal rate is minimum.
- ❑ Tissue contact time is maximum.

Absorption : Maximum absorption.

Bioavailability

As it is in ointment form, tissue contact time and bioavailability is increased.

- ❑ Acts as subconjunctival injections.
- ❑ Permeability through sclera: Acts on posterior segment disorders.
- ❑ Anjana contain arsenic and antimony compounds which have large molecular size which can enter scleral circulation but cannot cross blood aqueous barrier if administered systemically.

Hence Anjana is indicated in a variety of systemic diseases.

Gandusha and Kavala

Gandusha and Kavala generally mean gargle. The only difference is that in Gandusha the mouth is completely filled with medicated liquid so that it cannot be moved in the mouth, while in Kavala it is filled in lesser extent so that it can be moved in the mouth as in gargle. For Gandusha unctuous substances, oil, milk, honey, warm water, wine, etc. are used.

Indications of Gandusha

In healthy person daily Gandusha of oil promotes the health of the teeth, gums, lips and all parts of the oral cavity as well as their functions. It may prevent the disorders of these organs. The Gandusha with ghee is indicated in ulcer and burning sensation of mouth.

Types of Gandusha

- ❑ Snigdha Gandusha – Vatahara, e.g. Mansarasa.
- ❑ Shamana Gandusha – Pittahara, e.g. Gritha.
- ❑ Shodhana Gandusha – Kaphahara, e.g. Madhu.
- ❑ Ropana Gandusha – Vranahara, e.g. Yashtimadhu ksheerapaka

Sheetada

- ❑ Ksheeri Vriksha Kashaya
- ❑ Takshya, Nagara, Triphala, Shunthi, Priyangu and Musta.
- ❑ Arjuna Twak Kvatha
- ❑ Baboola Twak kashaya
  - Gingivitis – Katphala Kashaya, Ksheeri Vriksha Kashaya
  - Pyorrhea alveolaris – Ksheeri Vriksha Kashaya, Madhu, Gritha
  - Tundikeri- Triphala, Trikatu, Yavakshara, Daruharidra, Chitraka Rasanjana, Patha, Nimba, Gomutra
  - Mukha Roga - Arimedadi Taila

Kavala

Kavala is a procedure in which medicated oil is filled into the mouth till half of its capacity and followed by gargles after that. It is having the properties which are similar to Gandusha in many ways and is of four types:

1. **Snehi kavala:** Oil or decoctions which are indicated in Vataroga are used.
2. **Prasadi kavala:** Oil or sweet cool liquids which are indicated in Pittaja Roga are used.
3. **Shodhi kavala:** Warm irritant oil or liquids are used. It is indicated in Kaphaja Mukharoga.
4. **Ropana kavala:** Oil or liquids prepared from Madhur, Katu, Tikta and Kashaya Rasa medicines are used for kavala. It is indicated in Mukhaja vrana.

- ❑ Tonsillitis – Yasti, Jatipallava, Dadima pallava.

Dalhana- Ksheeri vriksha kashaya.

- ❑ Talu paka- Vasa, Nimba twak , Patola.
- ❑ Gala shundi- Vacha, Ativisha, Patha, Rasna, Katuki,
- ❑ Sheetada- Priyangu, Triphala, Mustha
- ❑ Saushira- Lodhra, Mustha, Rasanjana, Madhu
- ❑ Mukha paka- Jathi pallava kalka, Nimba pallava kalka

Indications of Kavala

Kavala is indicated in the pain of sides of neck, headache, diseases of ear, eye and throat, excessive salivation, dryness of mouth, nausea, anorexia, chronic cold and torpor.

Dhumapana

Definition

जत्रूर्ध्वकफवतोत्थविकाराणामजन्मने। (A.H.Su.21/1)

According to VS Apte, the literary meaning of Dhumapana is inhalation of smoke or vapor. It is also mentioned as a part of Dinacharya. It is used for both curative especially in Urdhvajatrugata rogas, preventive diseases of provoked Kapha and Vata.

Types

a. According to different authors:
   1. Charaka: 3 types, i.e.
      i. Prayogika
      ii. Snaihika
      iii. Shirovairechanika
   2. Sushruta: 5 types
      i. Prayogika [Regular]
      ii. Snaihika [Unctuous]
      iii. Vairechanika [Evacuative]
      iv. Kasaghna [Antitussive]
      v. Vamaniya [Emetic]

3. Ashtanga sangraha: 2 types
   i. 1. Shamana- Prayogika or Madhyama
      2. Bhrihana- Snaihika or Mridu
      3. Shodhana- Vairechanika or Tikshna
   ii. a. Kasaghna
      b. Vamaniya
      c. Vranadhupana
4. Ashtanga hridaya: 3 types

   स्निग्धोमध्यः सतीक्ष्णस्यवातेवातकफेकफे॥ (A.H.Su.21/1)

   1. Snigdha- for Vataja rogas
   2. Madhyama- for Vata-kaphaja rogas
   3. Tikshna- for Kaphaja rogas

1. Snigdha/mridu/prayogika
- Mild
- Lubricating
- In vata-disorders

  Drugs used- Sarja rasa, Bee-wax, Chandana, Ushira, etc.

2. Madhya/shamana
- Palliative
- Medium
- In vata - kapha disorders

  Drugs used—Eladi Ghana except Kushta and Tagara.

3. Tikshna
- Virechana / purgative
- Shodhana / purifactory

  Drugs used—Maricha, Pippali, Manashila, Jyothishmati, etc.

Contraindications

1. रक्तपित्त– Raktapitta
2. विरिक्त– Who have undergone purgation
3. उदर– Enlargement of abdomen
4. मेहिषु– Diabetes
5. तिमिर– Blindness
6. ऊर्ध्वानिला– Upward movement of Vata
7. आध्मान– Flatulence
8. रोहिणी– A throat disease
9. दत्तबस्तिषु– Who have been administered enema
10. शिरस्याभिहते– Injured in the head
11. पाण्डुरोगे–Anemia
12. जागरितेनिशि– Who have kept awake at night

13. Who have eaten, मत्स्यं (fish), मद्य (alcohol), दधि (curd), क्षीर (milk), क्षौद्र (honey), स्नेह (fat), विषाशिशु (poison).

Indications

1. Akshishula
2. Ardhavabedaka
3. Atitandra
4. Moha
5. Kandu
6. Kamasrava
7. Kasa
8. Shvasa
9. Netrasrava
10. Khalitya and Palitya
11. Vata-kaphaja vikaras

अकाल अति पीत धूमः

Dhumapana done at improper time or in excess leads to,

रक्तपित्तान्ध्बाधिर्यत्रुणमूर्च्छामदमोहकृत्। धूमोअकालेअतिपीतोवातत्रशीतोविधिर्हितः॥

1. रक्तपित्त – Bleeding diseases
2. अन्ध्य – Blindness
3. बाधिर्य – Deafness
4. तृड् – Thirst
5. मूर्च्छा – Fainting
6. मद – Intoxication
7. मोहकृत – Delusion

Chikitsa : Cold regimen is the ideal treatment for above conditions.

Proper Time for Dhuma/inhalation

1. **मृदुधूम : क्षुतजृम्भितविण्मूत्रस्त्रीसेवाशस्त्रकर्मणाम्। हासस्यदन्तकाष्ठस्यधुममन्तेपिबेन्मृदुम्॥**

   At the end of

   1. क्षुत – Sneezing
   2. जृम्भित – Yawning
   3. विण् – Defecation
   4. मूत्र – Micturation
   5. स्त्रीसेवा – Coitus
   6. शस्त्रकर्मणाम् – Surgery
   7. हासस्य – Laughing
   8. दन्तकाष्ठस्य – Tooth brush

2. **मध्यमधूमः कालेष्वेषुनिशाहारनावनान्तेचमध्यमम्।**

   At the end of

   1. निशा – Night
   2. आहार – Food
   3. नावना – Nasya/ nasal medication

3. **तीक्ष्णधूमः निद्रानस्योन्जनस्नानच्छर्दितान्तेविरेचनम्।**

   At the end of

   1. निद्रा – Sleep
   2. नस्य – Nasal medication
   3. अञ्जन – Collyrium
   4. स्नान – Bath
   5. छर्दि – Vomiting

Dhumapana Instrument

The pipe which is used for the Dhumapana is called as Dhumanetra. The Dhuma is to be inhaled by pipe because the structure of pipe provides safe for movement of smoke. Due to this, smoke will not enter directly into the sense organs.

a. धूमनेत्र/Nozzle: बस्तिनेत्रसमद्रव्यंत्रिकोशंकारयेत् ऋजु मूलाग्रेअन्गुष्ठकोलास्थि–प्रवेशंधूमनेत्रकम्।

1. बस्तिनेत्रसमद्रव्यं – From same materials as बस्तिनेत्र or enema nozzle
2. त्रिकोशं – With three chambers
3. ऋजु – Straight
4. Permitting entry of अन्गुष्ठ (thumb) and a कोलास्थि or stone of jujube fruit through orifices at its root मूलम् (root) and अग्रं (tip) respectively.

Dhumanetra is made up of same material {Gold, silver, copper, etc.} as that of Bastinetra. Length of Dhumanetra varies according to the opinions of different authors, i.e.

b. Dhumanetra Pramana

प्रमाणः तीक्ष्णस्नेहमध्येषुत्रीणिचत्वारिपञ्च अङ्गुलानांक्रमात्पातुः प्रमाणेनाष्टकांदकनितत्॥

(A.H.Su. 21)

Types	*Charaka*	*Sushruta*	*Asangraha*	*Ahridaya*	*Sharan gadhara*
Vairechanika	24	24	24	24	24
Snaihika	32	32	32	32	32
Prayogika	36	36	40	40	40
Kasaghna		16	10	8 to 10	16
Vamaniya		16	10		10
Vranadhupana		8	8	10	

c. Method of preparation of Dhumavarti

A reed of Kaasha, 12 Angula in length, soaked in water for day and night should be wrapped in five layers with a ribbon of cloth, smeared with thin paste of drugs. Its thickness should be that of the middle portion of the thumb. It should be dried in shade and the reed should be removed before use.

d. Dose

It is depend on the type of Dhumapana adopted. Charaka mentioned that it should be done thrice three puffs each time (Ch.Su.5/35). Chakrapani comments on it by saying Dhumapana should be taken three puffs at each time. One should require little interval after smoking once.

Sushruta says, three puffs should be taken each time through mouth and nose in Prayogika type and it is repeated for 3-4 times. Snaihika Dhumapana should be done until tears begin to flow in the Vairechanika Dhumapana until Dosha appears.

Mode of Dhumapana Inhalation

ऋजूपविष्टविवृतास्यस्त्रिपर्ययम् पिधायच्छिद्रमेकैकंधूमंनासिकयापिबेत्।

1. ऋजूपविष्ट – One should sit straight and should be attentive
2. विवृतास्य – Mouth should be kept open
3. Inhale smoke through each nostril alternatively by closing 1 nostril while inhaling through other inhalation should be done thrice, {i.e. 1 bout = sucking the smoke and letting it out together each time - 3 such bouts}.

Sushruta opines that:

a. Prayogika Dhumapana: Should be done through nose.
b. Snaihika Dhumapana : Should be done through both mouth and nose.
c. Vairechanika Dhumapana : Should be done through nose.

Precautions

The inhaled Dhuma from nose or mouth should be let out only through mouth. If it is made to let out through the nose, then it may destroy the vision. (Ch.Su.5/47)

Samyak Yoga

1. Lightness of chest, throat, head
2. Liquefaction of Kapha
3. Clarity of mind, sense organs, and head, etc. (Ch.Su.5)

Ayoga

a. Impairment of voice
b. Presence of Kapha in the throat and heaviness of head
c. Doshotklesha takes place.

Atiyoga

1. Dryness of palate
2. Increased thirstiness and later unconsciousness
3. Excessive bleeding leads to fainting.

Thalapothichil

Thala in malayalam vocabulary refers to Shiras and Pothichi refers to Lepana. So Thala pothichil refers to Shiro Lepana itself.

It has similar Gunas to that of Takra Dhara.

Preparations

Two methods of preparation have been explained in text Shirasekadi Vidhi by different authors.

- ❑ Boiling the drugs
- ❑ Triturating the dry medicinal powders in buttermilk.

Method 1

One Kudava (192 g) of dry, de seeded fruits of Amalaki is boiled with two Kudava (384 ml) of buttermilk mixed with an equal quantity (384 mL) of water.

When the water gets evaporated, the vessel is removed from the fire and the contents are ground to smooth paste.

Method 2

तक्रधाराविधानेन सिद्धे प्रस्थार्धसम्युते। तक्रे चतुष्पलमितम् शुष्कधात्रीफलत्वचम्।।
मृत्पात्रे वासितम् रात्रौ पिष्ट्वा च अथ अपरेअह्नि। निरबुघनम् सम्यक् द्रवस्यन्ध्यपि नैव वा।।

(Keraliya Panchakarma/Shirolepa 1-2)

- ❑ Half Prastha (384 mL) of buttermilk (prepared as in Takra Dhara) is taken. In this 4 Pala (In g) of dry, pericarp of Amalaki is soaked overnight preferably in a clay pot.
- ❑ The next morning the mixture is well triturated till a fine smooth paste is obtained, which is neither too liquid nor too solid.
- ❑ If it is too liquid, it will easily ooze down the head.
- ❑ If it is more of solid consistency of butter it may cause Vidaha.

Application

The method of application can be divided into 3 steps:

1. Purva Karma
2. Pradhana Karma
3. Pashchata Karma

Purva Karma

अभ्यज्य मूर्धनि सुदिने कालेप्यायवेष्टय वासना। (Keraliya Panchakarma/Shirolepen 3)

- ❑ Abhyanga of head is done prior to the procedure.
- ❑ A strap of cloth is tied all around the forehead to prevent any leakage of the substance downwards.
- ❑ Patient is made to sit on a stool.

Pradhana Karma

पिष्ट्वादल्पम् चोन्चभागे शिरश्शस्तु पुरस्ततः। भागे तु दक्षिणे प्रिष्टे वामे च पुनरन्चके।।
एवम् क्रमात् शिरस्सम्यगासमन्तात् समाव्रतम्। धात्रीकल्केन लेपस्स्यान्नोनाम्गुल घनस्ततः।।
म्लानेन रम्भापत्रेण पद्मपत्रेण वा क्वचित्। कर्णपालि सरण्याथ सादम् सम्वेष्टय युक्तितः।।
बध्नियादूर्ध्वतस्सम्यक् पत्रमौलि यथातुरः। अभ्यन्जयेद्वा सर्वानामासीनस्य यथा सुखम्।। (Shirasekavidhi)

- The medicinal paste is applied first at the center of the head, then front, right side, back and finally in the left side.in the respective order. In this manner, the paste is applied over the whole of the scalp.
- The thickness of the paste should be about 1/4, 1/3, 1/2 anguli based on Doshaghna, Vishaghna and Varnya lepa, respectively
- The head is then covered with a plaintain leaf which is made pliant by heating. A lotus leaf or other suitable leaves can also be used for this purpose.
- An opening is made at the center, and the patient is made to sit unmoved for the period of half Yama (1.5 hours) or for 1 Muhurta.
- There is also a custom of placing Taila at the center of the opening while doing this procedure.

Pashchat Karma

- At the end of the procedure, the medicinal paste is wiped off.
- Abhyanga is done on the head.
- Patient is asked to take bath.

Benefits

तक्रधाराफलम् चास्मदेकदेशम् समश्नुयात्। (Keraliya Panchakarma/Shirolepen 10)

It cures diseases like Klama, Apachi, etc. imparts strength to sight induces sleep. It has effects similar to Takra Dhara.

Contraindication

It should never be performed in Vata predominant disorders.

Other Drugs

अभ्यङ्गमाचरेन्नित्यं स जराश्रमवातहा। दृष्टिप्रसादपुष्टयायुः स्वप्रसुत्वक्तवदार्ढ्यकृत्॥
शिरः श्रवणपादेषु तं विशेषेण शीलयेत्॥ (A.H.Su.2/8-9)

Balamula, Yashtimadhu, Panchagandha Churna, Tugakshiri or Dashamoola which is triturated either in milk, buttermilk or cold water as per the need of the condition may also be used.

DESCRIPTION OF ABHYANTARA SNEHA ACCORDING TO ACHARAYA CHARAKA IN VARIOUS DISEASES

S. No.	Name of Sneha	Name of disease	Reference
		Ghrita	
1.	Amrit ghrita	Visha chikitsa	Ch. Chi. 23/241-242
2.	Amritprasha ghrita	Kshatkshina chikitsa	Ch. Chi. 11/35-43
3.	Aamlaka ghrita	Rasayanadhikara	Ch. Chi. 1-2/4-6
4.	Deepaniya ghrita for Amatisara	Grahani chikitsa	Ch. Chi. 15/202
5.	Deepaniya ghrita	Udara roga chikitsa	Ch. Chi. 13/111

Contd...

Contd...

S. No.	*Name of Sneha*	*Name of disease*	*Reference*
		Ghrita	
6.	Purana ghrita	Unmada chikitsa	Ch. Chi. 9/57-59
7.	Katukadi ghrita	Pandu chikitsa	Ch. Chi. 16/47-49
8.	Kantakari ghrita	Kasa chikitsa	Ch. Chi. 18/35
9.	Kalyanaka ghrita	Unmada chikitsa	Ch. Chi. 9/35-41
10.	Kasherukadi ghrita	Trimarmiya chikitsa	Ch. Chi. 26/94
11.	Kulatthadi ghrita	Kasa chikitsa	Ch. Chi. 18/129
12.	Dashmula ghrita (kevala vatahara)	Vatavyadhi chikitsa	Ch. Chi. 28/119-121
13.	Kolalakshadi ghrita	Kshatakshina chikitsa	Ch. Chi. 11/34
14.	Jeevaniya ghrita	Kasa chikitsa	Ch. Chi. 18/140
15.	Kshara ghrita	Grahani chikitsa	Ch. Chi. 15/171-172
16.	Ksheer shatpala ghrita	Gulma chikitsa	Ch. Chi. 5/147-148
17.	Guduchyadi ghrita	Kasa chikitsa	Ch. Chi. 18/161-162
18.	Tilvak ghrita	Gulma chikitsa	Ch. Chi. 5/ 147-148
19.	Chandanadi ghrita	Grahani chikitsa	Ch. Chi. 15/125-128
20.	Chavyadi ghrita	Arsha chikitsa	Ch. Chi. 14/104
21.	Changeri ghrita	Atisara chikitsa	Ch. Chi. 19/43
22.	Chitrak ghrita	Shotha chikitsa, Udara chikitsa	Ch. Chi. 12/58-59 & Ch. Chi. 13/113
23.	Chitrakadi ghrita	Shotha chikitsa. Arsha chikitsa	Ch. Chi. 12/55-56 & Ch. Chi. 28/122
24.	Vasadi ghrita	Jeernajvara chikitsa	Ch. Chi. 3/222-223
25.	Jeevantyadi ghrita	Rajyakshma chikitsa	Ch. Chi. 8/111-113
26.	Tiktashatpala ghrita	Kushtha chikitsa	Ch. Chi. 7/140-143
27.	Tejovatyadi ghrita	Hikka Shvasa chikitsa	Ch. Chi. 17/141-144
28.	Traymanadi ghrita	Gulma chikitsa	Ch. Chi. 5/118-121
29.	Tryushnadi ghrita	Grahani chikitsa, Trimarma chikitsa, Kasa chikitsa	Ch. Chi.15/87, Ch. Chi. 26/87-89 & Ch. Chi. 17/39-42
30.	Danti ghrita	Pandu chikitsa	Ch. Chi. 16/51
31.	Dashmula ghrita	Rajyakshma chikitsa	Ch. Chi. 8/97
32.	Dashmuladi ghrita	Rajyakshma chikitsa Grahani chikitsa Kasa chikitsa	Ch. Chi. 8/168, Ch. Chi. 15/82-86 & Ch. Chi. 17/140
33.	Dashmuli ghrita	Gulma chikitsa	Ch. Chi. 5/142
34.	Dadimadi ghrita	Pandu chikitsa	Ch. Chi. 16/44-46
35.	Darvyadi ghrita	Atisara chikitsa	Ch. Chi. 19/80-81
36.	Duralabhadi ghrita	Rajyakshma chikitsa	Ch. Chi. 8/106-110

Contd...

Contd...

S. No.	Name of Sneha	Name of disease	Reference
		Ghrita	
37.	Draksha ghrita	Pandu chikitsa	Ch. Chi. 16/52
38.	Drakshadi ghrita	Gulma chikitsa	Ch. Chi. 5/123-125
39.	Dvipanchmuladi ghrita	Kasa chikitsa	Ch. Chi. 18/158-160
40.	Nagadanyadi ghrita	Visha chikitsa	Ch. Chi. 23/241
41.	Nagradi ghrita	Udara chikitsa Arsha chikitsa	Ch. Chi. 13/115 Ch. Chi. 14/110-112
42.	Neelini ghrita	Gulma chikitsa	Ch. Chi. 5/105
43.	Neelinyadi ghrita	Gulma chikitsa	Ch. Chi. 5/106-109
44.	Panchkola ghrita	Udara chikitsa	Ch. Chi. 13/112-114
45.	Panchkoladi ghrita	Rajyakshma chikitsa	Ch. Chi. 8/169
46	Panchgavya ghrita	Apasmara chikitsa	Ch. Chi. 10/17
47.	Panchmuladi ghrita	Grahani chikitsa	Ch. Chi. 15/88-96
48.	Pathya ghrita	Pandu chikitsa	Ch. Chi. 16/50
49.	Padmakadi ghrita	Vatarakta chikitsa	Ch. Chi. 29/146
50.	Palankashadi ghrita	Apasmara chikitsa	Ch. Chi. 10/34-36
51.	Parushaka ghrita	Vatarakta chikitsa	Ch. Chi. 29/58-60
52.	Pippalimuladi ghrita	Grahani chikitsa	Ch. Chi. 15/170
53.	Brihat shatavari ghrita	Yonivyapad chikitsa	Ch. Chi. 30/64-68
54.	Brahmi ghrita	Apasmara chikitsa	Ch. Chi. 10/25
55.	Bhallatakadi ghrita	Gulma chikitsa	Ch. Chi. 5/143-146
56.	Madhuyashtyadi ghrita	Trimarmiya chikitsa	Ch. Chi. 26/179
57.	Manah shiladi ghrita	Hikka shvasa chikitsa	Ch. Chi. 17/145
58.	Maha kalyanak ghrita	Unmada chikitsa	Ch. Chi. 9/42-44
59.	Maha khadira ghrita	Kushta chikitsa	Ch. Chi. 7/142-156
60.	Maha tiktaka ghrita	Kushta chikitsa	Ch. Chi. 7/144-150
61.	Maha panch gavya ghrita	Apasmara chikitsa	Ch. Chi. 10/18-24
62.	Maha paishachika ghrita	Unmada chikitsa	Ch. Chi. 9/45-48
63.	Maha mayura ghrita	Trimarmiya chikista	Ch. Chi. 26/166
64.	Mayura ghrita	Trimarmiya chikitsa	Ch. Chi. 26/163
65.	Kharjuradi ghrita	Rajyakshma chikitsa	Ch. Chi. 8/95-96
66.	Rasnadi ghrita	Rajyakshma chikitsa	Ch. Chi. 8/170-172
67.	Rohinayadi ghrita	Gulma chikitsa	Ch. Chi. 5/115-117
68.	Vachadi ghrita	Apasmara chikitsa	Ch. Chi. 10/27
69.	Vajikarana ghrita	Vajikarana pada	Ch. Chi. 2/1-33-37
70.	Tryushnadi ghrita	Gulma chikitsa	Ch. Chi. 5/104

Contd...

Contd...

S. No.	Name of Sneha	Name of disease	Reference
		Ghrita	
71.	Vasa ghrita	Gulma chikitsa	Ch. Chi. 5/126-127
72.	Vasa shatavari ghrita	Rajyakshma	Ch. Chi. 8/105
73.	Vipadikahara ghrita	Kushta chikitsa	Ch. Chi. 7/120-121
74.	Nilini ghrita	Gulma chikitsa	Ch. Chi. 5/152
75.	Vrishya ghrita	Vajikarana pada	Ch. Chi. 2/2-21-23
76.	Vrishya shatavari ghrita	Vajikarana pada	Ch. Chi. 2/3-18
77.	Vyoshadi ghrita	Pandu roga chikitsa	Ch. Chi. 16/119
78.	Shatdhota ghrita	Dvivraniya chikitsa	Ch. Chi. 25/64
79.	Shatavari ghrita	Atisara chikitsa	Ch. Chi. 19/78
80.	Shatavaryadi ghrita	Raktapiita chikitsa	Ch. Chi. 4/95-96
81.	Shvadanshtradi ghrita	Trimarmiya chikita	Ch. Chi. 26/74
82.	Shatapala ghrita	Gulma chikitsa	Ch. Chi. 5/7
83.	Samsaktu ghrita	Kshatkshina chikitsa	Ch. Chi. 11/48-49
84.	Sidharthaka ghrita	Unmada chikitsa	Ch. Chi. 9/73
85.	Snuhiksheera ghrita	Udara roga chikitsa	Ch. Chi. 13/138
86.	Sthiradi ghrita	Trimarmiya chikita	Ch. Chi. 26/175
87.	Hapushadi ghrita	Gulma chikitsa	Ch. Chi. 5/71-73
88.	Haridradi ghrita	Pandu chikits	Ch. Chi. 16/53
89.	Haritakyadi ghrita	Trimarmiya chikita	Ch. Chi. 26/83
90.	Higusauvarchaladi ghrita	Gulma chikitsa	Ch. Chi. 5/69-70
91.	Hriberadi ghrita	Arsha chikitsa	Ch. Chi. 14/230
		Taila	
1.	Agurvadi taila	Jvara chikitsa	Ch. Chi. 3/267
2.	Amritadi taila	Vata vyadhi chikitsa	Ch. Chi. 28/157
3.	Ashtakatavara taila	Vata Rakta chikitsa	Ch. Chi. 29/103
4.	Arnaladi taila	Vata Rakta chikitsa	Ch. Chi. 29/122
5.	Eranda taila	Udara roga chikitsa	Ch. Chi. 13/172
6.	Udumbara taila	Yonivyapad chikitsa	Ch. Chi. 30/77
7.	Katbhyadi taila	Apasmara chikitsa	Ch. Chi. 10/33
8.	Kanaksheeri taila	Kushta chikitsa	Ch. Chi. 7/111-116
9.	Kampillakadi taila	Dvivraniya chikitsa	Ch. Chi. 25/70-71
10.	Kampilladi taila	Visarpa chikitsa	Ch. Chi. 21/37
11.	Kushtadi taila	Visarpa chikitsa	Ch. Chi. 21/137
12.	Kshara taila	Urusthambha chikitsa	Ch. Chi. 27/43-44
13.	Khadiradi taila	Trimarmiya chikita	Ch. Chi. 26/206

Contd...

Contd...

S. No.	Name of Sneha	Name of disease	Reference
		Taila	
14.	Khuddaka padmak taila	Vata Rakta chikitsa	Ch. Chi. 29/114
15.	Gandha taila	Trimarmiya chikita	Ch. Chi. 26/224
16.	Guduchyadi taila	Vata Rakta chikitsa	Ch. Chi. 29/121
17.	Chandanadi taila	Jvara chikitsa	Ch. Chi. 3/258
18.	Tiktekshavaku taila	Kushta chikitsa	Ch. Chi. 7/108-110
19.	Tail panchak	Gulma chikitsa	Ch. Chi. 5/96
20.	Trikantkadi taila	Prameha chikitsa	Ch. Chi. 6/38-39
21.	Tvgadi taila	Trimarmiya chikita	Ch. Chi. 26/184
22.	Durva taila	Dvivraniya chikitsa	Ch. Chi. 25/96
23.	Devdarvadi taila	Vata vyadhi chikitsa	Ch. Chi. 26/223
24.	Dhatakyadi taila	Yonivyapada chikitsa	Ch. Chi.30/78-81
25.	Nirgundi taila	Vata vyadhi chikitsa	Ch. Chi. 28/134
26.	Pathadi taila	Trimarmiya chikita	Ch. Chi. 26/145
27.	Punarnavadi taila	Trimarmiya chikita	Ch. Chi.26/82
28.	Piluparanyadi taila	Urusthambha chikitsa	Ch. Chi. 27/41-42
29.	Prapoundirkadi taila	Trimarmiya chikita	Ch. Chi. 26/276
30.	Bala taila	Vata vyadhi chikitsa	Ch. Chi. 28/148
31.	Baladi taila	Vata vyadhi chikitsa	Ch. Chi. 28/126
32.	Bhallatak taila	Rasyana pada	Ch. Chi. 1/2-15
33.	Bharangyadi taila	Trimarmiya chikita	Ch. Chi. 26/153
34.	Madhuka taila	Vata Rakta chikitsa	Ch. Chi. 29/115
35.	Madhuyashtayadi taila	Vata Rakta chikitsa	Ch. Chi. 29/91-92
36.	Mahanila taila	Trimarmiya chikita	Ch. Chi. 26/268
37.	Mahapadma taila	Vata Rakta chikitsa	Ch. Chi. 29/110
38.	Mulaka taila	Vata vyadhi chikitsa	Ch. Chi. 28/136
39.	Mulakadi taila	Vata vyadhi chikitsa	Ch. Chi. 28/167
40.	Rasna taila	Vata vyadhi chikitsa	Ch. Chi. 28/165
41.	Rasnadi taila	Trimarmiya chikita	Ch. Chi. 26/160
42.	Laghu panchmula taila	Vata vyadhi chikitsa	Ch. Chi. 28/138
43.	Pinda taila	Vata rakta chikitsa	Ch. Chi. 29/123
44.	Vidangadi taila	Sneha vyapat siddhi	Ch.Si.4/8-22
45.	Vidarigandhadi taila	Trimarmiya chikita	Ch. Chi. 26/263
46.	Vrishamuladi taila	Vata vyadhi chikitsa	Ch. Chi. 28/170
47.	Shatpaka vasa taila	Vata Rakta chikitsa	Ch. Chi. 29/119

Contd...

Contd...

S. No.	*Name of Sneha*	*Name of disease*	*Reference*
		Taila	
48.	Shatpaka madhuka	Vata Rakta chikitsa	Ch. Chi. 29/117
49.	Shvadanshtra taila	Vata vyadhi chikitsa	Ch. Chi. 28/146
50.	Shveta karvira pallvadi taila	Kushta chikitsa	Ch. Chi. 7/106-107
51.	Shveta karviradi taila	Kushta chikitsa	Ch. Chi. 7/105
52.	Sahacharadi taila	Pandu chikitsa	Ch. Chi. 16/264
53.	Sahasrapaka bala taila	Vata Rakta chikitsa	Ch. Chi. 29/119
54.	Sahachara taila	Vata vyadhi chikitsa	Ch. Chi. 28/144
55.	Sukumara taila	Vata Rakta chikitsa	Ch. Chi. 29/98-102
56.	Sandhavadi taila	Sneha vyapad siddhi	Ch. Chi. 4/13-16

CHAPTER 3

Svedana

INTRODUCTION

Out of the two important Purva karma modalities mentioned in the texts in reference to Panchakarma is Svedana. Svedana karma is generally administered after Snehana and precedes Vamana and Virechana.

Principally, Svedana (hot fomentation) is designed to induce sweating. Acharya Charaka very clearly states that the Svedana Karma is the procedure which relieves Stambha (stiffness), Gaurava (heaviness), Sheetata (cold) and which induces Sveda (sweat). It is also termed as sudation therapy or fomentation therapy. While describing what is Svedana, Ayurvediya Shabdakosha says, application of agni or niragni sveda to increase the temperature is Svedana. While vagbhatta (A.H. su. 17/1) says inducing Svedana in Snigdha person is Svedana.

स्निग्धस्य स्वेदनं कार्यमिति स्वेदोविधीयते। (A.H. Su. 17/1)

Mala in spite of being waste product have got very useful functions in the body. Sveda arises out of the effect of Ushma. Actually, Sveda or sweating is a normal physiological function of the body. However, the application of artificial means to induce or aggravate sweating is known as Svedana karma and is included amongst the Purva karma of the Panchakarma. Sveda, as mala of the body helps in maintaining the klinnata of body in balanced state. Vagbhatta says Sveda helps in holding kelda (A. H. Su. 11/15)

स्वेदस्य क्लेद विधृति। (A. H. Su. 11/15)

Svedana is a major preparatory procedure for Panchakarma therapy which is administered to liquefy the vitiated Doshas, which have achieved Snigdhata (by earlier Snehana) spread in the system in order to make it convenient to expel them out with the help of Pradhana Karma such as Vamana, Virechana, Basti and Shirovirechana etc. Moreover, Svedana Karma is also an important therapy for a number of disorders, where it works as Pradhana Karma e.g. vatavyadhi. Acharya Charaka had included Svedana under Shadupakramas and thus has given importance to Svedana as a principle method of treatment. Acharya Charaka has mentioned that Svedana therapy is the best treatment for vitiated Vata and Kapha dominant disorders.

लङ्घनं बृंहणं काले रुक्षणं स्नेहनं तथा। स्वेदनं स्तम्भनं चैव जानीते यः स वै भिषक्॥ (Ch. Su. 22/4)

स्नेहपूर्व प्रयुक्तेन स्वेदेनावजितेऽनिले। पुरीषमूत्ररेतसि न सज्जन्ति कथंचन॥ (Ch. Su. 14/4)

स्वेदासाध्याः प्रशाम्यन्ति गदा वातकफात्मकाः। (Ch. Su. 14/3)

ETYMOLOGY

The word Sveda is derived from the root 'Swid' (स्विद्) with 'Ghan' (घञ्) Pratyaya with addition of Bhava Vachaka 'Nich' (णिच्) and 'Ach' (अच्).
The word svedana is Napunsaka linga which is produced by 'Nich' and 'Lyut' Pratyaya.

DEFINITION

स्वेद इति स्वेदभवे धर्मे (Chakrapani)

Sveda word refers to Bodily sweat or Perspiration through the body.

स्तम्भ गौरवं शीतघ्नं स्वेदनं स्वेदकारकम्।। (Ch.Su.22/11)

The procedure, which induces Sveda (sweat), reduces Stambha (stiffness), gaurava (Heaviness) and Sheeta (cold) is called as svedana.

CLASSIFICATION OF SVEDANA

Dvividha Bheda of Svedana

इत्युक्तो द्विविधः स्वेदः संयुक्तो अग्निगुणैर् न च।। एकाङ्ग सर्वाङ्गगतः स्निग्धो रूक्षः तथैवं च।
इत्येति त्रिविधं द्वन्द्वं स्वेदम् उद्दिश्य कीर्तितम्। (Ch.Su. 14/65-66)

Charaka has mentioned 3 sets of opposite Sveda which are as follows:

1. Agni - Niragni
2. Ekanga - Sarvanga
3. Snigdha - Ruksha

I. Classification of Sveda According to Agnibheda

Based on Sanyoga of Agni it is of 2 types:

A. Niragni Sveda
B. Sagni Sveda

A. Niragni Sveda

In this method there is no direct contact with Agni (fire). These are of 10 types:

व्यायाम उष्णसदनं गुरुप्रावरणं क्षुधा। बहुपानं भय क्रोध उपनाह आहव आतपः।।
स्वेदयन्ति दशैतानि नरम् अग्निगुणाहृते।। (Ch.Su.14/64)

1. Vyayama	Exercise
2. Ushnasadana	Residing in a warm chamber
3. Gurupravarnam	Covering with thick or heavy clothing
4. Kshudha	Hunger
5. Bahupanam	Excessive drinking
6. Bhaya	Fear

7. Upanaha	Application of poultice
8. Krodha	Anger
9. Ahava	Wrestling
10. Aatapa	Exposure to sun's rays

B. Sagni Sveda

In this method of Svedana, there is direct contact with Agni (fire). These are of 13 types:

सङ्करः प्रस्तरो नाडी परिषेको अवगाहनम्। जेन्ताको अश्मघनः कर्षूः कुटी भूः कुम्भिक एव च॥
कूपो होलाक इत्येते स्वेदयन्ति त्रयोदश॥ (Ch.Su.14/39)

1. Sankara	2. Prastara
3. Nadi	4. Parisheka
5. Avagaha	6. Jentaka
7. Ashmaghana	8. Karshu
9. Kuti	10. Bhu
11. Kumbhika	12. Kupa
13. Holaka	

II. Classification of Sveda Based on Guna

वातश्लेष्मणि वाते वा कफे वा स्वेद इष्यते। स्निग्ध रूक्षस्तथा स्निग्धो रूक्षश्च अप्य उपकल्पितः॥ (Ch.Su.14/8)

Based on the Guna of the Dravya used for the Svedana Karma it is of 3 types:

S.N.	*Types*	*Beneficial in*
1.	Snigdha	Vata disorders
2.	Ruksha	Kapha disorders/Conditions with amavastha
3.	Snigdha-Ruksha	Vata-Kapha disorders

आमाशयगतेवाते कफेपक्वाशय आश्रिते। रूक्षपूर्वो हितः स्वेदः स्नेहपूर्वः तथैव च॥ (Ch.Su.14/9)

When Vata is localised in Amashaya, first Ruksha Sveda should be administered and when Kapha is localised in Pakvashaya, first Snigdha Sveda should be administered.

III. Classification of Sveda According to the Extent of Fomentation/Area of Application

Based on the area of fomentation it is of 2 types:

1. **Ekanga sveda:** Fomentation is done to a single part of the body.
2. **Sarvanga sveda:** Fomentation all over the body.

IV. Based on the Intensity of Fomentation

व्याधौ शीते शरीरे च महान् स्वेदो महाबले। दुर्बले दुर्बलः स्वेदो मध्यमे मध्यमो हितः॥(Ch.Su.14/7)
वृषणो हृदयं दृष्टि स्वेदयेत् मृदु न एव वा। मध्यमं वंक्षणौ शेषं अङ्गावयवं इष्टतः॥ (Ch.Su.14/10)

Based on the level of intensity Sveda is of 3 types :

S.N.	*Types of Sveda*	*Types of person*	*Part of the body*
1.	Mridu	Durbala	Vrishana, Hridaya, Drishti
2.	Madhyama	Madhyama Bala	Vankshana
3.	Mahan	Sheeta Vyadhi, Mahabala	Rest other place

V. According to Sushruta and *Vagbhatta*

Both Acharya's have mentioned 4 types of Sveda :

S.N.	*Name*	*S.N.*	*Name*
1.	Tapa Sveda	2.	Ushma Sveda
3.	Upanaha Sveda	4.	Drava Sveda

चतुर्विधः स्वेदः; तद्यथातापस्वेद, ऊष्मस्वेद, उपनाहस्वेदो, द्रवस्वेदइति; अत्र सर्वस्वेद विकल्प अविरोधः॥ (Su.Chi.32/3)

तपनं तापः, ऊष्मा बाष्पः, उपनह्यते इति उपनाहो बन्धनम् इत्यर्थः, द्रवती इति द्रवः कषाय क्षीरादिः॥

1. Tapa Sveda (Dry Heat)

तत्र तापस्वेदः पाणि कांस्य कन्दुक कपाल वालुका वस्त्रैः प्रयुज्यते, शयानस्य च अङ्ग तापो बहुशः खदिर अङ्गारैंदकइति॥ (Su.Chi.32/4)

It comprises of using dry heat such as making the patient to stay in hot room. Hot and dry substances such as sand, brick, metal ball wrapped in a piece of cloth are directly applied on the affected part of body. Hot water bag may also be used for this purpose.

2. Ushma Sveda (Steam Bath)

ऊष्मस्वेदस्तु कपाल पाषाण इष्टिका लोह पिण्डान् अग्नि वर्णान् अद्भिर आसिञ्चेद् आम्लद्रव्यैर्वा तौर् आर्द्रालक्तक परिवेष्टि तैर अङ्ग प्रदेशं स्वेदयेत्॥ (Su.Chi.32/5)

Ushma means vapours and the sudation done mainly through vapours is known as Ushma Sveda. Nadi and Bashpa (steam) Svedana are the examples of this type of sveda.

3. Drava Sveda

द्रवस्वेदे परिषेक अवगाहाव अन्तर्भवत॥ (Su.Chi.32/3.Dalhana)

Sudation done by using hot liquids in a tub or pouring them on the body comes under Drava Sveda.

4. Upanaha Sveda (Poultice)

उपनह्यते इति उपनाहो बन्धनम् इत्यर्थः (Su.Chi.32/3.Dalhana)

In this process a paste of the hot drugs is applied on the affected part. It may be bandaged to keep it at a proper place.

VI. Dalhana has classified Sveda into two types

1. **Sanshamniya sveda:** When svedana is done as independent therapy for pacification of dosha's in various disorders as pradhana karma.
2. **Sanshodhananga sneha:** When svedana is done as a purvakarma for purification of dosha's in shodhana chikitsa.

VII. Classification According to Other Acharyas

S.N.	*Harita*	*Bhela*	*Kashyapa*
1.	Loshta	Sankara	Hasta
2.	Ashpa	Prastara	Pradeha
3.	Agnijwala	Seka	Nadi
4.	Ghati	Nadi	Prastara
5.	Jala	Droni	Sankara
6.	Phala	Jala	Upanaha
7.	Baluka	Udakoshta	Avagaha
8.	–	Kuti	Parisheka

GENERAL SVEDA DRAVYA, PROPERTIES OF SVEDA DRAVYAS, SVEDOPAGA DRAVYAS

Properties of Svedana Dravya

उष्णं तीक्ष्णं सरं स्निग्धं रूक्षं सूक्ष्मं द्रवं स्थिरम्।
द्रव्यं गुरु च यत् प्रायः तद्धि स्वेदनम् उच्यते।। (Ch.Su.22/16)

S.N.	*Guna*	*Equivalent meaning*
1.	Ushna	Hot
2.	Teekshna	Sharp
3.	Sara	Tendency of flow
4.	Snigdha	Unctuous
5.	Ruksha	Rough
6.	Drava	Liquid
7.	Sthira	Stable
8.	Guru	Heavy

स्वेदने उष्णः (Hemadri)
Ushna guna induces sveda
शोधने तीक्ष्णः (Hemadri)
Tikshna guna helps in shodhana of dosha and removes srotorodha
यस्य प्रेरणे शक्तिः स सरः (Hemadri)
Sara guna induces movement in morbid dosha
यस्य क्लेदने शक्तिः स स्निगधः (Hemadri)
Snigdha guna induces kleda
शोषणे रूक्षः (Hemadri)
Ruksha guna removes extra fluids and induces dryness
यस्य विवरणे शक्तिः स सूक्ष्मः (Hemadri)
Sukshma guna helps in reaching micro channels
यस्य विलोडने शक्तिः स द्रवः (Hemadri)
Drava guna helps in liquefaction of morbid doshas
धारणे स्थिरः (Hemadri)
Sthira guna helps in inducing stability
यस्य द्रव्यस्य बृहणे शक्तिः स गुरु (Hemadri)
Guru guna helps in vriddhi of doshas and also it helps in brihana.

Svedopaga Dravya

शोभाञ्जन एरण्ड अर्क वृश्चीर पुनर्नवा यव तिल कुलत्थ माष बदराणी इति दशेमानि स्वेदोपगानि भवन्ति। (Ch.Su.4/13)

S.N.	Dravya	Botanical Name
1.	Shobhanjana (Fig. 3.1A)	*Moringa oleifera*
2.	Eranda (Fig. 3.1B)	*Ricinus communis*
3.	Arka (Fig. 3.1C)	*Calotropis gigantica*
4.	Vrischira (Shweta punarnava) (Fig. 3.1D)	*Boerhavia diffusa*
5.	Punarnava (Fig. 3.1E)	*Boerhavia diffusa*
6.	Yava	*Hordeum vulgare*
7.	Tila (Fig. 3.1F)	*Sesamum indicum*
8.	Kulattha	*Dolichos biflorus*
9.	Masha	*Phaseolus mungo*
10.	Badara	*Zizyphus jujuba*

SOME SVEDOPAGA DRAVYA

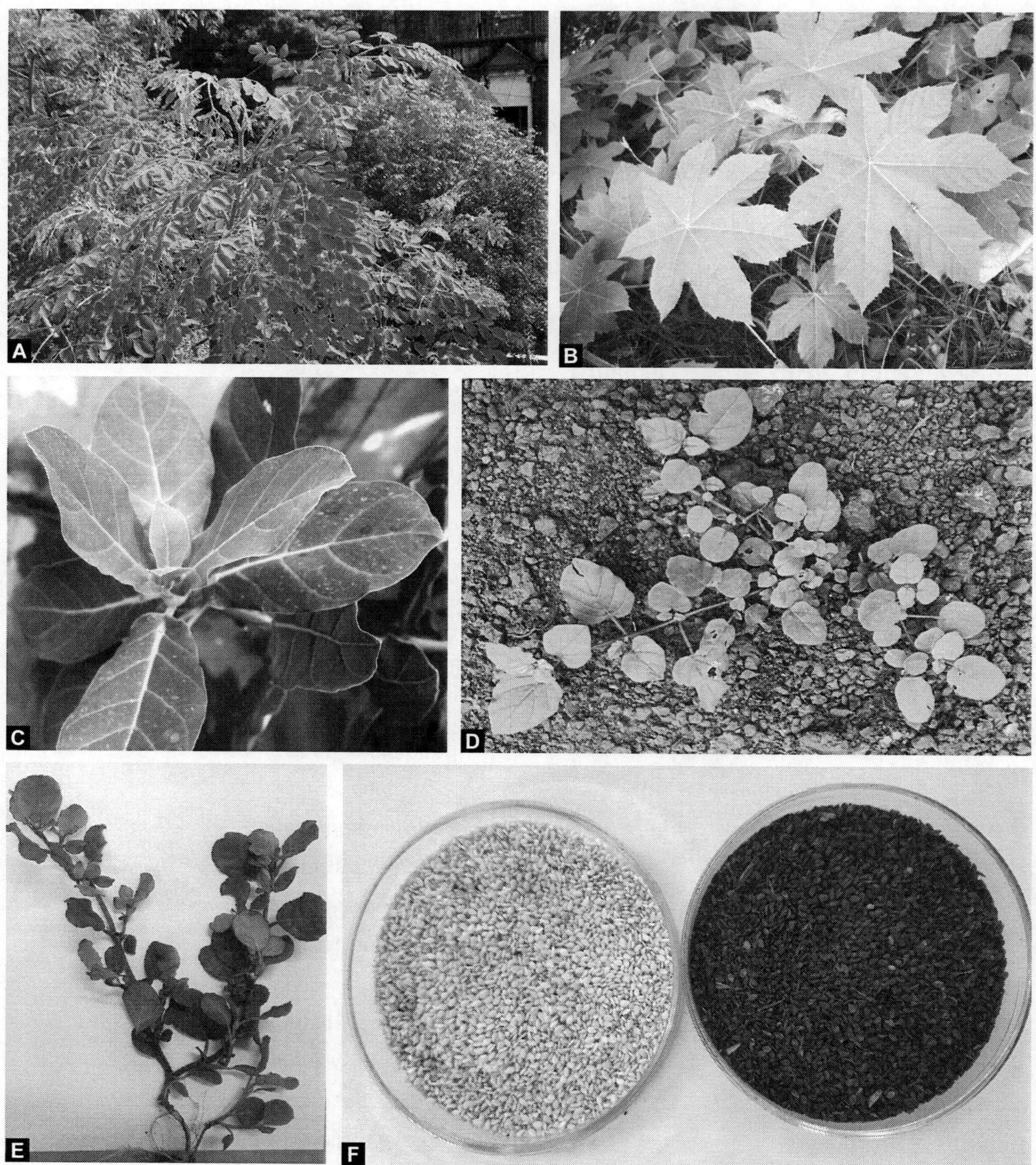

Fig. 3.1A to F: (A) Shobhanjana (B) Eranda (C) Arka (D) Vrishchira (E) Punarnava (F) Tila

INDICATIONS

Svedana is indicated in Vata and Kapha disorders and is a must prior to the performance of Shodhana therapy. In the following diseases svedana is regarded as an effective treatment.

प्रतिश्याये च कासे च हिक्का श्वासेषु लाघवे। कर्ण मन्या शिरः शूले स्वरभेदे गलग्रहे॥
अर्दितैर् एकाङ्ग सर्वाङ्ग पक्षाघाते विनामके। कोष्ठानाह विबन्धेषु मूत्राघाते विजृम्भके॥
पार्श्व पृष्ठ कटी कुक्षिसङ्ग्रहे गृध्रसीषु च। मूत्रकृच्छ्रे महात्वे च मुष्कयोर् अङ्गमर्दके॥
पाद जानू उरु जङ्घार्ति संग्रहे श्वयथावपि। खल्लीषु आमेषु शीते च वेपथौ वातकण्टके॥
सङ्कोच आयाम शूलेषु स्तम्भ गौरव सुप्तिषु॥ सर्वाङ्गेषु विकारेषु स्वेदनं हितमुच्यते॥ (Ch.Su.14/20-24)

S.N.	Disease	S.N.	Disease
1.	Rhinitis	2.	Cough
3.	Pharyngitis	4.	Dyspnoea
5.	Hiccups	6.	Pain in ears
7.	Disease of neck and head	8.	Distension of abdomen
9.	Constipation	10.	Ama disorders
11.	Colicky pain in abdomen	12.	Feeling of heaviness
13.	Cold	14.	Body-ache
15.	Stiffness of flanks	16.	Stiffness of back
17.	Stiffness of waist	18.	Stiffness in foot and knee
19.	Osteo-arthritis	20.	Sciatica
21.	Contracture	22.	Hardness
23.	Stretching stiffness	24.	Numbness
25.	Cramps	26.	Tremors
27.	Facial paralysis	28.	Dysarthria
29.	Monoplegia	30.	Hemiplegia
31.	Dysuria	32.	Anuria
33.	Inflammation		

Sushruta has Mentioned Trividha Svedavacharana

येषां नस्यं विधातव्यं बस्तिश्चैव हि देहिनाम्। शोधनीयाश्च ये केचित् पूर्वम् स्वेद्यास्तु ते मताः॥
पश्चात् स्वेद्या हृते शल्ये मूढगर्भाऽनुपद्रवा। सम्यक् प्रजाता काले या पश्चात् स्वेद्या विजानिता॥
स्वेद्यःपूर्वम् च पश्चाच्च भगन्दर्यर्शसस्तथा। अश्मर्या चातुरो जन्तुःशेषाज्छास्त्रे प्रचक्ष्महे॥
(Su.Chi.32/17-19)

Before procedure (As a Purva karma)	*After procedure (As a Pashchat karma)*	*Before and After (As a Purva and Pashchat karma)*
• Nasya	• Hrita Shalya (After removal of foreign body)	• Bhagandara
• Basti	• Anupadrava Mudagarbha	• Arsha
• Shodhana	• Samyak prajata kala	• Ashmari

CONTRAINDICATIONS (SVEDANA KARMA)

As the Svedana involves heating of the body parts, it may provoke the Pitta Dosha and hence, is harmful in certain delicate states of health. For the same reason in specific conditions that are listed below, Svedana is contraindicated.

Svedana Karma should not be administered in those who have taken too much alcohol, pregnant woman, those suffering from Raktapitta, Kamala (Jaundice), Udara roga (abdominal diseases), Timira, Atisara (diarrhea), Prameha (diabetes mellitus), inflammatory condition, prolapse of the rectum and toxic conditions.

It is contraindicated in fatty, thirsty, hungry, having Paittika constitutions and in those having dry skin. In a state of anger and anxiety. Those who are weak and dried up and whose Ojasa has been reduced.

कषायमद्यनित्यानां गर्भिण्या रक्तपित्तिनाम्। पित्तिनां सातिसाराणां रूक्षाणां मधुमेहिनाम्॥
विदग्धभ्रष्टब्रध्नानां विषमद्यविकारिणाम्। श्रान्तानां नष्टसंज्ञानां स्थूल्यानां पित्तमेहिनाम्॥
तृष्यतां क्षुधितानां च क्रुद्धानां शोचतामपि। कामल्युदरिणां चैव क्षतानामादयरोगिणाम्॥
दुर्बलातिविशुष्काणामुपक्षीणौजसां तथा। भिषक् तैमिरिकाणां च न स्वेदमवतारयेत्॥

(Ch. Su. 14/16-19)

स्विन्नेऽत्यर्थ सन्धिपीडा विदाहः स्फोटोत्पत्ति पित्तरक्तप्रकोपः।
मूर्च्छा भ्रान्तिर्दाहतृष्णे क्लमश्च कुर्यात्तूर्ण तत्र शीतं विद्यानम्॥ (Su. Chi. 32/24)
पाण्डुर्मेहा पित्तरकी क्षयतिः क्षामोऽजीर्णी चोदरार्तो विर्षतिः।
तृच्छर्द्यातो गर्भिणी पीतमद्यो नैते स्वेद्या यश्च मर्त्योऽतिसारी॥
स्वेदादेषां यान्ति देहा विनाशं नो साध्यत्वं यान्ति चैषां विकाराः।
स्वेदैः साध्यो दुर्बलोऽजीर्णभक्तः स्यातां चेद् द्वौ स्वेदनीयौ ततस्तौ॥ (Su. Chi. 32/25)
न स्वेदयेदतिस्थूलरुक्षदुर्बलमूर्च्छितम्॥
स्तम्भनीयक्षतक्षीणक्षाममद्यविकारिणः। तिमिरोदरवीसर्प कुष्ठशोषादयरोगिणः॥
पीतदुग्धदधिस्नेहमधून् कृतविरेचनान्। भ्रष्टदग्धगुदग्लानिक्रोधशोक भयार्दितान्॥
क्षुत्तष्णाकामलापाण्डुमोहिन पित्तपीडितान्। गर्भिणी पुष्पितां सूतां मृदु चाप्ययिके गदे॥

(A. H. Su. 17/14-5)

Parts Contraindicated For Svedana

Svedana Karma should not be administered over testicles, heart and eyes. Even if it is very necessary to administer, it should be of mild type, over scrotum it should be moderate fomentation and other parts of the body could be according to the individuals need.

NIRAGNI SVEDA

Fomentation can be done without the application of external heat and such types of sudation are termed as Niragni Sveda. Following ten types of Niragni Sveda are mentioned:

1. **Vyayama (Exercise)**- Muscular exercise produces sweating in the body.
2. **Ushna Sadana (Warm room)**- A room without ventilation particularly in the summer season may produce the sweating.

3. **Guru Pravarana (Covering with thick or heavy clothes)**- If a person lies by covering the body with thick cloths or woollen sheet then it may lead to sweating due to the non-conduction of body heat to the external environment.
4. **Kshudha (Hunger)**- Excessive hunger produces sweating.
5. **Bahupana**- Consumption of excessive alcohol produces sweating.
6. **Bhaya (Fear)** and
7. **Krodha (Anger)**- In emotional conditions such as fear and anger, sweating occurs.
8. **Upanaha (Poultice)**- Poultice produces sweating by preventing the loss of body heat. The poultice is applied on the affected part and is covered or bandaged with a cloth. If the poultice is applied in the night it should be removed in the morning and if it is applied in the day it should be removed in the night, so that irritation to the skin may not occur. However, the period of application of poultice may be prolonged in the cold season.
9. **Aahava (Wrestling)**- Wrestling and fighting lead to sweating.
10. **Atapa (Sun bath)**- Direct exposure to sun rays leads to perspiration.

KNOWLEDGE OF 13 TYPES OF SAAGNI SVEDA

1. Sankara Sveda

तत्र वस्त्रान्तरितैर् अवस्त्रान्तरितैर् वा पिण्डैर् यथोक्तैर् सङ्कर स्वेद इतित विद्यात्।। (Ch.Su.14/41)

It is a type of Pinda Sveda. Fomentation using bolus (Pinda) prescribed drugs with or without being wrapped cloth.

Drugs used

तिलमाष कुलत्थ आम्ल घृत तैल आमिष ओदनैः। पायसैः कृशरैर् मांसैः पिण्ड स्वेदं प्रयोजयेत्।।
गोखर ओष्ट्र वराह अश्व शकृद्भिः स तुषैर् यवैः। सिकता पांशु पाषाण करीष आयस पूटकैः।।
श्लैष्मिकान् दयेत् पूर्वैर् वातिकात् समुपाचरेत्। (Ch.Su.14/25-27)

I. **Ruksha (dry) Sankara Sveda**: In this type of Sveda, hot solid substances such as sand, brick, and stone are used. It is a mild type of Sveda and may be done by the patient himself in Kapha and Ama disorders affecting joints or muscles.
   Drugs for Kapha : Shakrit of Go, Khara, Ushtra, Varaha, Ashva, Satusha Yava, Sikata, Panshu, Pashana, Kareesha.
II. **Snigdha (Unctuous) Sankara Sveda**: Thick gruel is prepared from the substances like sesame, black gram, horse gram, citric fruits, ghee, oil, rice and milk pudding. This type of Sveda is more useful in the conditions of Kevala Vata. Shashti Shali Pinda Sveda and Nirgundi Patra Pinda Sveda are its varieties.

Drugs for Vata : Tila, Masha, Kulattha, Amla, Ghrita, Taila, Amisha, Odana, Payasa, Krishara.

2. Prastara Sveda (Fig. 3.2)

Materials used

Shuka Dhanya, Shami dhanya, Pulaaka (Kudhanya), Veshavara, Payasa, Krishara, Utkarika.

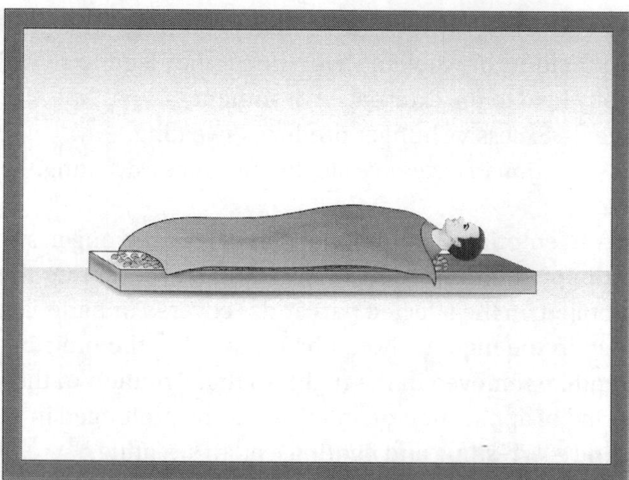

Fig. 3.2: Prastara sveda

Covering material

Kousheya (Silk), Avikottara Pracchada (woolen cloth), leaves of Panchangula (Eranda), Arka.

Method

- A slab of stone measuring about 7 ft × 2 ft is used as a bed.
- On it, hot gruel prepared with cereals, milk pudding, etc. is spread.
- It is covered either by a sheet of silken cloth or leaves of eranda.
- The patient, after a proper sarvanga abhyanga is asked to lie down on the stone after which, his body is covered with a thick cotton sheet, till he gets proper perspiration.

3. Nadi Sveda (Fig. 3.3)

It is a type of Agni Sveda in which Svedana is by vapours obtained by boiling liquids in a vessel through Nadi (pipe).

Materials Required

Mula or phala of different herbs like Eranda, Shigru, Amla, Lavana, Mutra, Sneha, ete. according to Dosha (Ch.Su. 14/33). Commonly, Dashamula are used to generate Sveda.

Method

Take the prescribed medicine and prepare the Kashaya in a pressure cooker with a capacity of 5- 10 litres, or in any other vessel in such a way that the vapour does not leak out. The individual well massaged with Vatahara Taila should get exposed to vapour through the curved pipe. Curvature of the pipe helps in preventing spillage of condensed drops coming out of the tube directly on the body of the patient. A pressure cooker may also be used and in that case the tube should be attached to the nozzle where normally the weight is attached. Other vapour producing instruments may also be used with required modification.

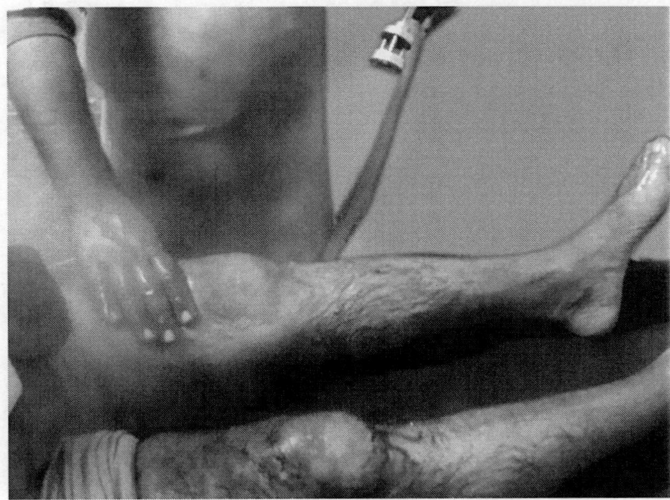

Fig. 3.3: Nadi sveda

Precautions

1. The pressure cooker/ steam generator vessel is filled properly to prevent damage to equipment.
2. The vessel is heated on the stove and when vapour starts coming out of the tube, exposed to the individual who has undergone Abhyanga already.
3. The tube should be kept at one feet distance, and may be adjusted according to the heat tolerance of the patient.
4. Care must be taken that the condensed drops coming out of the tube should not fall on the patient.
5. Condensed water drops will get collected in the curvature and it should be periodically emptied around five minutes.
6. Nadi sveda is done once in the morning, and if necessary, may be repeated in the evening depending upon the response of the patient and the disease.

4. Parisheka Sveda (Fig. 3.4)

The procedure in which hot liquids (oils, decoction etc.) are poured over the body of a patient is known as Parisheka sveda.

Materials

Dravya

Mulaadi (Patra, Twak, Phala etc.), which alleviates Vata, Vata-kapha.

Instruments

Kumbhi (pitcher), Varshanika (small pot with many openings), Pranadi.

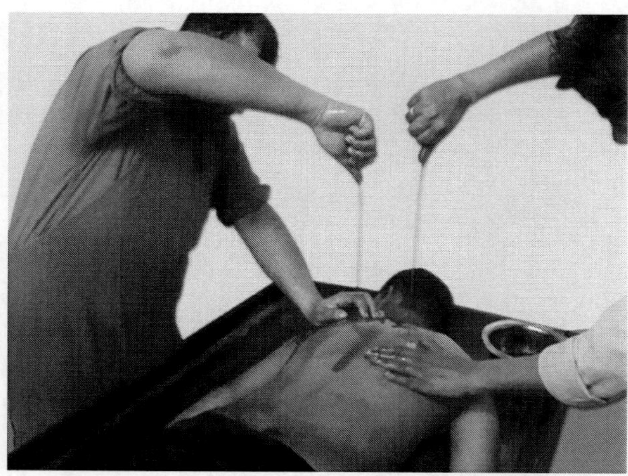

Fig. 3.4: Parisheka sveda

Method

- Decoction of the prescribed drugs is prepared and luke warm decoction is filled into a pot. On the prescribed oil cand also be used.
- Individual who has undergone Abhyanga with suitable oil should take Parisheka.
- This type of fomentation is called Parisheka Sveda.
- Nowaday's modified Parisheka Sveda is done under the name of Pizhichil.

5. Avagaha (Hot Tub Bath) (Fig. 3.5)

इति दोषपीडावशात्परिषेक स्वेदमाख्याय अवगाह स्वेदं द्रव भेदमाह तैरेव वा द्रवैः पूर्णं कुण्डं सर्वाङ्गगे अनिले।

अवगाह्य आतुरस्तिष्ठेतद् अर्शः कृच्छ्रादिरुक्षु च॥ (A.H.Su.17/11)

वातहरो उत्क्वाथ क्षीर तैल घृत पिशितरस उष्ण सलिल कोष्ठक अवगाहस्तु यथोक्त एव अवगाहः॥ (Ch.Su.14/45)

Immersion of the affected part in a tub filled with suitable warm liquid is known as Avagaha Sveda (tub bath). It can be carried out for the whole body in Sarvanga vyadhi and locally in disease such as painful Arsha (Hemorrhoids).

Materials

Dravya

Vatahara Kvatha, Ksheera, Taila, Ghrita, Pishita Rasa, Ushnajala.

Instruments

Jala Koshtha (tub)

जलकोष्ठः अवगाहार्थ कृत महत् जलपात्रम्॥ (Chakrapani)

Chakrapani comments that, Jalakoshta is a large tub like vessel which is used for the purpose of Avagaha.

Method

- The hot decoction prepared from Vata relieving drugs, hot milk, ghee, oil or water as per feasibility may be used.
- After proper massage the patient is asked to sit or lie down in the tub filled with liquid by keeping the head above.
- In case of sitting position, the level of the liquid should be up to chest and the warm liquid may be poured continuously on the shoulder.
- For lying position, it should be sufficiently filled so that the body remains immersed in the liquid.
- The patient may remain for 48 minutes in the tub. Thereafter the patient is allowed to come out from the tub and the liquid is cleaned with a towel.
- The patient should be advised take light meal after taking hot bath.

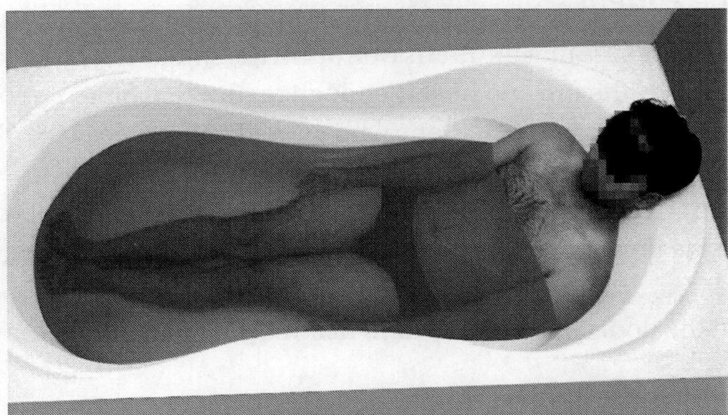

Fig. 3.5: Avagaha Sveda

Indications

Sarvanga Vata, Arsha, Kati-prishtha shula, Gridhrasi etc.

6. Jentaka Svedana (Figs 3.6A and B)

Svedana performed in a specially prepared kuti is known as Jentaka Sveda. Many specifications have been mentioned in the classics regarding the building used for the purpose of Jentaka Sveda.

Selection of Land

- Physician should examine the land before construction. Land should be selected in Eastern or western side.
- Land should be fertile with proper mist, sunlight and the soil should be sweet black (कृष्णमधुर) or golden colour (सुवर्ण मृत्तिक).
- It should be on the southern or eastern bank of a water reservoir like small or a big pond.

- The level of land should be uniformly plain and it should be situated at a distance of 7 -8 Aratni (1 Hasta = 24 angula = 18 inches), i.e. about 12 feet from the water reservoir.

Construction of Building

- The height and diameter of the building should be 6 Aratni.
- The building should be uniformly circular, well plastered with mud and should have many windows to facilitate ventilation.
- A bench of one Aratni height and one Aratni width is then to be prepared all around the wall up to the door.
- An oven of clay should be prepared in the centre of the room. Its diameter should be 4 Hasta and height should be equal to the height of an individual. It should be circular in shape and should have many fine holes and a lid.
- It should be filled with the fuel of Khadira and Ashwakarna etc and should be ignited.

Preparation of the Patient

- When the physician is sure that the fuel is well burnt the smoke has completely disappeared, the room is heated by the fire and heat is enough to produce fomentation.
- Then physician should ask the patient who is well massaged with Vatahara taila and covered with a cloth to enter the room.
- Physician should advice, "Oh noble one! Enter the room for the sake of your well being and cure of disease. Lie down there and keep changing your sides comfortably".
- Also if you faint/ feel drowsy owing to heat do not leave the bench as it may not be possible for you to reach the door. This may result in death owing to fainting due to heat.

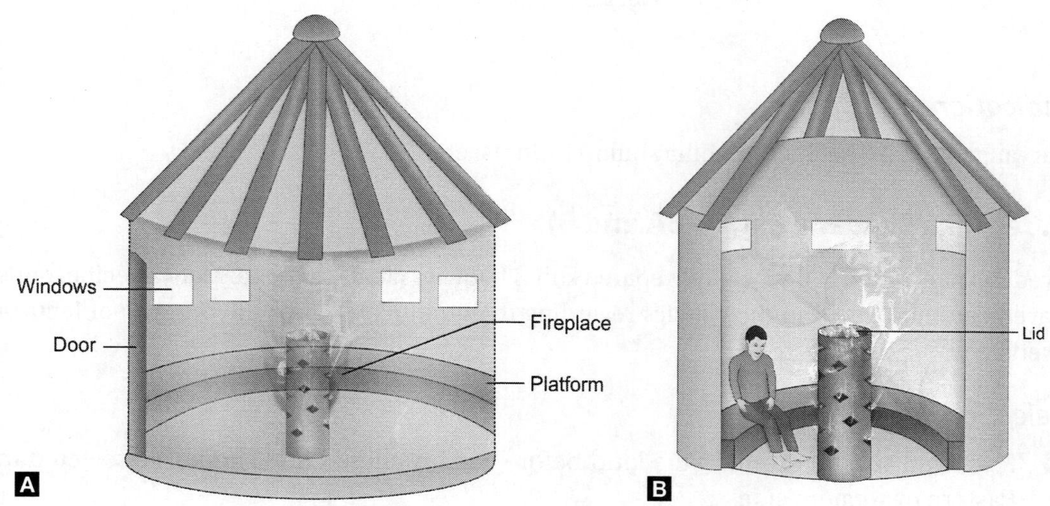

Figs 3.6A and B: Jentaka Svedana

Pashchat Karma

- When person feels that he is free from all obstructions, the sweat along with its sticking portion (Piccha) is completely drained out, all channels are light and free from all obstructions, there is no stiffness, numbness, pain, heaviness then he should move towards the door.
- One should not sprinkle cold water to eyes after coming out as it may affect eyes.
- After heat and exertion are over he should take bath with luke warm water after one Muhurta. Then he should be asked to consume laghu ahara.

It is indicated in Kapha disorders and in the very cold season and climate. It is also very useful where the Svedana is done to large number of patients in one day like in mass treatment camps because at such a time two or three people can be send inside the room for Svedana.

7. Ashmaghna Sveda (Fig. 3.7)

This is a kind of fomentation where the perspiration is induced by making the person to lie down over a preheated slab of stone.

Materials Required

- Compact slab of stone measuring the length of a man
- Sticks/fuel having Vatahara property
- Hot water
- Silk/woollen sheets

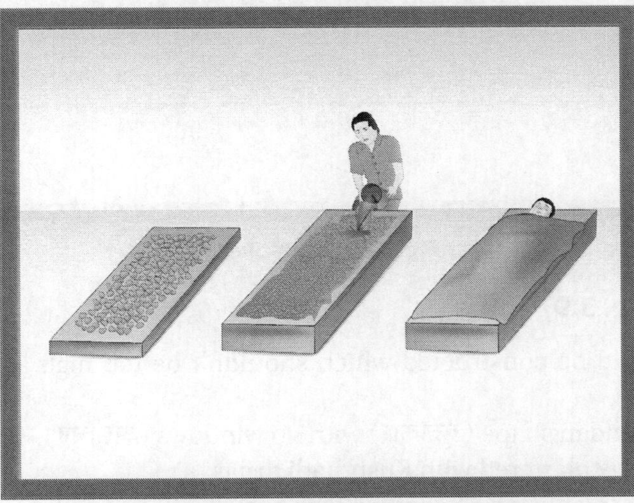

Fig. 3.7: Ashmaghna Sveda

Method

- Firewood having Vatahara properties should be burnt over a compact slab of stone.
- When stone gets heated firewood should be removed and hot water should be sprinkled over the slab.
- Stone should be covered with silk/woollen sheets.

- Person who has undergone Sarvanga abhyanga should lie on the stone and should be covered with a sheet.
- Patient should be made to lie till symptoms proper fomentation occurs.

8. Karshu Sveda (Fig. 3.8)

कर्षूः अभ्यन्तरविस्तीर्णः स्वल्पमुखो गर्तः। (Ch.Su.14/50.Teeka)

Karshu is a pit containing a large space inside and a narrow opening at the top (shape of flask).

- For this type of Sveda, a small kit of 5 feet × 1.5 feet × 2 feet is dug and is filled with smokeless burning coal.
- A cot covered with bed sheet is spread on it.
- The patient, after proper Abhyanga is asked to lie down on the cot by covering the body with bed sheet till he gets good perspiration along with other symptoms of proper Svedana.

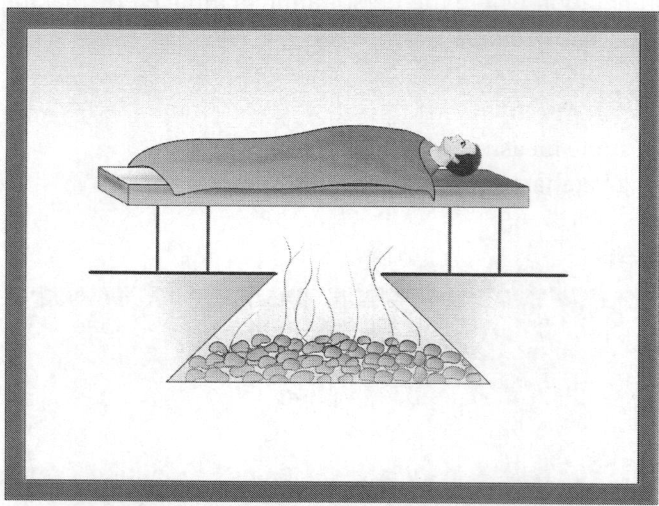

Fig. 3.8: Karshu Sveda

9. Kuti Sveda (Fig. 3.9)

- Kuti (hut) should be constructed which shouldn't be too high and too wide (अनति उत्सेधविस्तारा).
- It should be round in shape (वृत्ताकार) with no windows (अलोचन). The inner wall of the cottage should be plastered with Kushthadi drugs.
- In the centre of the hut a bed covered with cotton, silk, deer skin, woollen should be placed.
- The bed should be surrounded with the furnace, filled with fire wood brimming without shape.
- The patient who has taken the Abhyanga is asked to lie down on the cot by covering his body with a cotton sheet till he gets perspiration and other symptoms of proper Svedana.

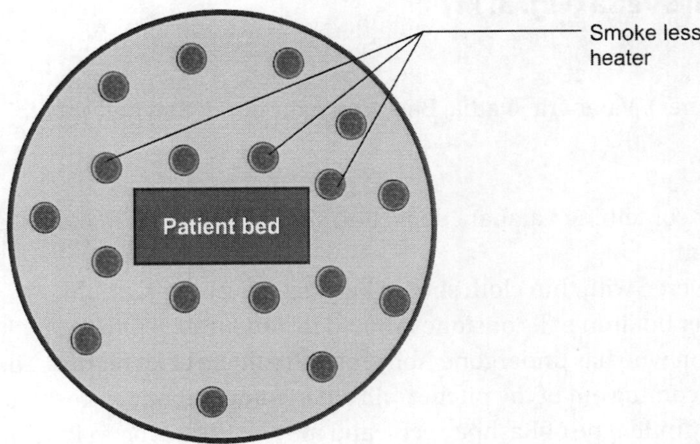

Fig. 3.9: Kuti Sveda

10. Bhu Sveda (Fig. 3.10)

- On the ground (Bhu), a suitable area measuring about 7' × 3' is well cleaned. The process mentioned in Ashmaghana Sveda is repeated. The only difference between these two is that: in Ashmaghana Sveda a stone slab is used while in Bhu Sveda the same process is done on the ground.
- An auspicious area, which is free from excessive wind, should be selected for this purpose.

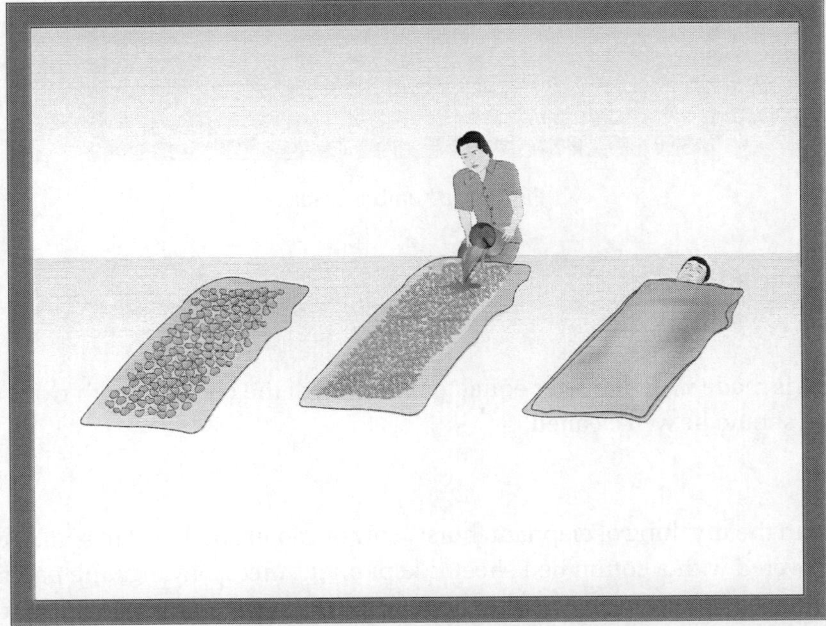

Fig. 3.10: Bhu Sveda

11. Kumbhi Sveda (Fig. 3.11)

Materials

Kumbhi (pitcher), Vatahara Kvatha, Bed, iron ball, stone, thin bed sheet.

Method

- A pitcher containing Vatahara decoction should be buried in earth upto half or one third of its length.
- A bed covered with thin cloth should be placed over the Kumbhi.
- There after hot iron balls or stones should be put into the pitcher.
- The person who has undergone Abhyanga should lie or sit on the bed.
- The heat coming out of the pitcher will aid in fomentation.
- It is a very mild type of Bashpa Sveda and may be used even in Pitta disorders.

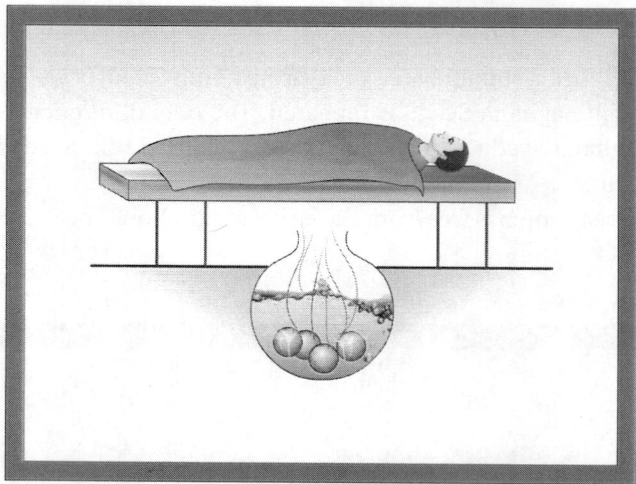

Fig. 3.11: Kumbhi Sveda

12. Kupa Sveda (Fig. 3.12)

Materials

A well like pit is made with diameter equal to the width of the cot and depth twice of it. Inner side of the pit should be well cleaned.

Method

Pit is filled with the dry dung of elephant, horse, cow or camel and burnt to smokeless coal. Then a cot covered with a cotton bed sheet is kept on it. After Abhyanga the patient is asked to lie down on the cot by covering his/her body with cotton sheet. The patient starts sweating with ease.

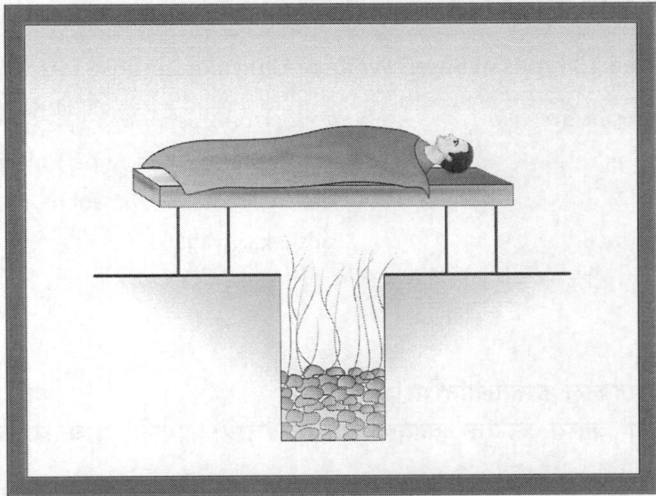

Fig. 3.12: Kupa Sveda

13. Holaka Sveda (Fig. 3.13)

Materials

Dry dung (करीष), bed, cloth/thin sheet.

Method

A heap of dung equal to the size of a bed should be made and ignited. When it is well burnt and becomes smokeless, a bed covered with thin cloth is kept over it. Person who has undergone abhyanga is asked to lie down on the cot by covering his body with a bed sheet.

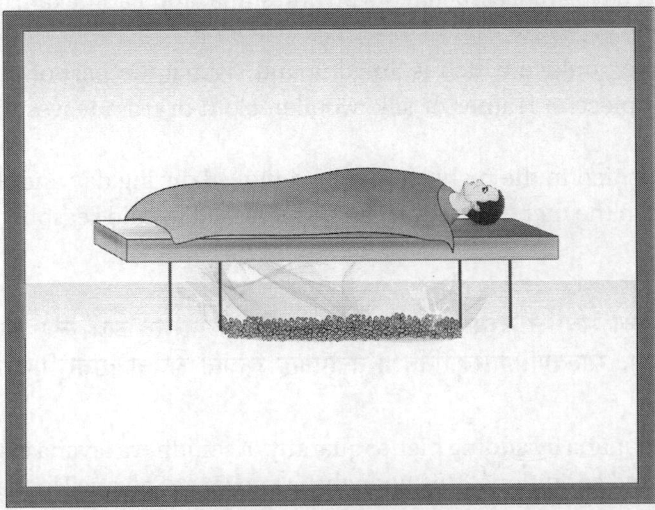

Fig. 3.13: Holaka Sveda

CHATURVIDHA SVEDANA

Dalhana has included 13 types of Sagni sveda of Charaka in these four types.

S.No.	Type of Chaturvidha Svedana	Inclusion of 13 Sagni sveda
1.	Tapa sveda	Jentaka, Karshu, Kuti, Kupa, Holaka
2.	Ushma sveda	Sankara, Prastara, Ashmaghna, Nadi, Kumbhi, Bhu
3.	Drava sveda	Parisheka, Avagaha
4.	Upanaha	

1. Tapa Sveda

तापो अग्नि तप्त वसनफाल हस्ततलादिभिः।
तत्र तापस्वेदः पाणि कांस्य कन्दुक कपाल वालुका वस्त्रैः प्रयुज्ते, शयनस्य च अङ्गतापो बहुशः खदिराङ्गरैर् इति॥ (A.H.Su.17/1)

Tapa Sveda is done by patting the body with heated cloth, metal plate, palm of the hand, sand etc.

2. Upanaha Sveda

The word upanaha means "bandha" or "to tie". It can be done with or without heating the medicine.

उपनाह् वचा किण्वा शताह्वा देवदारूभि। धान्यैः समस्तैर् गन्धैश्च रास्ना एरण्ड जटा आमिषैः॥
उद्रिक्त लवणैः स्नेह चुक्र तक्र पयः आप्लुतैः। केवले पवने, श्लेष्म संसृष्टे सुरसादिभिः॥
पित्तेन पद्मकाद्यैस्तु साल्वणाख्यैः पुनः पुनः॥ (A.H.Su.17/2-3)

Upanaha is the application of poultice prepared with Vacha, Kinva, Shatahwa, Devadaru, any kind of Dhanya, dravyas with a pleasant smell, roots of Rasna, Eranda or meat; each one added with higher amount of Lavana, Sneha, Takra, ksheera in the disease of only Vata. Drugs of Surasadi gana for vata associated with Shleshma, and Padmakadi gana drugs for vata associated with pitta.

After applying the poultice which is Snigdha and Ushna, the part of the body should be bandaged with soft piece of leather or silk, woollen cloth or from leaves of the plants which alleviate Vata.

Upanaha which is tied in the night should be removed during day and that tied in the day should be removed in the night. Duration can be increased in cold season.

Salvana Upanaha

काकोल्यादिः सवातघ्न सर्वाम्ल द्रव्यसंयुतः। स आनूप औदकं मांसस्तु सर्व स्नेह समान्वितः॥
सुखोष्णः स्पष्टलवणः साल्वणः परिकीर्तितः॥ तेनोपनाहं कुर्वीतं सर्वता वातरोगिणाम्॥

(Su.Chi.4/14-15)

Preparation of upanaha by adding higher quantity of saindhava lavana is specially indicated in Vata Dosha afflicted conditions. This upanaha is known as Salvana Upanaha.

In this type of Upanaha, Vatahara dravyas are used for preparation like Kakolyadi gana, amla dravya, Anupa-Audaka mansa, sneha etc. This Upanaha which is prepared with more quantity of lavana is made into a warm paste and applied to the affected part.

3. Ushma Sveda

ऊष्म तू उत्कारिका लोष्ट कपाल उपला पांसुभिः। पत्रभङ्गेन धान्येन करीष सिकता तुषैः।।
अनेक उपाय सन्तप्तैः प्रयोज्य देशकालतः।। (A.H.Su.17/6-7)

Ushma (steam) may be obtained by Utkarika (boiling grains, pulses, seeds etc. and allowing that steam over the part of the body) and stone potsherd, pebbles, mud, cuttings of leaves, grains, dried dung of animals, sand, husk etc., heated well in different ways and administered according to place and time.

4. Drava Sveda

Drava or liquid is prepared by boiling leaves of Shigru, Varanaka, Eranda, Karanja, Surasa, Arjaka, Shirisha, Vasa, Vansha, Arka, Malati, meat of animals of marshy land and of those living in water, drugs of Dashamoola, each one separately or all together, mixed with fats, sura, sukta, water and milk.

This medicated liquid should be filled into a pot jug with spout, or a tube and poured comfortably over the painful part.

KNOWLEDGE OF DIFFERENT SVEDANA PROCEDURE

Sankara/Pottali Sveda: Ruksha and Snigdha Sveda

Patra Pottali Sveda

The word "patra Pottali" is made of two words, patra means leaves and Pottali means bundle. Patra Pottali sveda refers to the svedana performed using bundle of vatakaphahara patra and it is a form of Ushma sveda.

शिग्रु चिंचार्क निर्गुण्डिवरण एरण्ड पल्लवैः। अन्यैर्वा तत्समैः स्विन्नैस्तैलस्विन्नैः स केरकैः।।
कार्पास पिण्डिकाः कृत्वा ताभिः तप्ताभिर् एव वा। सस्नेहपात्रे संतप्ते निक्षिप्ताभः मुहुः मुहुः।।

(Arogya raksha kalpadruma/Vatavyadhi chikitsa)

Materials required

Leaves (chopped into pieces) - 300 grams

Nirgundi (Fig. 3.14A)	*Vitex negundo*	75 g
Eranda (Fig. 3.14B)	*Ricinus communis*	75 g
Chincha (Fig. 3.14C)	*Tamarindus indica*	75 g
Dhatura (Fig. 3.14D)	*Datura metel*	25 g
Shigru (Fig. 3.14E)	*Moringa oleifera*	25 g
Arka (Fig. 3.14F)	*Calotropis procera*	25 g

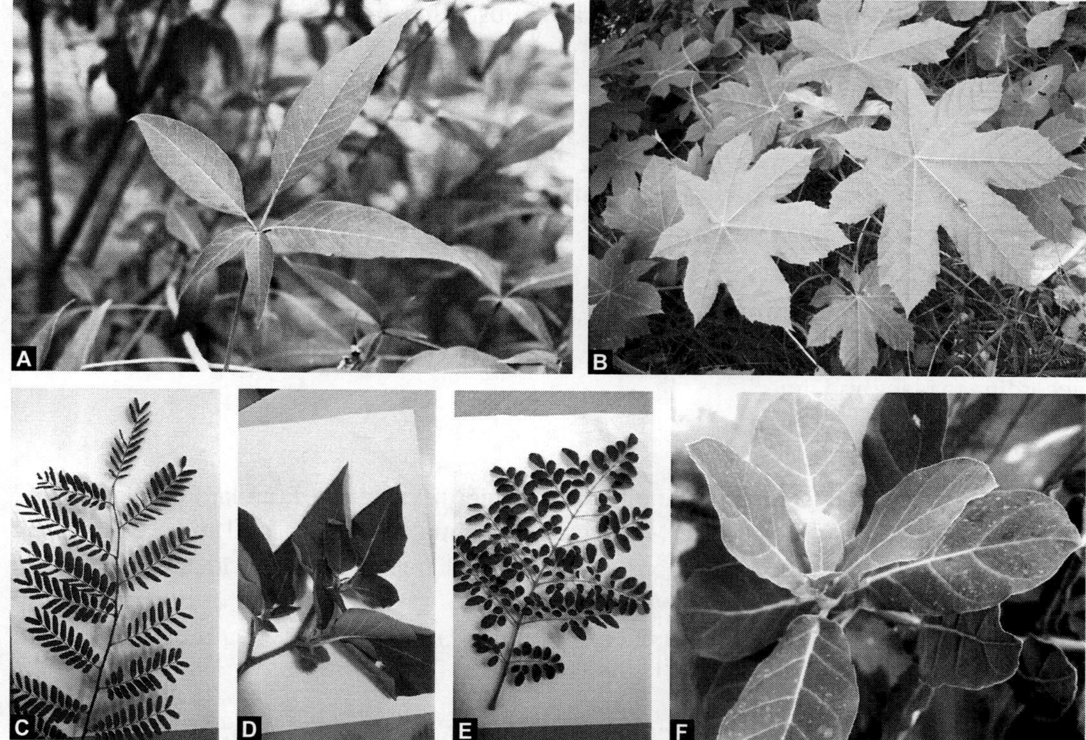

Figs 3.14A to F: Leaves use in PatraPottali Sveda

Grated coconut	150 g
Lemon	4 cut into 8 pieces each
Cotton cloth (45cm X 45cm)	2 pieces
Tags	2
Vessels (for frying leaves and for heating Pottalis)	1
Oil	100 mL
Saindhava, Rasna, Shatapushpa.Devadaru, Kushtha	each 10 g
Masseurs	2 /4

Preparation of Pottali (Figs 3.15A to J)

Fresh leaves should be cleaned and chopped finely. First add 50 mL of prescribed oil into frying pan, to this add grated coconut and sliced lemon and fry till it turns to light tinged brown. Add chopped leaves one by one; first add drugs which have thick leaves followed by thin. Then mix thoroughly and fry together till coconut scrapings attain a brown colour. It should be divided into two equal parts and made into 2 Pottalis (Average weight of a standard Pottali is 300–350 g).

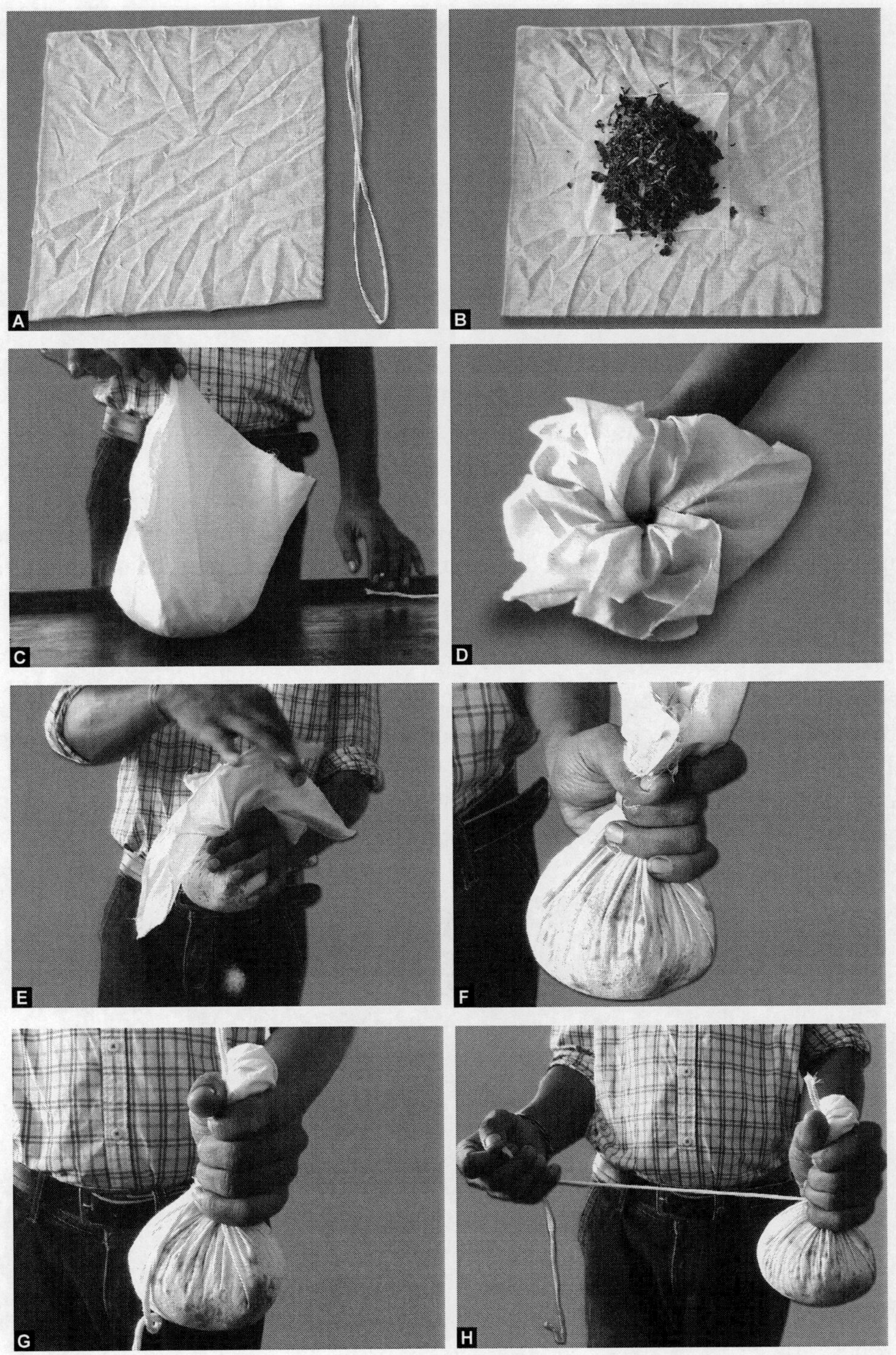

Figs 3.15A to H

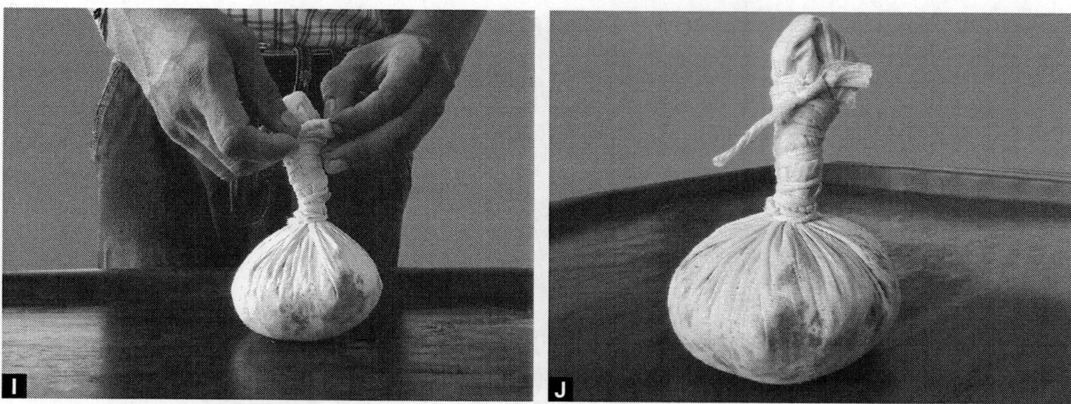

Figs 3.15 I and J

Figs 3.15 A to J: Steps for tying a Pottali

Purva Karma

The patient should be seated with leg extended over the droni facing East. Abhyanga should be performed with prescribed medicated oil all over the body for 20 minutes. Talam with suitable oil should be applied if procedure is to be done in summers/long duration.

Pradhana Karma (Fig. 3.16)

The prepared Pottali should be heated with suitable oil in a hot iron pan up to 42°-46°C. It should be applied only after checking the temperature over dorsum of hand. Then it should be applied throughout the body with mild pressure in seven prescribed positions by two attendants standing on both sides of the droni. Care should be taken to maintain the temperature throughout the procedure by reheating the Pottalis.

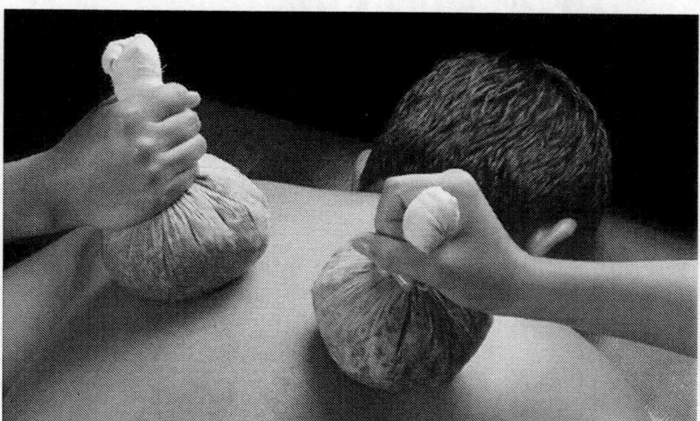

Fig. 3.16: Patra Pottali Sveda procedure

Pashchat Karma

Wipe off the oil from the body using clean dry towel. Remove talam and apply Rasnadi Churna. Patient should be advised to take hot water bath. This is followed by administration of Gandharvahastyadi kashaya.

Duration

45 minutes.

Precautions

1. Care should be taken to prevent charring while frying leaves and also while reheating the Pottalis.
2. Every time the therapist should ensure the temperature of the Pottali by placing it over their own dorsum of hand. Also enquire with the patient whether the temperature is bearable.
3. If the patient feels any discomfort or attains good perspiration at any time during the treatment, the therapy should be stopped.
4. Ideal time to perform the procedure is between 7–11 am and 3–6 pm.
5. One can use the same Pottali for three days.

Complications

Burns, skin allergy and fainting.

Management

- ❑ Rashes are the common complication which can be treated by the application of Sheeta veerya dravya like Shatadhauta, Sahasradhauta Ghrita, Yashtimadhu taila, Kumari pulp and Haridra with Ghrita over the affected part.
- ❑ Giddiness and fainting can be managed by providing Sharkarodaka to the patient for drinking after sprinkling cold water over the patients face.

Jambeera Pinda Sveda

Jambeera pinda sveda is performed with the bolus of Jambeera (lemon) pieces. This is mainly applied in Vata-kapha predominant conditions. It is usually done in frozen shoulder, plantar fascitis and traumatic conditions. It is Shophahara, Ruksha and Tikshna.

Materials required

Materials	*Quantity*
Jambeera (around 20 in number and chopped into pieces)	750 g
Saindhava	30 g
Rasona	200 g
Haridra	60 g
Cotton cloth (45 cm × 45 cm)	4
Threads	2
Vessels for heating	2
Suitable oil for Talam	10 mL
Rasnadi churna	5 g
Suitable oil for Abhyanga	100 mL
Oil for reheating the Pottali	Q.S.

Preparation of Pottali

First add 50 mL of prescribed oil into frying pan. To this add crushed garlic and lemon pieces and fry till it turns to light tinged brown. Later on add Saindhava and turmeric powder and mix well. It should be divided into four equal parts and made into Pottalis.

Purva Karma

The patient should be seated with leg extended over the droni and talam is applied with suitable oil.

Pradhana Karma

Abhyanga should be performed with suitable medicated oil. Out of the four Pottalis, the two Pottalis should be heated up to 40°C-45°C by keeping on the hot pan containing suitable oil. This Pottali should be applied to the patient as per the general procedure for about 45 minutes.

Pashchat Karma

After the procedure body should be wiped with clean towel, talam should be removed and Rasnadi churna should be applied. The patient should be advised to take rest for half to one hour.

Precautions

1. Tie the Pottalis firmly to avoid leaking of the contents during the procedure.
2. The therapists on either side should apply the bolus simultaneously in a synchronized manner.

Complications and Management

Same as that of Patra pinda Sveda

Valuka Sveda (Fig. 3.17)

Valuka sveda is one of the Ruksha sveda. It can be done over whole body or locally on a specific part. It relieves pain and inflammation. Commonly used as Ekanga sveda in Sandhigata vata, Amavata etc.

Materials

Materials	*Quantity*
Sand	1 kg (River sand is preferred. It should be clean and devoid of stones)
Cotton cloth (45 cm × 45 cm)	2
Tag	2
Vessel (iron)	1
Rasnadi churna	5 g

Preparation of Pottali

Clean sand, devoid of waste materials, collected from a neat place is used for this purpose. It should be washed dried and sieved. A vessel preferably of iron is placed on a stove and sand is heated. Pottali's are made using this sand.

Procedure

The patient should sit comfortably exposing the area where Svedana is to be given. The hot Pottali should be gently applied over the body, after confirming the temperature. Gentle pressing of the body with Pottali is advised; no need of kneading. The Pottali's should be used alternately or reheated to maintain uniform temperature throughout the procedure. For the whole body, it should be done for about 30 minutes in the prone and supine positions.

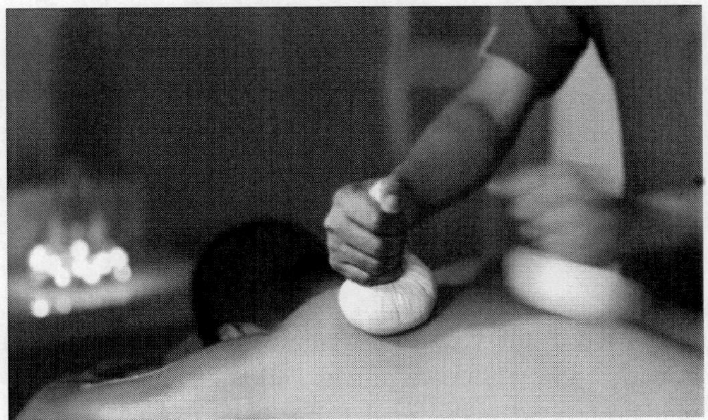

Fig. 3.17: Valuka Sveda

Pashchat Karma

After the procedure, Rasnadi churna should be applied over murdha. Patient should take complete rest for at least half an hour and should take bath with hot water.

Precautions

1. The sand used should be neat, clean and devoid of waste materials.
2. Temperature must be kept optimal to prevent burns.
3. Ensure there is no small hole in the Pottali through which sand may leak.

Complications and Management

Common complication is burns for which application of Murivenna and Shatadhauta Ghrita can be advised.

भृष्ट पटस्थित काञ्जिक संसिक्ता वालुका स्वेदः। शमयति वातकफ आमयमस्तह शूल अङ्गभङ्गादीन्॥
स्त्रोतसां मार्दवं कृत्वा नीत्वा पावकम आशयम्। हत्वा वातकफस्तम्भं स्वेदो ज्वरमणेहन्ति॥ (Bha.Pra)

The Valuka heated and tied into Pottalis can be applied directly or by dipping into Kanji. This is very useful in alleviating Vata and Kapha diseases, Shula, pain all over body etc. This brings about smoothness in the channels of body and also increases agni.

Churna Pinda Sveda (Ruksha)

Churna pinda sveda is one among Ushma sveda. lt is done with the boluses of various churnas (usually Methika, Sarshapa, Shatapushpa, Jatamansi, Atasi etc). It can be done as Snigdha or Ruksha according to the condition. In Snigdha pinda sveda, oil is applied over the body as well as the Pottali's are heated in oil. Whereas in Ruksha pinda sveda, Pottali's are heated without using oil.

The Pottali can be heated over the steam of boiling drava dravyas like Dhanyamla in specific conditions.

Materials Required

1. Suitable churna (coarse/fine)	1 kg
2. Cotton cloth (45 cm × 45 cm)	4
3. Tags	4
4. Rasnadi churna	5 g

Purva Karma

The powder should be fried in the vessel till it attains a golden brown colour. It should be divided into 4 equal parts and tied into 4 Pottalis. Patient should be seated on the table and Rasnadi churna should be applied on the head. Other Thalam like Navaneetha + Bala, Amalaki + Takra etc should be considered according to condition.

Pradhana Karma

The hot Pottali should be gently applied over the body, after confirming the temperature by applying Pottalis on dorsum of hand of therapist (42°C–45°C). Pressing the body with Pottalis followed by of kneading and massaging with the Pottali. Both Pottalis are used alternately after reheating to maintain uniform temperature throughout the procedure (Reheating is done either by keeping Pottali in vessel or by steam of dhanyamla or water). Same Pottali can be used for three days. For whole body, it should be done for about 30–45 minutes in the 7 positions. It can be applied locally also. Samyak svinna lakshanas must be observed.

Pashchat Karma

After the procedure, talam should be removed and Rasnadi churna should be applied over murdha. Patient should take complete rest for at least half an hour and should take bath with hot water.

Precautions

1. Care should be taken to prevent charring while frying churna's and also while reheating the Pottali.
2. If the patient feels any discomfort or attains good perspiration at any time during the treatment, the therapy should be stopped.
3. Ideal time to perform the procedure is between 7–11 am and 3–6 pm.

Complications and Management

1. Shivering: May occur due to uneven distribution of temperature or if body is exposed to cold breeze immediately after the procedure. In such condition, cover the body with thick cloth, give warm liquid for drinking or give hot fomentation.
2. Fainting: Due to increased temperature. Sprinkle cold water and apply Talam.
3. Rashes: Apply Madhu and Ghrita.

Shashtika Shali Pinda Sveda

Shashtika Shali pinda sveda is performed as Ekanga or Sarvanga with the bolus of boiled Shashtika shali with Balamula kvatha and Ksheera. The main properties of Shashtika are Snigdha, Guru, Sthira, Sheeta and Tridoshaghna. Though a Sveda karma, it has Brihana guna.

Materials Required

1. Shashtika shali – 250 g
2. Balamula – 250 g
3. Water – 4 lit
4. Cow's milk – 1 lit
5. Kora cloth (45 cm × 45 cm) – 4 pieces
6. Threads(75 cm) – 4
7. Vessels
   a. For preparing Kvatha
   b. For cooking rice
   c. To heat the boluses in mixture of Kvatha and milk during the procedure (5 litres capacity with wide mouth made of bronze).
8. Oil for talam – 10 mL
9. Rasnadi churna – 5 g
10. Suitable oil for abhyanga – 100 mL
11. Masseurs – 2

Preparation of the Medicine

Balamula Kvatha: 250 g of Balamula is cleaned, crushed and boiled in 4 litres of water and reduced to 1 litre (1: 16 parts and reduced to 1/4th).

Shashtika Rice Cooking: In 0.5 litre of Balamula kashaya and 0.5 litre of milk, 250 g of Shashtika rice should be added and boiled till it becomes thick and semisolid. Sufficient quantity of hot water can be used for proper cooking of the rice.

Another method is that the Shashtika rice can be semi cooked in cooker also.

Preparation of the Boluses

कृत्वाऽष्टौ च ततः पिण्डान् भक्तात् तुल्यविभागतः। वस्त्रखण्डैस्सुनूत्नेऽथ पिण्डमेकैकमेव तत्॥
समं बद्ध्वा चाष्टमूतीर्गोलाकारोः सवृन्तकाः। सुदृढलश्क्ष्णसूत्रेण नातिश्लथघनाः क्रमात्॥
कुर्यात् साधु विशेषेण सुग्रहाः सुकरा यथा। (Keraliya Panchakarma. Pinda Sveda. 12-14)

The cooked rice should be divided into 4 equal parts and put into 4 pieces of Kora cloths. Three corners should be folded together so that they come under the fourth corner and the fourth fold is used to cover the other three corner folds underneath. One end of the thread is held tight with left hand and the other end is wound around the folds. In short, the boluses should be tied in such a way that the mouth of the sac leaves a tuft at the top of the bundle, for holding it with ease.

Purva Karma

The patient should be seated with leg extended over the droni and talam should be applied with suitable oil. Abhyanga should be then performed with prescribed oil for about 20 minutes. Out of 4 Pottalis, 2 are kept in the mixture of Bala Mula kvatha and Milk (0.5 litres of each was already kept for this purpose), which should be put on a stove with moderate heat.

Pradhana Karma (Fig. 3.18)

Two warm Pottalis should be gently applied in a synchronised manner by the two therapists on two sides of droni. It is followed by a gentle massage with other hand. They should ensure that the heat of the boluses is bearable to the patient by touching them over the dorsum of their hand. The temperature of the boluses should be maintained throughout the procedure by continuous relay of the four boluses after reheating by dipping in ksheerapaka. The process should be continued till the patient gets samyak svinna lakshana or until the contents of the boluses exhausts.

Duration

45 minutes or the procedure can be stopped if the medicine in the boluses or the ksheera-paka is exhausted.

Pashchat Karma

At the end of the procedure, the paste remained over the body should be scraped off and the body is wiped dry with tissue paper or soft towels. After that medicated oil should be applied. Talam should be removed and Rasnadi churna applied over the head. Gandharvahastadi kashaya can be given for drinking. The patient should take complete rest for at least half an hour, and then the patient is allowed to take warm water bath.

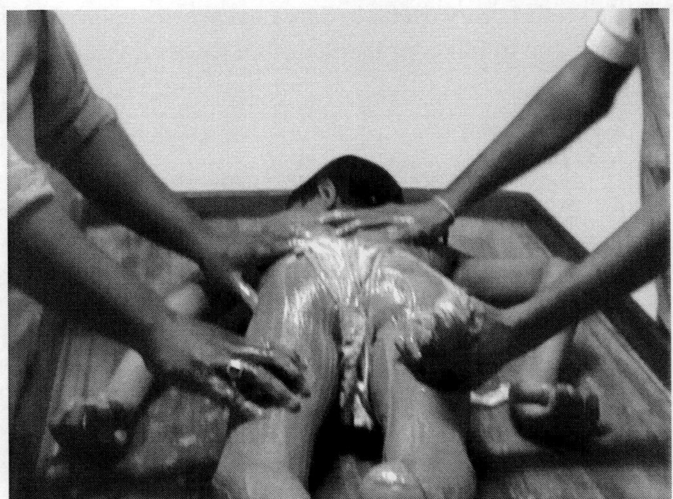

Fig. 3.18: Shashtika Shali Pinda Sveda

Precautions

1. During the preparation of the rice, care should be taken to avoid over/under cooking and should be stirred frequently for the better extraction and cooking.
2. Tie bolus firmly to avoid leaking of contents during rubbing.
3. The therapists on both the sides of the patient should massage with the bolus in a synchronised manner.
4. Ensure uniformity of pressure and temperature on all the body parts.
5. Boluses should be applied with sufficient warmth (40°C–45°C).
6. Therapy should be stopped at any time if the patient gets good perspiration or shivering.

Complications and Management

1. **Shivering**: It usually occurs due to the uneven distribution of temperature or prolonged time gap in between the taking up of new boluses; or if body is exposed to cold breeze 'immediately after the procedure. Allow the patient to take rest, cover with a blanket and give warm liquid diet.
2. **Fainting**: Due to increased body temperature or low heat threshold of the patient or atiyoga of kriyakrama. Sprinkle cold water over the face and body, and put talam with appropriate medicated oil and Churna. Drakshadi kashaya can be given internally.
3. **Rashes**: Due to heat intolerance of the patient of pitta prakriti. Apply madhu and ghrita, preferably Shatadhouta Ghrita or Murivenna.

Benefits of Shashtikashali Pinda Sveda

सर्वांगैकांगशोषे वा घोरेष्वप्यानिलार्तिषु। आयामाक्षेपसंकोच स्तम्भपक्षवधादिषु॥
चिरकाल भवेष्वेवं गुल्मशूलादिकेष्वपि। स्वेद्यामयेषु सर्वेषु यथावस्थं प्रयुज्यते॥

(Keraliya Panchakarma. Pinda Sveda. 6-7)

Shastika shali pinda sveda is very useful in Sarvanga ashrita balayukta vataroga's. It is also beneficial in diseases due to Rakta prakopa and in diseases which decreases the Bala of the Sharira.

Bashpa Sveda (Fig. 3.19)

Bashpa refers to steam. This is the most commonly used Sveda for the administration of sarvanga Sveda due to case of use, cost effectiveness, minimal therapist effort. Uniform and persistent Sveda can be administered using Bashpan sveda.

Features of Steam Chamber

It is meant for the steam bath of the whole body. For this purpose a special wooden/fibre cabin of 5 feet height, 2.5 feet wide and 3 feet long width size is prepared. It is covered from all the sides with one door. At the top of the steam chamber, an opening is made so that the patient may keep his head on it comfortably. It is covered with cotton bed sheet.

A small sized adjustable revolving chair is kept inside steam chamber, so that based on the patient height the chair can be adjusted. After vatively lying down type may also be used.

Procedure

Patient who is indicated for Bashpa sveda should undergo the Abhyanga using prescribed oil. Then he/she is made to sit inside the steamed chamber by adjusting the height of the chair.

This type of sudation is very appropriate where the whole body fomentation is indicated such as ployarthritis, hemiplegia and sciatica or as Purva karma in Vamana and Virechana.

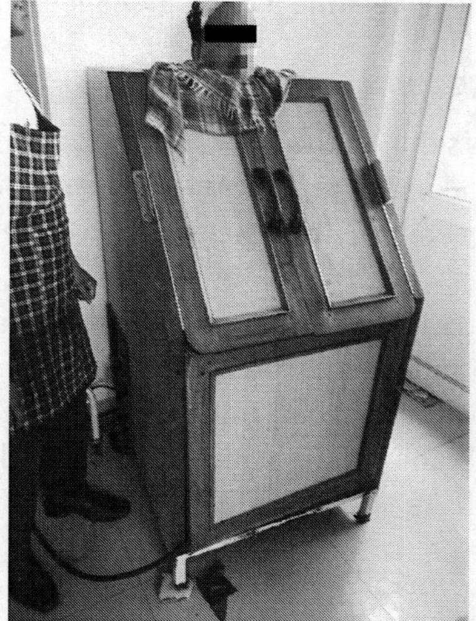

Fig. 3.19: Bashpa Sveda

Kayaseka with Oil (Pari Sheka)

Kayaseka is a snigdha sveda in which the warmed oil is poured all over the body/specific part for a stipulated period, in a specific manner. It has the advantage of producing Snehana and Svedana simultaneously. Pizhichil is a modified form of Kayaseka widely practiced in Kerala.

Materials Required

1.	Suitable oil	5 L
2.	Cotton cloth (40 cm × 40 cm)	2 pieces
3.	Vessels(5 liters)	3
4.	Rasnadi churna	5 g
5.	Gauze (60 cm)	1
6.	Earplugs	2
7.	Gandharvahastyadi Kashaya	20 mL
8.	Masseurs	2

Purva Karma

Patient should be made to sit on the droni with legs extended, with minimum cloths. Talam is applied with suitable oil, and then Abhyanga is performed. Gauze should be tied around the head above the eyebrows. Ears should be plugged with cotton and Mridu Abhyanga to be performed.

Pradhana Karma (Fig. 3.20)

The oil for Seka should be heated in a vessel kept in a hot water bath. The temperature of the oil must be 42°C–45°C.The cotton pieces are dipped in the warm oil and should be squeezed with one hand of masseurs such that the oil should flow, in a uniform stream from the thumb facing downwards, from a height of 6–9 inches (12 angula as per the condition. The process should be carried out in:

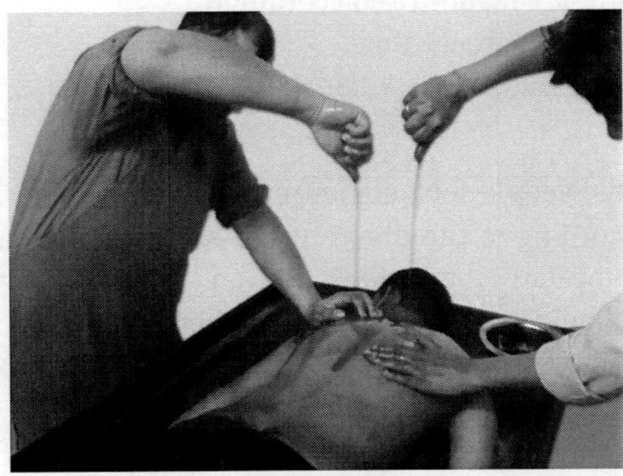

Fig. 3.20: Kayaseka

1. Supine
2. Prone positions.

Oil flowing out should be collected and used after reheating. A gentle massage should be given along with the stream. Same oil may be used for 3 days after removing sediments. This should be preserved after removing moisture and small quantity of fresh oil should be added to this to maintain the quantity.

Kayaseka can also be done using kindi. In this, oil should be filled in the kindi (Tea kettle like pot) and poured on the body after checking the temperature by pouring on the dorsum of therapist's own hand. Modern equipment with auto temperature regulation is also available.

Pashchat Karma

The oil is wiped off with the help of coconut leaves/smooth wipers. Body should be cleaned with soft towel. Talam should be removed and appropriate churna like Rasnadi is applied on the head. Gandharvahastyadi Kashaya should be given for drinking. Patient is asked to take rest for an hour and then allowed to take warm water bath.

Duration

45 minutes for 7, 14 or 21 days.

Time of Procedure

7–10 am or 4–6 pm.

Precautions

1. Temperature should be maintained at the same level throughout the procedure.
2. Stream should be uniform and continuous.

Complications

1. Fainting- stop the procedure and treat accordingly.
2. Fever-stop the procedure and treat accordingly.
3. Hypotension, Giddiness, Fatigue-treat accordingly.
4. Burns- Shatadhauta Ghrita application

Ksheera Dhuma

Ksheera Dhuma is a Nadi Sveda, which comes under Ushma sveda. The therapeutic efficacy of Nadi sveda varies according to the dravya used. Ksheera Dhuma is a snigdha sveda. In Nadisveda, a tube of appropriate length attached to an apparatus containing dravya is used to direct the steam appropriately to the area which is to be fomented. In Ksheera Dhuma, steam is generated by boiling milk and Balamoola, Dashamula, Vacha kvatha.

Indication

It is mainly practised in the management of Ardita, jihvastambha, Hanustambha and Swarabhanga.

Materials Required

1. Milk	–	500 mL
2. Bala Kvatha	–	500 mL
3. Oil for abhyanga	–	50 mL
4. Rasnadi churna	–	5 g
5. Blanket	–	1
6. Nadi sveda apparatus	–	1
7. Eye pad	–	1
8. Chair	–	1

Preparation of Medicine

Bala kvatha: 500 g of crushed Balamula is boiled with 2 litres of water, 500 mL of milk and reduced to 500 mL. This is used to generate steam for the therapy.

Purva Karma

Patient should be seated in a chair and talam should be applied with suitable oil. Abhyanga should be done over face, forehead, neck, shoulder and chest. Eyes should be covered with cotton cloth after placing lotus petals over both lids. The head and neck portion is covered from the back with a blanket.

Pradhan Karma

The patient should sit comfortably for the procedure. Then steam from the apparatus is directed over face, neck, chest and shoulder. Special care should be taken to avoid burns and to get uniform steam. The procedure should be continued up to the appearance of sweat. It is done for about 15 minutes. Intermittent opening of the mouth is to be done.

Pashchat Karma

Eye pads are removed from the eyes and sweat is wiped off. Talam is to be removed and Rasnadi churna should be applied. Kavala or Gandusha should be done with proper medicines. The patient should take complete rest.

Precautions

1. Eyes should be covered to protect them from heat.
2. Move the pipe of svedana apparatus frequently to avoid burns.
3. Ideal time to perform the procedure is between 7–10 am and 4–6 pm.

Avagaha Sveda

The word 'Avagaha' means to immerse. Avagaha sveda is a type of sudation therapy which is included under Drava sveda. In this Sveda, the patient is made to sit/lie in a tub containing medicated drava-dravya to produce sveda.

Materials Required

1.	Bath tub (6ft × 2.5 ft × 1.5 ft)	1
2.	Vessels	2
3.	Suitable drava-dravya's	40–60 litres (sarvanga)/10–15 litres (adhaha kaya)
4.	Oil for talam	10 mL
5.	Churna for talam	5 g
6.	Attendant	1

Preparation of Medicine

According to the disease condition suitable drava dravya is selected. It should be poured into the tub with a temperature preferably around 42°C–46°C.

Purva Karma

Talam should be kept over the head with suitable oil and churna. Abhyanga should be performed with prescribed medicated oil around the umbilicus up to the thighs or all over the body according to the condition. It can be performed without Abhyanga in certain conditions where Ruksha Sveda is indicated.

Pradhana Karma

The patient should be seated comfortably in the tub containing medicated drava-dravya in such a way that the lower part of his/her body should be submerged till the level of umbilicus. Sarvanga avagaha sveda is performed by submerging the body up to neck.

When the temperature of the medicated drava-dravya comes down, some amount should be replaced by warm drava-dravya, thus keeping the temperature uniform.

Pashchat Karma

After the prescribed time, patient is asked to come out and body is wiped with tissue paper or towel. Talam should be wiped off using dry towel and apply prescribed churnas like Rasnadi churna/ Karcchuradi churna etc. He/she is advised to take rest for half to one hour, and then to bath with warm water.

Precautions

1. Therapy should be stopped at any time if the patient gets good perspiration.
2. The temperature of the drava-dravya should be maintained.

Complications and Management

Fainting- May occur due to increased body temperature or low heat threshold of patient or Atiyoga of Kriya Krama. Sprinkling cold water on face and body; providing sufficient water supplement or Drakshadikashaya are useful in this condition.

Burns– Burns may occur due to heat intolerance of patient or excessive heat of drava dravya. Application of madhu and ghrita preferably Shatadhauta Ghrita is advisable in this condition.

Indications

इति दोष पीडावशात् परिषेक स्वेदमाख्याय अवगाह स्वेदं द्रव भेदमाह तैरेव वा द्रवैः पूर्ण कुण्डं सर्वाङ्गगेऽनिले। अवगाह्य आतुरस्तिष्ठेत् अर्शः कृच्छ्रादिरुक्षुच॥ (A.H.Su.17/11)

Sarvanga Vata, Arsha, Mutrakricchra etc.

Benefits of Taila Avagaha

सिरामुखै रोमकूपैर् धमनीभिः च तर्पयेत्। शरीरे बलमाधते युक्तः स्नेहोऽवगाहने॥ (Sha.Ut. 2/31)

Taila Avagaha nourishes the Sira, Romakupa, Dhamani and gives strength to body.

Dhanyamla Dhara

It is a type of Kayaseka, included under Drava sveda. Dhanyamla is included under Sandhana kalpana. It is used in Vataroga, especially with Kaphanubandha.

Materials Required

1.	Dhanyamla	5 L
2.	Vessels	4
3.	Oil for Abhyanga	100 mL
4.	Rasnadi Churna	5 g
5.	Dharapatrn	2
6.	Masseurs	2

Purva Karma

Patient should be made to sit/lie down on the droni; talam should be kept on head and Sarvanga Abhyanga should be done. In some conditions it is done without Abhyanga. Gauze should be tied around the head above the eyebrows. Ears should be plugged with gauze. The patient should be covered with a thin cloth below the neck. This procedure may also be practiced without covering the body.

Pradhana Karma

Warm Dhanyamla is poured with Kindi by two attendants standing on either sides of the droni. Temperature should be around 42°C. Dhara should be poured at a medium speed and from a height of 6–12 cm. It can be done hot or cold according to the condition. Fresh Dhanyamla should be used every day.

Pashchat Karma

After dhara, the body and head are cleaned using a soft towel. Ear plugs and gauze are removed and Rasnadi Churna is applied to the head. Rest is advised for 1 hour and then asked to take bath. Abhyanga before bath is optional.

Duration

45 minutes per day for minimum of seven days. It is preferably done in morning hours in moderate climate.

Complications and Management

Chills and Rigors: It usually occurs due to uneven maintenance of the temperature of Dhanyamla or prolonged time gap between the changing up of fresh warm Dhanyamla or if body is exposed to cold breeze immediately after the procedure. In this condition, body is covered with thick cloth and warm liquid is given for drinking. Even hot fomentation can be given.

Qualities of Dhanyamla

धान्याम्लं धान्ययोनित्वात् जीवनं दाहनाशनम्। स्पर्शात् पानात् तु पवन कफ तृष्णाहरं लघु।।
तैक्ष्ण्यात् च निर्हरेद् आशु कफं गण्डूष धारणात्। मुखवैरस्य दौर्गन्ध्य मलशोष क्लमापहम्।।
दीपनं जरणं भेदि हितम् आस्थापनेषु च। समुद्रम् आश्रितानां च जनानां सात्म्यम् उच्यते।।

(Su.Su.45/214-216)

Dhanyamla is very helpful in relieving Daha (burning sensation). It alleviates Vata and Kapha by internal or external use and relieves excessive thirst. Gandusha dharana with Dhanyamla removes Kapha, Mukhavairasya, Daurgandhya, Klama etc. It is Deepana, Jarana and Bhedi in nature. It can be used in Niruha basti as Avapa dravya.

Pizhichil

The whole body is bathed in streams of lukewarm medicated oil with simultaneous soft massage. Pizhichil literally means squeezing same as that of Kaya Seka.

Method

The patient with minimum cloth is asked to lie down on the Droni. Ideally five masseurs are required, two (one for upper and one for lower limb) for each side and one helper for collecting, heating and supplying of the oil.

18" × 18" cloth piece is taken by each masseur and dipped in the hot oil kept in a bowel placed in the Droni within the reach of the masseurs. The oil soaked cloth is squeezed from the fist with the help of thumb and simultaneously massage is done with the other hand. The oil is poured from the height of about 9 inches (12 angula) and it is advisable to squeeze the oil from right hand and do massage simultaneously with left hand.

It is started from upper side and continuously done towards the lower side without interruption. The helper collects the oil, reheat it and refills the bowl. It should be done in the seven positions mentioned for Abhyanga about 5 minutes in each position.

The temperature of oil should be kept at 40°C to 42°C depending upon the tolerance of the patient. The oil is continuously collected and reheated for the use on the same day. It is done daily or on alternate days for 21 days and after the gap of 3 weeks other course may be repeated.

It is advisable to change the oil daily, if the patient is affordable, otherwise same oil can be reused for a maximum period of 7 days by adding the lost quantity of oil during the process daily. However, on the eighth day it has to be replaced by the new oil.

Pizhichil is indicated in hemiplegia, paraplegia, post-polio paralysis, low backache, sciatica, pain in abdomen, colic and other painful conditions involving many parts of the patient.

Upanaha Sveda (Poultice Sudation)

Nirukti

Etymologically the word Upanaha is derived by adding the upasarga 'upa' to 'nah' dhatu which means "bandhana" or "to tie".

Types of Upanaha Sveda

Chakrapani classifies Upanaha Sveda into 2 types:

a. Sagni type
b. Niragni type

He describes that the recipes that are mentioned in Ch.Su.3rd chapter for thick application on the body belongs to Niragni type of Upanaha Sveda. The one, in which there is a direct contact of Agni can be called as Sagni type. In Niragni type the powder form of the drugs are applied directly on the body parts by mixing them with suitable Drava dravya' to form a paste. They are applied without exposing them into Agni for heating.

Duration of Upanaha Sveda

बद्धं रात्रौ दिवा मुञ्चेत् मुञ्चेद् दिवाकृतम्। (A.H.Su. 17/2-5)

If the bandage is applied at night it should be removed in the morning and the one applied in the morning should be removed during night.

According to the opinion of Dalhana (Su.Chi. 32/12), there are 3 possible varieties of Upanaha Sveda. They are:

1. **Pradeha:** Here the roots and leaves of the drugs which have Vatashamana properties are made into a Kalka form by grinding with Kanji or Amla. Then it is applied on the body parts in a thick paste form after adding Saindhava. It is removed soon after drying by washing with luke warm water.

   The thin cold application of herbal paste is called as pralepa. This application may remain wet or even allowed to dry. Alepa falls in between pradeha and pralepa, i.e. of medium thickness. It can be applied hot or cold. It should be removed soon after drying or can be allowed to remain for some time even after drying.

2. **Sankara/Pinda Sveda**: Here the drugs of Kakolyadi or Surasadi or Eladi gana are selected along with other drugs like Atasi, Tila etc and made to Kalka form like the above procedure. Pottalis are prepared to perform Svedana Karma by applying a firm pressure over body parts.
3. **Bandhana**: The drugs mentioned in the above two procedures are heated after powdering and applied over the body parts and then Bandhana is done with cotton cloth.

Some drugs used in the application are mentioned below

- Kola
- Kulattha
- Suradaru
- Masha
- Atasi
- Eranda

When the patient is suffering from Vata diseases, the above drugs must be powdered and mixed with sour drugs made warm and applied.

Duration of Upanaha Sveda

The opinion of Acharya Charaka and Vagbhatta holds same that if the bandage is applied at night it should be removed in the morning and if applied in the morning should be removed at night.

Procedure of Upanaha

Purva Karma

It includes preparatory measures like preparation of the patient, preparation of medicine and collection of materials required for the smooth conduction of the procedure.

a. Atura Pariksha: The patient is examined in relation to Prakriti, Vikriti etc. by dash righa of examination and by applying Pratyaksha, Anumana and Aptopadesha to assess Vyadhi and Deha Bala. Then, the affected area should be examined properly and mark the tender region. Examine for scars, wounds if any at the joint.

b. Atura Siddhata: Patient is asked to sit erect by extending lower limbs on the table. Expose the affected area properly. Support the limbs, so that they are placed horizontally and comfortably.

Pradhana Karma

The prescribed medicines will be made into paste form by adding sufficient amount of Godhuma. Then Upanaha is prepared by heating it over medium flame. When it is half cooked around 30 mL of prescribed medicated oil is added and stirred well. It should be stirred continuously to prevent formation of lumps. Once it is cooked well it should be taken out of flame.

The part to which Upanaha is to be applied is exposed. Sthanika Abhyanga with prescribed oil is optional. The prepared medicine is applied in Pratiloma gati (Upward direction) over the affected part. It should be of thickness of Mahisha ardra charma or about 0.5 cm. Then it is covered with preheated and softened vatahara leaves like Eranda patra or plantain leaves and bandaged with the help of gauge roll.

Pashchat Karma

Upanaha can be retained for around 12 hours then removed and the part should be cleaned with warm water. In summer season it can be retained up to 6 hours.
According to Doshas pradhanata, Vagbhatta and Sushruta mentions:

- In Pittanugata vata: Kakolyadigana dravyas or padmakadi gana dravyas.
- In Kaphanugata vata with: Surasadigana dravyas.
- In Kevala vata with: Krishara, Veshavaram, Salvanopanaha.

Anna Lepana

Anna means cooked rice and Lepa is application. In this process the gruel is prepared from the cereals and is directly applied to the body of the patient without wrapping in cloth. It is a classical Kerala procedure. It is believed to have same benefits of Shashtika Shali pinda Sveda.

Before doing Anna lepana, Sarvanga Abhyanga should be performed. Here Lepana is for individual muscle or group of muscles. Luke warm Anna should be applied gently over parts with slight Mardana pressure. Entire procedure may be finished within an hour.

It is very useful in Shosha, loss of function, shula, vata and rakta dushti. It is specially indicated in Daha pradhana Vyadhi's.

LOCAL BASTI

Basti literally means "to stay" or "to reside for some time". Therefore, in some local applications where oil is kept on external parts of the body for prescribed time is named as Basti by adding adjective of the name of that region. For instance, if the oil is kept on Kati (lower back) then it is named as Kati Basti and if on Janu (knee), then it is named as Janu Basti and so on.

For this purpose an artificial pit is made with the help of dough prepared preferably with masha. Into this pit, tolerable heated oil is poured. The temperature of oil should be maintained by frequently replacing cooled oil with warm oil. It is allowed to retain for about 30 minutes. After completion of the process, the oil is taken out followed by dough and the part is massaged gently. The process is done once daily for two to three weeks, if necessary its courses may be repeated after the gap of one or two weeks.

Vagbhatta has described four types of oil application on head under Murdha Taila, which are Shiro-Abhyanga, Shiro-Seka, Shiro-Pichu and Shiro-Basti. In Shiro-Basti the head is immersed with oil by putting a cap on the head. As one of the meanings of Basti is to fill and reside, therefore the word Basti has been added to Shiro. Shiro-Basti, where oil is kept on head by making an artificial pit for prescribed time. Local Basti procedures are described from this reference.

Kati Basti (Fig. 3.21)

It is a procedure in which, retaining of warm medicated oil with in a specially formed frame in the lumbo-sacral region is done. It performs the combined action of Snehana and Svedana. Effective as applied to site of lesion.

Indication

Painful low back conditions like:

- Lumbar Spondylosis
- Spondylolisthesis
- Disc prolapse
- Ankylosing spondylitis
- Sacroileitis.

Contraindications

Acute inflammatory conditions and in a patient who are unable to lie in prone position for 30 minutes.

Prescription: Any of the 4 Maha snehas are used as per the condition.

Selection of oil on doshic dominance. Examples:

- Mahanarayana taila
- Mahamasha taila
- Dhanwantara taila
- Vishagarbha taila
- Karpasastyadi taila
- Nirgundi taila

Materials

Black gram flour	–	250 g
Medicated oil	–	200 mL
Vessel	–	2
Spoon	–	1

Preparation of Basti

Add sufficient quantity of water and prepare dough from the black gram flour. Make a round pit of about 15–20 cm, thickness of 3 cm and height of 5 cm.

Preparation of patient

Patient should lie in a comfortable prone position exposing the lumbosacral area; draping should be done to the remaining part of the body. Prepared dough is fixed on the area to be treated in a circular shape, steel or plastic rings can be used. Ensure proper sealing to avoid leaking of oil

Procedure

The prescribed medicated oil should be warmed by keeping the vessel on hot water bath. After ensuring the tolerable temperature, oil should be poured inside along the sides of the dough.

The temperature of the oil should be maintained at 40°C– 48°C by replacing a small quantity after reheating on hot water bath.

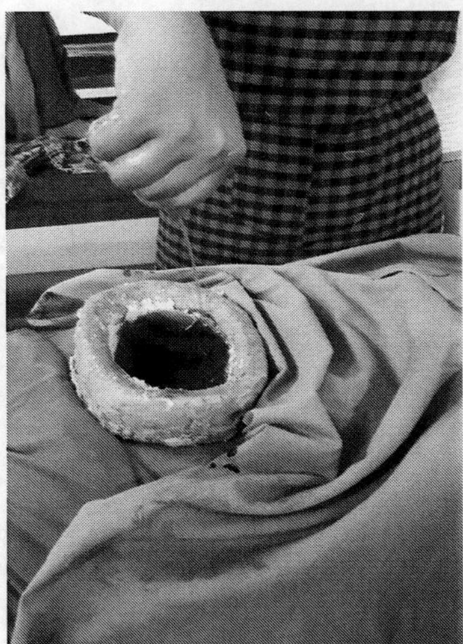

Fig. 3.21: Kati Basti

Precautions

Uniform temperature is maintained throughout the procedure.
Be cautious about temperature of oil to avoid accidental burns.
Ensure proper sealing to avoid leaking of oil.

Duration

30 min, usually done for a period of 7–14 days.

Pashchat Karma

After removing the dough, the part is massaged with circular and linear strokes. The part is given fomentation either with Nadi sveda, Patrapinda sveda, Parisheka Sveda if needed.

Complications and Management

Accidental burns is the common complication. If there are burns, stop the procedure and do Agni dagdha chikitsa, like application of Aloevera gel, Haridra mixed ghrita, Shatadhautha ghrita etc.

Greeva Basti (Fig. 3.22)

It is similar to kati basti. The procedure in which, warm medicated oil is retained within a specially formed frame in the cervical region is Greeva Basti.

Indication

- ❑ Musculoskeletal manifestations of neck
- ❑ Cervical spondylosis
- ❑ Spondylolisthesis

- Disc prolapse
- Ankylosing spondylitis.

Contraindications

- Acute inflammatory conditions
- Unable to lie in prone position.

Materials

Black gram flour	–	250 g
Medicated oil	–	200 mL
Vessel	–	2
Spoon	–	1

Preparation of Basti

Add sufficient quantity of water and prepare dough from the black gram flour. Prepare round pit of about 10–15 cm, thickness of 3 cm and height of 5 cm. Oil is selected as per the condition.

Preparation of Patient

Patient is made to sit on a knee high stool, with his arm and head resting on a chest high table kept in front of him or in a prone position with forehead resting on flexed arms. Prepared dough is fixed to the area in circular shape, steel or plastic rings can be used. Ensure proper sealing to avoid leaking of oil. After natively patient can be asped to lie in prone position.

Procedure

The prescribed medicated oil should be made warm after ensuring the tolerable temperature; oil should be poured inside along the sides of the dough. The temperature of the oil should be maintained at 40°C- 48°C by replacing a small quantity after reheating.

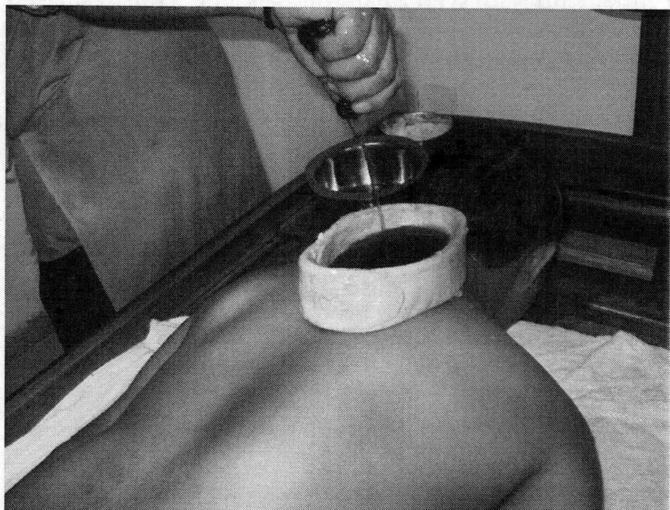

Fig. 3.22: Greeva Basti

Duration

30 min, usually done for a period of 7–14 days.

Pashchat Karma

After removing the dough, the neck and shoulder are massaged with circular and linear strokes. The part is given fomentation with a towel dipped in hot water.

Complications and Management

Accidental burns: Stop the procedure and perform Agnidagdha Chikitsa mentioned under kati Basti.

Janu Basti (Fig. 3.23)

The procedure in which, retaining of warm medicated oil is retained within a specially formed frame over the knee region.

Indication

Painful knee conditions like, osteoarthritis, ligament injuries, meniscal tear and rheumatoid arthritis.

Contraindications

Acute inflammatory conditions of knee.

Materials

Black gram flour	–	400 g
Medicated oil	–	300 mL
Vessel	–	1
Bowl	–	1
Spoon	–	1

Preparation of Basti

Add sufficient quantity of water and prepare a dough from black gram flour. Prepare a round pit of about 10–15 cm, thickness of 3 cm and height of 5 cm.

Preparation of Patient

Janu Basti can be carried out in four different locations of knee joint. Supine position of patient with knee extended is ideal for treating anterior part of knee joint. Popliteal area in prone, medial and lateral part of knee in lateral positions. For comfort a pillow can be supported below knee and prepared dough is fixed to the area in circular shape, steel or plastic rings can be used. Ensure proper sealing and to avoid leakage of oil.

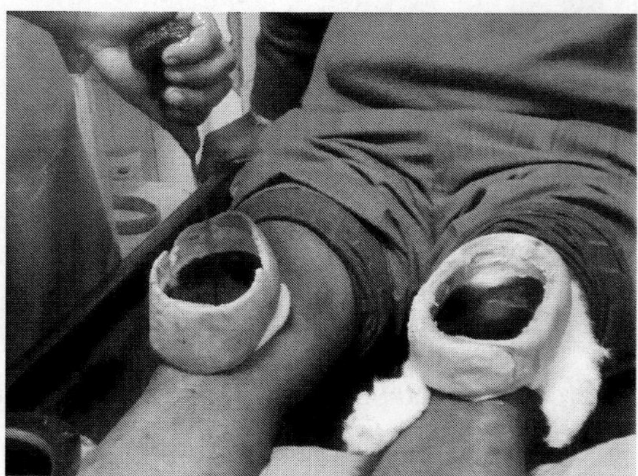

Fig. 3.23: Janu Basti

Procedure

The prescribed medicated oil should be made warm by keeping the vessel on a hot water bath. After ensuring the tolerable temperature, oil should be poured inside along the sides of dough. The temperature of the oil should be maintained at 40°C– 48°C by replacing a small quantity after reheating on hot water bath.

Duration

30 min, usually done for a period of 7 days.

Pashchat Karma

After removing the dough, the part is massaged with circular and linear strokes.
The part is given fomentation with a towel dipped in hot water.

Complications and Management

Accidental burns: Stop the procedure and perform Agnidagdha Chikitsa as mentioned under Kati Basti.

Uro Basti (Fig. 3.24)

It is also called as Hridaya or Hrid Basti. It is a special technique aimed at providing relief around chest area. The procedure in which, warm medicated oil is retained within a specially formed frame over the chest is known as Hrid Basti.

Indication

Regulates vata dosha in the chest region, improves blood circulation, muscular chest pain, strengthens heart muscle, useful in asthma, myocardial dystrophy, cardiomyopathy, etc. conditions.

Hrid Basti is very much effective in the rehabilitation from heart attacks with tachycardia, arrhythmias angina, etc.

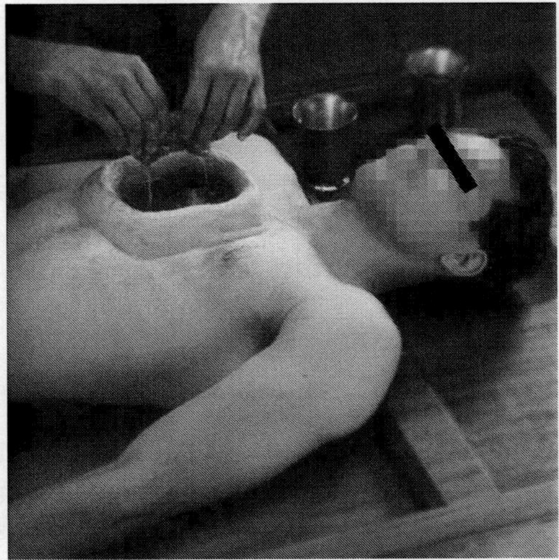

Fig. 3.24: Uro Basti

Mode of Action

- Bahya shamana chikitsa
- Bahya snehana and svedana
- Different actions as per selection of oil
- Local rise in temperature

Local increase in circulation due to dilation of capillaries at terminal region leads to contraction of internal vessels. Thereby blood is drawn towards periphery finally promoting phagocytosis and also combating inflammatory process.

Drainage of excessive fluid through lymphatics also takes place.

GENERAL PRECAUTIONS DURING SAGNI SVEDANA AND METHODS TO PROTECT VITAL DURING SVEDANA

General Precautions During Sagni Sveda

General precautions, which are necessary while performing any type of Svedana Karma, are :

1. Prior to svedana it is necessary to perform abhyanga. In cases where abhyanga is contraindicated, then ruksha sveda can be used.
2. The svedana should be done at a place which is devoid of direct air entry.
3. The temperature must be tolerable to the patient.
4. After completion of the svedana process, advice to take warm water bath followed by light meal as per the disease.
5. Svedana is generally done in empty stomach or, the previously taken meal must be digested.
6. Generally, svedana is done once daily preferably in the morning hours in empty stomach for maximum of 30 days.

सुशुद्धैर् नक्तकैः पिण्डया गोधूमान् अथापि वा। पद्म उत्पल पलाशैर् वा स्वेद्यः संवृत्य चक्षुषी।।
(Ch.Su.14/11)

Eyes should be covered with clean cloth, Godhuma Pinda or with leaves of Padma, Utpala, Palasha etc before Svedana for covering parts.

मुक्तावलीभिः शीताभिः शीतलैर् भाजनैर् अपि। जलार्द्र जलजैर् हस्तैः स्विद्यतो हृदयं स्पृशेत्।।
(Ch.Su.14/2)

Heart should be touched repeatedly with Muktavali (pearls), Sheeta Bhojana, Jalaja, Jalardrahasta.

Factors to be Considered before Svedana

व्याधि व्याधित देश .... वशात् मध्य अवर आवरम्।। (A.H.Su.17/12)
रोग ऋतु व्याधित आपेक्षो नात्युष्णो आतिमृदुर्नच। द्रव्यवात् कल्पितो देशे स्वेदः कार्यकरोमतः।।
(Ch.Su.14/6)

Svedana may be mild, moderate or strong depending upon the condition of the disease, patient, habitat and season.

Pashchat Karma

स्यात् शनैर् मृदितः स्नातः ततः स्नेहविधिः भजेत्। (A.H.Su.17/15)

After svedana light Mardana should be done followed by Ushna jala Snana. Regimens mentioned for Sneha Vidhi like taking light food, avoiding exposure to cold breeze or open air and contact with cold water etc are to be followed.

SAMYAK YOGA, AYOGA AND ATIYOGA OF SVEDANA

Samyak Yoga

सम्यक् स्विन्न लक्षणः
शीत शूल व्युपरमे स्तम्भ गौरव निग्रहे। संजाते मार्दवे स्वेदे स्वेदनाद्विर् अतिर्मता।। (Ch.Su.14/13)
स्वेदास्त्रावो व्याधिहानिर् लघुत्वं शीतार्थित्वं मार्दवं च आतुरस्य। सम्यक् स्विन्ने प्राहुरेत् मिथ्यास्विन्ने अत्ययेन् एतद् एव।। (Su.Chi.32/23)

Sheeta uparama - reduction of cold
Shula uparama - reduction of pain
Stambha nigraha - reduction of stiffness
Gaurava nigraha - reduction of heaviness

Dalhana had classified Svedana into two types viz., Shamananga and Shodananga svedas based on their effects or action.

Benefits of Sanshamana Sveda

अग्नेर् दीप्तिं मार्दवं त्वक् प्रसादं भक्त श्रद्धां स्त्रोतसां निर्मलत्वम्।
कुर्यात् स्वेदो हन्ति निद्रां सतन्द्रां सन्धीन् स्तब्धांश्च चेष्टयेद् आशु युक्तः।। (Su.Chi.32/22)

Agnidipti	–	Increased digestive capacity
Twakprasada	–	Imparts lustre to skin
Bhaktashraddha	–	Increased desire towards food
Sroto nirmalatva	–	Cleansing of body channels
Tandrahanti	–	Removes stupor
Nidrahanti	–	Reduces excessive sleep
Stabdhasandihanti	–	Reduces stiffness

Benefits of Shodhananga Sveda

स्नेहक्लिन्ना धातुसंस्थाश्च दोषाः स्वस्थानस्था ये च मार्गेषु लीनाः।
सम्यक् स्वेदैरश्र् योजितैस्ते द्रवत्वं प्राप्ताः कोष्ठं शोधनैरन्त्यशेषम्।। (Su.Chi. 32/22)

Shodananga Sveda when performed after Snehana helps in liquefaction of the Doshas which are situated deeply in Dhatu's. Shodhananga sveda helps in preparing Doshas for expulsion through shodhana.

Atiyoga

The administration of heat by improper assessment results in excessive fomentation. If the person develops the signs and symptoms indicative of excessive svedana during the procedure, then immediately one has to stop fomentation procedure. Following are the signs and symptoms indicative of excessive Svedana:

पित्तप्रकोपो मूर्च्छा च शरीरसदनं तृषा। दाहः स्वर अङ्गदौर्बल्यम् अति स्विन्नस्य लक्षणम्।। (A.H.Su.14/14)
पित्तास्त्राकोप तृट् मूर्च्छा स्वर अङ्गसदन भ्रमाः। सन्धीपीडा ज्वरः श्याव रक्त मण्डल दर्शनम्।।
स्वेद अतियोगच्छर्दिश्च ....। (A.H.Su.17/16)

Pitta and Rakta Prakopa	Increase in Pitta and Rakta
Murccha	Unconsciousness
Shareerasadana	Weakness of body parts
Trishna	Excessive thirst
Daha	Burning sensation
Svaradaurbalya	Weakness of voice
Angadaurbalya	Weakness in body parts
Sandhipeeda	Pain in joints
Sphototpatti and Shyava	Rakta Mandala Darshana multiple erruptions all over body
Bhrama	Giddiness
Jvara	Fever
Cchardi	Vomiting

Ayoga

The causes of inadequate sudation are—amount of heat is less or duration of heat is less. In such conditions the Svedana should be continued till the appearance of Samyak sveda lakshanas.

वातस्य अप्रगुणत्वं च गुरुत्वं स्तब्धगात्रता।
मन्द स्विन्नेन च ग्लानि तृष्णादीनां च विभ्रमः॥ (Ka.Sam)

- Improper anulomana of Vata
- Guruta: Heaviness of body
- Stabdha Gatrata: Stiffness throughout the body
- Glani and Trishna Vriddhi: Increase in thirst and weakness.

COMPLICATION OF SVEDANA AND THEIR MANAGEMENT ACCORDING TO AYURVEDA AND MODERN SCIENCE

Sveda Atiyoga Chikitsa

स्वादु शीतं द्रवं स्निग्धम् अन्नपानं तदा हितम्। शीतम् सशर्करं मन्थं जाङ्गलान् मृगपक्षिणः।
घृतं पयः सशाल्यान्नं भजन् ग्रीष्मे न सीदति॥ (Ch.Su.6/27)
.... तत्र स्तम्भनम् औषधम्। विष क्षार अग्नि अतीसार च्छर्दि मोहातुरेषु॥ (A.H.Su.17/16-17)

In case of excessive Svedana Grishma Ritucharya should be adopted. The following procedures should be followed :

1. The food which is Madhura, Sheeta, Drava, Snigdha is to be given.
2. Juice made of cold water and sugar should be drunk.
3. Lavana, Amla, Ushna, Katu dravyas should not be used.
4. The patient should be kept in Sheeta graha (air condition room)
5. His body should be smeared with paste of Chandana.
6. The treatment for pittashamana and raktashamana should be adopted
7. Cold water should be sprinkled.
8. Head low position maintained.
9. Cold water to drink.
10. Management of dehydration.
11. In case of excessive sveda which may cause Bhrama (giddiness), Murccha (fainting), Daha (thirst) etc. The treatment for respective disease should be immediately administered.
12. In case of sphota (blisters) or vrana (ulcers) fomentation should be stopped immediately and jatyadi taila, jatyadi malham, shatadhauta ghrita, jatyadi ghrita, ropana ghrita, etc. Should be applied.

DIET AND REGIMEN DURING AND AFTER SVEDANA

Purvakarma of Svedana

सर्वान् स्वेदान् निवाते च जीर्णान्नस्य अवचारयेत्। स्नेह अभ्यक्त शरीरस्य शीतैराच्छाद्य चक्षुषी॥
(Su.Chi.32/27)

It is advisable for snigdha person that after svedana they follow pathya ahara and should not do vyayama from that very day.

Acharya Sushruta adds that after samyak svedana, one should undergo light mardana and should drink warm or luke warm water only. A person should remain in nivata sadana, and have food which is not abhishyandi in nature.

Nivata-sthana: the place should be devoid of direct entry of wind.
Jeernanna: previously taken meal should be digested.
Snehabhyakta Ṣhareera: Bahya Snehana should be performed.
Sheeta chhadna over Chakshu. Eyes should be covered with sheeta dravya.

Beneficial Effect of Svedana

शुष्काण्यपि हि काष्ठानि स्नेहस्वेदोपपादनैः। नमयन्ति यथान्यायं कि पुर्नर्जीवतो नरान॥ (Ch. Su. 14/5)
अग्नेदीप्ति मार्दवं त्वक्प्रसाद भक्तश्रद्धां स्तोतंसा निर्मलत्वम्।
कुर्यात्त् स्वेदो हन्ति निद्रा सतन्द्रां सन्धीन स्तब्धाश्चेष्टयेदाशु युक्तः॥ (Su. Chi. 32/22)

- **Vatahara:** Svedana corrects imbalance of Vata dosha if any. The procedure is more effective in conjunction with Snehana treatment.
- **Mardava:** Svedana reduces the stiffness and hence improves the flexibility of the body parts.
- **Agnidipti:** Svedana causes increased digestion as well as metabolism.
- **Tvakmardava:** By subjecting to Svedana Karma skin becomes soft.
- **Tvakprasada:** Svedana improves the functioning of skin and leads to excellence of the dermis.
- **Bhaktashraddha:** Interest to consume the food is increased by Svedana Karma.
- **Srotoshuddhi:** By way of inducing perspiration, Svedana clears the body channels at all levels.
- **Nidramtandram Hanti:** As Svedana improves the activity of sense organs and hence reduce sleep and drowsiness.
- **Sandhistabdhan Hanti:** Svedana relieves the stiffness in the joints and thus improves range of the joint movements.
- **Shulahara:** Svedana is an early method to get quick relief from pain.

SVEDANA KARMUKATA (MODE OF ACTION)

Sveda Karma has four major actions over the body:

1. Stambhaghnata
2. Gauravaghnata
3. Sheetaghnata
4. Svedakarakata

Stambhaghnata

Stambha means stiffness. This attribute is a resultant of excess Sheeta Guna and also the influence of factors such as Samanavata, Sleshakakapha, Mansa, and Medas. All the above all factors are contributory to the production of Stambha.

Samanavata is Ruksha Gunapradhana and hence if vitiated does excessive Shoshana of Shareera, thereby producing contractures and stiffness. Sleshakakapha is Snigdha and Picchila and hence if decreased, results in less lubrication of joints causing stiffness.

Svedakarma being Snigdha and Ushna and it corrects both these deranged Dosha Ghataka and relieves stiffness. Acharya Chakrapani has stated that Stambha also means obstruction or block. Therefore, Svedana not only relieves stiffness, but also clears blockage of passages (Srotorodha).

Srotas as a structural entity is Kaphapradhana. Ayana or transport is the most important function of Srotas. This is under the control of Vata. Thereby it is evident that there is a predominant influence of Vata and Kapha over the Srotas. Vitiation of these two hampers the structural and functional aspects of the Srotas. We know that, Svedana has opposite qualities to that of Vata and Kapha, thereby producing a palliative effect on them and thus leading to normalcy of Srotas. It is well known that, unless there is a Srotodushti there is no disease. Thus, it is evident that Svedana clears the Srotodushti or Sanga thereby curing disease.

Gauravaghnata

Heaviness of the body is relieved by Svedana. By means of Svedana, fluids in the body are excreted through the Sveda (sweat) and hence a feeling of lightness in the body occurs. Svedana stimulates the nerve endings and promotes muscle strength.

Sheetaghnata

Sheetaghnata can be understood as the patient is relieved of the coldness existing prior because of the Ushna Guna Pradhana Sveda Karma. In other words, by the excretion of sweat, the heat in the body is being transmitted out.

Svedakarakata

Svedana induces Sveda and it is a Mala (excretory product) which includes the wastes of all the layers of skin, muscles, nerves, rasa, rakta, meda etc. Therefore, it is a mechanism of excreting the metabolic wastes in the body tissues.

Apart from these major actions, Svedana also produces the following effects:

Dosha Dravikarana

Svedana makes the Dosha Mridu and eradicates the Mala Sanga, penetrates to each channel in the body and liquefies the Dosha. These liquefied Dosha have to be eliminated from the body by the help of Shodhana Karma.

Vata Shamana

Snigdha Sveda pacifies Vata Dosha, thereby curing the Purisha-Mutra-Shukra Sanga. By its properties opposite to that of Vata, it pacifies the Vata. Svedana is also one of the Upakrama of Vata.

Gatra Vinamana

Acharya Charaka says that by application of oil and heat, even dry wood can be bent and so does the Sharira. It cures Ruk, Ayama, Shopha, Stambha, Graha and produces Mardava, thereby permitting normal flexible body movements.

Agnidipana

As Svedana is Ushna Guna Pradhana, it does the Ama Pachana thereby promoting Agni in the body.

Tvak Mardava and Prasadana

Mechanism of Sweating involves the skin, where in hair follicles, the Moola of Svedavaha srotas are situated. Due to sweating and excretion of wastes, skin becomes soft and pleasant.

Srotoshuddhi

Due to the production of sweat in the body, there will be dilatation of Srotas and the channels of the body will be cleared. Thus, Srotoshuddhi takes place, by which the Vata is regulated, which in turn regulates the movement of urine, faeces and flatus.

Sandhicheshtakara

Svedana relieves Stambha and Graha thereby promoting joint movements.

Acharya Sushruta stated that out of the four Tiryak Dhamanis, each divides gradually hundred and thousand times and thus become innumerable. It covers the body like a network and their openings are attached to Romakupa. Through them the Veerya of Abhyanga, Parisheka, Avagaha, Alepa enter into the body after undergoing Paka with Bhrajaka Pitta in skin.

In Sutrasthana, he explains lepa like Bahirparimarjana treatments yield result by entering to Romakupa thereby circulating through Svedavaha Srotas.

Svedana drugs by Ushna and Tikshna Guna are capable of penetrating the microcirculatory channels (Srotas) where they activate the sweat glands to produce more sweat. After dilatation of micro channels, Laghu and Sara guna of these drugs enables them to act on the Snigdha Dosha in the channels and direct them to move towards Koshtha or excrete them through microspores of the skin in the form of sweat, resulting in Srotoshodhana. The Dosha brought in Koshtha are expelled out of the body with the help of Shodhana Chikitsa.

Sveda is the by-product of Meda Dhatu which is dominant with Jala Mahabhuta. Sveda produces Kleda in the body which is also Apa Mahabhuta Pradhana. The Udaka Dhatu is present in the body in various forms like faeces, urine, sweat, skin, lymph and blood etc. It performs important functions like Jivana, Tarpana, Malashodhana etc. When Svedavaha Srotas is vitiated, it leads to presentation of various symptoms like irregular sweating, roughness of the skin, burning sensation all over the body etc.

Sweat consists of sodium chloride, water, urea, lactic acid, potassium, calcium etc. All these substances are present in extracellular fluid also, which provide nutrition to cells. Excessive sweating in the body leads to depletion of contents of extracellular fluid. Sodium chloride is one of the major substances, which is lost during sweating. Due to its loss, feeling of exhaustion or weakness in the body occurs.

Svedana by its qualities like Ushna, Tikshna etc. does stimulation of the body. It increases the metabolic rate in the body. Ushna Guna of Sveda dilates the capillaries thus it increases circulation. Increased circulation leads to more elimination of waste products and more absorption of Sneha or drugs through the skin. It also stimulates muscles and nerves which promotes its renovation.

Heat administration in Svedana may produce hypno-analgesic effect by diverted stimuli. Sweating controls the heat production, water and electrolyte balance in the body. Sweat glands are controlled by central nervous system. Hypothalamus is the centre of heat regulation in our body. Though the signals generated by the temperature receptors of the hypothalamus are extremely powerful in controlling body temperature, receptors in other parts of the body also play an important role in the temperature regulation.

The temperature control system employs two important mechanisms to reduce heat, when the body temperature is too hot during Svedana Karma.

1. **Vaso Dilation**: Due to Svedana, in almost all areas of the body, the blood vessels of skin become intensely dilated. This is caused by inhibition of the sympathetic centres present in the posterior hypothalamus that causes vasoconstriction. Full vasodilatation can increase the rate of heat transfer to the skin as much as eight folds. So it can be inferred that the Ushna Guna of Svedana Karma leads to stimulation of Sympathetic Nervous System and there is vasodilation. Ushna Guna also increases the circulation of Rasa and Rakta in the body.
2. **Induction of Sweating**: An additional one degree increase in body temperature causes enough sweating to remove ten times of the basal rate of body heat production. During Svedana karma the body temperature rises to more than 2–3°C. It results in increased Sweating by the above said mechanism. Due to the effect of 'Sara' and 'Sukshma' Guna of Svedana Dravya, the Leena Dosha are also liquefied in the body and they come out through micro pores which are present over the skin as pores of sweat glands. As there is extreme vasodilatation due to production of heat. It results in more excretion of liquefied vitiated Dosha from the body resulting in Sroto Shodhana. Thus, Svedana Dravya induces cleansing effect in the body.

GENERAL KNOWLEDGE ABOUT CURRENT SUDATION TECHNIQUES LIKE SAUNA BATH, STEAM BATH

Steam Bath

Background

The history of the steam bath can be traced far back into the mists of time. Popular with the ancient Greeks, the steam bath was subsequently adopted by the Romans as the "Sudatorium" which almost invariably formed part of the Roman baths of the period throughout the entire sphere of influence of the Roman Empire. In Turkey, the steam bath, or "Hamam" has survived thousands of years, and with it our continued use of the term.

"Turkish bath". The practice spread to northern Russia too, where it was known as the "Banja". While steam baths were also built in Europe, their expansion was probably limited in the first instance by technical problems (chiefly in regulating the steam temperature) and because of the high investment costs involved. Today though, new developments in steam generating technology have made it possible to install steam baths almost anywhere at reasonable cost.

What is a Steam bath ?

Not unlike a sauna in which it induces sweating, but with entirely different atmospheric conditions, the steam bath not only helps in relaxing and renewing energy, but also promotes health and beauty as well. It is operated most effectively at temperatures of between 43°C (110°F) and 46°C (116°F) and a relative humidity above 100%. In a steam bath, steam (or to be more scientifically correct, MIST) should be permanently present. This requires an efficient steam generator, a precise control system and a steam-tight cabin to prevent steam from escaping and damaging the fabric of the surrounding room.

Scientific Research

Between 1983 and 1986, at the University of Munich's Institute of Medical Balneology and Climatology, a comprehensive series of comparative tests were conducted to determine the effects of the sauna, steam bath and whirlpool bath on the human body in view of a considerable uncertainty which had previously surrounded the steam bath. Steam baths should not be recommended or prescribed to patients with known cardiac pathology. Steam baths are recommended wherever generalized moist heat applications are indicated.

Physical agents act directly with a physical effect; that is, radiant energy becomes heat when absorbed by living cells. Physical agents may in addition indirectly influence the **autonomic and endocrine systems as well as the electrolyte balance**. The **biologic response to the "push"** of physical stimulation of the **vegetative hormonal system** is an adaptive reaction to stress, which involves the adrenal cortex and increases blood steroids.

In fact, the interrelationship between adrenal and blood steroids may be an important factor in the hit-and-miss success of this form of hydrotherapy. If so, the intensity (or dose) of physical stimulation will determine the "stress" of this hydrotherapy program.

Physiological Effects

The body tries to increase its heat loss through all possible avenues-especially the skin and lungs. If the environmental temperature exceeds that of the body, the only way to lose heat is through sweating. The body cannot maintain a constant temperature when the environmental temperature is as high as that reached in a steam bath or sauna, and so the body temperature begins to rise.

As the cutaneous circulation increases, heat is accepted more readily by the body from the environment. A reduced skin circulation would reduce the rise of body temperature, but this is not possible. The rise in body temperature depends mainly on:

a. The temperature and humidity content of the steam bath
b. The sweating capability of the bather, and
c. The bathing time. Body temperatures have been found to range from 37.6°C (99.6°F) to 40°C (104°F).

Thus, the physiologic changes that occur during the bath are due in part to the rise in body temperature and in part to the influence of the reflexes of the hormonal and nervous systems, which attempt to increase the heat loss. The research results revealed that, given the correct choice of temperature and duration, a steam bath produces the same thermal effect on the body as a sauna and is equally beneficial.

Effects of Steam Bath

A steam bath is health giving as well as enjoyable. As a supportive activity, a steam bath is especially recommended to alleviate the conditions listed below by virtue of its high steam content and the general benefits of moist heat. The list was confirmed by the research carried out at the Institute of Medical Balneology and Climatology at the University of Munich: Bronchial asthma, bronchitis, catarrh of the upper respiratory tract, coughs, hoarseness, expectoration (particularly with the assistance of essential oils) non-acute rheumatic complaints and restricted or painful movements of the joints. In addition, again as a supportive measure the steam bath is beneficial for persons suffering from:

Sleeping disorders, particularly through overexcitability, Poor skin circulation, Dry, chapped skin, Muscular tension, Muscular weakness in the subcutaneous blood vessels, Sensitivity to sudden changes of temperature.

The moist heat stimulates the subcutaneous blood flow and cleanses the skin intensively, opening the pores, removing dead skin and impurities and leaving the skin feeling soft, clean and silky smooth.

The Correct Way to take Steam bath

The method that has proved successful for the Sauna applies to the steam bath.

- ❑ Patient should be subjected to Shower before first session.
- ❑ Time of stay in the steam bath in accordance with personal sensitivity of the patient.
- ❑ Do not exceed 15–20 minutes
- ❑ Cool off with cool fresh air and cool water without shocking the system and avoid shivering
- ❑ Subject patient to warm foot bath if the patient has cold feet.

Sauna Bath

A sauna is a small room or building designed at a place to experience dry or wet heat sessions, or an establishment with one or more of these facilities. The steam and high heat make the bathers perspire. Saunas can be divided into two basic types—a. conventional saunas that warm the air or b. infrared saunas that warm objects. Infrared saunas may use a variety of materials in their heating area such as charcoal, active carbon fibers, and other materials.

How to Give Sauna Bath?

- ❑ Ask the patient to undress in Dressing room.
- ❑ Ask patient to drink 1–2 glass or any Sport drink (avoid caffeine) which has electrolytes. Ask the patient to shower first, as this is to moisten the skin and to remove any possible body or fragrant odours, which do not belong to the Sauna.
- ❑ Do not give a sauna bath for over 10–15 minutes.
- ❑ Ask patient to exit Sauna bath if patient feels uncomfortable or become sleepy.
- ❑ Cool off with cool fresh air and cool water without shocking the system and to avoid shivering-give a warm foot bath if patient has cold feet and then repeat the session. Do not give more than 3 sessions at a time in the Sauna bath.

What are the Benefits of Sauna Bath?

In sauna bathers, blood vessels become more flexible and there is increased circulation to the extremities. During sauna bath, blood flow to the skin increases to as high as 50–70% of cardiac output (compared to the standard 5-10%). This brings nutrients to subcutaneous and surface tissue resulting in glowing healthy skin. Sauna provides a cardiovascular workout which helps condition the heart.

Sauna heat puts the body into an artificial fever state (hyperthermia). Fever is part of the body's natural healing process. This "fake fever" stimulates the immune system resulting in an increased production of disease fighting white blood cells and antibodies. While the growth of bacteria and virus is forced to slow down.

Athletes use Saunas to loosen tight muscles after a hard workout.

Sauna bath makes you feel rejuvenated and have increased energy levels. The Sauna helps to get a more restful sleep.

In the hydrotherapeutic tradition used at European and America spas, sweat therapy is used in preparation for massage as a means of increasing the suppleness of the muscles and creating a deep sense of relaxation in body and mind.

A sauna bath opens skin pores, soothes sore muscles, and increases circulation. However, more than common metabolic waste products are secreted through the skin.

What are the Precautions for Sauna Bath?

Do not use alcohol prior to or during a Sauna bath, alcohols (dehydrates your body) can cause drowsiness and alter the ability to detremine the effects of the Sauna bath.

After a workout, give the body adequate time to cool down, before exposing it to the heat of a sauna to avoid heat stroke. Patient must rest for at least 20 minutes.

Ask patient to drink plenty of water before and after the Sauna bath to replace fluid lost during the treatment.

Limit sauna/steam time to 15 minutes. The sweat glands can secrete up to 30 grams of sweat per minute, or almost one pint per 15 minutes, so dehydration is a very real possibility, if you are not careful. Fatigue and other indications of dehydration can occur with as little as 1 to 2% loss in body weight. Symptoms of too much dehydration include dizziness, vertigo, rapid heartbeat, or excessive thirst.

Also, make sure patient has not eaten any large meals beforehand.

Person with low blood pressure (as Sauna bath decreases blood pressure).

Pregnant women should not use a Sauna. High temperatures can harm foetus or cause fainting. Children's ability to tolerate heat is limited, since their skin area/body mass-ratio is high, sweating system is immature and fat layer is thin. Children can, however, take sauna baths totally safely, if some precautions are taken into account.

The Sauna should not, of course, be used as a weight loss aid by itself, but when used with a good diet and exercise program, a Sauna can help burn more calories. Weight is lost in a Sauna, but most of it is water loss from sweating.

CHAPTER 4

Vamana Karma

INTRODUCTION

Ayurveda as a science of life has evolved through its branches over a long period as its primary objective is to maintain health and avoiding and curing of diseases. As all the classics refer to the main reason of knowledge of Ayurveda being transferred from brahma down to the different Acharya's was not only preservation of health and prevention of diseases, but also rescuing the mankind from the clutches of diseases. Logically, therefore, there has been a constant research on therapeutic agents that keep the body fit, increase its capacity to combat a disease and bring it back to normal.

दोषाः क्षीणा बृंहयितव्याः, कुपिताः प्रशमयितव्याः, वृद्धा निर्हर्तव्याः, समाः परिपाल्या इति सिद्धान्तः ।

(Su.Chi.33/3)

According to Sushruta, basic philosophy of Ayurveda is to induce balanced state of the body by augmenting the deficiencies, suppressing the aggravation and eliminating the increment of doshas and also maintain the equilibrium of doshas in the state of health.

For achieving this purpose, Ayurvedic chikitsa has a two fold strategy which comprises of 1) Sanshodhana or Biopurification by Panchakarma therapies and 2) Sanshamana or Pacification of imbalanced conditions by appropriate diet, drug, and life style interventions.

While defining Sanshodhana therapy, Acharya Hemadri has said that the method by which the vitiated doshas are eliminated out of body is known as Shodhana Chikitsa.

''यत् दोषान् बर्हिनिष्कासयेत् तत् शोधनम्''॥ (Hemadri on A.H.Su 14/5)

When describing the Panchakarma's all the acharya's have considered Vamana as the first amongst the Pradhana Karmas. Vamana, is a process of expelling out contents of the stomach through oral route. Here contents such as Kapha, Kapha's conjunction with one dosha (sansarga) or both other doshas (sannipata) and mala which are toxic to body are eliminated through upper channels (urdhvabhaga), i.e. Mukha. The general meaning of Vamana is therapeutically induced vomiting of the stomach contents, which is indicated for the purification of urdhvabhaga of the body. The main place of Kapha is urdhvabhaga and especially Amashaya. It is a general principle to expel vitiated doshas from the nearest route, while the oral route is the nearest route for expelling Kapha dosha in the form of Vamana karma.

According to Charaka, it is meant for purification of upper part of the body. But according to Sharangadhara and Bhavaprakasha, the word Vamana is used to denote the removal of "Apakwa Kapha and Pitta" forcibly outside. It is important to understand that the Vamana karma is indicated for elimination of Kapha dosha not only in diseased states but also in healthy individuals in states where Kapha dosha is aggravated within normal limits, e.g. in Vasanta Ritu for preservation of health and prevention of disease. For this reason Vamana karma is specifically indicated in Kaphaja disorders, where Kapha is predominant. (Ch.Su.25/40).

ETYMOLOGY

वमनं, स्त्री, (वम्+भावे ल्युट्। छर्दनम् । यथा सुश्रुते
वम् उद्गारे, यक् सेत्, वमति अवमित्!
वमनंदक वमने ल्युट् (पु.) मर्दने छर्दनेः निःसारणे स स्वर्गाभिष्यन्दं वमनम्।।
वमि वम इन् च्छर्दो च्छर्दि शब्दे। वमथुः वमंदकअथुं च।। (Vachaspathyam)

The word Vaman is derived from the Sanskrit root,
Vam+ bhave + Lyut- Chhardanam. (Sushrut)
Vami vam in chhardo chhardi shabde. Vamathuh vam athun cha. (Vachaspatyam)
The exact functioning of the procedure can be sensed through the various terms which are harmonious with the word "Vamana", Etymology of Vamana sheds a light over them, viz.

A. When the suffix 'Yak set' is added to the root verb 'Vama,' it can be used in the forms of the verbs like 'Vamati' or 'A vamit' which hints about the tense of the verb. 'Vamati'means the act of voming and 'A vamit' means not vomited or sticked. The root word 'Vama' means 'Udgare.' It is derived from the root verb 'Udgtu,' conveys the exact interpretation through the meanings like-ejecting, giving out, oozing, stream, eruptations, echo and hissing sound. But according to Monnier William, 'Vama'means ejecting, spitting out, vomiting, giving out, emitting, saliva, belching, sound, roaring, echo, flowing out, sending forth, issuing out, etc.
B. By applying 'Lyut' suffix to the root verb "Vamane", the word Vamana (Masculine gender) is derived. It accords four meanings as Mardane, Chhardane, Nihsarane and Swargabhishyanda. To apprehend the concept of Vamana in relevant fashion all the four meaning should be screened watchfully.
   1. Mardane: Means destroying, crushing, grinding, laying waste or breaking up.
   2. Chhardane: Derived from the root verb "Chhard" meaning Vamane.
   3. Nihsarane: Exhibits the expressions like running away from, flowing out, Nirgama like going out, expelling, driving or turning out.
   4. Swargabhishyanda: The prefix 'Swarga' is appended to word 'Abhishyanda'

   The meaning of both are:
   (i) Swarga:- Gati, Gamana (VS Apte's Dictionary)
   (ii) Abhishyanda:- Oozing, flowing, running at, great increase, enlargement, surplus (VS Apte's Dictionary)

   In Kautilya, the word "Swargabhishyanda Vamanam" is used which means drawing off the surplus population, i.e. by emigration.
C. The words 'Vami' and 'Vamathu' are also used.
   1. The word "Vami" (Feminine gender) is derived from the root verb 'Vama' by adding suffix 'In,' means vomiting, nausea, an emetic or a thorn apple.

2. The word "Vamathu"(Masculine gender) is derived from the root verb 'Vama' by applying suffix 'Athuch' meaning nausea or water ejected from an elephant's trunk or a cough.

D. The word "Aahrutau" also intimates about Vamana through the meanings like to bring or fetch, to bring near, to take away or attract (as mind), to separate, to use as food or drink. (VS Apte's Dictionary)

According to Monnier William, it means the cotton shrub, the act of vomiting or ejecting from the mouth, emission, emiting, causing vomiting, an emetic, offering oblations to fire and pain or paining.

* Vaidyaka Kalpa Sindhu says that 'Vamana' means 'Urdhvamukha Doshaharana'.

* Likewise Amara Kosha says that 'Vama' means 'Udgirana'.

At last it is obvious from the foregoing that the word Vama - Vamana Vami-Vamathu means the act of vomiting.

DEFINITION

तत्र दोषहरणम् ऊर्ध्व भागं वमनसंज्ञकम्। (Ch.Ka.1/4)

It is a process in which waste products, i.e. vitiated doshas are eliminated out through the upper channels, i.e. through the mouth (Ch.Ka.1/4). Chakrapani mentions that Urdhvabhaga should be considered as Urdhvamukha. While Sharangadhara describes the same in other words as:

अपक्व पित्तश्लोष्माणौ बलादूर्ध्वं नयेत्तु यत् वमनं तद्धि विज्ञेयं मदनस्य फलं यथा॥ (Sh.Pu.4/8)

It means the process in which, 'Apakva' Pitta and Kapha are forcibly expelled out through the upward route or channel is known as Vamana. Likewise Acharya Charaka has said that:

वमनं श्लेष्म हराणाम्। (Ch.Su.25/40)
प्रतिमार्ग च हरणं रक्तपित्त विधीयते। (Ch.Chi.2/17)
स्नेह स्वेदावनभयस्य यस्तु संशोधनं पिबेत्। दारु शुष्कमिवानामे देहस्तस्य विशीर्यते॥ (Su.Chi. 33)

Vamana is the best treatment to eliminate out the vitiated Kapha dosha from the body. So in this way all are well concerned that Vamana helps to remove all sorts of derangements regarding Kapha. But the question arises that why Pitta is also mentioned emphatically along with Kapha while defining Vamana (Sha.Samhita 4). What might be the reason that for the treatment of Apakwa Pitta, Vamana takes the leading seat ahead of Virechana?

"Apakwa" literally means "undigested or unriped". When Pitta is undigested or unriped, it metamorphoses into 'Vidagdha Avastha' which is one of the sets of Ajirna. Vamana is said to expel vitiated Kapha and Kaphasthanagata doshas and as told by Acharya Charaka that Pitta resides at Amayashaya (Adhoamashaya as clarified by Chakrapani) utility of Vamana in eliminating Apakwa Pitta is illuminate. Futher Acharayas elucidate that Vamana is helpful in eliminating Apakwa doshas, whereas Virechana is use to expel Pakwa dosha. Thus Virechana is said to be best procedure for expelling out Pitta, but if Pitta is Apakwa or Vidagdha then Vamana is most appropriate Panchakarma procedure.

This can be more firmly solicited by viewing Vamana as the first nomination for treating Vidagdhajirna (A.H.Su.8/27), Pittaja Grahani (A.S.Chi.12) or Grahani (Ch.Chi.15/74-75) and Amlapitta (Bh.Pr. Amlapitta/12-13).

Thus, Vamana remains the best treatment for Apakwa Kapha as well as Apakwa Pitta.

Synonyms

Vama, Vamana, Vami, Vamathu, Virechana, Vireka, Chhardi, Chhardana, Ullekhana, Lekhana, Shodhana, Sanshodhana, Udgirana and Urdhvamukha Doshaharana.

वमथुर् वमनं वान्ति च्छर्दिर् उद्गिरणं वमिः।
प्रच्छर्दिक उल्लेखनं स्यात् ....। (Sh.Pr.4/8)

Predominance of Vamana karma in Panchakarma therapy: Vamana occupies the top place among all the elimination therapeutic techniques and requires special care during the process. It must be conducted under the supervision of practically trained physician; otherwise a number of complications will arise. For which Vamana has been kept ahead of Virechana in Panchakarma therapy. Because if Virechana is administered without Vamana, the provoked Kapha descends to Grahani and covers it, which will cause the heaviness or will produce Pravahika (Su.Chi. 33/18).

IMPORTANCE OF VAMANA KARMA

Reason Behind Administering Vamana before Virechana

विरेचनमपि स्निग्धस्विन्नाय वान्ताय च देयम्, अवान्तस्य हि सम्यग्विरिक्तस्यापि सतोऽधः स्रस्तः श्लेष्मा ग्रहणी छादयति; गौरवमापादयति, प्रवाहिकां व जनयति॥ (Su. Chi. 33/39)

Sushruta has clarified that a person who is supposed to undergo sanshodhana, after undergoing snehana and svedana should undergo vamana first and then only virechana because if a person is induced virechana before undergoing vamana, Kapha travels towards grahani and covers it leading to mandagni and leads to gaurava and pravahika.

Vamana has been kept ahead of Virechana in Panchakarma therapy because if Virechana is administered without Vamana, the provoked kapha descends to grahani and covers it which will cause heaviness or will produce pravahika.

Benefits of Vamana

1. वमनं श्लेष्म हराणां (Ch.Su.25/40)

   Vamana karma, the first measure amongest Panchakarma has been considered as the best line of treatment for the kaphaja disorders.

2. वमनं तु सर्व उपक्रमेभ्यः श्लेष्मणि प्रधानतमं मन्यन्ते भिषजः, तत् यत् इति एवम् आमाशयं अनुप्रविश्य उरोगतं केवलं वैकारिकं श्लेष्ममूलं ऊर्ध्वं उत्क्षिपति, तत्र अवजिते श्लेष्मणि अपि शरीर अन्तर्गताः श्लेष्म विकाराः प्रशान्तिं आपध्यन्ते, यथा भिन्ने केदारसेतौ शालि यव षष्टिकादीन् अनभिष्यन्ध्यमानात् अम्भसा प्रशोषं आपध्यन्ते तद्वत् इति। (Ch.Su.20/19)

Vamana karma is considered as the best for treating Kaphaja rogas. Acharya Charaka gives an example of Kedara setu. Here Acharya says that as Shaali, Yava, etc. yields gets dried out when water is removed from their roots, in the same way Kaphaja rogas cannot get provoked when Kapha is removed through Vamana karma.

3. **छिन्ने तरो पुष्प फल प्ररोहा यथा विनाशं सहसा व्रजन्ति।**
तथा हृते श्लेष्माणि शोधनेन तज्जा विकाराः प्रशमं प्रयान्ति॥ (Su.Chi. 13/33)

Sushruta asserts that as flower, fruits and branches are destroyed as soon as the mother tree is uprooted. Similarly diseases originated due to excessive Kapha are unresponsive after elimination of Kapha through the process of Vamana.

4. **कास उपलेप स्वरभेद निद्रा तन्द्रा आस्यदौर्गन्ध्य विषोपसर्गाः।**
कफप्रसेक ग्रहणीप्रदोषा न सन्ति जन्तोर्वमतः कदाचित्॥ (Su.Chi.33/12)

Disease like cough (kasa), stickiness in the throat (upalepa), hoarseness of voice (swarabheda), hypersomnolence (sleepiness), tandra, foul smell through mouth, secretions of kapha, afflictions' produced because of toxins and diseases produced in Grahani will be unable to cause any harm to the patient after Vamana karma.

Prabhava of Vamana

ननु वमनं कथं अतिसारघ्नं? उच्यतेद्रवश्लेष्मणः क्षयात् विपरीत मार्ग चिकित्सा प्रभावात् वा॥
(Su.Ut.40/106 Dalhana teeka)

Dalhana explained the effect of Vamana in 'Atisara' as Vamana works in it in the following three ways:

i. It reduces Drava and Shleshma,
ii. It works in the opposite direction as that of Atisara,
iii. By its self action (Chikitsa Prabhava).
    1. "Bahu" doshasavastha, i.e. when doshas are accumulated in 'large' quantity, Vamana can be advised (Ch.Su.16).
    2. More specifically Vamana may assist the body in the following conditions as:
        a. Aggravation of Kapha in its own sites or place.
        b. Kapha combined with Pitta which is present in a small proportion.
        c. Vata or Pitta invading the sites of Kapha.
        d. Excessive increase in the levels of Kapha. (A.S.Su.27/5)

INDICATIONS AND CONTRAINDICATIONS FOR VAMANA

Indications

विशेषतस्तु पीनस कुष्ठ नवज्वर राजयक्ष्म कास श्वास गलग्रह गलगण्ड श्लीपद
मेह मन्दाग्नि विरुद्धाजीर्णान्न विसूचिकालस विष गर पीत दष्ट दिग्ध विद्धाधः
शोणितपित्त प्रसेक हल्लास अरोचक अपच्य अपस्मार उन्माद अतिसार शोफ
पाण्डुरोग मुखपाक दुष्टस्तन्यादयः श्लेष्मव्याधयो विशेषेण................ (Ch.Si.2/10)

Indications	
Pinasa (chronic rhinitis)	Visha dashta (poisonous bites)
Kushtha (skin diseases)	Adhah Shonita pitta
Nava Jvara (acute fever of duration less than 7 days)	Praseka (excessive salivation)
Rajayakshma (tuberculosis)	Hrillasa (nausea)
Kasa (cough)	Arochaka (loss of taste)
Shvasa (dyspnea)	Apachi (lymphadenitis)
Galagraha (pharyngitis)	Apasmara (epilepsy)
Galaganda (goiter)	Unmada (psychosis)
Shleepada (elephantiasis)	Atisara (diarrhea)
Prameha (diabetes)	Shopha (edema)
Mandagni (low digestion)	Panduroga (anemia)
Viruddha anna (antagonistic diet)	Mukhapaka (stomatitis)
Ajeerna anna (indigestion)	Stanya Dushti (galactic disorders)
Visuchika (Gastroenteritis)	All the disorders due to vitiated Kapha
Alasaka (Distension of abdomen not associated with vomitting or passing of stools),	Visha (acute poisoning)
Garapeeta (chronic poisoning)	

तत्र उत्कृष्टे श्लेष्मणि पित्तसंसृष्टे वा ततः स्थानगते वा पित्तेऽनिले वा श्लेष्मोत्तरे वमनं आचरेत्॥

(A.S.Su. 27/4)

A. According to doshas, Vamana should be conducted when Kapha is vitiated; Pitta occupies the place of Kapha and Vata predominant Kapha state.
B. Diseases requiring Vamana, due to "Marga Virodhatwa", e.g. Adhoga Raktapitta.
C. Diseases having "Kapha Dominance", e.g. Shvasa, Kasa, Ajeerna, Agnimandya, Pinasa, Shleepada, etc.

Indication of Vamana Karma in Ayurvedic Texts

S.No.	*Diseases*	*Ch.*	*Su.*	*A.H.*	*A.S.*	*Ka.S*	*Bh.S.*	*Sha.S.*	*C.D.*
1.	Pinasa	+	+	+	–	–	–	+	–
2.	Nava Jvara	+	+	+	+	–	+	+	–
3.	Kushtha	+	–	+	+	–	–	+	–
4.	Shvasa	+	+	+	+	+	–	+	–
5.	Kasa	+	+	+	+	+	+	+	–
6.	Rajyaksma	+	+	+	+	–	–	–	–
7.	Galagraha	+	–	–	–	+	–	–	–
8.	Shleepada	+	+	+	+	–	–	+	–
9.	Galaganda	+	–	–	+	+	–	–	–
10.	Prameha	+	–	+	+	+	–	+	–

Contd...

Contd...

S.No.	*Diseases*	*Ch.*	*Su.*	*A.H.*	*A.S.*	*Ka.S*	*Bh.S.*	*Sha.S.*	*C.D.*
11.	Mandagni	+	+	–	+	–	–	+	–
12.	Viruddhajirna	+	+	–	+	+	–	+	+
13.	Visuchika	+	–	–	+	+	–	–	–
14.	Alasaka	+	–	–	+	–	–	–	–
15.	Vishapita	+	+	+	+	+	+	+	+
16.	Vishadagdha	+	–	+	–	–	–	–	–
17.	Viddha	+	–	–	+	–	+	–	–
18.	Adhoga Raktapitta	+	+	+	+	+	–	–	–
19.	Mukha Praseka	+	+	+	+	+	–	–	–
20.	Durnama (Arsha)	+	–	–	–	–	–	–	–
21.	Hrillasa	+	+	+	+	+	–	+	–
22.	Aruchi	+	+	+	+	+	–	+	–
23.	Avipaka	+	–	–	+	–	–	–	–
24.	Apachi	+	–	+	+	–	–	+	–
25.	Granthi	–	–	+	+	–	–	–	–
26.	Apasmara	+	+	+	+	–	+	+	–
27.	Unmada	+	+	+	+	–	–	+	–
28.	Atisara	+	+	+	+	+	–	+	–
29.	Shopha	+	–	–	–	–	–	–	–
30.	Pandu	+	–	–	+	–	+	–	–
31.	Mukhapaka	+	+	–	+	–	–	–	–
32.	Stanya Dushti	+	+	+	+	+	–	+	–
33.	Arbuda	–	–	+	+	–	–	+	–
34.	Vidarika	–	+	–	–	+	–	+	–
35.	Medoroga	–	+	+	+	–	–	+	–
36.	Hridroga	–	+	–	–	+	+	+	–
37.	Visarpa	–	+	+	+	–	+	+	–
38.	Chitta Vibhrama	–	+	–	–	–	–	–	–
39.	Vidradhi	–	+	–	–	–	–	–	–
40.	Kanthapaka	–	+	–	–	–	–	–	–
41.	Karnasrava	–	+	–	–	–	–	+	–
42.	Adhi Jihwika	–	+	–	–	–	–	+	–
43.	Galashundika	–	+	–	–	–	+	+	–
44.	Putinasa	–	+	–	–	–	–	–	–
45.	Kaphaja Vyadhi	+	+	+	+	+	+	+	+

Classification of Indications of Vamana Acoording to Marga, Dosha and Srotasa

Diseases	*Marga*	*Dosha*	*Srotas*
Pinasa	Madhyama	Kaphapradhana	Rasavaha
Kushtha	Bahya	Tridoshapradhana	Rasavaha
Nava Jvara	Abhyantara	Pittapradhana	Rasavaha
Rajyaksma	Madhyama	Tridoshapradhana	Rasavaha
Kasa	Abhyantara	Vatapradhana	Prana and Rasavaha
Shvasa	Abhyantara	Vata + Kapha	Pranavaha
Galagraha	Bahya	Kaphapradhana	Asthivaha
Galaganda	Bahya	Kaphapradhana	Medovaha
Shleepada	Bahya + Abhayantara	Kaphapradhana	Medovaha
Prameha	Madhyama + Bahya	Kaphapradhana Tridoshaja	Medovaha
Mandagni	Abhyantara	Kaphapradhana	Annavaha
Viruddhanna	Abhyantara	Kaphapradhana	Annavaha
Ajirnanna	Abhyantara	Kaphapradhana	Annavaha
Visuchika	Abhyantara	Kaphapradhana Tridoshaja	Annavaha
Alasaka	Abhyantara	Kaphapradhana	Annavaha
Vishapita	Abhyantara + Madhyama	Tridoshapradhana	Rasavaha
Garapita	Madhyama	Tridoshapradhana	Rasavaha
Durnana	Bahya	Tridoshapradhana	Mansavaha
Vidhradhi	Bahya	Tridoshapradhana	Mansavaha
Visarpa	Bahya	Tridosapradhana	Mansavaha
Adhahshonita	Madhyama	Pittapradhana Vataja	Raktavaha
Pitta Praseka	Abhyantara	Pittapradhana	Raktavaha
Hrillasa	Abhyantara	Kaphapradhana	Annavaha
Arochaka	Abhyantara	Kaphapradhana	Annavaha
Avipaka	Abhyantara	Kaphapradhana	Annavaha
Apachi	Bahya	Kaphapradhana	Medovaha
Apasmara	Madhyama	Tridoshapradhana	Manovaha
Unmada	Madhyama	Tridoshapradhana	Manovaha
Atisara	Abhyantara	Vatapradhana Tridoshaja	Rasavaha
Shopha	Abhyantara + Bahya	Kaphapradhana	Rasavaha
Panduroga	Madhyama	Kaphapradhana	Rasavaha
Mukhapaka	Abhyantara	Pittapradhana	Raktavaha
Dushtastanya	Bahya	Tridosapradhana	Rasavaha
Shleshmaja Vyadhi	All the marga	Kaphapradhana	Rasa and Pranavaha
Shosha	Madhyama	Tridoshapradhana	Rasa, Rakta and Prana

Thus the indications for Vamana can be categorized according to dosha dominance in disease and the site in which provocation of doshas is taking place (Indu on A.S.Su.27/3). Thus, to judge the efficacy of Vamana procedure more clearly, the diseases can be classified as:

A. Diseases having "Bahudoshavastha", e.g. Kushtha, Prameha, Unmada, Apasmara, etc.

From this classification, the following conclusions can be drawn viz:

1. Vamana is more effective in Abhyantara and Bahya roga marga.
2. Vamana proves to be more fruitful in the diseases having Kapha dominance.
3. Vamana primarily acts on Rasavaha srotasa, Annavaha srotasa and Pranavaha srotasa, while it also acts on Medovaha srotasa and Mansavaha srotasa.

Contraindications

क्षत क्षीण अतिस्थूल अतिकृश बाल वृद्ध दुर्बल श्रान्त पिपासित क्षुधित कर्म भार
अध्वहत उपवास मैथुन अध्ययन व्यायाम चिन्ता प्रसक्त क्षाम गर्भिणी सुकुमार।
संवृतकोष्ठ दुश्छर्दन उर्ध्वरक्तपित्त प्रसक्तच्छर्दिर् उर्ध्ववात आस्थापित अनुवासित
हृद्रोग उदावर्त मूत्राघात् प्लीह गुल्म उदर अष्ठीला स्वरोघात तिमिर शिर शङ्खः
कर्ण अक्षि शूलार्ताः॥ (Ch.Si.2/8)

S. No.	Diseases	Ch.	Su.	A. H.	A. S.	Ka.S.	Bh. S.	Sha. S.	C.D.
1.	Atibala	+	+	+	+	+	–	+	–
2.	Ativriddha	+	+	+	+	+	–	+	+
3.	Atisthula	+	+	+	+	+	+	+	+
4.	Atikrisha	+	+	+	+	–	+	+	+
5.	Sukumara	+	–	–	+	+	+	–	–
6.	Kshama	+	–	–	–	–	–	–	–
7.	Durbala	+	+	+	+	–	+	–	–
8.	Shranta	+	+	–	+	–	–	–	–
9.	Kshudhita	+	+	+	+	–	–	+	–
10.	Pipasita	+	+	+	+	+	–	–	–
11.	Karmahata	+	–	–	–	–	+	–	–
12.	Bharahata	+	–	–	+	–	–	–	–
13.	Upavasita	+	–	–	+	–	–	–	–
14.	Maithuna prasakta	+	–	–	+	–	–	–	–
15.	Adhyayana prasakta	+	–	–	+	–	–	–	–
16.	Garbhini	+	+	+	+	+	+	+	–
17.	Vyayama prasakta	+	–	–	+	–	–	–	–
18.	Chinta prasakta	+	–	–	+	–	–	–	–
19.	Samvrita koshtha	+	+	–	+	–	–	–	–
20.	Duschhardana	+	+	+	+	+	–	+	–

Contd...

Contd...

S. No.	*Diseases*	*Ch.*	*Su.*	*A. H.*	*A. S.*	*Ka.S.*	*Bh. S.*	*Sha. S.*	*C.D.*
21.	Kshatakshina	+	+	+	+	+	–	+	+
22.	Krimi koshtha	–	+	+	+	+	–	+	+
23.	Urdhva raktapitta	+	+	+	+	+	–	+	+
24.	Urdhva Vata	+	+	+	+	–	–	–	–
25.	Asthapita	+	+	+	+	+	–	+	–
26.	Anuvasita	+	+	+	+	+	–	–	–
27.	Hridroga	+	+	+	+	–	–	–	–
28.	Udavarta	+	+	+	+	–	–	+	–
29.	Mutraghata	+	+	+	+	–	–	–	–
30.	Pleeha dosha/roga	+	+	+	+	+	–	–	–
31.	Gulma	+	–	+	+	+	–	+	+
32.	Udara roga	+	+	+	+	+	–	+	+
33.	Ashthila	+	+	+	+	–	–	–	–
34.	Timira	+	+	+	+	–	–	+	+
35.	Shankhaka	+	+	–	+	–	–	–	–
36.	Akshishula	+	–	–	+	+	–	–	–
37.	Karnashula	+	–	–	+	+	–	–	–
38.	Arsha	–	–	+	+	–	–	–	–
39.	Parshwashula	–	–	+	+	–	–	–	–
40.	Nitya rogi	–	–	–	–	–	–	–	–
41.	Adhwahata	+	–	–	–	–	–	–	–
42.	Prasakta chhardi	+	+	+	–	–	–	–	–
43.	Svaropaghata	+	+	+	–	–	–	–	–
44.	Bhrama	–	–	+	–	–	–	–	–
45.	Vatavyadhi	–	+	+	–	–	–	–	–

Reason for Contraindications

Contraindications	*Reasons for contraindications*
क्षत (Koch's disease)	क्षणनात् रक्तातिप्रवृत्ति If subjected to emesis, due to further strain, profuse hemorrhage may occur
क्षीण (Debilitated), अतिस्थूल (Obese), कृश (Underweight), बाल (Children), वृद्ध (Old age), दुर्बल (Weakness)	औषधबल असहात्वात् प्राणोपरोध। There will be danger to their lives because of their inability to tolerate the action of medication and also strain of the procedure. May cause death.
श्रान्त (Exhaustion), पिपासित (Afflicted with thirst), क्षुधित (Hungry)	Same as above

Contd...

Contd...

Contraindications	*Reasons for contraindications*
कर्म (Excessive physical exercise), भार (Lifting heavy weights), अध्वहत (Excessive walking), उपवास (Observation of fast), मैथुन (Indulging in excessive sex), अध्ययन (Continous reading), व्यायाम (Excessive exercise), चिन्ताप्रसक्त (Excessive thinking), क्षाम (Physical weakness)	रौक्ष्यात् वातरक्तच्छेदक्षतभयं On account of their ununctous (Rukshata in shareera) condition there will be provocation of Vata, hemorrhage or ulceration
गर्भिणी (Pregnanacy)	गर्भव्यापद् गर्भभ्रंश Complications of pregnancy, abortion or fetal anomaly and incidence of fatal diseases
सुकुमार (Person of delicate constitution)	हृदयापकर्षणादूर्ध्वामधो वा रुधिरातिप्रवृत्ति Due to strain of the procedure, they may suffer from discomfort in chest region; severe hemorrhage may take place through upper and lower channels
संवृतकोष्ठ (Vayuvyapta Koshtha or Vata dominant koshtha), दुश्छर्दित (Poor response to emetics)	Causes Dosha utklesha leading to विसर्प, स्तम्भ, जाड्य, वैचित्य, मरण, morbid doshas get stimulated but do not get eliminated. These accumulate in the alimentary tract and cause internally acute spreading infections, stasis, dullness, fainting or even death
ऊर्ध्वरक्तपित (Bleeding tendency from upper channels)	उदानमुत्क्षिप्य प्राणान् हरेद्रक्तं चातिप्रवर्तयेत् It may provoke Udana Vata and take away life or cause profuse bleeding
प्रसक्त छर्दि (Person suffering from persistent vomiting)	Same as above
ऊर्ध्ववात (Reverse course of Vata)	ऊर्ध्ववातातिप्रवृत्ति
आस्थापित (The person subjected to Niruha basti), (person subjected to Anuvasana basti), अनुवासित	Increase in upward movement of Vata
हृद्रोग (Heart diseases)	हृदयोपरोध There will be impairement in cardiac function
उदावर्त (Upward movement of Vata)	घोरतर उदावर्तः स्यात् शीघ्रतरहन्ता Aggravation of condition which may quickly cause death
मूत्राघात (Obstructed micturition), प्लीहा (Splenic enlargement), गुल्म (Abdominal pain), उदर (Ascitis), अष्ठिला (Prostate enlargement)	तीव्रतरशूलप्रादुर्भाव Manifestation of acute pain
स्वरोपघात (Hoarseness of voice)	Same as above
तिमिर (Progressive cataract)	तिमिरातिवृद्धि Aggravation of the condition
शिरःशूल (Headaches), कर्णशूल (Ear ache), अक्षिशूल (Pain in eyes)	शूलातिवृद्धि There is an increase in the intensity of pain

After having a look at the diseases which are described in contraindications, we can say that Vamana should not be given in:

1. Diseases with acute onset, e.g. Hridgraha, Udavarta.
2. Diseases in which body is largely emaciated, e.g. Kshatakshina.
3. Diseases in which doshas move in upward direction, e.g. Urdhvaga Raktapitta.
4. Very weak, delicate and aged individuals.
5. Diseases involving vital organs (Marma).

Vamana Mentioned in Contraindicated Disesase

Although there are many disorders which are contraindicated for Vamana, even then the acharyas have at time of describing chikitsa of specific subtypes and conditions advocate use of vamana, following are some examples:

1. **Udara roga:** Though contraindicated by Charaka, Gangadhara advised it in Kaphaja type (Gangadhara on Ch.Chi.13/41) and Harita did the same in Jalodara (Harita/3rd Adhyaya).
2. **Gulma:** In Kaphaja Gulma (Ch.Chi.5/48-52, 60-61, 137, 186, A.S.Chi.16, A.H.Chi.54/76).
3. **Hridroga:** Vataja Pittaja and Kaphaja types of Hridroga (Vangasen/Hridroga/ 6-8, 15-16, 25-26).
4. **Vata Vyadhi:** Vamana is advised in several types of Vatavyadhi, viz:
   i. **Gridhrasi:** Bh.Pr.Chi. 24/133, 134
   ii. Vakshagata, Trikagata, Skandhagata, Manyagata Vata (Vangasen/Vata)
   iii. Pratyadhmana (Su.Chi. 5/26)
   iv. **Ardita:** When associated with Shopha (Vangasen/Vata)
   v. **Paksaghata:** Mild type of Sanshodhana after Snehana and Svedana (Su.Chi.5/19). Dalhana mentions that Vamana is encouraged first followed by Virechana (after 15 days) (Dalhana on Su.Chi.5/19).
   vi. **Amashayagata Vata:** (Su.Chi. 4/3, Ch.Chi.28).

Vamana in Various Contexts

1. Effect over Agni

i. **Grahani:** Ahara gets 'Vidagdhatwa' when vitiated by 'Weakened Agni' (Mandagni) and symptoms of Vishtabdhajirna are produced. The whole matter can be cured by expelling it through Vamana by luke warm water (Gangadhara on Ch.Chi.15/30).

ii. **Prameha:** Patients of Prameha have 'Abhishyanda' in the body which suppresses Agni leading further to the production of vitiated Meda and Mutra though one consumes all the five types of diet. So to augment Agni and to passify Kleda and Meda, Sanshodhana is advocated in Prameha (A.S.Chi.Prameha).

2. Effect over Pitta

Grahani: Pitta having liquid property (Drava Guna) and possessing the ability to subdue Agni, when provocated or excited at its own site, Vamana or Virechana might be the first choice of treatment (Ch.Chi.15/122).

3. Effect over Ama

i. **Atisara:** If the symptoms like shula, anaha and praseka are produced due to 'Ama', Vamana is administered to combat with the condition. (A.S.Chi.Atisara)
ii. **Grahani:** When the symptoms of Ama associated with chief symptoms of Grahani, Ama is removed by means of Vamana (Ch.Chi.15/75).
iii. **Visarpa:** The disease Visarpa when having involvement of Ama, Vamana is advised (Ch. Chi. 21/44).
iv. **Udavarta:** When Anaha is produced due to presence of Ama in 'Udavarta', Vamana is advised (Ch.Chi.26/26).
v. **Amajirna:** Vamana is advised in 'Amajirna' (Bh.Pr.Chi.6/39-40, Harita 3rd. 4th Adhyaya). Harita advised to do so, as Vamana will purify Koshtha and remove all the vitiated Rasa in it and thus preventing the body from complications those are produced due to this vitiated Rasa.

Vamana in Pakwa Condition

Atisara

Vamana is indicated in Pakwa condition of Atisara (Dalhana on Su.Ut.40/106).

Vamana and Udaka Dhatu

i. **Grahani:** It is advised in "Shleshmaja Grahani" as it will remove the increased or excessive 'Ab Dhatu'which is pacifying 'Teja (Agni)' and helps to augment the Agni to perform Pachana and Deepana' (A.S.Chi.12).
ii. **Atisara:** Dalhana raised the question in Atisara that if the disease is produced due to Agnimandya, then why Vamana is suggested which also produces the same? He further resolves the same that it is advised to prevent the excessive loss of 'doshas' from the body (Dalhana on Su.Ut. 40/25, 26). Here doshas are associated with Udaka dhatu.

Vamana on Hridaya and Manovaha Srotas

i. **Apasmara:** Tikshna (Strong) Vamana should be administered in Apasmara to stimulate Manovaha srotasa and heart for further motivation which are obstructed due to Vata (Avritavata). It normalizes the function, i.e.'Prabodhanam'of Mana (Ch.Chi.10/14,15).
ii. **Unmada:** It is administered in 'Kaphaja type'. After the proper purification by Vamana, the organs like heart, head, abdominal region and sense organs get rid off the vitiated doshas and mind gets refreshed with one's Smriti (Memory) and Sangya (Ch.Chi.9/28). Mild Vamana should be given when Vata is encircled or obstructed (Avrita) by Kapha or Pitta (Gangadhara on Ch.Chi. 9/28).
iii. **Sanyasa:** When the patient is in very much delirious state and going to be in the comatose condition, one should be kept alert by the means of fear, happiness or through the means of 'Vamana'. Thus Vamana helps the individuals by preventing from further attack (A.S.Chi.9/62).

Vamana in 'Santarpanotha' Conditions

i. **Jvara:** If Jirna Jvara is produced due to Santarpana (Santarpanotha Jvara), then Vamana is indicated in them. If it is associated with burning sensation and thirst, Vamana given by water mixed with sugar and honey (A.S.Chi. 2) can cure the condition.
ii. **Raktapitta:** Vamana is given in "Adhoga Raktapitta", when the main cause is the Santarpana (Indu on A.S. Chi./Raktapitta). So it is given in "Santarpanotha Adhoga Raktapitta".

Vamana: In Relation with Strength of the Patient

i. Vamana should be ventured by the individuals who are having good strength, in the diseases like Prameha, Shvasa, Hikka (Bh.Pr.Chi. 13/16), Gulma (Gangadhara on Ch.Chi.5/88, Dalhana on Su. Chi. 11/7).
ii. **Yakshma:** If one administers Vamana or Virechana drug without judging the strength of the patient, the patient will certainly die because expulsion of excess doshas from the body will take away the strength of the patient with it. (Ch.Chi. 8/87, 88).
iii. **Chhardi:** In Kaphaja type, stronger individuals are advised to undergo Vamana and weaker ones for 'Shamana' (Indu on A.S. Chi./Chhardi).

Types of Vamana → Mridu and Tikshan

According to Acharya's, Vamana is of two types (explained in various diseases), viz.
(A) Mild Vamana (Mridu Vamana) and
(B) Strong Vamana (Tikshna Vamana)

A. Mild Vamana (Mridu Vamana)

i. It is advocated in Gulma (Gangadhar on Ch. Chi. 5/3, 7and88), Yakshma (Ch.Chi. 8/87,88) and Vatarakta.
ii. If Vata is obstructed or encircled (Avrit) by Kapha or Pitta, one can administer mild Vamana or Virechana with unctous material for the same. (Ch.Chi. 9/9).
iii. Dalhana advised to administer mild Vamana in 'Pandu' after judging season (ritu), place (desha), constitution, time (Kala) and body status (Dalhana on Su. Ut. 44/14-15).
iv. If Shvasa and Hikka are associated with coughing, vomiting, spasm in cardiac region, laryngitis, then Vamana can be given (A.S. Chi./Shvasa).

B. Strong Vamana (Tikshna Vamana)

i. **Prameha Pidaka:** It is suggested as the disease is turned to 'Durvirechya stage' due to spread to 'Medasthana' throughout the body (A.S.Chi.4).
ii. **Unmada:** Sushruta advised to give strong Vamana (Su.Ut.62/14-15) in Unmada. Commentators claim to.give repeated Vamana (Yathasankhyam, Aruna Dutta on A.H.Chi. 6/11 and 20) if doshas are present in excessive quantity (Yatha dosham, Ch.Chi.9126-27).
iii. **Pandu:** Charaka suggested to give strong Vamana (Ch.Chi.16/40). Indu mentioned the purpose of it as to remove the soil (Mrittika) present in the Koshtha (Indu on A.S.Chi.8) that causes Mrittika bhakshanajanya Pandu.
iv. **Murccha:** Tikshna Vamana is advised (Vangasen on Murccha / 29) here.

Indication of Vamana According to the Adhishthana of Disease

In Kaphadhishthana

1. Amashaya

i. **Chhardi:** Vamana is advised in chhardi where doshas are secreted and accumulated in amashaya region (Ch.Chi.20/20). In Kaphaja condition, it is advocated as it purifies amashaya (Ch.Chi. 20/34).

ii. When excessive Pitta moves upwards and stays in Kaphashaya, it should be removed by Vamana (Ch.Chi.20/21).

iii. **Visarpa:** Vamana is advised when humors move into the sites of Kapha (Ch.Chi, 21/44).

iv. **Visha:** When poison enters amashaya, Vamana is advised (Ch.Chi. 27/122).

v. **Madatyaya:** When Kapha and Pitta get provoked in amashaya and having symptoms of excessive humors, burning and thirst, Vamana is immediately administered (Ch. Chi.24/141,142).

vi. **Vrana:** If 'Sadyovrana' is in 'Amashaya' and there is accumulation of blood in the same, later on Vamana is advised (Chakradatta/Vrana).

vii. **Vatavyadhi:** Vamana is advised in Amashayagata Vata (Su.Chi.4/3, Ch.Chi.28).

2. Hridaya

Vamana is advised in Kaphaja Marmaroga (Ch.Chi. 26).
Vangasena advised it in all the three types of Hridroga (Vangasen / Hridroga).

3. Other Sites

i. **Mukharoga:** Vamana is advised in Paridara (Chakradatta/Mukharoga), Rohini (Su.Chi. 23/59, 60), Sarvasara (Chakradatta/Mukharoga) and Pittaja Oshtharoga (Vangasen/ Mukharoga/18, 212).

ii. **Karnaroga:** Vamana is also advised in Karnapaka (Chakradatta and Vangasen) and Karnapali roga (Su.Chi. 25/13).

iii. **Danta galaroga:** To combat local Kapha present in the oral cavity Vamana is advised (Dalhana on Su.Chi. 22/19) in 'Upakusha' involving chiefly Rakta and Pitta.

iv. **Nasaroga:** It is advised in Kaphaja Pratishyaya, Nava Pratishyaya, Vataja Pinasa and Kaphaja Pinasa (Chakradatta and Vangasen/Nasaroga).

v. **Vatarakta:** Dalhana mentions that Vatarakta if manifested in upper limbs, it generally has the involvement of Kapha and Pitta. So Vamana and Virechana are advised there. (Dalhana on Su.Chi. 5/7).

Vamana in Visha Chikitsa

i. Vega No. / References

Vega No.	References
I	A.H.Ut. 35/17
II	A.H.Ut. 35/18
III	Ch.Chi. 23/48

ii. In Kaphaja Visha type (Ch.Chi. 23/171).

iii. Bites of several poisonous insets like:

a. Darvikara snake bite (A.H.Ut. 36/74, 76, 77)

b. Scorpion bite (A.H.Ut.37/39, 40)

c. Luta bite (A.H.Ut 37/175, 76)
d. Mouse poison (A.H.Ut. 38120)
iv. In the treatment of dushivisha (A.H. 35/38)

Vamana to Pacify Shula

i. **Atisara:** If symptoms like shula, anaha and praseka are there, Vamana is administered by hot water mixed with rock salt to pacify the symptoms.
ii. **Shula:**
   a. In generalized treatment of shula, Vamana is indicated. (Bh.Pr.Chi.shula/30).
   b. In 'Shleshmika shula', when it is getting aggravated after having a meal, Vamana is advised (Su.Ut. 42/109,110)
   c. In other types of shula including 'Bastishula', Vamana is recommended as an immediate remedy along with Svedana, Niruha and Snehabasti (Su. Ut.42).
iii. **Vilambika:** Vamana is suggested to fight with shula (Su.Ut.42).
iv. **Parinama shula:** (Harita 16th Sthana 17th Adhyaya)
v. **Pittaja shula:** (Vangasen - 241 Shula)
vi. **Annadravashula:** Vamana pacifies the pains quickly. Vangasena advised to give Vamana in 'Pittaja' Annadravashula and Virechana in Kaphaja one (Vangasen Parinamashula).

Role of Vamana in Srotorodha

Vriddha Vagbhatta points out that, in the pathogenesis of Shvasa and Hikka, flow of Vata is interrupted or obstructed by Kapha (Avrita) which further aggravates Vata. Hence to clear this pathway, Sanshodhana through both ways is advised (A.S.Ch./Shvasa).

Regarding Tamaka Shvasa (Asthma)

Various activities have been carried out regarding effect of Vamana over Shvasa, viz.
i. The results of study regarding Vamana karma suggest that Vamana reduces tolerance to stimulants which reflects restoration of the airway responsiveness.
ii. Vamana does not only cause histamine dialysis to washout the existing histamine from the system rather it also stabilises the histamine production mechanism. These humoral changes occurring after Vamana were found to be proportionately accompanied by symptomatic relief (Prof RH Singh).

Prabhava of Vamana

Dalhana explained the effect of Vamana in 'Atisara', as Vamana works in it in the following three ways:
i. It reduces Drava and Shlesma.
ii. It works in the opposite direction as that of Atisara.
iii. By its self action (Chikitsa Prabhava) (Dalhana on Su.Ut.40/160).

Vamana in Purvarupa

i. **Visarpa:** Vriddha Vagbhatta advised to give Vamana when the prodromal symptoms of Visarpa are being manifested (A.S.Chi.20).
ii. **Jvara:** In the Purvarupa of 'Kaphaja Jvara', "Mridu Vamana" is advised (Su.Ut.39/98).

Miscellaneous

i. **Pandu:** Strong Sanshodhana is advised in "Mridbhakshanajanya Pandu" (A.S.Chi.18). Indu clarifies as one cannot cure the disease, if Mrittika (Soil) remains in Koshtha. So it has to be removed for the further treatment (Indu on A.S.Chi.18).
ii. **Prameha:** Vamana is contraindicated in the individuals who are having excessive Rukshata in them (Dalhana on Su.Chi.11/7).
iii. **Cchardi:** Vamana is advised in the individuals in whom Chhardi is produced due to 'sudden withdrawal of satmya things' (Su.Ut.9/ 24-26, Vangasen/Chhardi 1/64).
iv. **Kshayaja Trishna:**
   a. It is not indicated here due to 'Kshinadhatu' condition in the body (Dalhana on Su.Ut.8/16).
   b. It is prescribed in the type of Trishna which is produced due to 'consumption of heavy food' (Su. Ut. 49/29).
v. **Vrana:** In Sadhya Vrana when doshas are in provoked condition, Vamana is advised (Vangasen/Agantuja Vrana).
vi. **Udavarta:** If 'Udavarta' is produced by suppressing the urge of vomiting, Vamana is advised there. (Bh. Pr. Udavartta 31/29).
vii. **Shleshmavyadhi:** (Bh.Pr.Chi. 29/6)
viii. **Kardamaka Visarpa:** It is indicated as 'the quickest remedy' (Shighrataram, A.S.Chi. 20) to remove the humors completely.

Vamana a Remedy as 'Pratimarga Harana'

i. **Raktapitta:** Vamana is advised in "Adhoga Raktapitta only" and not in "Urdhvaga Raktapitta" (Ch.Chi./54-60).
ii. **Atisara:** When feces with a lots of liquid are passed frequently in Atisara, Vamana is administered, followed by Langhana and pachana. Dalhana explains that 'Udakadhatu' will be expelled through oral route which will ultimately stop the flow from the opposite direction (Dalhana on Su.Ut.40/32). It works there just in the same mechanism like that in Raktapitta.

Explanations

In the context of Raktapitta, commentator Chakrapani says that due to 'Vyadhi mahima', Pratimarga harana is the treatment (Ch.Ni. 2/19 Chakrapani). Here doshas are vitiated in excessive quanity ('Bahudoshanam', Ch.Chi. 4/54).

If doshas are accumulated in the body in 'Bahudoshavastha', they should be removed at first by Sanshodhana (Ch.Su.16/16). So Sanshodhana will be the prime treatment. Now if

Sanshodhana has to be done, it should be done in any of the routes available, i.e. Urdhvaga or Adhoga. In Raktapitta, Rakta is oozing out due to damage in Raktadhara Kala or in the organ like stomach. So if the bleeding is appearing in upper region, the site of the lesion may be in any region from stomach up to oral cavity. So in this condition if Vamana is done, it will become fatal within a few bouts producing or augmenting the previously started bleeding. Vamana will cause friction in that site which will increase the bleeding (Ch.Si.2/9). On contrary, the ulceration produced in colons or hemorrhoids may be tore due to continuous friction produced due to Virechana (if given in Adhoga Raktapitta) and ultimately lead to more bleeding. So to remove the vitiated humors from the body, opposite way is chosen through the means of Vamana and Virechana in Raktapitta.

Vamana and Rasayana

Vamana directly as such is not mentioned in the main texts anywhere as preparatory procedure before Rasayana. But Charaka (Ch.Chi.1/1/18-24), (Ch.Chi.2/1/50, 51) clearly indicates to purify the body before leading to Rasayana and Vajikarana, respectively. Chakrapani mentions that Vamana, Virechana, Asthapana and Shirovirechana must be done. Similar references can be obtained in (A.H.Ut.39/ 3, 4, 8,12,13,14, 113, 114 and 174), Ashtanga Hridaya where Vagbhatta instructs the physician to perform Rasayana by removing vitiated humors completely. Sushruta did the same thing by allowing "Srotas Sanshodhana" before administering several Rasayana like Vidangatandula (Su.Chi.27/8), Avalguja (Su.Chi.28/3), Mandukaparni (Su. Chi.28/4), Brahmi (Su.Chi.28/5) and recommended Vamana before 'Vajikarana' (A.S.Ut.9/10, A.S.Ut.50/73). Thus, Vamana might be helpful before leading to Rasayana.

Vamana and Ritu

Vamana is advised in Vasanta Ritu to combat with the exaggerated Kapha. (Ch.Su.7/46). Vasanta Ritu comprises of two months, viz. Phalguna and Chaitra (Ch.Si.6). So if one removes doshas in Phalguna, there remains the fear of increasing humors in Chaitra. So it is better to remove them in Chaitra only. (Chakrapani on Ch.Su. 7/46).

ROLE OF KOSHTHA IN VAMANA

In the context of Vamana, Koshtha means :

श्लेष्म अधिक्येन मृदुत्वं, श्लेष्म मध्यत्वेन मध्यत्वं, श्लेष्म हीनत्वेन क्रूरत्वं वमने कोष्ठस्य बोध्यम्॥

(A.H.Su. 19. Arunadatta)

Arunadatta has mentioned three types of Koshtha in relation to Vamana. Dominance of Kapha in Koshtha is considered as Mridu Koshtha for Vamana. Similarly, Madhya shleshma gives rise to Madhyam Koshtha and slight kapha in Koshtha is Krura Koshtha.

By implication, it can be said that the patient who has a dominance of Kapha in Koshtha requires less dose of Vamaka dravya, while those having slight Kapha need more dose of the drug.

VAMANA DRAVYA

They are mainly divided into two main sections, i.e.

A. **Vamana drug:** Vamana drugs are the drugs which initiates or produces the act of vomiting, e.g. Madanaphala.

B. **Vamanopaga drugs:** vamanopaga drugs are the supportive drugs in the process of vomiting. They help in proceeding the act of vomiting, e.g. milk, juice of sugar cane, hot infusion or decoction of *Glycyrrhiza glabra*. All vamaka drugs have vamaka prabhava and hence irrespective of all other properties, they induce the act of vomiting. The function of vamanopaga drugs can be judged by the properties which they possess. Most of the vamanopaga drugs are having madhura (sweet) taste, sheeta virya and madhura (sweet) vipaka. Vamanopaga drugs are the drugs which are used for "akanthapana". Thus they remain in the body for a quite long time. This time may be prolonged if a complication like ayoga occurs. Thus they should possess such properties with which they can be retained in the body with large quantity and for much more time without causing harm to the individual. Supportively if possible, they should supply energy to body to bear strain. The drugs having Ushna and Tikshna properties cannot be consumed in a large quantity. They also cannot be beared for a longer period. So the drugs selected which will have the qualities like Madhura rasa, Sheeta virya, vipaka and Brihana property along with their tendency to produce vomiting after ingestion, are termed as "Vamanopaga drugs".

Vamaka Dravya (Figs 4.1A to F)

मदनं मधुकं निम्बं जीमूतं कृतवेधनम्। पिप्पली कुटज इक्ष्वाकून् एलां धामार्गवाणि च॥ (Ch.Su.2/7)

मदन मधुक लम्बा निम्ब बिम्बी विशाला त्रपुस कुटज मूर्वा देवदाली कृमिघ्नम्।
विदुल दहनचित्राः कोशवत्यौ करञ्जः कण लवण वच एला सर्षपा च्छर्दनानि। (A.H.Su.15/1)

मदन, मधुक, निम्ब, जीमूतक, कृतवेधन, पिप्पली, कुटज, इक्ष्वाकू, ऐला, धामार्गव।

मदन, मधुक, लम्बा (अलाबु), निम्ब, बिम्बी, विशाला (इन्द्रवारुणी), त्रपुस कुटज, मूर्वा, देवदाली, कृमिघ्न (विडङ्ग), विदुल (जलवेतस), दहन (चित्रक), चित्रा (मूषिकपर्णी), कोशवत्यौ (कोशातकी, राजकोशातकी), करञ्ज, कण, लवण, ऐला, सर्षप।

Charaka has explained 6 Vamana dravyas in Kalpasthana. In total he has mentioned 355 Vamana yogas in Kalpasthana. Dravyas are as follows :

फल जीमूतक इक्ष्वाकु कल्पो धामार्गवस्य च। पञ्चमो वत्सकस्योक्तः षष्ठश्च कृतवेधने।

(Ch. Su. 30/62)

S.No.	*Vamana Dravya*	*Botanical name*	*Number of Yogas*
1.	मदनफल	*Randia dumetorum* (Fig. 4.1A)	133
2.	जीमूतक	*Luffa echinata* (Fig. 4.1B)	39
3.	इक्ष्वाकु	*Lagenaria vulgaris* (Fig. 4.1C)	45
4.	धामार्गव	*Luffa cylindrica* (Fig. 4.1D)	60
5.	वत्सक	*Holarrhena antidysentrica* (Fig. 4.1E)	18
6.	कृतवेधन	*Luffa acutangula* (Fig. 4.1F)	60

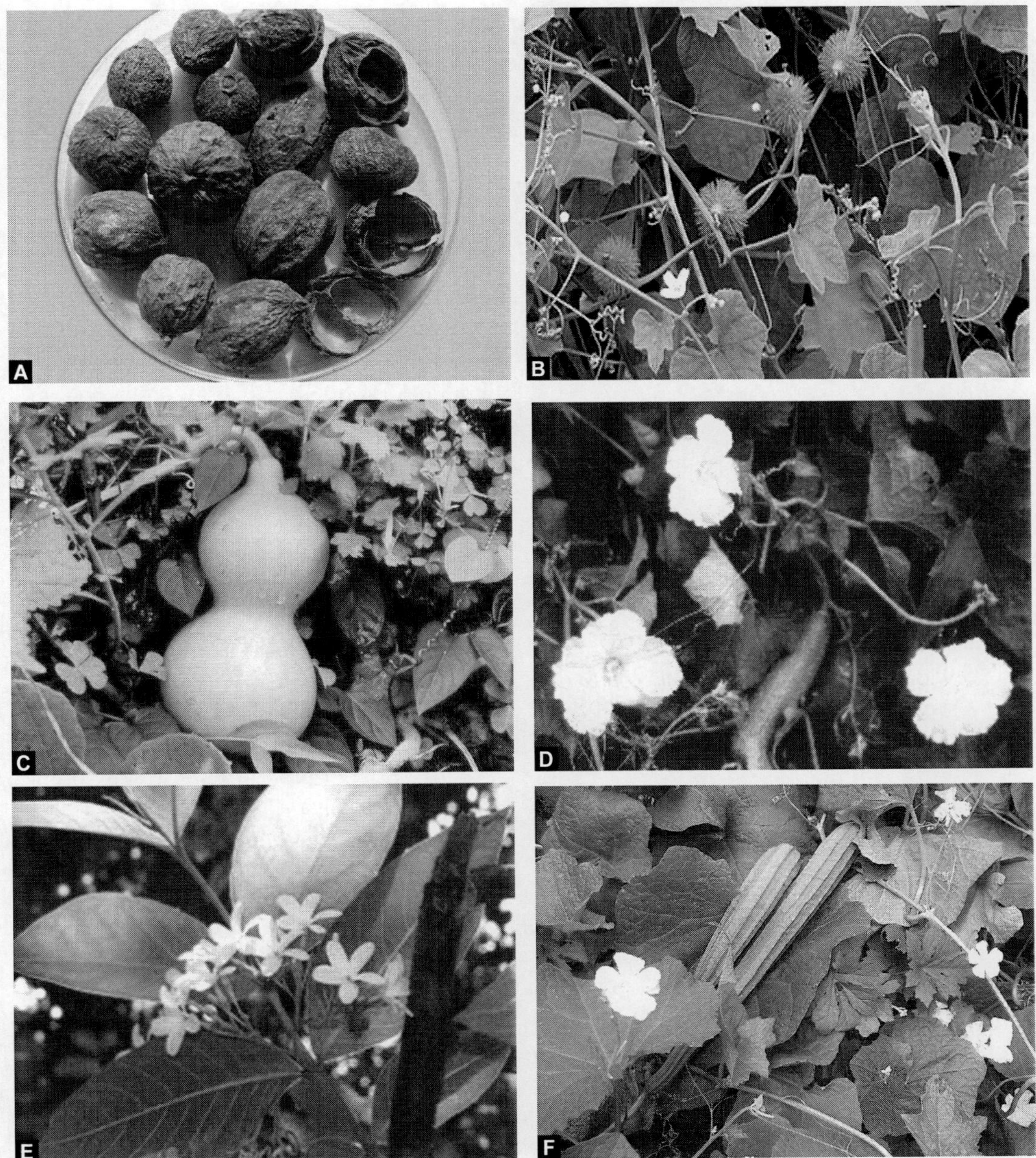

Figs 4.1A to F: Vamaka Dravya

Vamanopaga Dravyas (Figs 4.2A to I)

मधु मधुक कोविदार कर्बुदार नीप विदुल बिम्बी शणपुष्पी सदापुष्पी प्रत्यक्पुष्प्येति दशेमानि वमन उपगानि भवन्ति।। (Ch. Su. 4/23)

Vamanopaga drugs are supportive drugs to the process of vomiting (क्रियायां सहायत्वेनोप गच्छन्तिति Ch.Su.4/8 teeka). They help in aiding the act of vomiting as well as minimize the complications which may arise during the course of vamana.

बमनोपगानीत्यत्र मदनफलादीनां वमनद्रव्याणां मधुमधुकादीनि सहयानि भवन्ति।। (च.सू. 4/8 चक्र.)
क्रियायां सहायत्वेपगच्छन्तीति।।

S.No.	Vamanopaga	Botanical name	Properties
1.	Madhu	–	• Rasa : Kashaya, Madhura • Veerya : Sheeta • Guna: Guru, Sheeta, Ruksha
2.	Madhuka (Fig. 4.2A)	*Glycyrrhiza glabra*	• Rasa : Madhura • Vipaka : Madhura • Veerya : Sheeta • Guna : Guru, Snigdha
3.	Kovidara (Fig. 4.2B)	*Bauhinia purpurea*	• Rasa : Kashaya • Veerya : Sheeta • Vipaka : Katu • Guna : Ruksha, Laghu
4.	Karbudara (Kanchanara) (Fig. 4.2C)	*Bauhinia variegata*	• Same as above
5.	Neepa (Kadamba) (Fig. 4.2D)	*Anthocephalus cadamba*	• Rasa : Madhura, Kashaya, Lavana • Vipaka : Katu • Veerya : Sheeta • Guna : Guru, Ruksha
6.	Vidula (Fig. 4.2E) (Vetasa)	*Salix caprea*	• Rasa : Tikta, Katu • Vipaka : Katu • Veerya : Ushna • Guna: Laghu, Ruksha
7.	Bimbi (Fig. 4.2F)	*Coccinia indica*	• Rasa : Tikta • Vipaka : Katu • Veerya : Ushna • Guna : Laghu, Ruksha, Tikshna
8.	Shanapushpi (Fig. 4.2G)	*Crotalaria verrucosa*	• Rasa : Tikta, Katu, Kashaya • Vipaka : Katu • Veerya : Ushna • Guna : Laghu, Ruksha, Tikshna
9.	Sadapushpi (Arka) (Fig. 4.2H)	*Calotropis gigantea*	• Rasa : Katu, Tikta • Katu : Vipaka • Veerya : Ushna
10.	Pratyak pushpi (Apamarga) (Fig. 4.2I)	*Achyranthes aspera*	• Rasa : Katu, Tikta • Katu : Vipaka • Veerya : Ushna • Guna: Laghu, Ruksha, Tikshna

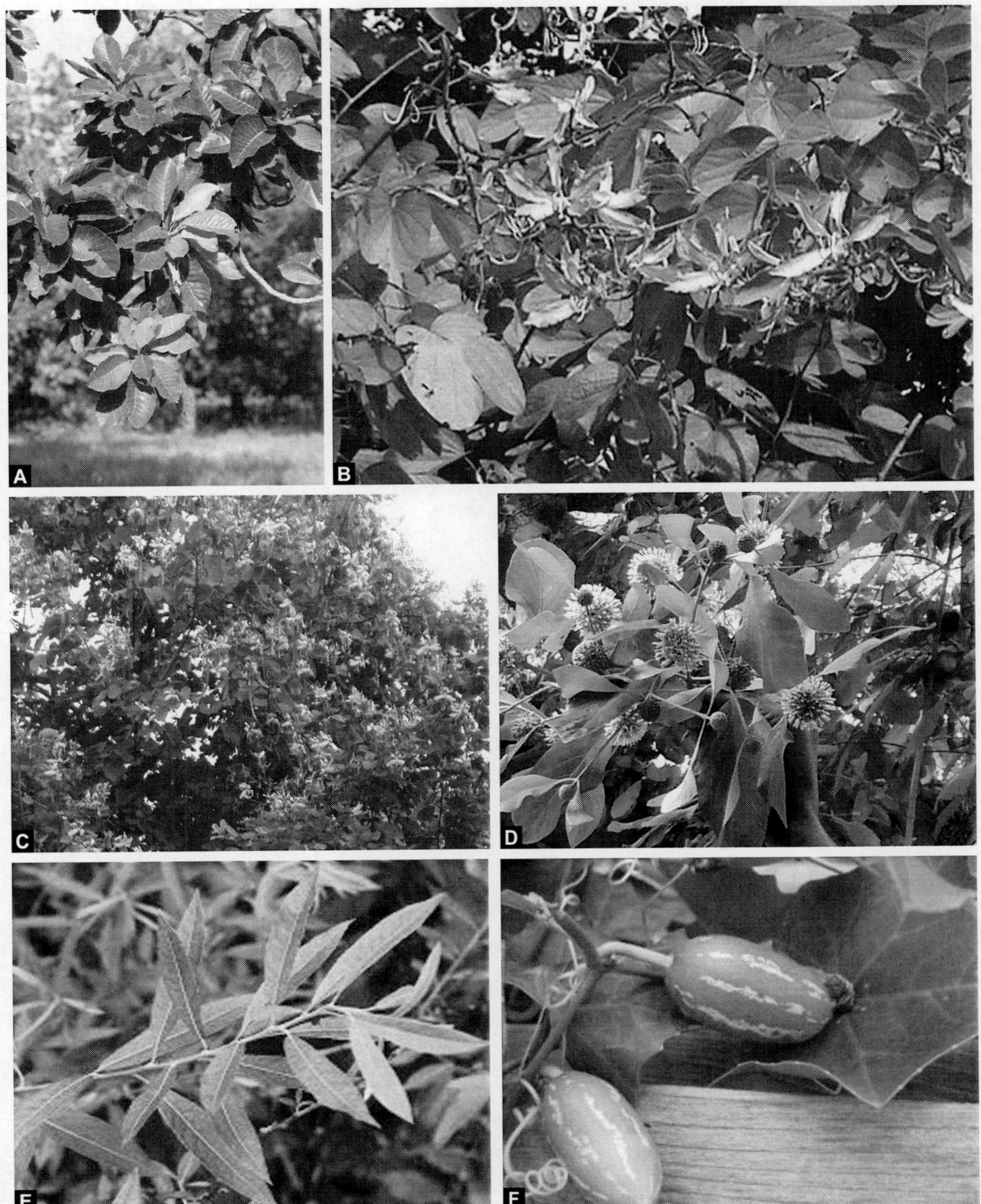

Figs 4.2A to F: Vamanopaga Dravyas

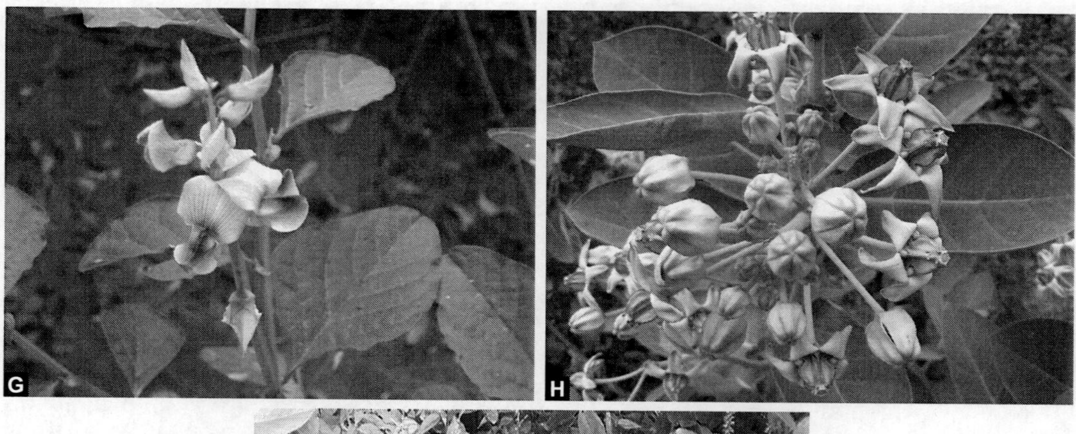

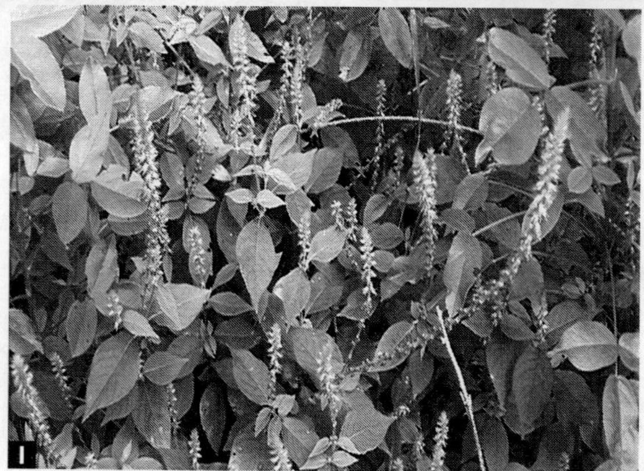

Figs 4.2G to I: Vamanopaga Dravyas

1. Madanaphala (Fig. 4.3)

Botanical Name	:	*Randia dumentorum/Rospinosa Poir*
Family	:	Rubiaceae
Synonyms	:	मदनः करहाटश्च राठः पिण्डीतकः फलम्। श्वसनश्चेति पर्यायैरुच्यते तस्य कल्पना।। (Ch.Ka.1/27) Madana, Karahaata, Raatha, Pinditaka, Phala, Shvasana.

Collection

- Madanaphala should be collected in between Vasanta (spring) and Greeshma (summer) in Pushya, Ashvini or Mrigashira Nakshatra (constellation) in Maitre Muhurtha.
- Fruits which are Pakwa (ripened), not green but are yellowish, neither touched by insects, rotten or bitten by insects, not small in size should be collected.
- It should be cleaned and bundled up in sacred grass (Durva), smeared with cow dung and kept for 8 days in a heap of Yava, Tusha, Masha, Shali, Kulattha or Mudga.

Preservation

- When the fruits have become soft (मृदुभूत) sweet and pleasant smelling (मध्विष्टगन्ध) they should be taken out and dried.
- When they are well dried, their seeds (फलपिप्पली) should be taken out.
- Seeds should be soaked and macerated with Ghrita, Dadhi, Madhu, Palala and dried again.
- (Tilapishta) Then they should be filled up to the neck in a new pot which is clean and free from dust, well closed with lid, well protected and placed securely in a swing.

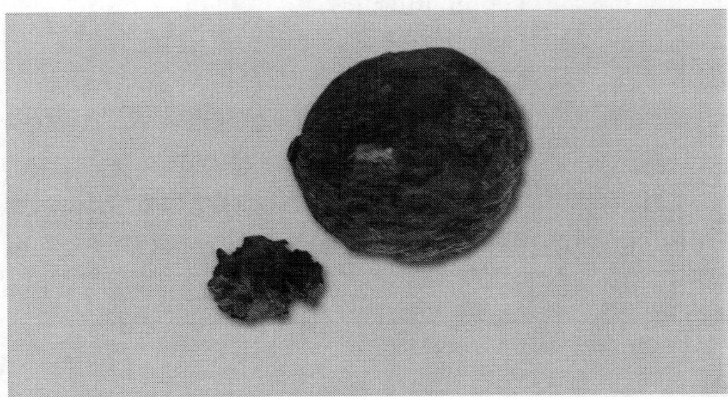

Fig. 4.3: Madanaphala

Properties

मधुरं सकषाय तिक्तकं तदरूक्षं सकटूष्ण विज्जलम्।
कफपित्तहृद आशुकारि च अपि अनपायं पवन अनुलोमि च॥ (Ch.Si. 11/14)

Rasa	:	Madhura, Tikta
Guna	:	Ruksha, Laghu
Veerya	:	Ushna
Vipaka	:	Katu
Karma	:	Kaphapittahara, Vatanulomana, Ashukari, Anapayatvam

..................., मदनं सर्व गदाविरोधि तु।

It is also said that madanphala can be given in all the diseased conditions because it does not oppose or aggravate any condition and helps in purification of all the doshas.

Yogas

Total : 133 yogas.

Kashaya : 9	Phanita : 1	Varti : 6	Utkarika : 20
Matra : 8	Churna : 1	Leha : 20	Shashkuli : 16
Payaghrita : 5	Ghreya : 1	Modaka : 20	Pupa : 16
Shadava : 10			

2. Jeemutaka

Botanical Name	:	*Luffa echinata*
Family	:	Cucurbitaceae
Synonyms	:	गरागरी च वेणी च तथा स्यात् देवताडकः। (Ch.Ka.2/3) Garagari, Veni, Devatadaka

Properties

Rasa	:	Katu, Tikta
Guna	:	Laghu, Ruksha
Veerya	:	Ushna
Vipaka	:	Katu
Karma	:	Tridoshagna
Indications	:	जीमूतकं त्रिदोषघ्नं यथा स्व औषध कल्पितम्। प्रयोक्तव्यं ज्वर श्वास हिक्कद् येषु आमयेषु च।। (Ch.Ka.2/4)

Jeemutaka is Tridoshanghna (pacifies 3 doshas). It is especially useful in Jvara, Shvasa, Hikka, etc. diseases.

Yogas

Total : 39 yogas

Ksheera : 6	Varti : 8
Madira Manda : 1	Jeevakadi : 4
Guduchyadi : 12	Ghrita : 1
Argavadhad : 7	

3. Ikshvaku

Botanical name	:	*Lagenaria vulgaris ser.*
Family	:	Cucurbitaceae
Synonyms	:	लम्बाऽथ कटुकालाबू तुम्बी पिण्डफला तथा। इक्ष्वाकुः फलिनी चैव प्रोच्यते तस्य कल्पना।। (Ch.Ka. 3/3) Lamba, Katukalabu, Tumbi, Pindaphala, Ikshvaku, Phalini

Properties

Rasa	:	Tikta
Guna	:	Laghu, Ruksha
Veerya	:	Sheeta
Vipaka	:	Katu
Karma	:	Kaphapittahara

Indications

कास श्वास विष च्छर्दि ज्वरार्ते कफकर्षिते।
प्रताम्यति नरे चैव वमनार्थ तदिष्यते।। (Ch.Ka. 3/4)

Ikshvaku is useful in Kasa, Shvasa, Visha, Chhardi, Jvara, Kaphakarshita persons.

Yogas

Total : 45 yogas

Paya : 8	Vardhamana : 6
Sura : 1	Ghrita : 1
Manda : 1	Kashaya : 9
Takra : 1	Varti : 8
Ghreya : 1	Leha : 5
Palala : 1	Mantha : 1
Taila : 1	Mansa rasa : 1

4. Dhamargava

Botanical Name	:	*Luffa cylindrica*
Family	:	Cucurbitaceae
Synonyms	:	**कर्कोटकी कोठफला महाजालिनिर् एव च।** **धामार्गवस्य पर्याया राजकोशातकी तथा।।** (Ch.Ka.4/3) Karkotaki, Kothaphala, Mahajaalini, Dhamargava, Rajakoshataki.

Properties

Rasa	:	Tikta
Guna	:	Laghu, Ruksha Teekshna
Veerya	:	Ushna
Vipaka	:	Katu
Karma	:	Kaphapittahara

Indications

गरे गुल्म उदरे कासे वातेश्लेष्म आशयस्थिते।
कफे च कण्ठ वक्रस्थे कफ संचयजेषु च।।
रोगेषु एषु प्रयोज्यं स्यात् स्थिराश्च गुरवश्चये।। (Ch.Ka. 4/4)

Gara, Gulma, Udara, Vata situated in Shleshmasthana, kapha in Kantha and Vaktra and in Kapha Sanchayavastha.

Yogas

Total : 60 yogas

Pallava : 9	Kashaya : 20	Anna : 1	Ghrita : 1
Ksheera : 4	Kalka : 2	Ghreya : 1	Vishananshaka : 1
Surasava : 1	Shakritrasa : 10	Leha : 10	

5. Kutaja

Botanical Name	:	*Holarrhena antidysenterica*
Family	:	Apocyanaceae
Synonyms	:	वत्सकः कुटजः शक्रो वृक्षको गिरिमल्लिका। बीजानि इन्द्रयवा स्तस्य तथोच्यंते कलिङ्गकाः॥ (Ch.Ka.5/4) Vatsaka, Kutaja, Shakro, Vrukshaka, Girimallika. Its seeds are called as Indrayava, Kalingaka.

Collection and Preservation

काले फलानि संगृह्य तयोः शुष्काणि निक्षिपत्। (Ch.Ka.5/7)

Fruits should be collected in their proper season and should be dried and stored.

Properties

Rasa	:	Tikta, Kashaya
Guna	:	Laghu, Ruksha
Veerya	:	Sheeta
Vipaka	:	Katu
Karma	:	Kaphapittahara
Indications	:	रक्तपित्त कफघ्नस्तु सुकुमारेषु अनत्ययः। हृद्रोग ज्वर वातासृग् विसर्पादिषु शस्यते॥ (Ch.Ka.5/6)

Raktapitta, Sukumara, Hridroga, Jvara, Vatarakta, Visarpa.

Yogas

Total:18 yogas

Kashaya : 9 Salila : 3

Churna : 5 Krishara : 1

6. Kritavedhana

Botanical Name	:	*Luffa acutangula*
Family	:	Cucurbitaceae
Synonyms	:	क्ष्वेडः कोशातकी चोक्तं मृदङ्गफलमेव च॥ (Ch.Ka.6/3) Kshveda, Koshataki, Mridangaphala.

Properties

Rasa	:	Tikta
Guna	:	Laghu, Ruksha, Teekshna
Vamana	:	Ushna
Vipaka	:	Katu
Doshaghnata	:	Kapha pitta hara

Indications

अत्यर्थ कटुतीक्ष्ण उष्णं गाढेषु इष्टं गदेषु च।
कुष्ठ पाण्ड्वामय प्लीह शोफ गुल्म गरादिषु॥ (Ch.Ka.6/4)

Diseases which are deeply seated like Kushtha, Pandu, Pleeha, Shopha, Gulma, Garavisha etc.

Yoga

Total: 60 yogas

Ksheera : 4	Varti : 6
Sura : 1	Leha : 8
Kashaya : 22	Mansa : 7
Piccha : 10	Ikshurasa : 1
Ghrita 1	

7. Yashtimadhu

Botanical Name	:	*Glycyrrhiza glabra (Linn.)*
Family	:	Fabaceae
Synonyms	:	Madhuka, Madhuyashti, Yashti, Jalaja Klitaka

Properties

Rasa	:	Madhura
Guna	:	Guru, Snigdha
Veerya	:	Sheeta
Vipaka	:	Madhura
Karma	:	Tridoshahara, Rasayana, Vrishya

8. Nimba (Fig. 4.4)

Botanical Name	:	*Azadirachta indica*
Synonyms	:	Arishta, Subhadra, Pichurarda

Properties

Rasa	:	Tikta, Kashaya
Guna	:	Laghu, Ruksha
Veerya	:	Sheeta
Vipaka	:	Katu
Karma	:	Deepana, Kaphapittahara, Krimighna
Indications	:	Jvara, Prameha, Kushtha

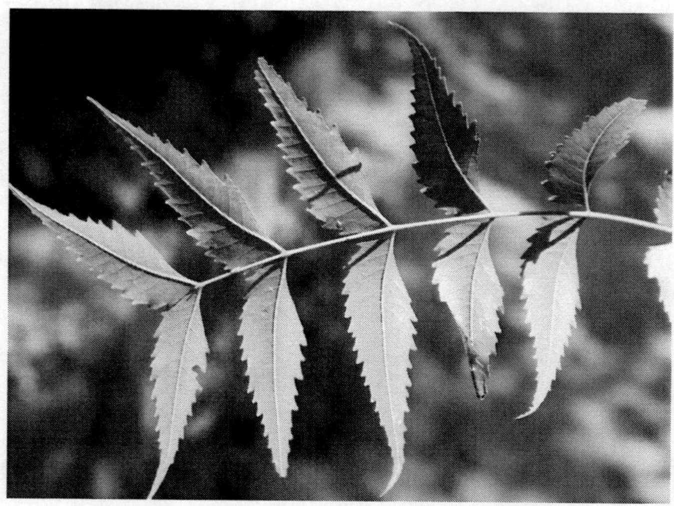

Fig. 4.4: Nimba

9. Vacha (Fig. 4.5)

Botanical name	:	*Acorus calamus*
Family	:	Araceae
Synonyms	:	Ugragandha, Shadgrandha, Golomi, Shataparvika

Properties

Rasa	:	Tikta, Katu
Guna	:	Laghu
Veerya	:	Ushna
Vipaka	:	Katu
Karma	:	Vibandhahara, Adhmanahara, Shulaghni, Shakritmutra vishodhini and Vatnulomaka.

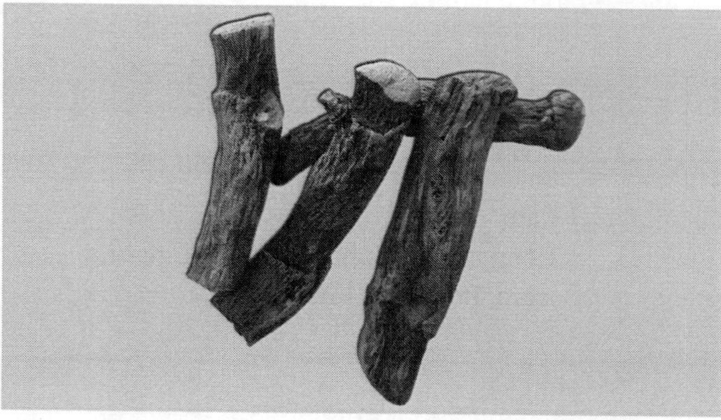

Fig. 4.5: Vacha

Bhavana Dravya According to Dosha

तानि यथादोषं प्रयुञ्जीत सुरां-सौवीरक-तुषोदक-मैरेयं-मेदक-धान्याम्ल-फलाम्ल-दध्यम्लादिभिर् वाते।
(Ch.Ka.1/12)

In vata predominant disorders emetic drugs should be given bhavana with Tushodaka, Maireya, Dhanyamla, Phalamla, Amla Dadhi, Sura, Sauveeraka, etc.

मृद्वीका आमलक-मधु-मधुक-परूषक-फाणित-क्षीरादिभिः पित्ते। (Ch.Ka.1/12)

In pitta predominant disorders emetic drugs should be given bhavana with Draksha, Amalaki, Madhu, Madhuka, Parushaka, Phanita, Gokshira, etc.

श्लेष्मणि तु मधु-मूत्रं-कषाय आदिभिर् भावितानि आलोडितानि च; इत्युद्देशः। (Ch.Ka.1/12)

In kapha predominant disorders emetic drugs should be given bhavana with Madhu, Mutra Varga and decoctions prepared with Kaphahara drugs.

PURVA KARMA OF VAMANA

Vamana should always be preceded by suitable Purva Karmas in order to mobilize the Doshas from the discreate parts of the body (Shakha). It is believed that imbalanced Doshas spread from the Koshtha to the Shakha and thus are able to produce various types of diseases depending upon the Dosha Dushya -Adhishthana pattern.

To eradicate the imbalanced Doshas, it is essential to mobilize the vitiated Doshas in the shakha to the Koshtha so that they may be easily expelled out by Vamana Karma. Snehana softens the Doshas and Svedana helps in mobilization and liquification of these Doshas. By snehana and Svedana doshas gets liquefied and move back to the Koshtha.

Therefore, appropriate Purva Karma in the form of Snehana and Svedana is always necessary.

Purva Karma

It includes

A. Sambhara sangraha (i.e. Collection of materials)
B. Atura pariksha (i.e. Examination of the patient)
C. Matra nirnaya (i.e. Deciding the dose of an emetic)
D. Atura siddhata (i.e. Preparation of the patient) includes
   A. Pachana and deepana
   B. Vamana purva bhojana vyavastha (i.e. Dietic regimen before the emetic therapy)
   C. Snehana and svedana (oleation and sudation therapy)
   D. Manasa upachara (counseling)

A. Sambhara Sangraha (i.e. Collection of Materials)

Charaka advocated to get ready for preparing Vamana karma by collecting the necessary equipments at first to which he used the term "Sambhara Sangraha". (Ch.Su.15/5).

Importance

1. He advised to do the collection of materials so well in advance, so that Vamana can be carried out safely (Samyak Yoga Pratibhogarthan) and if any complication arises during the therapy, then it can be combated immediately (Vyapatsu Vyapt Pratikararthan Cha). (Gangadhara on Ch.Su.15/5).
2. The equipments should be kept ready as it is not easy to get them immediately. This storage will be helpful in the event of emergency even if the means to buy them are available. (Ch. Su.15/3).

Collection

1. Wash basins, tubs, measuring flasks, measuring glass, towel, bowls, rubber catheter, spoons, hot plate, pitchers (small and big) etc. (Su. Chi. 33/7) Should be made available.
2. Weighing machine, glass test tubes, test tube stand, glass rod, sphigmomanometer, strips of pH paper, stethoscope, thermometer and gloves should be arranged.
3. Stalk of eranda (*Ricinus communis*) or neem (*Azadiracta indica*) and medicines to treat complications should be kept ready.
4. Similarly, the drugs to be used for vamana karma and diet articles required for the previous night and for sansarjana karma should also be kept in reservoir.

Drugs used for Vamana

Refer Vamana dravya to page no. 206.

Vamana Drugs

The description about Vamaka drugs is available throughout Samhitas at a plenty of places, which are given as follows:

Treatise	*Reference*	*Context*
Sutrasthana	1/78	Mulini drugs
Sutrasthana	1/79	Phalini drugs
Sutrasthana	1/88-89	Vamaka Lavana drugs
Sutrasthana	4/24	Vamanopaga drugs
Sutrasthana	1/114	Kshira use
Sutrastahana	2/7,8	Vamana drugs
Sutrasthana	4/5	Number of Yoga
Vimanasthana	8/139	Several drugs with several parts to be used for Vamana karma
Charaka		
Kalpasthana	1-6	Drugs described as Vamaka kalpa
Sushruta		
Sutrasthana	39/2	Vamaka drugs

Vagbhatta		
Sutrasthana	15/1	Vamaka drugs
Kalpasthana	2	Vamaka drugs (वमनविरेचन कल्पाध्याय)

Drugs used in Vamana Karma

Name of the Herbs	*Botonical name*	*Part used*
1. Madanaphala	*Randia dumetorium*	Fruit
2. Jeemutaka	*Luffa echinata*	Fruit
3. Ikshvaku	*Lagenarea vulgaris*	Fruit
4. Dhamaragava	*Luffa cylindrica*	Fruit
5. Kutaja	*Hollarrhena antidysenterica*	Root-bark, seeds
6. Kritvedhana	*Luffa acutangula*	Fruit
7. Vacha	*Acorus calamus*	Rhizome
8. Sarshapa	*Brassica campestris*	Seeds
9. Nimba	*Azadirachta indica*	Leave, fruit, bark, root.
10. Pippali	*Piper longum (Linn)*	Fruit

B. Atura Pariksha (Selection and Examination of the Patient)

Criteria

A. Vamya/Avamya - At first, one should carefully check the patient and rule out the condition whether the individual is "Vamya" (indicated for Vamana) or "Avamya" (Contraindicated for Vamana). Ch. Si. 2/8-10, Su.Chi.33/14-15, Su.Chi. 33/18, A.H.Su.18/1-6).

B. Analysis of other factors—
   1. Before leading to any karma, Charaka advised to scrutinize the difference in variations regarding dosha (bio-humors), desha (place), kala (time), bala (strength), sharira (body), satmya, satva (mind), prakriti (constitution) and vaya (age). These factors have a great potency to influence the disease and thus having ability to confuse the vaidya having great intellect (Ch.Su. 15/5).
   2. Sushruta advocated Vamana in the patients who are having augmented appetite, good strength, humors exaggerated excessively, inexorable disease and his ability to bear strainous procedure of Vamana.

C. Doshavastha—Charaka advocated "Sanshodhana treatment" in the conditions where doshas are aggravated in an excessive proportion. (Ch.Su. 16/13).

D. Inspection of Acharya—Acharya Bhela suggests that Vaidya should execute Vamana in the proper individual after watchful monitoring of the ashaya (Bh.Sa.Su.21/9). Indu comments (Indu on A.S.Su.27/3) as indications for Vamana can be categorized according to dosha dominance in disease and the site in which provocation of doshas is taking place.

E. Other criteria—
   a. Patient should be examined by 'Ashtavidha and Dashavidha Pariksha.'
   b. In present era, patient should also be examined with modern clinical examinations like git examination, respiratory system examination, cardio vascular system examination, central nervous system examination, and special examination of diseases for which vamana is being done.
   c. Pulse, blood pressure, temperature, respiratory rate and weight should be monitored during the procedure.
   D. The tests like pathological, biochemical investigations, ECG should be used for including the diseases whether vamana is contraindicated.

Caution

1. The patient must be hospitalized for Vamana karma.
2. If the patient is having some other disease or complications arised from Snehana or Svedana, then it should be treated first.(Gangadhara on Ch.Su.15/8).

C. Matra Nirnaya (Dose of the Vamaka Drugs)

The dosage of Vamaka drug has to be determined according to principles laid down in Ayurvedic classics. The quantity of the drug which produces the desired effects in the form of elimination or adequate elimination of vitiated doshas is to be regarded as the proper dose for the patient. Charaka says that the dose by which the appropriate, but not the excessive (Atiyoga) or too less (Ayoga) proportion of vitiated humors will be expelled out, can be considered as the dose for Sanshodhana. This dose will differ in every patient accordingly (Ch.Su.15/10). While illustrating the process of Vamana, Charaka elucidated the dose of Madanaphala pippali as the bulk of the same which can be kept inside the fist of an individual, i.e. Antarnakha Mushti pramana (By patient's own hand) (Ch.Ka.1/14).

The dosage of Vamana drug should be determined according to the principles laid down in Ayurvedic classics.

तत्र सर्वाण्येवौषधानि व्याध्याग्नि पुरुष बलान्याभिसमिक्ष्य विदध्यात्। (Su. Su. 39/10)

According to Sushruta, dosage of all the aushadhi shall be decided according to vyadhi bala, jatharagni and rogi bala.

अल्पमात्रं महावेगं बहुदोषहरं सुखम्।
लघुपाकं सुखास्वादं प्रीणनं व्याधिनाशनं॥
अविकारी च व्यापत्तौ नातिग्लानिकरं च यत्।
गन्ध वर्ण रसोपेतं विध्यान्मात्रावदौषधं॥ (Ch. Si. 6/15-16)

Charaka says that the dose by which the appropriate, but not the excessive (Atiyoga) or too less (Ayoga) proportion of vitiated humors will be expelled out, can be considered as the dose for Sanshodhana. This dose will differ in every patient accordingly. He has recommended the following properties for the selection of the drug for inducing emesis (Ch.Si. 6/15-16):

1. The best medicine is that which removes maximum doshas from the body with minimum dose.
2. It should produce Vegas in good manner.
3. It should be digested properly.
4. It should alleviate the disease process.
5. It should not produce any complications as well as exhaustion.
6. Its smell, color and taste should be palatable.

The quantity of the drug which produces the desired effects in the form of elimination or adequate elimination of vitiated doshas is to be regarded as the proper dose for the patient. Sushruta repeats in other words as the dose of the Kvatha, churna, avaleha, kalka can be determined after analyzing the Vyadhi bala, Purusha bala (Body) and Agni bala, i.e. Koshtha of the patient. (Su.Su.39/10). Chandranandana has amplified the view. He used the knowledge of Koshtha to determine the dose of medicine as follows (Chandranandana on A.H.18/14).

Type of Koshtha	*Dose of Medicine*
Mridu Koshtha	Lesser dose
Madhyama Koshtha	Medium dose
Krura Koshtha	High (increased) dose

Sharangdhara advised to prepare a decoction using medicines having a quantity of one Kudava in the water having quantity of one Adhaka. After reducing it to half, the same can be used for Vamana (Sha.Sam.Ut. 3/23).

Doses of Vamana Drugs According to Sharangadhara

Kalpana	*Uttama Matra*	*Madhyama Matra*	*Kaniyasi Matra*
Kvatha	9 Prastha (576 Tolas)	6 Prastha (384 Tolas)	3 Prastha (192 Tolas)
Kalka	3 Pala (12 Tolas)	2 Pala (8 Tolas)	1 Pala (4 Tolas)
Avaleha	3 Pala (12 Tolas)	2 Pala (8 Tolas)	1 Pala (4 Tolas)
Churna	3 Pala (12 Tolas)	2 Pala (8 Tolas)	1 Pala (4 Tolas)

Adhamalla quoted that though the dose seems to be quite larger and cannot be consumed at a time, one can administer it in divided doses. He also says that if the Ayoga occurs, one can have it again after adding some water in it (Adhamalla on Sha.Sam. Ut. 3/14). Kashiram doubted about mentioning the opinion of Bhela, but he himself explain the same as the later is mentioned for "Akanthapana" in the cases of poisoning or the individuals having big constitution (Kashiram on Sha.Sam.Ut.3/14).

According to Adhamalla out of one Sarava, one Adhaka can be used for a single time. Adhamalla (Adhamalla on Sha.Ut.3/14) finally concludes the opinions of Jejjata and Charaka that the Sarava is filled completely for 'sacred purposes'.

Bhela discussed in detail about the dosages.

According to him (Bh.Sa.Si.1/5-12):

Condition of an individual	*Dose*
1. Young age, good strength, affected by poison, having skin disorder, swasa (Asthma)	Uttama
2. Diseases in moderate stage with moderate strength	Madhyama
3. Disease having involvement of lesser humors and lesser strength	Laghu

If someone does not follow this rule, diseases will not be cured but several afflictions will be occurred or sometimes there may be death of the patient. So referring to Magadhamana, he described the dose of Vamaka decoction as:

Pramana	*Dose*
Kaniyasi	3 Prastha (192 तोला)
Madhyama	4 Prastha (256 तोला)
Jyeshtha	9 Prastha (576 तोला)

In the person, underlying the Vamana process for the first time one must be administerd 'Kaniyasi dose' first. For them, dose schedule will be as:

Pramana	*Dose*
Uttama	3 Pala (12 Tola)
Madhyama	2 Pala (8 Tola)
Laghu	1 Pala (4 Tola)

D. Preparation of the Patient

1. Pachana/Deepana

अजीर्णे वर्धते ग्लानिर् विबन्धश्च अपि जायते। पीतं संशोधनं चैव विपरीतं प्रवर्तते॥ (Ch.Si 6/14)

Sanshodhana medicine if administered in the condition of Ajeerna will lead to Vibandha and Glani. On the contrary, it will produce Samyak Shodhana in the absence of Ama.

सर्वदेह प्रविसृतान सामान् दोषान् न निर्हरेत्। (A.H.Su.13/28)

Vagbhatta also opined that if one tries to remove doshas in the presence of Ama by Sanshodhana, they will destroy the body.

Hence, prior to snehapana, pachana karma should be carried out. Drugs like shunthi churna, agnitundi vati, chitrakadi vati, etc. are used for the purpose.

2. Snehana Svedana

स्निग्धात् पात्राद् यथा तोयम् अयत्नेन प्रणुद्यते। कफादयः प्रणुद्यते स्निग्धात् देहात् तथौषधैः॥

(Ch.Si. 6/11)

Here Charaka quotes that Kapha glides fluently towards Koshtha through the body which is kept ready by Snehana and Svedana, in the same manner as water moves easily through the vessel coated with a layer of sneha dravya.

Chakrapani elaborates it as Snehana helps to increase 'Drava Guna' needed for the transfer of vitiated Doshas.

स्नेह स्वेदावनभ्यस्य यस्तु संशोधनं पिबेत्। दारू शुष्कमिवानामे देहस्तस्य विशीर्यते॥ (Su.Chi 33/46)

Sushruta opines Sanshodhana administered without snehana and Svedana will destroy the body easily like the dried wood.

Thus, Snehana and Svedana should be done prior to Shodhana or preventing the body from hazardous afflictions produced due to sanshodhana.

Snehapana should be administered till the Samyak Snehana symptoms are produced, generally for 3 to 7 days.

There after one-day gap should be given during which the patient should be subjected to Abhyanga and Svedana. Chakrapani while elaborating Snehana and Svedana states that Abhyanga should be done along with Svedana (particularly of vashpa type) for 2 or 3 days, i.e. on the day on which Snehapana is completed, gap day (Vishrama Kala) and day on which Vamana is to be administered.

मलो हि देहाद् उत्क्लेश्य ह्रियते वाससो यथा। स्नेह स्वेदैस् तथ उत्क्लिष्टः शोध्यते शोधनैर् मलः॥
(A.H.Su.18/58)

Vagbhatta mentions that waste products are removed from the body by Snehana and Svedana in the same way, as dirt in the cloth is removed with the help of soap and hot water.

Management of One Gapday-Abhyanga And Svedana, Diet, Special Kapha Increasing Diet

Ahara Upakalpana

Dietic regimen of the subject before vamana should be considered in the following ways:

A. Diet during the days of Snehapana

भोज्योऽन्नं मात्रया पास्यन् श्वः पिबन् पीतवानपि। द्रव उष्णं अनभिष्यन्दि नाति स्निग्धम् असङ्करम्॥
(A.H.Su.16/25)

Food having the quality of Drava – Liquid, Ushna – Warm, Anabhishyandi – (not having 'Abhishyandi') property, Pramanayukta – Regulated quantity, Na Atisnigdha – Not too much Snigdha, Asankirna – Satmya should be consumed.

The food must not have too unctuous material mixed in it. Also it should not contain the articles which may provoke any other Dosha.

B. Diet for Night before Vamana Karma

Diet for previous night of Vamana: The individual should be instructed to take Milk, krishara (Khichdi) made up of rice, black gram (Urada), Sesame (Tila) and jaggery (Guda) in enough quantity along with curd or any sweets material like Shrikhanda, etc. or food which aggravate Kapha dosha.

Need for Dietetic Regimen

i. Arunadatta mentioned that this diet helps doshas which are provoked due to proper Snehana and Svedana to move towards Koshtha due to their similar nature with later. (A.D. on A.H.Su.18/9).
ii. This diet also has the property to excite Kaphadi doshas (Kaphotklesha). (Dalhana on Su.Chi.33/6) and to minimize the pain and produces the vomiting with much less efforts (Gangadhar on Ch.Su.15/5,6).
iii. Dalhana advised to inspect the doshas which are flowing freely after losing bonds with the channels and arrange the meals accordingly. (Dalhana on Su.Chi.33/5). He further mentioned that doshas which have already become provoked, if associated with new ones excited by this type of diet, they will produce "Samyaka Yoga" otherwise "Ayoga" will occur (Dalhana on Su.Chi.33/5).
iv. But Gangadhar stroke a brilliant string by stating that "this type of diet is served, so that Kapha should neither turn dissociated nor become dense or solidified. (Gangadhara on Ch.Chi.17/23). Thus to maintain the liquified stage of the humors achieved by Snehana and Svedana during Purva karma, this type of diet should be provided.

Properties of this Diet

i. Dalhana comments over the word "Sambhojayet" as the meal containing both Pathya and Apathya together (Samashana) (Dalhana on Su.Chi.33/5).
ii. Thus it should have the properties like heavy, liquid and ability to produce secretions (Abhishyandi).

Food articles described by different texts

i. The meat of the animals of gramya, anupa and audaka origin. (Ch.Si.1/8-9)
ii. The articles made up of milk (Ch.Si.1/8-9)
iii. Sesame, black gram, curd, milk, jaggery, fishes, mutton soup, etc. (A.H.Su.16)
iv. Above articles + shali rice (Arunadutta on A.H.Su.16)

C. Diet Just Preceding to Vamana Karma

ग्राम्य आनूप औदक मांसरस क्षीरंददधिंमाषंतिलंशाकादिभिः समुत्क्लेशित श्लेष्माणं व्युषितं जीर्णाहारं पूर्वाह्ने कृत बलि होम मङ्गल प्रायश्चितं निरन्नं अनतिस्निग्धं यवाग्वा घृतमात्रां पीतवन्तं....................॥ (Ch.Ka. 1/14)

- ❑ The patient should be on empty stomach. (Nirannam).
- ❑ The Vamanopaga drugs should not be too unctuous or one may add a little unctuous material in it.(Ishat snigdham)
- ❑ The diet taken on the previous night should be digested properly before proceeding to Vamana.
- ❑ Physician can provide Yusha, Ikshurasa, Ksheera, Mansarasa, Madhya, Tushodaka, Yavagu, and Manda in relation to one's condition and articles having food value in the patients who have less strength, aged, very young age, have fear of Vamana.
- ❑ To others, just before starting Vamana, Yavagu mixed with Ghrita can be given.

Preparation of the Patient on Morning of Vamana Day

Manasopachara : Counseling

Vamana is the process which depends much more upon the mental strength of the patient (Satva). It progresses effortlessly when the patient will be satisfied regarding several doubts in one's mind about the process and prepared mentally for the same.

This process can be divided in three sections:

A. **Counseling before Vamana:**
   i. Patient already has a lot of wrong information from other people. So mental counseling by the physician is much more important to carry out the procedure of Vamana smoothly.
   ii. Before Vamana, patient must be instructed about Snehapana, Svedana, dietary regimen, administration of Vamana and Vamanopaga drugs by the physician.
   iii. He should be informed about the whole procedure and proper understanding of each step and its benefits which will encourage him.

B. **Preparation of patient before Vamana:** charaka advised to carry out the process under auspicious constellation, day, karana, and muhurta. He also says that before Vamana, "Svastivachana" should be performed by brahmins and patient.

   ॐ ब्रह्मदक्षाश्विरुद्रेन्द्रभूचन्द्रार्कानिलानलः ।
   ऋषयः सौषधि ग्रामा भुतसङ्घाश्च पान्तु ते।।
   रसायनमिवर्षीणां देवानाममृतं यथा ।
   सुधेवोत्तमनागानां भैषज्यमिदमस्तु ते।। (Ch. Ka 1/14)

   Encourge the patient by allowing him/her to have a head bath, anoint his body with several essences, wear a garland and untorn clothes. He also advocated creating an atmosphere by performing holy rituals for well-being of patient before Vamana. Nowadays, all these things may not be possible practically. However, offering a prayer to God before beginning the procedur e of Vamana karma should be done.

C. **During Vamana:** During Vamana process, patient is advised to concentrate. on Vamana process, by keeping Kama, Krodha, Lobha, Irshya, etc. factors aside. Parmeshwara, commentator of Astanga Hridaya provided a reason behind all the auspicious proceedings as "Vyapat bahulatvat" that means Vamana has a plenty of complications with it.

PRADHANA KARMA

ततस्तं पुरुषं स्नेह स्वेदो उपपन्नं अनुपहृत मनसम् अभिसमीक्ष्य सुखोषितं सुप्रजीर्ण भक्तं शिरः स्नातं अनुलिप्तगात्रं स्त्रग्विणम् अनुपहत वस्त्रसंवीतं देवता अग्नि द्विज गुरु वृद्धवैद्यानर्चितवन्तमिष्टे नक्षत्र तिथि करण मुहूर्ते कारयित्वा ब्राह्मणान् स्वस्तिवाचनं प्रयुक्त अभिराशीर्भिरभिमन्त्रितां....................। (Ch. Su.15/9)

After the person has undergone abhyanga and svedana procedures, and has had a sound sleep with peaceful mind, has digested previous day's food well, anointed his body, taken head bath, worn a garland and untorn cloth, worshipped the Diety, fire, brahmana, Guru, elders and the physicians, he should be administered vamaka yoga's after being blessed by the chanting of the brahmins (svasti vachana) performed under an auspicious day, karana and muhurta. These are the procedures that reduce the anxiety of the patient about the treatment. Hence, by this the patient is likely to cooperate in a better way.

The whole process which is to be performed from the period of oral administration of Vamana drug up to the completion of Vamana Vega may be taken as Pradhana Karma. It can be classified under four headings as follows.

It can be classified under the following four divisions, viz:

A. Administration of Vamaka Yoga
B. Observations of the Patient
C. Observations regarding Shuddhi
D. Observations about Vamana Vyapadas

A. Administration of Vamana Yoga

This can be organized in the following way:

a. Vamana Room and Position of Patient

I. After performing all the regularities in Purva karma, patient is brought in Vamana room. Charaka portrayed Vamana room beautifully. Gangadhara elaborated his points as (Gang. on Ch.Su.15/6) follows :
   1. **Dridham:** It should be built by consulting the architect. The room built in such a way can be said as 'Dridh'.
   2. **Nivatam Pravat-ekdesham:** In the room, the space should be left with less air circulation where Vamana Karma would be performed and the rest of place should be with proper ventilation.
   3. **Sukha Pravicharam:** The room should be so spacious that one can carry out the activities comfortably. It should have enough outlets for proper light and air ventilation.
   4. **Anupatyakam:** It should not situated near mountain or Upatyaka.
   5. **Dhuma Atapa Rajasam Anabhigamaniyam:** It should be protected from external dust, air, light and disturbing sounds.

II. Then patient positioned in Vamana chair, Charaka used the word: Janu-tulyasanam and "Asankirnam" (Ch.Su.15/5). That means, Vamana seat (Vamana Pitha) should have a height upto the level of knee joint (Janu-tulya Samam) and it must be comfortable one (Asankirnam). A rolling chair having cushion is more comfortable as the patient can relax on it. He may be covered with a clean cloth so that the clothes may not be spoiled by vomitus. Towels may be provided.

b. Examination of Vital Data

1. Always the weight should be recorded before starting Vamana and after the completion of Vamana.
2. The pulse rate, blood pressure, respiration rate and temperature should be recorded prior to administration of Vamana drugs. It is advised to record pulse and blood pressure at regular intervals during Vamana.

c. Administration of Vamaka and Vamanopaga Drugs

i. Now the patient is asked to take Vamanopaga drugs mentioned previously up to the full stomach. It has been stated that yavagu along with some quantity of ghrita should be given to eat just before the administration of vamaka drug. Sushruta's opinion in this regard is that kshira, dadhi, takra, yavagu; mansa rasa, etc. Should be given to weak, child and old patients (Su.Chi.33/7). Vagbhatta mentions that ikshurasa, yusha, mansa rasa, madya and tushodaka can also be given just before administration of Vamana drug. Practically, now a days, milk, sugar cane juice or decoction/hot infusion of Glycyrriza are used as Vamanopaga drugs.

   Charaka explained that Madanphala pippali was taken in antarnakha musti pramana and powdered it. Then it is mixed in the decoction of anyone of the Vamanopaga drugs such as Yashtimadhu (*Glycerrhiza glabra*), Karbudara (white variety of *Bauhinia variagata*), Nipa (*Anthocephalus indicus*), Vidula (*Salix caprea*), Bimbi (*Coccina indica*), Shanapushpi (*Crotalaria verucosa*), Sadapushpi (*Calotropis gigantea*) and Pratyakpushpi (*Achyranthus aspera*) in previous night of Vamana karma. On the day of vamana karma, this processed Madanaphala pippali kashaya or Vamana kashaya should be stirred properly with hand and then filtered. The liquid thus obtained should be slightly warm and given along with saindhava (rock salt) and madhu (honey) (Ch.Ka.1/14). But nowadays after giving vamanopaga drugs up to full stomach, vamana yoga, a paste which is prepared by Madanaphala pippali churna = 4 parts, Vacha = 2 parts and Saindhava = 1 parts mixed with honey; is given to patient for swallowing at a time. Thenafter the vamanopaga drugs are again given up to end of the process. Lastly lavanodaka was given to to expel the remaining medicine and doshas present in abdomen.

ii. There are several opinions about the time of administration of drug since ancient times, viz:
   1. Charaka advocated to administer Vamaka drug (Madanaphala pippali) with the Vamanopaga decoction (Yastimadhu) till samyaka lakshanas appear (Ch.Ka.1/14).
   2. Later on, for weak and vriddha patients, Sushruta advised to use kshira, ikshurasa, etc. at first and then to have vamaka drugs.
   3. Arunadatta invented a new method for these patients. He discloses it as to administer milk, sugarcane juice, mansa rasa etc. after providing 'Bhavana' of Vamaka drugs. (A.D. on A.H.18/10-12).
   4. Nowadays, in some parts, a different method is followed. In this method, patient is given Vamaka drugs after a glass of Vamanopaga drug. Then Vamanopaga drug is administered after each Vega till Pitta comes out.

iii. Relation of Koshtha
   1. Arunadatta has mentioned 3 types of Koshtha (A.D. on A.H.Su.8/10-11). He considered dominance of Kapha to differentiate these 3 types as:
      - Mridu Koshtha - Kapha in more quantity.
      - Madhyama Koshtha - Kapha in medium quantity.
      - Krura Koshtha - Kapha in lesser quantity.

2. Chandranandana (Chand. on A.H.Su.18/1 0-12) used the knowledge of Koshtha to decide the dose of Vamaka drugs as:
   - Mridu Koshtha - Lesser quantity of drug.
   - Madhyama Koshtha - Medium quantity of drug.
   - Krura Koshtha - Maximum quantity of drug.

B. Observation of the Patient

After administration of Vamana drug, the patient should be watched carefully for a Muhurta (48 minutes). Symptoms expressed by patient help Vaidya to judge the activities of doshas progressing in the body. They are explained under the heading of dosha gati.

Observation During the Act of Vomiting

Sushruta states that when salivation starts, the patient should be instructed to sit in a comfortable position (Su.Chi.33/7). Intimate friends whose presence would not create any disturbance to the psyche of the patient should be allowed to stay near by the patients seat (Ch.Su.15/11).

For collecting vomitus, a vessel should be kept ready. Now the patient should be instructed to vomit without much straining. The urge may be excited by opening wide the lips, palate, throat and by slightly bowing the upper part of the body. The dormant urge may be excited by tickling the throat with two well manicured fingers or with stalks of blue lily, night lotus or white water lily (Ch.Su.16/12).

During the act of emesis when actual bout is being thrown out, the forehead and chest of the patient should be held by the friend or nurse. Charaka suggests that umbilical region of the patient should be pressed and back of the patient should be gently massaged. The direction of this gentle massage of the back by hands should be in the direction from below to upwards, i.e. "pratiloma"(A.S.Su.27/14).

In Ashtanga Sangraha, it has been stressed that patient should not bow down too much or lesser extent otherwise complications will occur. (A.S.Su.27)

Hemadri reveals the complications manifesting due to wrong posture (Hemadri on A.H.18/12). He says that:

1. Extreme stretched position of neck creates the pain in back and chest (Hridaya) region.
2. Extreme forward bending causes the headache and abdominal discomfort.
3. Extreme tilting on the lateral side produces the pain in the sides of chest, abdominal region, heart and upward region.

During the procedure, Vamana Kashaya or Vamapopaga dravya explained previously can be administered repeatedly till the appearance of bile in vomitus. If the urge is weak, it should be augmented by repeated administration of the paste of Pippali, Amalaka, Sarshapa and Vacha with Saindhava and hot water until bile comes out in the vomitus. For measuring the output of vomitus, one can use the bowl for collection. Afterwards it can be measured by measuring flask or jug. To analyze the changes in pH, strips of pH paper can be used and samples of the vomitus (after each Vega) are then collected in separate test tubes for further analysis.

Administration of Vamanopaga Dravya such as Milk, Sugarcane Juice, Yashtimadhu Decoction (Administration of Vamanopaga Drugs)

Yastimadhu Phanta (Hot infusion) is generally used as Vamanopaga. Charaka explained that Antarnakha mushti pramana of Madanaphala should be soaked in the Kvatha of Vamanopaga drugs such as Yastimadhu (Glycerrhiza glabra), Karbudara (White variety of Bauhinia Variagata), Nipa (Kadamba-Anthoecephalus indicus), etc. overnight. Next day it should be macerated well and this processed medicine of Madanaphala pippali should be given along with Saindhava and honey.

Lakshana Indicating Doshagati During the Process (Observation During Vamana Karma)

पीतवन्तं तु खल्वेनं मुहूर्तमं अनुकाङ्क्षेत्, तस्य यदा जानीयात् स्वेद प्रादुर्भावेण दोषं प्रविलयनमं आपद्यमानं, लोमहर्षेण च स्थानेभ्यः प्रचलितं, कुक्षि समाध्मापनेन च कुक्षिमनुगतं, हृल्लास आस्य स्त्रवणाभ्याम् अपि च उर्ध्वमुखीभूतम्, अथास्मै जानुसममसंबाधं सुप्रयुक्त आस्तरण उत्तर प्रच्छदोपधानं सोपाश्रयमासनमुपवेष्टुं प्रयच्छेत्, प्रतिग्रहांश्च उपचारयेत्, ललाटप्रतिग्रहे पार्श्वोपग्रहणे नाभिप्रपीडने पृष्ठोन्मर्दनेचानापत्रपणीयाः सुहृदोऽनुमताः प्रयतेरन्॥ (Ch.Su. 15/11)

पीतौषधं च पाणिभिरग्नितप्तैः प्रताप्यमानं मुहूर्तमुपेक्षेत। (Su.Chi. 33/7)

After administration of Vamana drug, the patient should be allowed to sit in the chair and during the whole process he should be watched carefully. In the beginning the physician should continue to apply his warmed palm to the face and back. Patient should be kept in this position for one Muhurta or till he/she gets the Vega of Vamana, whichever is earlier. It can be understood in the following ways also;

Symptoms appeared	*Process*	*Changes are produced due to*
Appearance of Sweating (Sveda Pradurbhava) (Fig. 4.6A)	Doshas are liquefied	Due to Ushna and Tikshna properties, the Doshas are fragmented and then exuded through Shthula and Anu Strotasas
Horripilation, (Romaharsha) (Fig. 4.6B)	Doshas moving towards Amashaya	Due to Ushna property, they exude and move towards Koshtha
Discomfort in abdomen (Kukshi adhmana) (Fig. 4.6C)	Enters the Amashaya	These Doshas enter the Amashaya by Anupravana bhava (ability to flow)
Nausea, salivation (Praseka and Hrillasa), pain in chest region (Fig. 4.6D)	Doshas marching towards mouth region in upward move in upward direction	Excited by Udana Vayu, due to their Agni and Vayu predominance and self tendency to move upwards, they start to move in upward direction

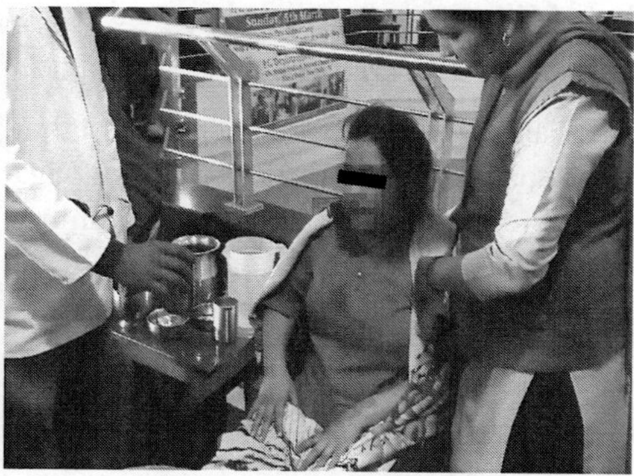

Fig. 4.6A: Sveda Pradurbhava

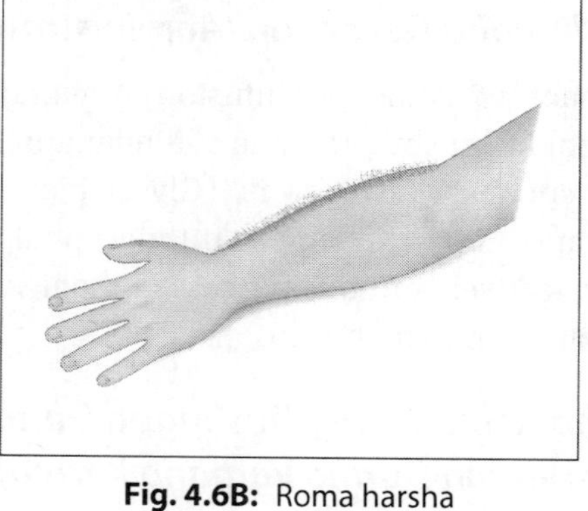

Fig. 4.6B: Roma harsha

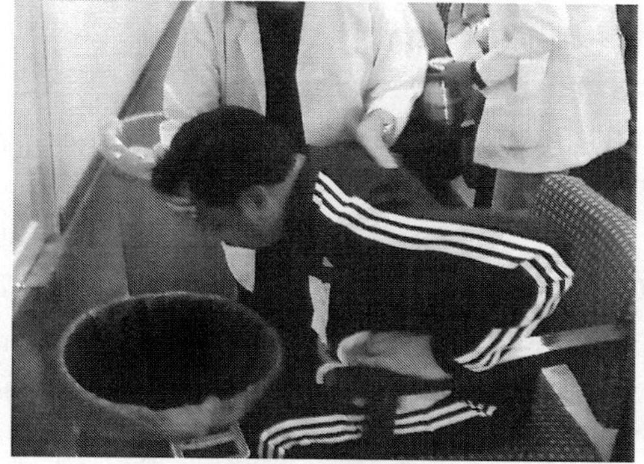

Fig. 4.6C: Kukshi adhmana and discomfort

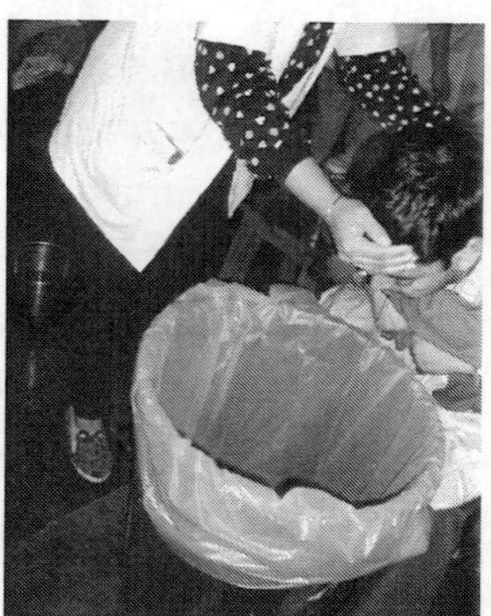

Fig. 4.6D: Hrillasa and praseka

Management During Vamana Karma and Observations (Care of the Patient During the Onset of Vamana Vega)

1. **Lalata pratigraha:** Holding at the forehead, when patient will bow down to expel vomitus. This will help to relax ones overstretched neck muscles and also prevent entry of vomitus into nose (Fig. 4.7A).
2. **Parshvopagrahana:** The muscles at the sides of the chest mainly originating from the back region and which help to keep the body straight should be supported to prevent spasm occuring due to force of vomiting.
3. **Prishthonmardana:** Gentle massage in the opposite direction over the muscles of the spine which is again a process to relax the same muscles (Fig. 4.7A).
4. **Nabhiprapidana:** This will help the abdominal muscles and diaphragm to move upwards and helps in effortless evacuation of vomitus (Fig. 4.7B).

**विवृतोष्ठ तालुकण्ठो नातिमहता व्यायामेन वेगान् उदीर्णान् अनुदीरयन् किञ्चिद्
अवनम्य ग्रीवामूर्ध्वं शरीरमुपवेगम प्रवृत्तान् प्रवर्तयन् सुपरिलिखित नखाभ्याम
अंगुलिभ्याम् उत्पल कुमुद सौगन्धिक नालैर्वा कण्ठम् अधिपृशन् सुखं प्रवर्तयस्वेति,
स तथाविधं कुर्यात्।**

(Ch.Su.15/12)

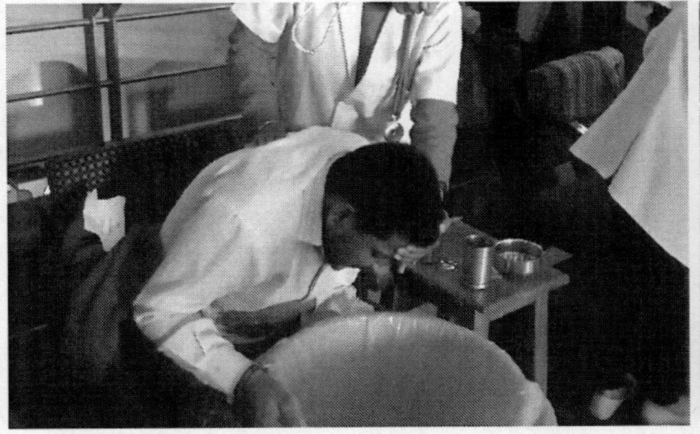

Fig. 4.7A: Lalata pratigraha and prishthonmardana

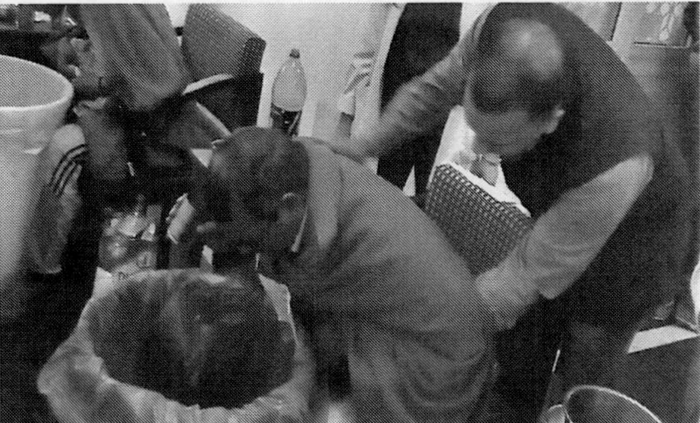

Fig. 4.7B: Nabhiprapidana

The patient should be instructed to open his mouth on feeling nauseuated and slightly bend forward, the neck and upper part of the body in the direction of vessel. The vomiting occuring without applying any force or external aid is considered best.

However, if patient needs any aid in vomiting then the root of tongue may be touched by means of finger with trimmed nails or Nala of Kamala, Eranda, etc. It has been stressed that patient should not bend down too much or lesser extent, otherwise complications may occur.

तत्र अति उन्नतस्य पृष्ठ हृदय पीडा भवति।
अति अवनतस्य शिरः कोष्ठ पीडा, पार्श्वं अपप्रवृत्तस्य पार्श्व कोष्ट हृदय ऊर्ध्व जत्रु पीडा॥
(A.S.Su.27/11 teeka)

उन्नतमूर्ध्वशिराः पार्श्वापवृत्तं तिर्यक् शिराः अवनतोऽधःशिरा॥ (A.S.Su.27/14, Ch.K.1/14)

Symptoms of Samyak Yoga, Ayoga and Atiyoga of Vamana Karma (Assessment of Vamana)

Chakrapani categorized them by naming as Aantiki, Vaigiki, Maniki and Laingiki criteria.

According to Dalhana, Vaigiki and Maniki Shuddhi may be discarded as patients have different types of Prakriti, Sara, Samhanana, Vaya and Bala, etc. and may not have Pravara Shuddhi only by 8 Vegas but may have Pravara Shudhi by more or less than 8 Vegas also.

Thus, more importance has been given to Laingiki Shuddhi. But the Shuddhi symptoms described by Charaka in Vaigiki and Maniki criteria should be considered after restricting them by Antiki criteria.

Here the Laingiki and Antiki lakshana are indicative of Samyak yoga or Ayoga of the Vamana. Where as Maniki, Vaigiki lakshanas are helpful to assess Pravara, Madhyama and Avara Shuddhi. These measures are also helpful in planning Sansarjana Krama.

Samyak Vamana Lakshanas

क्रमात् कफः पित्तम् अथानिलश्च यस्यैति सम्यग् वमितः स इष्टः।
हृत्पार्श्व मूर्ध इन्द्रिय मार्गशुद्धौ तथा लघुत्वेऽपि च लक्ष्यमाणे॥ (Ch.Si.1/15)
पित्ते कफस्यानु सुखं प्रवृत्ते शुद्धेषु हृत्कण्ठशिरः सु चापि।
लघौ च देहे कफसंस्त्रवे च स्थिते सुवान्तं पुरुषं व्यवस्येत्॥ (Su.Chi.33/9)
निर्विबन्धं प्रवर्तन्ते कफपितानिलाः क्रमात्। मनःप्रसादः स्वास्थ्यं चावस्थानं च स्वयं भवेत्।
वैपरीत्यमयोगाना न चातिमहती व्यथा॥ (A.H.Su.18/25)

Lakshana	*Meaning*	*Lakshana*	*Meaning*
Kale pravritti	Onset of Vegas on precise time	Srotasa shuddhi	Clarity in all the channels
Yathakrama dosha harana	Orderly elimination of Kapha, Pitta and Vata Dosha	Indriya Shuddhi	Clarity in all sense organs
Svayam avasthana	Stops by itself	Laghuta	Lightness
Hridaya shuddhi	Sensation of lightness in the chest	Karshya	Reduction in the body weight
Parshva shuddhi	Feeling of lightness in the sides of the body	Daurbalya	Sense of weakness
Murdha shuddhi	Lightness in the head	Kantha shuddhi	Clarity of the throat
Kapha sransrave cha stithe	Arrest of excessive salivation	Anatimahati vyatha	Not much Discomfort

Atiyoga Lakshana of Vamana Karma

तृणमोह मूर्च्छ अनिल कोप निद्रा बलादि हानिर् वमनेऽति च स्यात्। (Ch.Si.1/17)
पित्ताति योगं च विसंज्ञातां च हृत्कण्ठ पीडामपि चातिवान्ते।। (Su.Chi.33/8)
...............अतियोगे तु फेनचन्द्रकरक्तवत्।। वमितं क्षामतां दाहः कण्ठशोषस्तमो भ्रमः।
घोरा वायु आमया मृत्युर्जीवशोणितनिर्गमात्।। (A.H.Su.18/26)

Lakshana	*Meaning*	*Lakshana*	*Meaning*
Phenila vamana	Presence of froth in the vomitus	Nidrahani	Insomnia
Rakta chandrikayukta	Streaks of blood in the vomitus	Balahani	Marked reduction in the physical strength
Trisha	Excessive thirst	Hrit peeda	Chest pain
Moha	Altered state of consciousness or confused state	Kantha peeda	Pain in throat
Murccha	Transient loss of consciousness	Tamah pravesha	Darkness in front of eyes
Vata prakopa	Provocation of vata	Bhrama	Giddiness
Daha	Burning sensation	Pittati yoga	Excessive loss of pitta dosha
Mrityu	Death in extreme cases		

Ayoga Lakshana of Vamana Karma

दुश्छर्दिते स्फोटक कोठ कण्डू हृत् ख अविशुद्धिः गुरूगात्रता च। (Ch.Si 1/16)
कफप्रसेकं हृदय अविशुद्धिं कण्डूं च दुश्छर्दितलिंगमाहुः।। (Su.Chi.33/8)
प्रवृत्तिः सविबन्धा वा केवलस्यौषधस्य वा। अयोगस्तेन निष्ठीव कण्डू कोठ ज्वारादयः।। (A.H.Su.18/24)

Lakshana	*Meaning*	*Lakshana*	*Meaning*
Apravritti	Inadequate bouts of vomiting	Kevala aushadha pravritti	Vomitus containing only the medicine
Hridaya avishuddhi	Lack of clarity in chest	Vega vibandha	Obstructed bouts of vomiting
Srotasa avishuddhi	Lack of clarity in body channels	Kandu	Itching
Gurugatrata	Sense of heaviness in the body	Kapha praseka	Excessive salivation
Sphota	Different forms of eruptions in the skin	Jvara	Fever
Kotha	Different forms of eruptions in the skin	Pratiloma pravritti	Evacuation through anal route

C. Observations Regarding Shuddhi

Vamana and Virechana are the Sanshodhana processes carried out to remove the morbid doshas mainly Kapha and Pitta from body. Both these doshas have the nature of dravya, i.e. they have definite color, taste, odor, and consistency. To assess the quantity and nature of the vitiated doshas and to assess the effects achieved after Sanshodhana, Charaka at first, coined some definite parameters. Chakrapani categorized them by naming as Aantiki, Vaigiki, Maniki and Laingiki criteria (Ch.Si.1/14-16).

It seems that there remained a lot of controversies amongst the commentators for awarding one as "the best criteria" among these special four criteria. Adhering to that, a plenty of theories were put on and think over. Out of them some succeeded to achieve the conclusion. But till now, it remained one of the most fascinating points for debate among the learned scholars of Ayurveda.

Chakrapani and Dalhana both had a very comprehensive commentary about these 4 aspects and their intricate nature in assessing the Vamana. Chakrapani quotes the 4 criteria at first but later on counts 'Antiki Shuddhi' under 'Laingiki' one. (Chakr. on Ch.Si.1/14-16). Dalhana elucidates 3 criteria, viz. Laingiki Shuddhi/ Vaigiki Shuddhi/ Maniki Shuddhi and not explained 'Antiki Shuddhi' separately (Dal. on Su.Chi.33/9). At last, both of them clearly approve "Laingiki Shuddhi" is the most acceptable one and not the others.

Explanation by Dalhana (Dal. on Su.Chi.33/9)

Vaigiki Shuddhi— Vamana karma with the shuddhi in Vega that projected out in numbers of 4,6,8 is considered as 'Vaigiki shuddhi.' He puts aside Vaigiki criteria. While expounding the purpose to think so, he says that sometimes after expulsion of plaintive bouts through process of Vamana, complete purification may not be manifested. There is always a countless uncertainty in assessing the purification through Vamana concerning to number of Vega. The purification may occur in varying number of Vega which is influenced by the factors like body consistency, age and strength of an individual.

Maniki Shuddhi: Maniki shuddhi is defined as the shuddhi in which the proportions of Hina, Madhyama, and Uttama shuddhi are 1/2, 1 and 2 Prastha, respectively. He casts off 'Maniki Criteria' by saying that there is a huge diversification in the texture, consistency, composition of various individuals regarding the factors like tallness, dwarfism, obesity, emaciation, body consistency, prakriti, satva and by the fact that dosha, dhatu, mala have no dimensions.

Laingiki Shuddhi: The signs and symptoms featured in 'Samyaka Lakshana' can be considered under 'Laingiki Criteria.' After resoluting the various opinions, he concludes that the symptoms told in Samyaka Yoga should be recognized as 'Laingiki Shuddhi.'

Explanation By Chakrapani

Chakrapani says that 'Jaghanya, Madhyama and Utkrishta Shuddhi' are told to understand dosha proportion which is removed out through them. The Shuddhi regarding Vega is explained on the basis of observations which were frequently noticed during several processes of Vamana. Also the Shuddhi based on "Mana" is also relative. During Vamana, if 1 prastha vomitus is expelled through 4 Vega, it can be said a Jaghanya Shuddhi. In the similar fashion one can ascertain other two Shuddhi (Madhyama and Utkrishta) also. But the Shuddhi symptoms described by Charaka in 'Vaigiki' and 'Maniki' criteria should be considered after restricting them by "Antiki Criteria". That means, in both types of Shuddhi, the rule says that Pitta should arrive last, must be followed. Otherwise a lot of confusion will be created if someone claims of Jaghanya Shuddhi without finding Samyaka Shuddhi Lakshana and Pittantatwa, just on the basis of quantity expelled and Vega imparted under "Jaghanya Shuddhi" (Ch.Si.1/14,15). Further he comments about 'Anila Gamana,' after Pitta expulsion that it is indication of total expulsion of Kapha and Pitta and nothing is remained back in Amashaya (Chakrapani on Ch.Si.1/14-16).

Conclusion

When one goes through all the textual references regarding these criterias, there is a debate over the point that which criteria must be followed for assessment. But, if studied critically, all these four criteria have to be used by Vaidya while following the procedure which is as follows:

1. Charaka when explained the process of Vamana in Kalpasthana has mentioned to continue the procedure till Pitta comes out. So, Vaidya has to concentrate on Pittanta criteria while directing the process. At that time he does not emphasize on the quantity of doshas expelled or number of vegas occurred.
2. After completion of process when time comes to set "The sequence for Sansarjana", one should review the quantity of Doshas expelled (Maniki Pariksha) and counts the number of Vegas (Vaigiki Pariksha) expelled. Decision over the nature of Shuddhi is taken and Sansarjana krama is set upon.
3. After completion of "Sansarjana krama" when one has to decide the 'Treatment regime.' Now Vaidya should consider all the 3 parameters, correlate them with the proportion and placement or Doshas, observe the symptoms and set the treatment regime.

Vaigiki Shuddhi

The root word is 'Vij' and by conversion as "Vij Ghan", the word "Vega" is received. It denotes the meaning like impulse, speed, velocity, force, stream, activity, power, force and sudden impulse. It is also expressed as Pravaha, Odha, Veni, Dhara in Shabdakalpadruma (By Hemachandra). They all convey about the nature of bout. Thus, Vaikigi criteria is nothing but to contemplate the Vega for its nature, force, strength, speed, etc. The analysis of Vega regarding its several factors constitutes 'Vaigiki criteria' which are as follows:

1. Only Charaka emphasizes on the observations based on Vega. Sushruta and Vagbhatta have ignored the Vaigiki Pariksha completely. Charaka described 3 types of Shuddhi naming them as Hina, Madhyama and Pravara Shuddhi when 4, 6 and 8 no. of Vega come out respectively. (Ch.Si.1/14-16).
2. In Kashyapa Samhita, Kashyapa mentioned an opinion of another author named as "Kotsa" (Ka.Sam.Si. 3), who says that Shuddhi can be called as 'Kaniyasi' producing 2-3 Vega, Madhyama having 4-5 Vega and Uttama having 6-7 Vega. There is no direct reference available in Samhitas which will define the word "Vega". Indu, for the first time provides definition of Vega as **"सुखादागत: प्रतिग्राहप्राप्तो वेग उच्यते"** (Indu on A.S.Su. 27/16)
   Where 'Pratigraha' means a bowl in which Vega is collected. "The bout collected in a bowl after an effortless expulsion" is termed as 'Vega'. There is another word Upavega used by to Charaka which is defined by Chakrapani as **"उपवेगं वेग समीपम्"** (Chakrapani on Ch.Su.15/12), i.e. Upavega means nearer to Vega which can be explained as lesser in every aspect than Vega.

Explanation

While detailing the terms Vega and Upavega, one should provide much attention to the way in which both are produced and thrown out. There is a large variety observed in the production of Vega and Upvega by every patient.

Following factors are important to differentiate Vega and Upvega:

A. **Quantity**
   1. Vega and Upavega are 'relative' terms. The prime factor which marginates them is the difference in quantities.
   2. Mostly Vega counts more quantity than Upavega. It is expected that Vega will collect more doshas for removal than Upavega.

B. **Force**— Indu used the word 'Sukhaat Agatah' means Vega should be easily and effortlessly expelled out. When one uses the word 'force' of Vega. It means that the Vega produced against 'the force of gravity', the muscles helping to it; have to act against force of gravity when they throw the Vega out. So the bout which will require much force to expel the morbid material may be termed as "Mahavega/Vega" because doshas are accumulating in "the Amashaya" and to expel the material from the Amashaya, i.e. stomach will require much more force than those which will be thrown back through esophagus or oropharyngeal region.

C. **Time**

1. Most of the patients expel the bout at a sudden stroke using very little time. The force in it is more and the quantity is also more. So one can easily identify and define it as "Vega".
2. But some may produce less quantity in a bout which is coming from the bottom of the stomach, but duration for expulsion will be prolonged in a break less stream which can be nomenclatured as "Vega".

So while defining the term "Vega", the factor time/duration taken for expulsion should be taken in consideration.

So, one can easily define 'Vega' on the basis of the above 3 factors.

Acharya have also advocated to observe Upavega carefully, but not mentioned the number of Upavega while assessing Shuddhi. So one can include the Upavega expelled before and after the major Vega in one group of Vega and name them as one Vega. Thus, by counting these major Vega only, one can reach nearer to counting set by Acharyas as 4,6 and 8 Vegas in Hina, Madhyama or Pravara Shuddhi, respectively.

Importance of Assessing each Vega

1. Experts in assessment of Vamana observe each Vega carefully because they can intimate about Hina, Madhyama or Pravara Shuddhi through (after analyzing) it, which helps them for planning 'the Sansarjana Krama' (Gangadhara on Ch.Su.15/5,6).
2. Gangadhara explains that Vaidya can make prompt decisions after smelling any severe complication which is going to arrive, by keeping his mind alert and assessing each Vega carefully.
3. The quantity wise measurements of the vomitus after each Vega gives the clear idea about the drug which is residing inside.
4. One can observe the changes in color, pH and consistency occurring after each Vega.

Maniki Shuddhi

It is derived from the root verb "Man." The word holds the meanings like the measurement. The criteria assisting to count the magnitude of humors (removed in the vomitus) is named as "Maniki criteria". While narrating the Hina, Madhyama, Pravara Shuddhi, Charaka mentioned the quantities of the same as one, one and half, two Prastha, respectively. Chakrapani considered them under the term 'Maniki Pariksha' (Ch.Si.1/14).

Explanation

When Acharya indicated that Sanshodhana karma should be done in "Bahudoshavastha", the word "Bahu"indicates the increased Kapha or Pitta or vitiated matter. It is increased by all means, i.e. Gunatah (qualitatively), Karmatah (functionally) and Dravyatah (quantitatively) also.

So the Maniki Pariksha highlights the quantitative analysis of the vomitus, i.e. the quantity of Kapha or Pitta that is to be expelled out.

Note: According to Chakrapani:

1 Prastha = 13½ Pala = 54 Tola = 540 g or mL (If 1 Tola = 10 g/mL approx) = 648 g or mL (If 1 Tola = 12 g/mL approx.)

So according to Chakrapani, the magnitudes of humors expelled in terms of Shuddhis are:

Hina Shuddhi = 1 Prastha = 540 or 648 mL; 1 Prastha = 540 or 648 g

Madhyama Shuddhi = 1½ Prastha = 810 or 972 mL; 1½ Prastha = 810 or 972 g

Pravara Shuddhi = 2 Prastha = 1080 or 1296 mL; 2 Prastha = 1080 or 1296 g

But according to Magadha and Kalinga Maana (Which is told by Acharya Charaka) 1 Prastha = 16 Pala = 64 Tola = 640 g or mL (If 1 Tola = 10 g/mL approx.) = 768 g or mL (If 1 Tola = 12 g/mL approx.)

So according to Charaka, the probable magnitudes of humors expelled are - Hina Shuddhi = 1 Prastha = 640 or 768 mL 1 Prastha = 640 or 768 g

Madhyama Shuddhi - 1½ Prastha = 960 or 1152 mL, 1½ Prastha = 960 or 1152 g

Pravara Shuddhi - 2 Prastha = 1280 or 1536 mL, 2 Prastha = 1280 or 1536 g

Thus, during each type of purification, the matter in respective proportions should be expelled out.

Importance

1. It will help to know in better views about the nature of Kapha, Pitta present in the body.
2. It will help us to assess the differences or deviations getting after the usage of various types of Vamanopaga drugs.
3. It will help us to judge directly the quantity of Kapha and Pitta vomited during Vamana.

Antiki Shuddhi

The root word is 'Ant' derived as 'Ant An' meaning final or terminal. Thus, "Antiki" word points towards 'the criteria' needed in the final stages. The symptoms telling that Vamana has entered in the terminal phase can be considered as "Antiki Lakshanas" and Criteria as "Antiki Shuddhi or Antiki Criteria."

Description Available in Ayurvedic texts

1. Charaka set a feature to cease Vamana at a particular point. He advised to continue Vamana till bout of Pitta are not appeared (Ch.Ka.1). Later on, while describing "Ishta Vamana", he provided a clue that Vamana should be Pittanta and at last when time comes to reveal Samyaka Vamana Lakshanas", he confidently claimed that in "Samyaka Vamana", Kapha should be succeeded by Pitta. (Ch.Si.1/15).
2. Chakrapani while analyzing this, clearly advocated inclusion of Pittanta criteria in Laingiki Shudhi and proposed both of them by a single nomenclative as "Laingiki Criteria ", Thus, according to Charaka, "Antiki Criteria" is framed with "Laingiki Criteria".
3. Afterwards, Sushruta included the symptom, "Kapha followed by Pitta" in the "common symptoms of Samyaka Vamana" and ruled out any parameter such as Antiki Criteria (Su. Chi.33/8, 9).

4. But Vriddha Vagbhatta, for the first time, dissected this 'Antiki criteria' distinctly, aiming at its practical importance (A.S.Su.27). He arranged this criterion in a beautiful manner. He advised to continue Vamana till (a) Kapha Chheda: When Kapha will start to be diminised and will exude in a lesser quantity. (b) Kevalam Aushadha Pravritti: After curtailed Kapha, only medicine will begin to ooze out. (c) Pitta Darshanam Va: or till the appearance of Pitta.

Pittanta (Fig. 4.8)

"Appearance of Pitta" as:

Color: A greenish yellow

Taste: Bitter or Pungent taste, (Sour taste also) (Ch.Su.1).

Symptoms: It produces certain symptoms while coming through "Amashaya" like burning sensation in chest or throat or eyes (Urodaha, Kanthadaha, Netradaha, respectively). When all the aspects explained above or some of these begin to appear, Vaidya can conclude about achievement of "Pittanta criteria" and can end Vamana process. Thus "Antiki criteria" requires:

1. Vamana having Pitta as an end point.
2. The Symptoms telling about the Samyaka Vamana.

Importance

1. This is the most valuable criteria assisting Vaidya in making the decision whether to carry on or cease the process of Vamana.
2. It indicates about the complete expulsion of Kapha dosha.
3. It limits the Vamana process. That means, it warns the physician from proceeding further and creating 'Atiyoga' of Vamana.

Procedure

To decide "Pittanta Lakshana", one has to ask the patient about symptoms like pungent or bitter taste in mouth (Katukasyata or Tiktasyata), Netradaha, Kanthadaha, Urodaha, etc. for deciding whether Pitta is coming or not. One has to be very watchful about changes in color of vomitus also, because these are the criteria which will indicate about the arrival of Pitta in vomitus.

Laingiki Shuddhi

The word "Lingam" represents the meanings like a mark, sign, taken a badge, and symbol. Hence the term 'Laingiki' signifies the explanation as relating to a sign or mark depending on or inferred.Thus Laingiki criteria deals with the signs or markings presenting after proper Vamana (Samyaka Vamana). In other words, the Samyak, Hina and Atiyoga should be confirmed on the basis of the signs and symptoms described for this purpose and it is known as Laingiki Shuddhi.

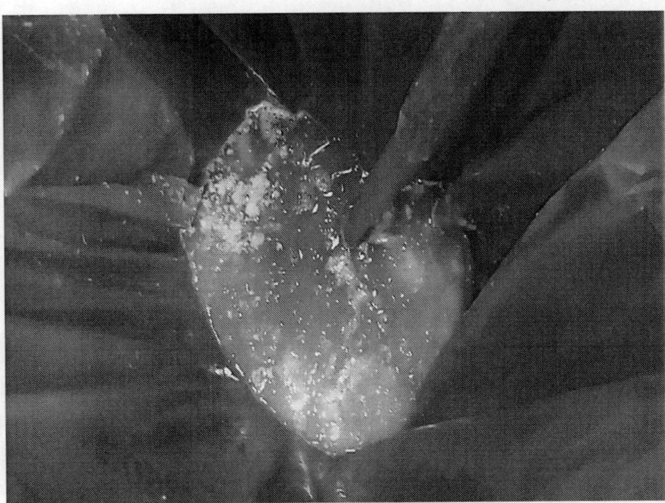

Fig. 4.8: Pittanta

Description available in Ayurvedic texts

1. Chakrapani undoubtedly declares that there is little existence of other Shuddhi except 'Laingiki one'. He moreover goes on claiming that Laingiki Shuddhi is the only Shuddhi.
2. Deliberately including Antiki criteria in this, he says there is little doubt about its importance. So, the symptoms described for Samyaka Vamana and Pittanta criteria both comprise "Laingiki criteria".
3. Sushruta has mentioned only Laingiki Shuddhi (Su.Chi.33/5). According to Dalhana Vaigiki and Maniki Shuddhi may be discarded as the patient having different types of Prakriti, Sara, Samhanana, Vaya and Bala, etc. may not have Pravara Shuddhi only by 8 Vegas but have Pravara Shuddhi by more or less than 8 Vegas also. Thus more importance has been given to Laingiki Shuddhi.

Laingiki Criteria has two Aspects, viz

1. Symptoms arising immediately after Vamana: Chakrapani and Dalhana both included Pittanta criteria in the Laingiki criteria.
2. Symptoms arising after some duration after completion of Sansarjana krama: So the goal behind the conduction of Vamana is to check the disease or minimize the symptoms in it. Hence, a Laingiki criteria is much more emphasized by all the commentators.

Importance

1. This decides when Vamana should be stopped (End point of Vamana).
2. Chakrapani says that Samyaka Vamana is portrayed to hold Vaidya back from preceding towards Atiyoga or from preventing him to cause Ayoga.
3. It helps Vaidya for prescribing correct regimen of medicine after Sanshodhana.

Symptoms

They can be divided into two categories:

A. The symptoms appearing immediately after Vamana—It includes Samyaka Yoga, Atiyoga and Ayoga Lakshanas. But Acharya Sushruta describes Atiyoga and Ayoga under 15 types of Vamana Vyapadas.
B. The symptoms occurring after a span of time which are as follows:
(1) Svasthata (2) Svara Vishuddhi (3) Ruchi (4) Laghava (5) Koshtha Tanutwa

PASHCHATA KARMA

सम्यग्योगेन वमितं क्षणमाश्वास्य पाययेत्। धूमत्रयस्यान्यतमं स्नेह आचारम् अथादिशेत्।। (A.H.Su.18/27)
ततः सायं प्रभाते वा क्षुद्वान् स्नातः सुखाम्बुना। भुञ्जानो रक्तशाल्यन्नं भजेत्पेयादिकं क्रमम्।। (A.H.Su.18/28)
ततोऽपराह्ने शुचि शुद्धदेहम् उष्णाभिरद्भिः परिषिक्तगात्रम्। कुलत्थ मुद्र आढकि जाङ्गलानां यूषै रसैवाऽप्युपभोजयेत्तु।। (Su.Chi 33/11)

After completion of Vamana, all types of care has to be taken, till the patient starts taking the normal diet, and it may be grouped under Pashchata Karma. It may be subdivided into four groups, viz. Dhumapana, Pariharya vishaya, Sansarjana krama and Santarpana chikitsa.

Dhumapana (Fig. 4.9)

सम्यग्वान्तं चैनमभि समीक्ष्य स्नेहन विरेचन शमनानां धूमानामन्यतमं सामर्थ्यतः पाययित्वाऽऽचारिकमादिशेत्।। (Su.Chi 33/10)

योगेन तु खल्वेनं छर्दितवन्तमभिसमीक्ष्य सुप्रक्षालित पाणिपादास्यं मुहूर्तमाश्वास्य,
स्नैहिकवैरेचनिकोपशमनीयानां धूमानामन्यतमं सामर्थ्यतः पाययित्वा, पुनरेवोदकमुपस्पर्शयेत्।। (Ch.Su 15/14)

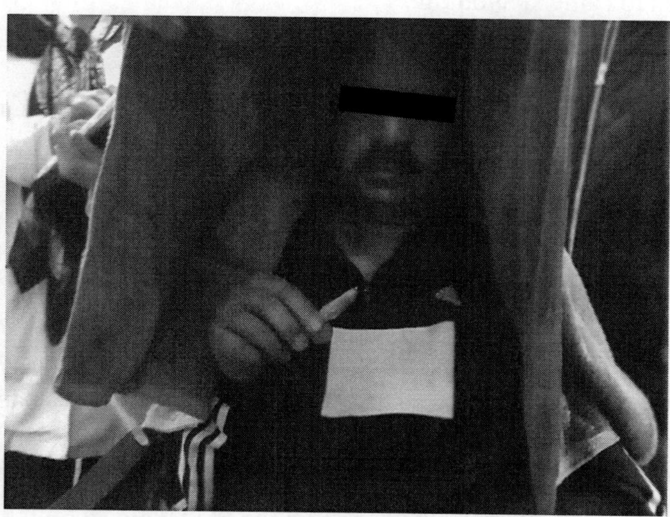

Fig. 4.9: Dhumapana

After completion of Vamana, hands, feet and face of the patient should be washed with Sukoshna Jala (Luke warm water). There after Dhumapana should be given. The type of Dhumapana, i.e. Snaihika, Vairechanika, Shamana depends upon the condition of the patient. After administration of Dhumapana, the patient should be asked to wash his feet and hand again.

Vagbhatta adds that the patient should be given tambula to eat and that the patient should be allowed to rest in a nivata griha with comfort. Although it is important that the patient should not lie down straight as it will lead to Kapha vriddhi, rather they should be rested in half lying position. It is also mentioned to follow all the regimen from Pashchat karma of Snehana.

Charaka adds that the patient shall be taken to Nivata griha and advised to not to undergo the Ashta mahadoshkara vishaya; avoid viruddha, apathya and guru ahara, also not to undergo vegodirana and vega vidharana.

Vangasena says that after Vamana karma, apart from all the above precautions sneha abhyanga too shall not be done.

वमनानन्तरं स्त्रोतोविलग्रकफहरणार्थं धूमपानमत्रोक्तम्॥
वातप्रकृतौ स्नैहिकं, कफपित्तप्रकृतात् उत्क्लिष्ट दोषे च वैरेचनिकं, समदोषप्रकृतात्
उपशमनीयं प्रायोगिकं स्वस्थवृत्तिकं इत्यर्थः। (Su.Chi. 33/10 teeka)

Dalhana is of the view that Pashchata karma is undertaken for removing the remaining Kapha Dosha. According to him, Dhumapana is very useful for Kapha which is still sticking to the Srotasa.

Further Dalhana mentions, Snaihika Dhumapana should be given to the patient who has Vata Prakriti. lf the patient is of Kapha or Pitta Prakriti and Utklesha of Dosha is present, Vairechanika Dhumapana should be prescribed. Shamaniya or Prayogika Dhumapana is indicated in the case of Sama Dosha Prakriti and Svastha person.

Peyadi Sansarjana Krama and Tarpanadi Krama with their specific Indications

Sansarjana Krama

The specific diet prescribed after Vamana Karma till the patient starts taking his normal diet is called as Sansarjana Krama. Due to the Shodhana done by Vamana, weakness, loss of weight, freeness of Sandhi Bandhana, decrease in the Agni and emptiness in respective Ashaya due to expulsion of Vata, Purisha, Mutra, Kapha and Pitta is observed. Therefore patients cannot tolerate any type of chikitsa or diet, other than prescribed for this purpose.

संशोधनाभ्यां शुद्धस्य हृतदोषस्य देहिनः। यात्यग्निर्मन्दतां तस्मात् क्रमं पेयादिमाचरेत्॥ (Ch.Si 6/24)

Due to Dosha elimination from the body after Sanshodhana Karma, Agni becomes hampered. In order to restore the strength of Agni and Prana, Peyadi sansarjana krama should be followed.

यथाणुरग्निस्तृण गोमयाद्यैः सन्धुक्ष्यमाणो भवति क्रमेण। महान् स्थिरः सर्व पचस्तथैव शुद्धस्य पेयादिभिरन्तरग्निः॥ (Ch.Si. 1/12)

Charaka reveals its importance by giving example that small sources of fire, if simulated by adding small and light fuel, later on become so big that it can burn anything. Similarly, by applying sansarjana krama, Jatharagni can be increased to such an extent that it can digest all types of food.

Sansarjana Krama According to Strength

बलं यत्त्रिविधं प्रोक्तमतस्तत्र क्रमस्त्रिधा। तत्रानुक्रममेकं तु बलस्थः सकृदाचरेत्॥
द्विराचेन् मध्यबल स्त्रीन् वारान् दुर्बलस्तथा। केचिदेवं क्रमं प्राहुर्मन्दमध्योत्तमाग्निषु॥ (Su.Chi 39/18)

Sushruta mentioned that Sansarjana sequence can be followed by considering the strength of the patient. He says 3 types of Bala exist; Sansarjana Krama should also be adopted accordingly. For the individuals having good strength, three Annakalas are advocated, two annakala for the individuals of medium strength and in the individuals with lesser strength only one annakala is advised.

Divisions of Sansarjana Krama: Charaka classified Sansarjana Krama into two divisions as:

(A) Peyadi Sansarjana Krama

अथैनं सायाह्ने परे वाऽह्नि सुखोदक परिषिक्तं पुराणानां लोहितशालितण्डुलानां
स्ववक्लिन्नां मण्डपूर्वां सुखोष्णां यवागूं पाययेद् अग्निबलं समीक्ष्य, एवं द्वितीये तृतीये चान्नकाले,
चतुर्थेत्वन्नकाले तथाविधानामेव शालितण्डुलानामुत्स्विन्नां विलेपी उष्णोदक द्वितीयाम्
अस्नेहलवणाम् अल्पस्नेहलवणां वा भोजयेत्, एवं पञ्चमे षष्ठे चान्नकाले,
सप्तमे त्वन्नकाले तथाविधानामेव शालीनां द्विप्रसृतं सुस्विन्नम् ओदनम् उष्णोदक
अनुपानं तनुना तनुस्नेहलवण उपपन्नेन मुद्गयूषेण भोजयेत् एवमष्टमे नवमे चान्नकाले,
दशमे त्वन्नकाले लाव कपिञ्जलादीनाम् अन्यतमस्य मांसरसेन औदकलावणिकेन
नातिसारवता भोजयेद् उष्णोदक अनुपानम्; एवमेकादशे द्वादशे चान्नकाले; अत
ऊर्ध्वमन्नगुणान् क्रमेणोपभुञ्जानः सप्तरात्रेण प्रकृतिभोजनमागच्छेत्॥ (Ch.Su 15/16)

After Vamana process (Sanshodhana Karma), the "Peyadi sequence" is advised as diet regimen as follows :

Days	*Annakala*	*Pravara Shuddhi*	*Madhyama Shuddhi*	*Avara Shuddhi*
I	1 morning	–	–	–
	2 evening	Peya	Peya	Peya
II	1 morning	Peya	Peya	Vilepi
	2 evening	Peya	Vilepi	Krita/ Akrita Yusha
III	1 morning	Vilepi	Vilepi	Krita/ Akrita Mansa rasa
	2 evening	Vilepi	Akrita Yusha	Normal diet
IV	1 morning	Vilepi	Krita Yusha	–
	2 evening	Akrita Yusha	Akrita Mansa rasa	–
V	1 morning	Krita Yusha	Krita Mansa rasa	–
	2 evening	Krita Yusha	Normal diet	–

Contd...

Contd...

Days	*Annakala*	*Pravara Shuddhi*	*Madhyama Shuddhi*	*Avara Shuddhi*
VI	1 morning	Akrita Mansa rasa	–	–
	2 evening	Krita Mansa rasa	–	–
VII	1 morning	Krita Mansa rasa	–	–
	2 evening	Normal diet	–	–

पेयां विलेपीमकृतं कृतं च यूषं रसं त्रिर्द्विरथैकशश्च। क्रमेण सेवेत विशुद्धकायः प्रधान मध्य अवर शुद्धि शुद्धः॥ (Ch.Si 1/11)

Peya—Rice is cooked by adding fourteen times of water and is boiled till the rice is almost dissolved to become liquid and that is known as Peya.

Vilepi— Rice is cooked by adding four times of water so that it becomes semi-liquid and it is termed as Vilepi (Sharnghadhara Madh. 2: 166-167).

Yusha— 6 times of water is added to anyone of the pulses and it is cooked properly so that it contains more liquid and little solid. When it is taken as such without adding any thing, then it is termed as Akrita Yusha, but when added with salt and condiment as well as prepared (Sanskarita) with ghee then it is named as Krita Yusha.

Mansa Rasa—Cleaned meat cut into small pieces and meat juice is prepared by adding water and then by cooking properly. When it is taken as such without adding any thing, then it is termed as Akrita Mansa Rasa; but when added with salt and condiment as well as fried with ghee then it is named as Krita Mansa Rasa.

(B) Tarpanadi Krama

कफपित्ते विशुद्धेऽल्पं मद्यपे वातपैत्तिके। तर्पणादि क्रमं कुर्यात् पेयाऽभिष्यन्दयेद्धि तान्॥ (Ch.Si 6/25)

Charaka advised to follow "Tarpanadi krama" as 'Sansarjana Krama' in these conditions:

I. When Kapha and Pitta are eliminated in a smaller quantity during Sansodhana.
2. In alcoholic subjects.
3. The patients having Vata, Pitta Prakriti.

This preffered against 'Peyadi Sansarjana Course' as Peyadi Sansarjana may produce 'Abbisyanda' (increase in the secretions) again in the srotasas (channels) of 'Vishodhita' (well purified) body.

Nature of Tarpanadi Krama

तर्पणादिक्रमे च पेयायाः स्थाने स्वच्छतर्पणं विलेप्याः स्थाने च घनतर्पणं देयम्। (Ch.Si.6/25 teeka)

According to Chakrapani, 'Swaccha Tarpana' can be served instead of 'Peya' and 'Ghana Tarpana' instead of 'Vilepi'.

Jejjata says due to similarities, Mudga Yusha and Mansa rasa can be given as Tarpana but commentators of vagbhatta mentioned the diet regimen clearly pertaining to 'Annakala'.

प्रथमेऽन्नकाले लाजसक्तवो द्वितीयेऽन्नकाले मांसरसौदनमित्येष तर्पणादिक्रमस्तेषां हितः॥

	I	*II*	*III*
Arunadatta	Laja + Saktu	Jirna, Shali Odana	Mansa rasa + Odana
Parameshwara	Laja + Saktu	Yusha + Anna Bhojana	Mansa rasa + Anna

Rasa Sansarjana Karma

During "Annasansarjana krama", there are chances of doshas getting excited due to augmented Agni. To prevent such increase, doshas are mitigated by arranging "taste of the recipes" in such a series that the chances of increase will be lessened. It is elaborated by "Dalhana" and Chakrapani.

संसर्गेण विवृद्धेऽग्नौ दोषकोप भयाद्व्रजेत्। प्राक् स्वादुतिक्तौ स्निग्ध अम्ल लवणान् कटुकं ततः॥
स्वाद्वम्ल लवणान् भूयः स्वादु तिक्तावतः परम्। स्निग्ध रूक्षान् रसांश्चैव व्यत्यासात् स्वस्थवत्ततः॥
(Su. Chi.39/19-20)

अग्निसंधुक्षणार्थं तु पूर्वं पेयादिना भिषक्। रसोत्तरेण उपचरेत् क्रमेण क्रमकोविदः॥
स्निग्ध अम्ल स्वादु हृद्यानि ततोऽम्ललवणौ रसौ। स्वादुतिक्तौ ततो भूयः कषाय कटुकौ ततः॥
अन्योऽन्यप्रत्यनीकानां रसानां स्निग्ध रूक्षयोः। व्यत्यासाद् उपयोगेन प्रकृतिं गमयेद्भिषक्॥(Ch.Si 12/6-8)

Taste Used		*Probable effect on Dosha and Agni*
According to Charaka	*According to Sushruta*	
Sweet, sour, pleasant to heart, unctuous.	Sweet and bitter	1. To pacify Vata Pitta and to balance Agni 2. To pacify Vata situated in Pakvashaya
Sour and Salty	Unctuous, Sour, Salty, Pungent	1. To increase Agni Bala 2. To pacify Vata and Kapha and to augment Agni in the Upper site
Sweet and bitter	Sweet, Sour, Salty	1. To pacify Pitta 2. To pacify Pitta and Vata
	Astringent and pungent Sweet, Bitter	To pacify Kapha Pitta situated in the upper region

Here, unctuous and dry properties should be used alternatively in 'appropriate manner. Chakrapani says that these properties can be planned through the means of taste (Rasa). When the taste having unctous property is applied, then the taste having dry property can be planned and the same pattern is followed; further unctuous and dry properties are mentioned here as representatives. One can arrange heavy and light properties and further more in the same manner.

Need for Sansarjana Krama

1. Helps to regularize the Agni which is weakened due to purificatory process.
2. To overcome Dosha Kshaya/Dhatu Kshaya.
3. By arranging in such plan, diet comprising of all the tastes can be served through 12 meals along with different qualities.

COMPLICATIONS OF VAMANA AND THEIR MANAGEMENT WITH AYURVEDA AND MODERN DRUGS

Observations about Vamana Vyapadas

Simply "Vyapada" are the symptoms which are produced other than "Samyaka Vamana Lakshana" causing harm to the patient and increasing the symptoms of the disease. The word

'Vyapada' originated from the root 'Vyapad' meaning to fall away, to fall into misfortune (Monier Williams). So the word 'Vyapada' indicates the meanings like destruction, ruin, death (MW) or Sankatam (Su. Chi. 34/1) and Anyatha Apatti (Su. su. 15/2).
Factors responsible for Samyak yoga:

स्नेह स्वेद उपपन्नेन जीर्णे मात्रावत् औषधम्। एकाग्र मनसा पीतं सम्यग्योगाय कल्पते॥ (Ch.Si.6/10)

Proper sneha and sveda
Jeerna: Proper digestion of previous day meal
Matravat Aushadha: Appropriate dosage
Ekagramanasapeeta: Taking the medicine with concentration.

Causes for Vyapat

अकाले अल्प अतिमात्रं च पुराणं न च भावितम्। असम्यक् संस्कृतं चैव व्यापद्यैतौषधं द्रुतम्। (Ch.Si 6/18)

Akala	Purana
Alpamatra	Not bhavita
Atimatra	Asamyak sanskrita

प्रेष्यभैषज्यवेद्यानां वैगुण्याद् आतुरस्य च॥ (Ch.Si. 6/30)

Improper functioning of:

प्रेष्य	–	परिचारक (Attendent)
भैषज्य	–	औषध (Medicine)
वेद्या	–	वैद्य (Doctor)
आतुर	–	रोगी (Patient)

Vamana Vyapat

आध्मानं परिकर्तिकश्च स्त्रावो हृद्रात्रयोर्ग्रहः। जीवादानं सविभ्रंशः स्तम्भः सोपद्रवः क्लमः॥
अयोगाद अतियोगाच्च दशैता व्यापदो मताः॥ (Ch.Si. 6/29)
वैद्यातुर निमित्तम् वमनं विरेचनं च पञ्चदशधा व्यापद्यते।
तत्र वमनस्याधो गतिरूर्ध्वं विरेचनस्येति पृथक्; सामान्यमुभयोदकसावशेषौषधत्वं,
जीर्णौषधत्वं, हीनदोषापहृतत्वं, वातशूलम्, अयोगो, अतियोगो, जीवादानम्, आध्मानं,
परिकर्तिका, परिस्त्रावः, प्रवाहिका, हृदयोपसरणं, विबन्धः, अङ्गप्रग्रह इति। (Su.Chi.34/3)
प्रतिकूला गतिः पाको ग्रथितत्वं सगौरवम्। दोषोत्क्लेशो भृशाध्मानं परिकर्तः परिस्त्रवः॥
प्रवाहिका हृद्ग्रहणं सर्वगात्रपरिग्रहः। सह धातुस्त्रवेणैता द्वादशोक्ताः ससाधनाः॥ (A.S.Ka.3/21)

1. Charaka explained them as Adhmana (distension of abdomen), Parikartika (Gripping pain), Srava (Excessive discharge), Hridgraha (Cardiac spasm), Gatragraha (Spasm of limbs), Jivadanam (Discharge of blood), Savibhramsa (Improper action of medication), Stambha (rigidity), Upadravah (Serious afflictions), and Klamah (Exhausion). These are considered to be the 10 complications due to under action or over action of the drug, due to the defects of attendent, medication, physician or the patient (Ch.Si.6/29, 30).
2. Sushruta mentioned 15 complications, out of which Adhmana, Parikartika, Jivadana, Hridayopasaranam and Parisrava are common. Saavasheshausadhatwam,

Jirnaushadhatvam, Vatashula, Ayoga, Atiyoga, Vibandha, Pravahika, Hina Doshaapahritatva (movement of the humors in opposite direction), Virechana and Vamana (of Virechana drug) are different in Sushruta which are included in the causes of complication by Charaka (Su.Chi.34/3).

3. Vriddha Vagbhatta explained 12 complications having some different afflictions like grathitatva, Gaurava, Doshotklesha, and Dhatusrava, etc. (A.S.Ka.3)

Factors

1. 4 elements which influence the occurrence of complaints during process of Vamana are: Paricharaka (Nurse), Bhaishajya (Medicine), Vaidya (Physician) and Rogi (Patient) himself (Ch.Si.6/30).
2. Before initiating anyone of the processes in Panchakarma, Charaka warned Physician to keep an eye on the aspects like Doshas (bio-humors), Ausadha (Medicine), Desha (Place), Kala (Ritu, time), Satva, Agni, Satya, Vaya (Age) and Bala (Strength) of the patient. (Ch.Si.3/6).1f one failed to judge any of this objects, as a result it will lead to Vyapada (Complications).

Types

While describing Vyapada or complications, Charaka categorized them into two broad divisions, viz, A) Ayoga B) Atiyoga. That means, whenever any complication will arise, it will be due to either Ayoga or Atiyoga of the process influenced by other factors. Ten Complications explained in Siddhisthana may be divided into these two broad categories. But Chakrapani ruled out the law of inclusion under these two, by a remark in which he says, "It is not mandatory that these symptoms should be produced after Ayoga or Atiyoga of Vamana (Explained in Ch.Si.1/16-17) but they may be produced as an 'Upadrava' of the act". Later on, he blended them in two divisions, i.e. Ayoga and Atiyoga (Chakr. on Ch.Si.6/29-30) as:

Ayoga

- Adhmana
- Srava
- Hridgraha
- Angagraha
- Stambha
- Upadrava
- Klama

Atiyoga

- Parikartika
- Jivadanam
- Vibhramsa (Gudabhramsa and Sanjnabhramsa)

Mithyayoga

1. While reasoning to exclude mithyayoga from the complications of Vamana, Chakrapani analyzed whole concept brilliantly. He explains, "though Ayoga-Atiyoga and Mithyayoga are described accordingly everywhere in the texts, but in the case of Vamana and Virechana there is no need to consider Mithyayoga as a separate entity". In these processes, expulsion occurs in four different ways as:

1. Ati pravritti - Excessive expulsion.
2. Asamyak pravritti - Expulsion by improper way.
3. Apravritti - Cessation of process of expulsion.
4. Alpapravritti - Expulsion in a lesser quantity.

Here, last 3 are covered under an umbrella of "Ayoga". As an "Asamyak Pravritti" means expulsion through opposite route, it indicates that expulsion of vitiated matter is not in a quantity which is expected. So it must be considered under the term of "Ayoga" and not "Mithyayoga" (Chakr. on Ch. Si.6/29, 30, Ch.Su.16/3,4).

2. On the verse Su.Chi.34/22 which divides 15 complications of "Vireka" into Atiyoga, Duryoga and Ayoga, Dalhana expresses the views as here Vireka includes both Vamana and Virechana. Vyapadas are again divided into 3 fractions, viz. Atiyoga, Duryoga and Ayoga.
    1. Atiyoga means excessive Vamana.
    2. Duryoga means wrongly medicated (Duryojanam) or wrongly administered (Dushprayoga or Mithyaprayoga). It further goes on dividing into 3 categores as:
        a. Vaidyaduryoga (Wrong medication by physician) causing Vamana Mithyaprayoga, Virechana Mithyaprayoga, i.e. Parikartika.
        b. Aturaduryoga (Wrong response by patient) producing Hridaya Upasarana and Vibandha.
        c. Ubhayaduryoga (Wrongly treated and wrongly responded) causing Pravahika and Valashula.
    3. Ayogaja: Administered in lesser quantity.

Ayoga

Vriddha Vagbhatta explains Ayoga means:

i. Apravritti, i.e. the ingested material does not come out absolutely.
ii. The medicine which is administered, that is coming out lonely.
iii. Vibandha, i.e. the vomitus coming out in small bouts slowly (A.S.Su.27/18).

Factors Initiating Ayoga

1. Status of bowel: Krura and Bahudosha
2. Medicine: Quality - dry (Ruksha), insubstantial (Alpagunaro), state - old or wasted (Jirnaro); Quantity - Inadequate (Alparo)
3. Status of individual: Not properly oleated (Snigdha) and sweated (Svinna)
4. Status of appetite: Increased appetite (Deeptagni), but medicine - Ruksha and leena.
5. Doshasthiti:
    1. Dosha in less excited (Utklishta) condition.
    2. If Doshas are in large quantity and accumulated in Koshtha having medicine with less potency and with a less appetite.

Symptoms

They can be divided into 3 groups:

A. Classically explained as 'Ayoga' (Ch.Si.1/15, A.S.Su.27/18, Su.Chi.33/7, and A.H.Su.18/23,24).
B. Described under ten complications produced as 'Upadrava' (Ch.Si.6/29-30)
C. Emerged after influenced by certain conditions. (Ch.Si.6/39, Su.Chi.34/6,8)

Group A	*Group B*	*Group C*
Cessation of Vega, Expulsion of medicine only, Srotoguruta, Vegavibandha, Gurugatrata, Hridya Ashuddhi, Sphota, Jvara (Sheeta), Shula, Kotha, Kandu, Kaphapraseka, Shopha, Alasya, Pratishyaya and Lomaharsha	Adhmana Srava Hridgraha Angagraha Sthambha Vibhransha Upadrava Hrillasa, Udgara Avishuddhi Klama	Vibhransha, Shotha, Hikka, Tamasah darshana, Pindika Udveshtana, Kandu, Urusaada, Vivarnata, Gaurava, Utklesha, Hridaya Ashuddhi, Arati, Vyadhi Vriddhi, Trishna, Parshvashula, Chhardi, Murccha, Parvabheda

Atiyoga

Atiyoga means explusion of vitiated matter in excessive quantity. Factors leading to Atiyoga (Ch.Si.6/4S, 46)

1. Status of bowel: Mild (Atimridu) or Madhyama Koshtha
2. Medicine: Quality = Penetrating (Tikshna), Hot (Ushna); Quantity = Large (Bahu) quantity
3. Condition of individual:
   1. With lesser strength
   2. Oleated and fomented excessively.
4. Status of Appetite: Kshudharttasya
5. Status of humors: Kapha in lesser quantity or excited (Utklishta Kapha) in lesser quantity.

Thus, symptoms produced due to Atiyoga can be explained in 3 groups:

A. Classically explained as 'Atiyoga' (Ch.Si.1/15 and Su 15/13, Su.Chi. 33/7, A.H.Su.15/25)
B. Included in 10 complications produced as "Upadrava"(Ch.Si.6/29, 30)
C. Appeared due to specific conditions (Ch.Si.6/46)

Group A	*Group B*	*Group C*
Phenila Vamana, Raktachandrika, Trishna, Moha, Daha, Murccha, Vataprakopa, Nidrahani, Balahani, Hritpida, Kanthapida, Tamah Pravesha, Bhrama, Pitta Atiyoga, Unmada, Death due to excessive bleeding, Svarakshaya, Kanthashosha, Karnashula. Jihwa Pravesha, Shirah Shunyata, Hridaya dhumayana, Supti, Gatrashula, Urdhvanilaprakopa, Ardita, Agnihani, Hanusanhanana, Jihwa shonitapravritti, Jihwanirgamana, Akshivyavrti, Vishamnjnata, Vaksanga	Parikartika Jivadanam Vibhransha Guda- Bhransha Sangya- Bhransha	Pitta Atipravrtti, Balahani, Vata- Prakopa, Jihwanirgamana, Shosha, Svarahani, Daha Kantha Bhransha, Trishna

Ten Vyapadas Explained by Charaka

1. Adhmanam (Distension of abdomen) :

A. Patient: Less appetite, misperistalsis
B. Medicine: Less in a dose
C. Physician: Has excess of morbidity, dehydrated
D. Pathogenesis: Will rouse the morbid humors and obstruct the body channels.
E. Signs and symptoms: Great distension of abdomen, pain in back, sides of the chest and head, serious obstruction to breath, feces, urine and flatus.
F. Treament: (1) Induction (2) Sudation (3) Suppository and similar treatment (4) Evacuative and unctous enema and all treatment curative of disorders of misperistalsis (Udavarta).

2. Parikartika (Gripping Pain):

A. Patient: Hard bowel
B. Medicine: Strong
C. Physician : Patient suffers from Ama morbidity, in a person who is emaciated soft bowel, exhausted and is poor of vitally.
D. Pathogenesis : Reaches the rectum and eliminates morbid matter along with chyme.
E. Signs and symptoms: Causes acute colic and gripping pain accompanied with slimy and bloody discharge.
F. Treatment:
   a. Patients with Chyme morbidity starvation:
      1. Digestive medication, diet should be dry, hot and light articles.
      2. In conditions of emaciation, measures of roborant therapy.
      3. Medications prepared with drugs of Madhura varga are recommended.
   b. If even after the digestion of Ama there is obstination medication with acid and alkali and light diet.

3. Srava (Discharge) :

A. Patient: Stools with abnormal excessive morbidity.
B. Medicine: In a small dose.
C. Physician: With excessive morbidity.
D. Pathogenesis: Rouses the humors
E. Signs and symptoms: Causes frequent and scanty elimination and gives rise to the pruritus, edema, dermatitis, heaviness of the body, impairement of gastric fire, nausea, stiffness, anorexia and anemia.
F. Treatment: Either treated with sedative drugs with emetics or giving oneself oleation. Again one should be administered a strong purgative and perfectly cleansed, may be given powders, medicated wines prepared with suitable medications.

4. Hridgraha

A. Patient: Suppression of urge after taking the emetic drug.
B. Medicine: Due to low dose of medicine
C. Pathogenesis: Vata and other humors getting provoked and reaching the heart causing severe cardiac spasm.

D. Signs and symptoms: The person becomes affected with hiccup, cough and pain in the sides of the chest. He gets depressed. There is dribbling from the mouth, agitation of the eyes, one bites the tongue, falls unconscious and gushes one's teeth.

E. Treatment:

a. If condition is serious (fainting) due to excess of Pitta, emesis should be given prepared with drugs of sweet group. If it is due to Kapha, drugs of pungent group can be used. Thereafter the residual morbidity should be digested away by digestive medications. Then one's body and vitality should be systematically rehabilitated. Also, if the person while vomiting excessively is afflicted in heart by Vata, one should be given unctous acid and salt articles and in conditions due to Pitta and Kapha, dry, pungent and bitter articles should be given.

5. Gatragraha (stiffness in body):

A. Patient: Suppression of the urges by a person who has taken the purificatory dose.

B. Medicine: Flow dose of medicine.

C. Pathogenesis: Owing to obstruction of Vata by Kapha or owing to purification done in excess. The provoked Vata seizes the limbs.

D. Signs and symptoms: Causes the stiffness, tremor, pricking pain, asthenia, cramps and churning.

E. Treament: Oleation, sudation, and all similar other measures curative of Vata should be carried out.

6. Discharge of occult blood (Jivadanam):

A. Patient: Soft bowelled

B. Medicine: Strong medication

C. Physician: Soft bowelled + slight morbidity

D. Pathogenesis: After eliminating the morbid matter and churning the system excessively.

E. Signs and symptoms: Causes the discharge of the pure blood.

F. Treatment: Measures curative of Pitta or treatment benificial in the over action of purificatory procedures. Give fresh blood of a live deer, cow, buffalo or goat. May be given blood churned with sacrificial gross in the form of an enema.

7. Vibhransha (Prolapse of Rectum):

A. Prolapse of rectum (Gudabhransha): Should be replaced after constricting it with astringent medication.

B. Unconsciousness (Sangyabhransha): Soothing songs and words should be uttered.

C. Symptoms due to agitation (Lakshanbhransha): If the purgative dose caeses to act immediately after elimination of fecal matter or the emetic dose is immediately vomited out, it causes only the agitation of the morbid humor but does not eliminate it. Provoked humors cause pruritus and other diseases. This called condition of wrongful action as medication in accordance with pathological features.

8. Stambha (Rigidity):

A. Patient: Undergone oleation procedures.

B. Medicine: An unctuous portion.

C. Pathogenesis: It gets covered up by the morbid matter which is in softened condition and will be unable to expel the morbid matter from its habitat. It even obstructs those that have been dislodged from their habitats.

D. Signs and symptoms: Causes scanty and frequent elimination accompanied with acute obstruction of Vata. Stambha (rigidity) and pain in the rectum.
E. Treatment: Strong enema or purgation preceded by lightening and digestive measures.

9. Serious afflictions (Upadrava):

A. Patient: Lacking in unctous property, debilitated.
B. Medicine: Ununctous purgative medication.
C. Pathogenesis: Will provoke the Vata quickly and give rise to severe complications.
D. Signs and symptoms: Causes rigidity and severe pain in all limbs and fainting.
E. Treament: Oleation, sudation. similar measures (treatment curative of Vata).

10. Klama (Exhaustion):

A. Patient: Undergone the oleation procedure and soft bowelled.
B. Medicine: Mild medication.
C. Pathogenesis: Rouses up the Kapha and Pitta and obstructs Vata.
D. Signs and symptoms: Heaviness, exhaustion.
E. Treatment: Vamana, Langhana (lightening), Pachana (Digestive remedies) should be given unctuous and strong purificatory measures.

Vamana Vyapada Lakshanas

Symptoms/Samhita	*Charaka*	*Sushruta*	*Vagbhatta*	*Bhela*	*Kashyapa*
Adhmana	+	+	–	–	–
Parikartika	+	+	+	+	+
Srava	+	–	–	–	–
Hridgraha	+	–	–	–	–
Gatragraha	+	–	+	–	–
Jivadanam	+	+	–	+	+
Vibhransha	+	–	–	–	–
Stambha	+	–	–	–	–
Upadrava	+	–	–	–	–
Klama	+	–	–	–	–
Aushadhasya Pratikula					
Pravritti	+	–	–	–	–
Savasheshausadhatva	–	+	–	–	–
Jirnaushadhatva	–	+	–	–	–
Hina doshapritasya	+	–	–	–	–
Vatashula	–	+	–	–	–
Ayoga	–	+	–	–	–
Atiyoga	+	–	–	–	–
Pravahika	–	–	–	–	–
Hridayopasaranam	–	+	–	–	–

Contd...

Contd...

Symptoms/Samhita	*Charaka*	*Sushruta*	*Vagbhatta*	*Bhela*	*Kashyapa*
Parisrava	–	+	+	–	–
Vibandha	–	+	–	+	+
Angamarda	–	+	–	–	–
Paka	–	+	–	–	–
Grathitatva	–	–	+	–	–
Gaurava	–	–	+	–	–
Doshotklesha	–	–	+	–	–
Brishadhmana	–	–	+	–	–
Sarvadhatusravana	–	–	–	+	–
Gudaparisrava	–	–	–	+	–
Hridroga	–	–	–	+	–
Shula	–	–	–	+	+
Pratishyaya	–	–	–	+	–

Vyapada of Vamana along with their Treatment

Vyapada	*Charaka*	*Sushruta*	*Treatment*
Adhmana	+	+	Abhyanga, Svedana, Phalavarti Prayoga, Niruha and Anuvasana Basti
Parikartika	+	+	Langhana, Pachana, Ruksha, Ushna, Laghu Ahara Sevana, Ghrita Manda Anuvasana Basti, Picchabasti Sheeta Jala Parisheka, Ghrita, Madhu, Madhura, Sheetala lepa, Madhura Ksheera Bhojana
Parisrava	+	+	Vamana or Tikshna Virechana, Asthapana Basti by Baladi Kvatha, Churna, Asava Arishta Prayoga
Gatragraha	+	+	Snehana, Svedana, Vatahara karma
Hridgraha	+	+	In Pitta Janya Murccha, use of Madhura dravya and in Kaphajanya Murccha, Katu dravya should be used for Vamana. Then for Sheshadosha, Pachana dravya should be given. If Vata is aggravated, Snigdha, Amla, Lavana dravya and if Pitta and Kapha are aggravated, then Ruksha, Tikta and Katu dravya; mainly Madhura dravya prayoga is beneficial.
Jeevadana	+	+	Pittaharakarma, Rakta Pana, Sheetala Piccha Basti, Ghrita Manda Anuvasana Basti
Vibhransha	+	–	Santavana, Samaveda pathana, Priyashabda Vachana.
Stambha	+	–	Langhana, Pachana, Tikshna basti, Tikshna Virechana
Klama	+	–	Langhana, Pachana, Snigdha Dravya, Tikshna -Shodhana
Upadrava	+	–	Snehana, Svedana, Vatahara Kriya
Vamanasya Adhogati	–	+	Snehana, Tikshna Vamana

Contd...

Contd...

Vyapada	*Charaka*	*Sushruta*	*Treatment*
Virechansya Urdhva Gati	–	+	Vamana, Virechana
Savashesha Aushadha Jeema	–	+	Give Ushna jala for Vamana
Aushadh Alpa Dosha	–	+	Tikshna Aushadha Prayoga
Harana	–	+	Snehana, Svedana, Virechana
Vata Shoola	–	+	Snehana, Svedana, Yashtimadhu taila anuvasana
Ayoga	–	+	Vamana with Madana Phala and Lavana Mishrita Laja, Anuvasana and Asthapana Basti
Atiyoga	–	+	Abhyanga, Sheeta Jala Snana, Avaleha Prayoga, Ksheera Bhojana
Pravahika	–	+	Snehana, Sanshodhana
Vibandha	–	+	Vamana, Avasthanusara Chikitsa (treatment according to condition)

PARIHARYA VISHAYA

After taking Dhumapana, patient is transferred to the ward. Thereafter, he should be instructed not to indulge in the following factors, which are collectively known as Pariharya Vishaya.

उच्चैर्भाष्यम् अत्याशनम् अतिस्थानम् अतिचंक्रमणं क्रोध शोक हिम आतप आवश्याय आतिप्रवातान् यानयानं ग्राम्यधर्ममस्वपनं निशि दिवा स्वप्नं विरूद्धाजीर्ण असात्म्याकाल प्रमितातिहीन गुरु विषमभोजन वेगसन्धारणोदीरणमिति............ (Ch.Su 15/15)

1. Speaking loudly
2. Eating too much
3. Standing for a long time
4. Moving for long time
5. Anger and grief
6. Exposure to sun and strong wind
7. Travelling by vehicles
8. Indulging in sexual intercourse
9. Vigil during night
10. Sleeping during day time
11. Ingestion of Viruddha, Asatmya, Guru type of food
12. Vegasandharana etc.

तत्र विहारो बहुविधोऽपि त्रिविध एव, काय वाक् मनो भेदात्; स त्रिविधोऽप्य युक्तो अप्यववर्ज्यश्च आतुरोपद्रवीये वक्ष्यते। (Su.Chi. 33/10 teeka)

Dalhana has reclassified the above-mentioned factors into three viz. Kayika, Vachika and Manasika.

VAMANA KARMUKATA (MODE OF ACTION)

Probable Mode of Action of Vamana Dravya

तत्रोष्ण-तीक्ष्ण-सूक्ष्म-व्यवायि-विकाशीन्यौषधानि स्ववीर्येण हृदयमुपेत्य धमनीरनुसृत्य स्थूलाणुस्त्रोभ्यः केवलं शरीरगतं दोषसङ्घातमाग्नेयत्वाद् विष्यन्दयन्ति, तैक्ष्ण्याद् विच्छिदन्ति, स विच्छिन्नः परिप्लवन् स्नेहभावितेकाये स्नेहाक्त भाजनस्थम् इव

क्षौद्रम् असज्जम् अणु प्रवण भावात् आमाशयम् आगम्य उदान प्रणुन्नौ अग्निवाय्यात्मकत्वाद् उर्ध्वभाग प्रभावात् औषधस्य उर्ध्वम् उत्क्षिप्यते, सलिल पृथिव्यात्मकत्वाद् अधोभाग प्रभावात् च औषधस्याधः प्रवर्तते, उभयतश्च उभय गुणत्वात्। इति लक्षणोद्देशः॥ (Ch.Ka.1/5)

Vamana Mode of Action

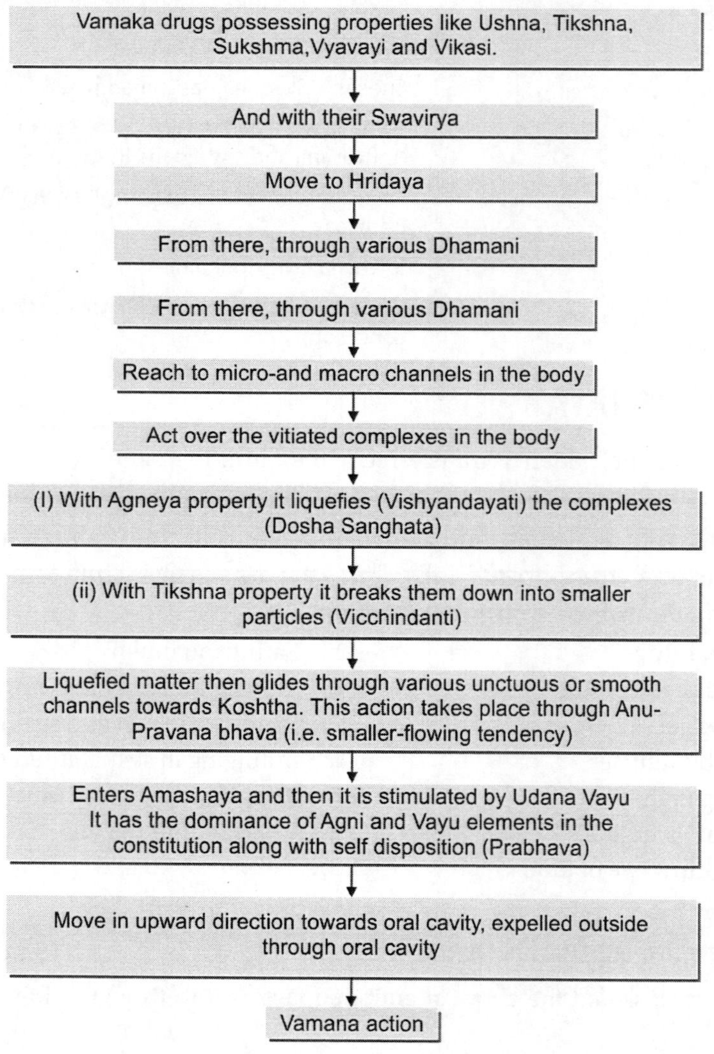

Descriptions

1. The Vamaka dravyas having the properties like Ushna, Tikshna, Sukshma, Vyavayi and Vikashi, get absorbed and reach to heart due to their Swavirya (Potency).

2. Due to Sukshma and Vyavayi properties, they move into dhamani to reach 'Sthula' and Suksma (macro and micro) channels throughout the whole body.
3. They work over the sites where "complex of the vitiated humors" is built. At first, they liquefy (Visyandayanti) these complexes by their "Ushna property". Increased liquidity will further help to flow through circulation. Afterwards these complexes are fragmented into smaller molecules due to "Tikshna property" which will help them to extricate (Vicchindanti) from the micro channels.
4. Then these liquefied and fragmented molecules are lead to Amashaya, flowing through "Anu srotas" (Anu Pravana Bhava) without adhering to them. This advancement takes place in the similar manner in which the water floats through the pot layered by unctuous material without sticking to the same.
5. Where from encouraged by "Udana Vayu" and due to the "Agni and Vayu mahabhautika constitution" and "Prabhava", they march in upward direction to expel the vitiated doshas, brought along with them.
   Properties: Ushna, Tikshna, Sukshma, Vyavayi, Vikasi.
   Sites: Hridaya, Amashaya
   Channels : Dhamani
   Stimulant : Udana Vayu
   Constitution : Agni + Vayu
   Prabhava : Urdhva bhagahar

Corelation with Modern View

Vamana karma is not merely a gastric lavage as done nowadays to empty the content of stomach, but it is a complete management of systemic diseases caused by Kapha. Amashaya particularly Urdva Amashaya is the seat of action of Kapha. The active principle of Vamana drug taken orally is absorbed from the stomach into circulatory system where from it is circulated to all over the body. On reaching at the site of lesion (Dosha Sanghata) which is at the cellular level, it breaks the association of doshas and bring back the toxic substances thus released into the stomach, where from they are expelled out of the body by the action of vomiting. Further, generally it is considered that the drug given orally cures the diseases originating from the stomach in better way, as it is the main seat of Kapha. Mild inflammation is must for purification action. It is noticed that most of the drugs employed in Vamana have mild irritation effect and produced mild inflammation facilitates the quick absorption of the active principles (Veerya) of the drug in the initial stage. Later on it facilitates the excretion of the morbid matters which generally are not supposed to be excreted out. It is possible only because inflammation increases the permeability of the capillaries which in turn allow the absorption as well as excretion of the substances which are not allowed in normal conditions. The softening (Vishyandana) action of the drugs may be understood from the example of fatty degeneration. In fatty degeneration, the saturated molecules are chemically inert and do not respond to any chemical reaction. But if the suitable catalytic agent is applied, then it will later on react to the other chemicals also to break them in smaller molecules. The smaller molecules thus formed can be driven out of the cell due to the normal function of the cell or by the action of drug and thus the cell is free from the harmful substance leading to the cure of the degeneration.

The Vamana drugs are given in full stomach when the pyloric end of stomach remains closed and all the local activities of the Vamana drugs are limited to the stomach only. As the drugs have irritant action, so a mild inflammation of the stomach mucosa is produced. It will increase the permeability of the capillaries of the stomach which in the beginning facilitated the absorption of the active principles of the drug and later on facilitates the excretion of the toxins and metabolites into the stomach where from they are thrown out of the body by the process of vomiting. The process of emesis therapy is considered complete as soon as the pyloric valve opens which is evident from the appearance of bile in vomitus due to the flux of antiperistalsis set during the process of vomiting.

Pharmacological Properties of Vamana Dravyas

1. **Ushna**— The property which produces "Sveda" is called as 'Ushna Guna' (Hemadri on A.H.1/15). Sushruta says, Ushna property has Pachana karma specifically (Su.Su.46/515), while Chakrapani says (Ch.Ka.1/5) Ushna means 'Ushna Veeryam'. Ushna Veerya possesses the functions like dahana, pachana, fomentation, vilayana and having ability to decrease Vata and Kapha dosha. (A.S.l7/1S). Dalhana opines as Ushna Guna owns the capacity to tone down the Saumya bhava (Dal. on Su.Chi.33/ 33). In the Vamana process, according to Chakrapani (Chakrapani on Ch.Ka.1/5). 'Visyandayanti' means "Viliyana Kurvanti". Accoding to Apte (1965), Viliyana means to dissolve or to liquefy. Gangadhara comments (on Ch.Su.1/13) that after the action of Teja, the complex built by "Apa" starts to liquefy (vilayana). Any molecule is made by compression of particles of Apa, when it comes in contact with 'Teja', the bonds made due to Apa start to be loosened leading to expansion of the space between the particles causing it to liquify. Thus, the process of "Viliyanam" is headed by Ushna property. Thus, Ushna property helps to separate the vitiated matter from Srotas and 'Tikshna property' also helps to fragment them. In modern idiom, it may be like the action of catalytic agents which may be converting the saturated compounds into the unsaturated one or in the form in which they are more reactive.
2. **Tikshna**— Sushruta defines "Tikshna" as the property producing Daha, Paka and Srava (Su.Su.46/515), whereas Charaka says 'Tikshna Guna' functions for 'Vicchindana' (Ch. Ka.1/5). Dalhana explains the action of oozing of vitiated humors through channels takes place due to Tikshna property (Dal. on Su.Chi.33/33). While Chakrapani clarified the word 'Viccindayanti' by wording that it is nothing but breaking down of the complex of morbid matter into smaller molecules (Chakr. on Ch. Ka.1/5). Tikshna, according. to Hemadri, carries out 'Shodhana' that means it is the basic property needed for Vamana (H. on A.H.Su.1/18). Thus, one can conclude that 'Tikshna Guna' carries the particles which are broken down and separted from all the micro and macro channels (Shakha) to Amashaya (Koshtha) due to 'the Anupravana bhava' of the drugs.
3. **Sukshma**— According to Dalhana, Sukshma property makes the pathway for the Vamana drugs to reach minute channels and remove the morbid matter from them to reach Amashaya in the process of Vamana (Dal. on Su.Chi.33/33). Hemadri quotes as Sukshma

property possessing the capacity to dilate the channel, helps them to pass into micro channels (H.on A.H.Su.1/18). The Agni, Vayu and Akasha Mahabhuta are dominant in its Bhautika constitution. Sharangdhara has also mentioned that Vamana drugs having this property can enter smallest Srotasa of the body (Sh.Pu.Kh.4/18).

4. **Vyavayi**— Vyavayi drugs when administered in the body initiate their actions immediately irrespective of their digestion by the body (Sha.Sam.Pu.4). Due to this property only, Vamana drugs get absorbed and spread for further action quickly. Dalhana mentions that due to this property Vamaka drugs spread into the body without changing their form. He also mentions that after reaching to cellular level, it affects the body like Madya (Alcohol) and Visha (Poison) (Dal. on Su.Su.46/523). Charaka also attributes Vyavayi property to Visha and Madya. (Ch.Chi. 23/23, Ch.Chi. 24/30). In Madatyaya, the word "Vyapaktva"is used to indicate the efficacy of Visha. So one can conclude that due to this property the drug spreads to every cell of the body. "Vyayayi property" is considered under 'Drava'property by Hemadri (H. on A.H.Su. 1/18). Indu quotes that Vyavayi property is considered as the 'extended form of Sara property', according to some authors. (Indu on A.S.Su.1/29). Thus, it can be said that Vyavayi property may need liquid property to spread throughout the body and Vamana drugs thus, due to their Vyavayi property spread quickly in the whole body and start the action before their Pachana.
5. **Vikasi**—According to Sharangdhara, the drugs having Vikasi property produce loosening in joints and especially in Oja (Sha.Sam.Pu.4). Sushruta opines that Vikashi drugs loosen the Dhatu Bandhana (Vimokshayet) (Su.Su.46/523). Dalhana explains that Vanaka drugs due to Vikashi property also pervades through the whole body without digestion like that of Vyavayi. Further he mentions that loosening of Dhatu Bandhana means 'Dhatu Shaithilya' (Dal. on Su.Su.46/523), Hemadri includes it under "Khara Property" (on A.H.Su.1/18). Vriddha Vagbhatta opines that it is extended nature of' Tikshna property' [A.S .Su.1/29]. Indu explains the function as 'Vikasi' property scraps dhatus (Vikasana, Hinsan), breaks the junctures between two joints, clears off the coatings and terminates the same (Indu on A.S.Su.1/29). Thus, from the above discussion, one can say that Vamana drugs reach rapidly to the cellular level due to 'Vikasi' property alongwith the 'Vyavayi' one; they penetrate the micro channels with their "Tikshna property" and scrap off the morbid matter due to "Khara property" to convey the same to Amashaya through circulation.
6. **Saratva**— Saratva is the property mentioned for Vamana drugs by Sushruta. Dalhana says that Saratva means 'Anulomatva'. Gayi expresses that Saratva means the tendency to spread (Dal. on Su.Chi.33/33). At another juncture, Dalhana describes that Anulomana is nothing but Vata and Mala Pravartanam (Dal. on Su.Su.46/529). Hemadri says that the capacity to stimulate comes under "the Sara guna" (on A.H.Su. 1/18). This property shows the tendency of the drug to be remained in active form. Due to this guna; Vamana drugs after administration, work continuously without any break (opposite to 'Sthira property'). It may be said that due to this guna, the Vamaka drugs lead to micro channels, bring doshas to koshtha and then expel them out.

Veerya

Vamana drugs have Ushna Veerya and due to this, Dalhana, Svedana, Vivarana and particularly Pachana occur. Drugs first enter the Hridaya by potency where from they are circulated through Dhamani to Sthula and Anu srotas of the body. (Ch.Ka.1/5) Thus Ushna Veerya helps the Vamana drugs in their circulation all over the body and also in breaking down the dosha sanghata.

Vipaka

Vipaka of Vamaka drugs seems not to play much role in Vamana karma because Vyavayi guna gets the drugs absorbed without their digestion.

Prabhava

The main action of Vamana is due to its Prabhava. "Urdhva Anulomikam yaccha tat Prabhava Prabhavitam", i.e. the actions of Vamana and Virechana drugs are mainly due to their Prabhava (Ch.Su.26/69). Elaborating Prabhava of Vamana drugs, Chakrapani says that due to dominance of Agni and Vayu Mahabhuta in their Panchabhautika constitution, there is a tendency of Urdhvagati of Vamaka drugs. It may be initiated by Udana Vayu. However, he says that it is the Prabhava of drugs that have important role in Urdhvagati (Chakr. on Ch.Ka.1/5).

Udana Vayu

While demonstrating the act of Vamana, Charaka has used the word, "Udana Pranunno" (Ch.Ka.on 1/5), on which Chakrapani (Ch.Ka.on 1/5) comments that Vamana drugs lead in the upward direction due to Udana Vayu. Udana Vayu has the prime role in conducting the whole Vamana process as the one occurs in its site. Charaka narrates the sites of Udana Vayu as Nabhi, Urah and Kantha. Vagbhatta also supports his view and adds new site like 'Nasa' in it (A.H.Su.12/5, 6). Sushruta awarding it the status of 'Pavanottamah' and says that it moves in upward direction. Thus it shares some of the vital functions of the body. Charaka and Vagbhatta described these functions as, production of words (Vakpravritti), help in efforts (Prayatna), to provide energy (Urjah), to keep the strength (Bala), to lighten the color of skin (Varna) and memory (Smriti) (A.H.Su.12/5-6, Ch.Chi.28/7). During the process of vomiting, it is totally stimulated and continuously working. It helps the Vamaka drugs to drag the vitiated matter from channels (Prayatna). It provides the energy to expel these things out (Urja). It maintains the courage and strength of the patient to bear this much strenuous process (Bala). Vriddha Vagbhatta adds the function like "Srotasa Prinan" (A.S.Su.17). During the process of Vamana, Udana keeps the Srotasa well perfused. It leads further saying that Udana helps to activate Dhi, Dhriti, Smriti, and Mana. The process of Vamana is the act to be ventured by courageous people. Continuous changes of "fight or flight" emotions are progressing in the mind which can be well combated by strengthened Udana. Thus, one can conclude that by every virtue, 'Udana Vayu' helps the Vamana drugs to remove the extracted matter through exhaustive process of Vamana.

Role of Udana Vayu in the Act of Vomiting through the Means of Pressure Changes

The cavities are comprised of Akasha element. They are infiltrated by Vayu element. Vata plays an important role in maintaining the pressure in any cavity of the body. Prana and Udana works in the province of thoracic cavity. So one can say that intrathoracic pressure is maintained by Prana and Udana Vata with the help of Vyana Vata. Abdominal region (Koshtha) is governed mainly by Samana Vata. So one can say that intraluminal pressure of the intestines and intra-abdominal pressure are guided by Samana and Vyana Vata. During Vamana, Udana Vata lifts the humors from the gastric cavity and throws them through the oral cavity to outer world. (Ch. Ka.l/5). To bring about this mechanism, it has to make sudden changes in the pressure gradient between these two cavities. It increases intra-abdominal pressure initially. Vyana Vata alongwith Samana Vata helps in it by the following way. If the intra-abdominal pressure is sufficiently high, the gastric contents may breach upper esophageal sphincter leading to vomiting. Abdominal pressure is increased due to abdominal muscle contraction and to the descent of diaphragm. The gastric, cardiac sphincters and other esophageal muscles relax. The pylorus usually, contracts to prevent any normal onward transport from the stomach. After that, when medicine starts to move upward, there is "gain change in the pressure gradient between these two cavities". Now "with the dilated esophagus and lower esophageal sphincter tone, intrathoracic pressure changes from negative to positive with upward diaphragm movement".

Vamana removes toxic Doshas especially from head region. Increased blood flow in any region encourages the transport activity there. To drag the wastes from upper channels, it takes the assistance of Vyana Vata.

वृद्धानुदानो व्यानसङ्गतः। (Su. U.T. 49/7)

What vomiting does is cause a huge increase in intrathoracic pressure. This intrathoracic pressure is transmitted to the blood vessels in the head and neck including eye vessels (which can be seen as "red sclera" during vomiting).

Explanation for contraindication of Vamana is specific.

Dhamani

Charaka used the word "Dhamani" through which Vamana drugs spread throughout the body (Ch.Ka. 1/5). These are the channels which carry some constituents with them. Definition of "Dhamani" by Charaka is, "Dhamnat Dhamanyah" that means "Dhamana"; is what which pulsates (Ch.Su.30/12). Thus, it is the structure resembling to artery. Chakrapani also comments that it provides nourisment to Paramanus. (Chakr. on Ch.Su. 30/12). So, in the Vamana process, Dhamani is the medium through which Vamaka drugs reach the cellular level for their purpose. But Chakrapani points out another aspect in this regard. He remarks that Vamaka drugs remain there themselves and pass the impulses towards several areas throughout the body by the way of Dhamani (Chakr. on Ch.Ka.1/5). This distinctly points to the conduction of impulses through the means of the nerves. Thus, one can conclude that during the act of Vamana, the process of Sanshodhana proceeds through both the systems, i.e. circulatory system and nervous system.

Amashaya

In Maharoga adhayaya, Charaka describes Amashaya as the part of both Kapha as well as that of Pitta. (Ch.Su.20/8). When one says that Kapha residing in Urah controls all other types of Kapha in the several sites of the body thus bestowing it the status of the chief site of Kapha, it is very obvious to collect the vitiated one from all over the body at the same site too. So, it is very much easy to expel the Kapha from Amashaya; the place nearer to its main site.

Charaka conveyed the same thing in Maharoga adhyaya, where he delivered the details of treatment for Kapha and Pitta. For Sanshodhana of both Kapha and Pitta, he mentioned the same site, i.e. Amashaya (Ch.Su.20/16, Ch.Su.20/19). Chakrapani made a note there by saying that Urdhva Amashaya is the site of Kapha and Adho Amashaya is the site of Pitta (Chakr. on Ch.Su. 20/8).

Now one can understand why Charaka has mentioned the word "Amashaya", as the receiving site of morbid doshas (especially Kapha and also in association with Pitta). While explaining Pittanta Vamana (Ch.Si.1/14-16), Chakrapani says that at the end, Pitta should come out from Amashaya, but not only from 'Urdhva Amashaya'.

Hridaya

The drugs due to their "Svaveerya" reach to the Hridaya from where they spread to all over the body. To reach the micro level throughtout the body in a very short time, there are two chief systems in the body, i.e. circulatory and nervous systems. As it is said that Vamaka drugs move into Dhamani after passing from Hridaya, One can say that; here the word "Hridaya" may have both the meanings showing the involvement of both the vital and chief organs, i.e. heart and brain.

Physiologic
Constipation
Gastric stasis/outlet obstruction
Brain metastasis
Increased intercranial pressure
Bowel intestinal obstruction
Hepatomegaly:
Oral thrush
Cough

Metabolic:
Uremia
Endocrine imbalance
Electrolyte imbalance:
- Hypercalcemia
- Hyponatremia

Treatment Related
Chemotherapy
Radiation therapy
(especially to brain or GI tract)

Medications
Initial opioid therapy
Antibiotics
Aspirin/NSAIDS
Carbamazepine
Steroids
Expectorants
Causes of nausea and vomiting

Vomiting Center of the of the Brain :
lower medula
Emotional/spiritual/psychological
Anticipatory Nand. V (prior to chemotherapy)

Meaning of Illness
Loss of person hood
Role change
Suffering
Anxiety/fear
Fatigue

Modern View

Vomiting is the oral expulsion of upper gastrointestinal contents resulting from contractions of gut and thoracoabdominal wall musculature. Vomiting is the means by which the upper GIT rids itself off from its contents when almost any part of the upper tract becomes excessively irritated, overdistended, or even overexcitable. Excessive distention or irritation of the duodenum provides an especially strong stimulus for vomiting.

Act of Vomiting (Physiology)

The act of vomiting is accompanied by a complex series of movements which are controlled by the vomiting center present in the dorsal portion of the lateral reticular formation in the medulla oblongata. The vomiting center is the final common pathway for the act of vomiting. It receives afferent impulses from chemoreceptor trigger zone (CTZ), vestibular apparatus, higher centers in the brain and peripheral structures including the GI tract, and nucleus tracts solitarius. Once the vomiting center has been sufficiently stimulated and vomiting act instituted, the first effects are:

1. A deep breath
2. Raising of the hyoid bone and the larynx to pull the upper esophageal sphincter open.
3. Closing of the glottis.
4. Lifting of the soft palate to close the posterior nares.

Next a strong downward contraction of the diaphragm comes along with simultaneous contraction of all the abdominal wall muscles. This squeezes the abdominal viscera including the stomach between the diaphragm and the abdominal muscles making the intragastric pressure to a high level. As a result the pyloric region also is firmly contracted and occluded, whereas the body and fundus of the stomach are relaxed. Cardiac sphincter is also relaxed and finally, lower esophageal sphincter opens completely. As a result of all these factors, the gastric contents are thrown upward into the esophagus and then into the mouth.

In short, pressure on the stomach increases (Due to descent of diaphragm, etc.) Gastric contents, therefore, forcibly ejected into esophagus to mouth to exterior. Vomiting is usually preceeded by the sensation of nausea and increased secretion of saliva, bronchial fluid and sweat. The muscles involved in the act of coughing take part in the act of vomiting, and the vagal, vomiting, and cough centers have a close functional relationship. Vomiting is also under the voluntary control and can be induced voluntarily, more easily by giving Vamaka and Vamanopaga drugs (As in Vamana procedure).

Antiperistalsis (The Prelude to Vomiting)

1. In the early stages of excessive gastrointestinal irritation or overdistention, antiperistalsis begins to occur often many minutes before the vomiting occurs.
2. The antiperistalsis may begin as far down in the intestinal tract as the ileum. The antiperistalsis wave travels backward upto the intestine at a rate of 2-3 cm/sec.
3. Then as the upper portions of GIT, especially the duodenum becomes overdistended. This distension becomes the excitating factor that initiates the actual vomiting act.

4. At the onset of vomiting, strong intrinsic contractions occur in both the duodenum and the stomach along with partial relaxation of the lower esophageal sphincter thus allowing the vomitus to begin moving into the esophagus.
4. Now, the gastric cardia herniates across the diaphragm and the larynx moves upwards to promote oral expulsion of vomitus. From here, a specific vomiting act involving the abdominal muscles takes over and expels the vomitus to the exterior.

Muscles and Musculature During Vamana

The whole process requires the proper junction of "a physiological anti-reflux barrier" which is located at gastroesophageal junction. The specialized smooth muscles of the wall of the lower esophagus and encircling fibers of the crural diaphragm make this barrier. The differences between the pressures of the cavities of abdomen and thorax controls this barrier. These structures exert a radial pressure over this barrier. During the process of vomiting this anti-reflux barrier must be lowered for expulsion from stomach to esophagus. (Whillis 1931)

Vomiting produced by the bursts of activity involving contraction of diaphragm, intercostals and abdominal muscles in a pattern distinct from that of a respiration. This activity is coordinated with the relaxation of the crural fibers around the esophagus. (Miller 1990).

Coordination of emesis

1. **Complex network:** Vomiting was coordinated by a single locus in the medullary reticular formation. However, further work has shown that no one "vomiting center" exists and that several brainstem nuclei initiate emesis including nucleus tractus solitarius, dorsal vagal and phrenic nuclei, Medullary nuclei that regulate respiration, and nuclei that conduct (control) pharyngeal, facial and tongue movements.
2. **Neurotransmitters:** Neurokinin NK1, serotonin, and vasopressin pathways are postulated.
3. **Muscular system:**
   i. Somatic and visceral muscles exhibit stereotypic responses during emesis.
   ii. Inspiratory thoracic and abdominal wall muscles contract producing high intrathoracic and intra-abdominal pressures that facilitate expulsion of gastric contents.
   iii. The gastric cardiac herniates across the diaphragm and the larynx moves upwards to promote oral expulsion of vomits.
4. **Visceral movements:** Under normal conditions, distally migrating upper gut contractions are regulated by an electrical phenomenon, the slow wave which cycles at 3 cycles/min in the stomach and 11 cycles/minute in the duodenum. With emesis, slow waves are replaced by orally propagating spike activity which induces the retrograde contractions that assist in the oral expulsion of small intestinal contents.

Activators of Emesis

Emesis stimulates at several anatomical sites. They are:

i. Emesis provoked by noxious thoughts or smells originates in the cerebral cortex.
ii. Whereas cranial nerves mediate vomiting after gag reflex activation.

iii. Motion sickness and inner ear disorders act on the labyrinthine apparatus by which the impulses are transmitted mainly by way of the vestibular nuclei into the cerebellum.

iv. Gastric irritants and emetogenetic anticancer drugs (e.g. cisplatin) stimulates gastroduodenal vagal afferent nerves.

v. Nongastric visceral afferents are activated by small intestinal and colonic obstruction and mesenteric ischemia.

vi. The area postrema, medullary nucleus respond to blood-borne emetic stimuli and termed as "chemoreceptor trigger zone".

vii. Many emetic drugs act on the area postrema as do bacterial toxins and metabolic disorders such as uremia, hypoxia and ketoacidosis. Neurotransmitters that mediate induction ofvomiting are selective for these anatomic sites.
   a. Labyrinthine disorders stimulate vestibular cholinergic muscaranic, muscaranic acetycholine receptor (M1) and Histaminergic (H1) receptors.
   b. Gastroduodenal vagal afferent stimuli activate serotorin 5 HT3 receptors.
   c. The area postrema is richly served by nerve fibers acting on diverse receptor subtypes including 5 HT3, M1, H1, and dopamine D2.

Alimentary Tract

Autonomic Stimulation of Secretions

a. Parasympathetic stimulation:
   i. This causes increase in the rates of glandular secretion.
   ii. This is especially true of the glands in the upper portion of the tract, innervated by the vagus and other cranial parasympathetic nerves including the salivary glands, esophageal glands, gastric glands, pancreas and Brunner's glands in duodenum.

b. Sympathetic stimulations: Sympathetic stimulation has dual effects
   i. It alone usually increases secretion (slightly).
   ii. If parasympathetic or hormonal stimulation is causing copious secretion by glands, superimposed sympathetic stimulation usually reduces the secretion. Sometimes significantly mainly because of reduced blood supply.

c. Hormonal regulation of gland secretions: The presence of Vamanopaga drug in gut lumen causes secretions of hormones. These hormones from GI mucosa get absorbed in the blood and carried to glands where they stimulate the secretions. This type of secretion is valuable in increasing the output of gastric juices and pancreatic juice, when Vamanopaga drug enters the stomach or duodenum. Hormone stimulation of gall bladder wall causes it to empty its stored bile into duodenum.

Stimulation for Secretions

The types of stimuli that do this are:

1. Tactile stimulation.
2. Chemical irritation.

3. Distension of the gut wall (P. 815–16, Guyton and Hall, 1996) When the 'Vamanopaga drug' strikes the mucosa of the stomach, the stimulation for gastric secretion through the nervous signals arises in the two ways.

↓

Either in brain (limbic system) (Long vasovagal reflxes) 112 of the nervous signals to the stomach	Stomach itself (short reflexes) Other ½ of the nervous secretory signals are generated by—
↓	↓
That cause gastric secretion	Local reflexes that occur entirely within the walls of the stomach itself in the entire nervous system
↓	↓
Originate in the "Dorsal motor nuclei of the vagus"	Gastric secretion from gastric glands
↓	
Pass by the way of 'vagus nerve'	
↓	
Enteric nervous system of stomach wall gastric glands	

Now, one can admire the vision of the great Acharyas for arranging the drugs having both Tikshna (Penetrating) property and Vikasi property (Vikasi property = 'Tikshna Prakarsha', A.S.Su.1). Tikshna property may be helpful in producing the short reflexes, while Vikashi property will help to carry the long vasovagal reflexes at the same time. The reflexes produced in the limbic system may be conferred to the Vyavayi Guna which directly reach the limbic system for the further action. From the above discussion, one can also remember the verse saying that Vamana dravya acts without the process of digestion. (Ch.Ka.12)

Secretions During Vamana

When medicine strucks the stomach, several secretions start to flow. To avoid any mechanical injury due to continuous vomiting, 'Gastroduodenal mucosal defence' also starts to secrete mucous. This mucosal defence system is composed of pre-epithelial, epithelial and sub-epithelial elements. First line of defence is a mucous bicarbonate layer which secretes as 'physicochemical barrier' to multiple molecules. It is secreted by gastroduodenal surface epithelial cells. Mucin is the constitutent glycoprotein that in combination with phospholipids forms a hydrophobic source with fatty acids into the lumen from the cell membrane.

To follow the qualitative and quantitative analysis of Kapha dosha, Hexosamine (one of the glycoproteins and mucopolysaccharide in nature) present in the mucous was analyzed in the viscous matter collected from the vomitus (P.1649, Harrisons). If the process is scrutinized watchfully, one may observe the involvement of almost every system in the same. Removal of provoked doshas during Vamana process from Amashaya may be taking place through the medium of different secretions exuding from the mucosa of stomach. The microvascular system within the gastric submucosal layer provides an adequate supply of micronutrients and oxygen while removing toxic metabolic byproducts (P.1649, Harrisons).

Basic factors that stimulate the gastric secretions are Acetylcholine, Gastrin, and Histamine which are said to be "the secretions" during Vamana.

(A) Acetylcholine

All the secretary nerves release Acetylcholine as the neurotransmitter at their endings on the glandular cells. (P. 821, Guyton and Hall, 1996).

(B) Gastrin

(One theory in Page-99, S.K.Chaudhuri, Concise Medical Physiology, 1993)
Overdistension of stomach (By Vamana Kashaya/Akanthapana/by food)

α noradrenergic stimulation	β noradrenergic stimulation
(Inhibition)	(Enhancement)

Gastrin secretion
↓
Parietal cell stimulation
↓
HCl secretion
↓
(Another theory in Page- 822, Guyton and Hall, 1996).
The nervous signals from the Vagus nerve. Those from the local enteric reflexes
Cause
(1) Direct stimulation of glandular secretions of stomach juices.
(2) Also, cause mucosa in the stomach antrum to secrete hormone Gastrin.
This hormone is secreted by gastrin cells ('G' cells) in the pyloric glands.
↓
'Gastrin' when absorbed in the blood
↓
Carried to oxyntic cells in the body of stomach
↓
Stimulate parietal and peptic cells strongly
to increase the rate of 'HCl secretion'.

"Thus, gastrin stimulation helps to produce more and more secretions through the stomach wall in which there may be the presence of morbid and provoked doshas."

(C) Histamine

A small amount of histamine is formed continuously in the gastric mucosa either in response to acid in the stomach or for other reasons. Histamine is a necessary 'cofactor' exciting the significant acid secretion.

(D) Secretin

During the process of Vamana, a gastrointestinal hormone, i.e. secretin is also produced by the cells of duodenal mucosa when come in contact with the HCl. The course of secretions continues to flow not only from the walls of stomach, i.e. Urdhva Amashaya but from the walls of duodenum, (i.e. Adhoamashaya) also. When the acid chyme (having pH 4.5 to 5.0) enters the duodenum from the stomach, it causes the release and activation of "Secretin" which is subsequently absorbed into the blood. It, in turn, causes pancreas to secrete large quantities of fluid, that contains a high concentration of bicarbonate ions (upto 145 mEq/L), but low concentrations of chloride ion which leads to further reaction as $HCL + NaHCO_3 \rightarrow NaCl + H_2CO_3$.

In the small intestine, thus neutralizing the acid from the stomach.

Bile

Bile is secreted by the liver normally between 600 and 1200 mL/day.

A. It plays an important role in fat digestion and absorption because of bile acids in the bile, that aid in the transport and absorption of the digested fat end products to and through the intestinal mucosal membrane.
B. About 80 percent of the cholesterol synthesized in the liver is converted into the bile salts which in turn are secreted into the bile.
   i. The active chemical medium of the liver is well known for its ability to detoxify or excrete into the bile by many drugs including sulfonamides, penicillin, ampicillin, erythromycin.
   ii. In a similar manner, several hormones secreted by endocrine glands are either chemicaly altered or excreted by liver including thyroxine and essentially all the steroid hormones such as estrogen, cortisol and aldosterone.
   iii. Finally one of the major routes for excreting calcium from the body is first secretion by liver into bile and then passage into the gut and loss in the feces. Thus, bile serves as means for excretion of several important "waste products" from "the blood". Here, one may recall the "Snehapana" done by an individual before proceeding towards the main karma. This Snehapana consumed in an excessive quantity, may lead to the collection of excessive cholesterol in the liver cells in which the waste products and denatured material already processed in the liver may be transferred which further may be thrown out of the body by the act of vomiting. Usually, these toxic materials or the vitiated substances pass through the feces. But as there lies a risk of reabsorption of the same through gut; the wise Acharyas might have planned this invaluable procedure.

Vamana in GIT

1. The process of Vamana is performed after 3 to 7 days of preparatory measures and is induced by certain emetics.
2. The process of emesis is central as well as peripheral by the distension of stomach by the decoction or hot infusion ingested in large amounts.
3. During the initial bouts of emesis, the content of upper GIT upto pylorus comes out. Repeated emesis creates a negative pressure gradient towards the lumen of upper GIT, while the decoction causes a positive osmotic gradient towards the lumen. Both of them cause forced extraction of easily detachable substances from the cells of the lumen and those containing waste metabolites situated nearby peripherally.
4. In this way excessive lipids which was consumed during the preparatory days blebs into the lumen with water soluble substances which are excreted out due to osmotic gradient.
5. Repeated emesis also causes the generation of a negative pressure gradient upto the second part of the duodenum, where the bile duct and pancreatic duct open into the ampulla of vater.

6. This negative pressure gradient causes forced expulsion of bile from the gallbladder and so eliminates some of the wastes with bile which have been transported to the liver via the bloodstream during the preparatory days of Sanshodhana.

Vamana Act in Other Ways

1. The osmotic gradient generated by the Vamanopaga drugs and the physical insult done to the luminal cells during the process causes loss of some of the integral proteins on the inner cell surface and other components of the cell.
2. Some old and degenerated cells are also shed into lumen due to this osmotic shock. This loss stimulates the cell machinary to recoup. This leads to the pacified anabolism in the luminal cells which means more effective absorption through GIT. In a nutsell, it can be said that every component in the body, right upto the micro level is connected to the rest of the body through a number of "Srotansi" which are vital for the being of its individual components. "Sansodhana procedures" make these communications effective, vital and prompt and thus make the tissues and ultimately the whole body more vital and viable.

Vamana : Mechanism of Action Through Nervous System

The process of Vamana proceeds through the way of nervous system.
Vamana karma occurs at three different levels in this mechanism. They are as follows:

A. Activation of emesis
B. Stimulation of vomiting center
C. Actual motor response through motor nerves

A. Activation of Emesis

I. Vomiting starts in the stomach or upper GIT, when it is full of contents (like Akanthapana during Vamana). It becomes overdistended and overexcitable afterwards.
It is told that it has same pathogenesis as that of 'Chhardi.'
According to Acharya Charaka:

अजीर्ण कट्वम्ल विदाह्य शीतैरामाशये पित्तमुदीर्णवेगम्। (Ch.Chi.20/10)

Here Udirana or excitation of Pitta to create Vega indicates the reflex from gastric mucosa. This excited stage stimulates both sympathetics and Vagal afferents leading to upward movements, where it stimulates the Mana (Hridaya) and produce the vomiting.

II. In another way, electrical stimuli or administration of certain drugs (which have Vamaka Prabhava) may stimulate chemoreceptor trigger zone directly to produce Vamana. It can be sensed in the similar way where Charaka says:

रसायनीभिर्विसृतं प्रपीडय मर्मोर्ध्वमागम्य वमि करोति। (Ch.Chi. 20/10)
व्यायाम तीक्ष्णौषध शोक रोग भयोपवासाद्यतिकर्शितस्य वायुर्महास्श्रोतासि सम्प्रवृद्ध उत्क्लेश्य दोषांस्तत्
ऊर्ध्वमस्यन्। आमाशयोत्क्लेशकृतां च मर्म प्रपीडयश्छर्दिमुदीरयेत् तु। (Ch.Chi. 26/7,8)

III. Emesis is provoked by several psychic stimuli or by noxious thoughts or smells that originate in the cerebral cortex. These types of stimuli directly stimulate the certain areas of the hypothalamus.

These types of causes create excessive increase in Vata, which otherwise̱ly expel the vitiated humors (Utkleshita doshas) as mentioned by Charaka.

उरः शिरोमर्म रसायनीः च सर्वाः समावृत्य वमि करोति॥ (Ch.Chi. 20/12)

And it also directly stimulate the higher centers प्रपीऽय मर्मोर्ध्वम्। (Ch. Chi. 20/10) to produce Chhardi. Thus, various types of stimuli work during the initial stages of Vamana.

B. Stimulation of Vomiting Center:

These all the types of vomiting stimuli directly stimulate bilateral vomiting center in the medulla like.

'वमि करोति'॥ (Ch.Chi. 20/10,12)

C. Actual motor response through motor nerves:

These stimuli further lead automatic motor reactions which further send direct motor impulses to be transmitted from vomiting center to:

i. 5th, 7th, 9th, 10th and 12th cranial nerves and then towards upper GIT.
ii. Spinal nerves which further progress to diaphragm and abdominal muscles.

D. Psychic Stimuli

(a) Upper GIT when full of contents
↓
Becomes
↓
Overdistended and overexcitable
↓
Both sympathetic and vagal afferents

(b) Electrical stimuli and administration of certain drugs "chemoreceptor trigger zone" stimulation

(c) Psychic stimuli and direct stimulation of the certain areas

Stimulates
bilateral vomiting center
in the medulla
↓
(Leading to)
↓
Automatic motor reactions
(Leading to)
Motor impulses are transmitted
from "vomiting center" through

↓ 5th, 7th, 9th, 10th, 12th Cranial nerves
↓
Upper GIT

↓ Spinal nerves
↓
Diaphragm and abdominal muscles

↓
Initiates "vomiting"

Action of Vamana Through Stress Mechanism

"Chhardi" is one of the synonyms used for "Vamana". Etymology of the word "Chhardi" itself indicates the mechanism of actual process exerting during Vamana.

छादयन्माननं वेगैरर्दयन्नङ्गभञ्जनैः। निरुच्यते छर्दिरिति दोषो वक्त्रं प्रधावितः॥ (Su. U.T. 49/6)

Thus, vomiting is the process that creates agony in the whole body during the expulsion of humors through the oral cavity which is flooded by them completely, where the word "Chhardayan", meaning "Putsyen" (Madhu on Ma.Ni.15/4), has the root word "Chad". It means to spread as a cover, to hide, to protect, etc. (Monier Williams). The word "Ardayan"(means Pidayan) is derived from root verb 'Ard' which has the meanings like to torment, to kill, to make agitated, distress, to do harm, strike, destroy (MW). "Madhukosha Teeka" provides further meaning of 'Ard' as Ard Hinsayam (Madhu on Ma.Ni.15/4), where "Hinsa"means injuring, hostile, mischievous (MW) Thus, it is the process in which the humors, which are accumulated (Purayan) in and covering (Chadayan) the whole Amashaya, inducing an injury or wound (root verb "Hins" (M.W.) in the covering of the stomach over which they have spread up and squeezing out from the stomach to be thrown out through oral cavity. It produces pains in the body or distresses it completely during the act (Ardayan). In short, "Physical and mental stress is produced in the whole body during the act of vomiting." Vomiting produces inflammation and mucosal damage secondary to insult to gastric mucosa.

"It is amazing that almost any type of stress, whether physical or neurogenic will cause an immediate and marked increase in ACTH secretion by the anterior pituitary gland followed within minutes by greatly increased adrenocortical secretions of cortisol". A wide variety of nonspecific stimuli can cause marked increase in the rate of cortisol secretion by adrenal cortex. (P. 963, Guyton and Hall, 1996).

Mental stress can cause rapid increase in ACTH secretion. This is believed to result from an increased activity in the limbic system, especially in the region of Amygdala and Hippocampus, both of them then transmitting signals to the posterior medial hypothalamus. The nucleus of hypothalamus receives many nerves connections from the limbic system and lower brainstem (P. 966, Guyton and Hall, 1996).

Secretions of cortisol took place during minor stress too 'such as a febrile illness, a laceration, severe exercise, bouts of gastroenteritis with vomiting and diarrhea and minor surgery, the normal adrenals respond by secreting about 100 mg of hydrocortisone per day'. (P. 882, Pharmacology and Pharmacotherapeutics, RS Satoskar, 15th edition). During vomiting when one administers a large amount of decoction of Vamanopaga medicine and afterwards Vamaka yoga to cause irritation in the gastric mucosa again and again to produce vomiting, it scraps the mucosal layer over the gastric mucosal surface.

This stimulates a series of several steps by the defense mechanism of the body, to protect, further damage through the means of inflammation as follows:

i. Chemical substances released from damaged cells activate the inflammatory process—chemicals such as histamine, bradykinin, prostaglandins, proteolytic enzymes and leukotrines.
ii. There will be an increased blood flow in that area.
iii. Leakage of large quantities of pure plasma out of the capillaries into the damaged areas.

iv. Infiltration of the area by leukocytes. Thus, these type of changes may compel cortisol to be secreted in large amounts during the process of vomiting.

"Actually cortisol is secreting to achieve immediate effect of blocking most of the factors that are promoting the inflammation. But in addition the rate of healing is also enhanced. This probably results from the same mainly the undefined factors that allow the body to resist many other types of physical stress when large quantities of cortisol are secreted".

Perhaps this results from the mobilization of amino acids and their use to repair the damaged tissues, perhaps it results from the increased gluconeogenesis that makes extra glucose available in critical metabolic system, perhaps it results from increased amounts of free fatty acids available for cellular energy. In fact, it has been shown that in a few instances that damaged tissues that are momentarily severely depleted of proteins can use the newly available amino acids to form new proteins that are essential for the lives of the cells (P. 964, Guyton and Hall, 1996).

So by this path, it might be helping to root out many ailments with the complex pathogenesis. Following are some examples to comprehend the action of Vamana through the medium of cortisol secretions.

IMPORTANCE OF PURVA KARMA BEFORE VAMANA

(1) Snehana

Majority of Sneha are of animal origin and so a possibility of similarity in chemical and physiological nature to that of the cell membrane cannot be ruled out. This, thus intensifies the penetration of Sneha substances through cell membrane. Cell membrane acts as a barrier to the passage of water soluble molecules, but provide free passage to lipids and lipid soluble substances.

Several studies shows that rapid diffusion of lipid soluble substances through cell membrane depend on the rate of diffusion as solubility in lipids has also been proved. By observing these facts, certain speculations can be drawn pertaining to the mode of action of preparatory measures in sanshodhana.

1. Lipid substances which are parallel to the cell membrane get directly incorporated into the cell membrane (as cell membrane is a dynamic structure this incorporation increase its surface areas).
2. Some of the lipids and lipid soluble substances directly reach the cytoplasm through the cell membrane.
3. Application of heat after Oleation causes the generation of a temperature gradient across the cell membrane. Besides facilitating the diffusion of lipid substances through cell membrane. This plays an important role in the formation of lipid vesicles from the drop outs in the membrane in areas of low temperature. This causes as expansion in the cell volume as well as surface area. But as the cell is not an isolated structure and is bound by other cells around, it is not allowed to expand freely especially in peripheral direction.

At the time of oleation and fomentation as every nearby cell expands peripherily, the blebbing of cell membrane is restricted tangentially.

- The only possibility that remains is a blebbing of the cell membrane inside.

The temperature gradient and pressure gradient caused by fomentation further helps blebbing in this particular direction.

These lipid vesicles or blebs detached from the cell membrane flow in a direction of low pressure gradient.

↓

Get attached to some other organelle or the other sides membrane and

↓

Remain there till a critical surface area reached.

↓

This membrane then blebs out and spreads further.

↓

The whole phenomenon of "The dropping of cell membrane vesicles and their incorporation into other membranous structures was described as "Membrane flow Hypothesis" by Palade (1959).

Now, while concluding it can be said that it is in this way that the Sneha reaches deep into the body tissues causing partial rejuvenation of cell organelles and cell membranes by replacing their older components with new ones and extracting the lipid soluble waste products from the cell to drain them into the bloodstream.

Thus, oleation causes the liquification, displacement, softening and smoothening of vitiated doshas (stagnated metabolic wastes) and makes their elimination possible.

The blood transports these wastes to specific areas like liver, lungs and kidneys from where they can be eliminated. The phenomenon again highlights the most precious principle in Ayurvedic management, i.e. elimination of vitiated doshas by dragging them to the major channels from the periphery, i.e. from Shakha to Koshtha.

(2) Svedana

Svedana has a vital role in carrying out the Vamana karma. It helps in the process by adapting the body so that Kapha can be emitted easily and effortlessly. Charaka narrated this in the treatment of Shvasa reasonably (Ch.Ch. 17/71-76). It functions away in the following fashion.

1. Srotah Su Abhiviliyate— It helps to dissolve shleshma which is in a dense stage (Grathita) stuck to the channels firmly. Further, it liquifies shleshma allowing it to move freely.
2. Khani Mardavam Ayanti— It makes the channels soften after which 'Vata' can flow through its normal direction (Anulomana).
3. Shleshma - Vishyandate— It increases the secretions of vitiated shleshma through the channels (Visyandana = Sravanam, Su.Chi. 4/33 = to secrete). During fomentation, heating the tissues result in rise in a temperature, the main reaction to which are as follows :
    a. Increased metabolism: So according to Vant Hoff's statement "any chemical change capable of being accelerated is accelerated by a rise in temperature". Consequently heating of tissues accelerates the chemical changes, i.e. metabolism. As a result of increased metabolism, there is an increased demand for oxygen and food stuffs and an increased output of waste products including metabolites.

b. Increased blood supply: The metabolised removed away from the cells act on the walls of capillaries and arterioles causing dilatation of these vessels. As a result of vasodilatation, there is an increased flow of blood through the area, so that the necessary O_2 and nutritive materials are supplied and waste products are removed. Thus, Svedana might be helping to melt the vitiated shleshma and let it move into the channels after dragging from the various sites.

Proper time for Vamana karma (Purvahane)

All the texts have mentioned to perform Vamana in the morning time, i.e. at the "Purvanha" when levels of Kapha are high. During this time (approximately 6.00 am to 10.00 am) Kapha is naturally in the provoked state. So it becomes easy to eliminate the deadly matter during this time.

As one has to bear some exhaustion or stress, it becomes easy to face physical exercise due to increased cortisol levels in the body during this period. "The secretory rates or CRH, ACTH and cortisol are high in the early morning but low in the late evenings. The plasma cortisol level ranges between a high of about 20 μg/dL an hour before arising in the morning and a low about 5 μg/dL around midnight".

If Vamana produced during the high levels of cortisol, further increase over this index may lead to the sufficient secretions of cortisol required for medicinal purposes in natural way, needed by the body. With these levels, it may combat the derangements present in the body.

Akanthapana

Once Akanthapana started, the drink engulfed moves forwards and function of 'Prana Vayu' starts. As the Prana and Udana working in the same area, they try to counter balance each other. Ingestion of the medicine (**अन्नप्रवेशकृत** A.H.Su.12/5) is the function of Prana Vayu. At the same time, it propagates several stimuli towards its higher centers working in the brain (**प्राणोऽत्र मूर्धग:** A. H. Su. 12/4) through the vagal afferent nerves. Till then, Udana Vayu with the help of its 'Prayatna and Bala' (A.H.Su 9/6) does not allow this highly irritant decoction to rebound back. Patient can engulf a lot of decoction till then. But at a certain stage, it becomes impossible for one to consume a single extra glass too. Thus one reaches then at the stage of feeling of fullness of stomach, i.e. "Akanthapana".

Until stage of Akanthapana is reached, several signals come into function. This type of regulation is called as "short term regulation". Following are the several types of signals that are important for this purpose.

1. **Gastrointestinal Filling:** When GIT becomes distended (especially stomach and duodenum), stretch inhibitory signals are transmitted mainly by the way of vagus to suppress the feeding center, thereby reducing the desire for food.
2. **Humoral or Hormonal factors that suppress feeding:**
   i. "Cholecystokinin" mainly released in response to fat entering the duodenum has a strong direct effect over feeding centers.
   ii. Presence of food in the stomach and duodenum causes the pancreas to secrete significant quantities of Glucagon or insulin, both of which also suppress the neurogenic feeding signals from the brain.

3. **Metering of food from the oral receptors:** Various oral factors related to the feeding such as chewing, salivation, swallowing and testing "meter" the food as it passes through the mouth and after certain amount has passed, the hypothalamic feeding center becomes inhibited. Thus all these signals stimulate "satiety center" (present in the ventromedial nuclei of the hypothalamus) and inhibit the feeding center.

Practical Application

One must refer to the first disease mentioned by Charaka in 'Nanatmaja disorders,' i.e. "Tripti" where Chakrapani defines it as (Chakr. on Ch.Su. 20/19). By treating with 'Vamana,' this center can be rearranged to its normal function through the way of alternate stimulation and inhibition.

Sweating

The process of sweating during the process of vomiting takes place in two different ways:

a. Stimulation of the anti-hypothalamus preoptic area either electrically or by the excess heat generate the impulses. They are transmitted through autonomic pathways to cord which initiates sympathetic outflow and reach skin everywhere in the body.
b. Sweat glands are innervated by sympathetic cholinergic nerve fibres. These glands can also be stimulated by epinephrine or norepinephrines circulating in the blood, even though the glands themselves do not have the adrenergic innervations.

It is important, during the strenous and exhaustive process of vomiting when the body needs to loose the extra heat produced by the active muslces, these hormones are secreted by adrenal medullae. Thus, when doshas started to liquify, (Pravilayanam Aapadyamanam) drava guna throughout the body increases due to "Doshasavghata", Bhedhana leading to 'Visyandana' because of Agneya guna. So the morbid matter situated in the skin may be drained to outside through Sveda Pravanana.

Salivation

The process of salivation occurs when salivary nuclei (situated in the brainstem) are stimulated by parasympathetic nervous signals or salivary nuclei are excited by both the taste and tactile stimuli from the tongue and the other areas of the mouth. The irritating foods are swallowed or when the person is nauseated, and reflexes are sent from the stomach and upper intestines. This swallowed saliva helps to remove the irritation factor in GIT by diluting or neutralizing the irritating substances. Saliva itself contains the two major types of secretions: serous secretion and mucous secretion (pH ranges between 6.0 and 7.0).

Thus, one can say the increased "Shleshita" from every site of the body starts to oozes out through the nearest route available, once the process of Vamana started.

Role of Antigravity Muscles

1. The process of vomiting itself is the mechanism carried out against specific gravity. During this act there are continuous changes arising in the muscles of neck, vertebral column, legs, abdomen, chest, etc. The abdominal muscles become flexed, muscles of back of spine become extended, extension and flexion of cervical muscles take place.

2. In the internal environment also, the oesophageal muscles and muscles of stomach move in opposite direction to throw the material upwards, i.e. the direction opposite to gravitational force.

To make equilibrium against this antigravitational force, body has to make some arrangements.

There are two types of reticular nuclei in the brain

Pontine reticular nuclei		Medullary reticular nuclei
↓		↓
Exciting the Antigravity Muscles	(Functioning antagonistic to each other)	Inhibiting antigravity muscles.

The "pontine reticular nuclei" has a high degree of natural excitability.

They also receive the strong excitatory signals from the vestibular nuclei as well as from the deep nuclei of cerebrellum.

For the process of Vamana the excitation of the antigravity muscles, i.e. the muscles of the neck, trunk and extensors of the legs is inevitable. But at the same time, for the smooth and effortless proceedings during Vamana, body activates the medullary reticular inhibiting system also. So that, during the process of Vamana, body muscles can be relaxed. Therefore, the excitatory and inhibitory reticular nuclei constitute a controllable system which is manipulated by motor signals from the cortex and elsewhere to provide the necessary muscle contraction during vomiting.

Acharyas having a great vision pointed out some specific suggestions regarding this process. While explaning the Vamana chair, Charaka advised to keep it with the height of "Janusamam". (Ch.Su.15/5). Sitting in this position, the muscles of the neck and those of the spine come more nearer to the earth and also remain parallel to the muscles of the legs. Thus, with this position, body can make the equilibrium regarding the changes in positions during Vamana (like stretching of the spine, making the neck muscles rigid, slightly extending the legs, bowing/ bending down to vomit; etc). Also, in the same context, Charaka suggests to help the individual during the procedure by lalata pratigraha, etc. as described on page no 230.

Thus, all these acts are advocated to assist the patient in this strenous procedure.

Agnimandya after Vamana

There is an Agnimandya after Vamana which has to be restored by Sansarjana course. Actually, after Vamana, the environments in the stomach got totally alkaline due to mucous secretions, bicarbonate flows and bile extraction. This ultimately hampers the pepsin activity. "Pepsin activity is significantly diminished at pH4 and irreversibly inactivated and denatured at a pH of >7. So, this might be the reason why diminution of Agni takes place after Vamana".

Vamana Yoga according to Disease

S. No.	*Name of Disease*	*Vamana Yoga*	*References*
1.	Jvara	Madanaphala Pippali with Lavanodaka	Ch.Ci.3/227-228
2.	Raktapitta	Madanaphala and Kutaja	Ch.Ci. 4/55-56
3.	Kustha	Kutaja, Madanaphala, Patola Nimba, Yastimadhu and Madhu	Ch.Ci.7/42
4.	Rajyakshama	Madanaphala kshira	Ch.Ci. 8/117-118
5.	Grahini	Madanaphala + Pippali + Sarshapa Kalka	Ch.Ci. 15/73-74
6.	Pandu	Tikshana Vamana	Ch.Ci. 16/39
7.	Hikka-Shvasa	Madanphala + Pippali + Saindhava Lavana + Madhu	Ch.Ci. 17/74,75,76
8.	Kasa	Madanphala + Yastimadhu Kvatha + Gambhari	Ch.Ci. 18/83
9.	Chhardi	Jimutaka Phala	Ch.Ci. 20/22
10.	Visarpa	Madana, Madhuka, Nimba, Kutaja Patola, Pippali, Kutaki.	Ch.Ci. 21/51,52
11.	Yonivyapada	Vacha, Priyangu, Yastimadhu, Kutaja Sarshapa, Nimba, Patola.	Ch.Ci. 30/251-252

CHAPTER 5

Virechana

INTRODUCTION

After Vamana karma, the next purification process is called Virechana. The general meaning of virechana is (induced or instantly induced) purgation of the stomach contents. It is a process of expelling out contents of the stomach through purgation. Virechana is one of the Pradhana karma among the Panchakarma and it is the ideal and best treatment in which Pitta, Pitta's conjunction with one dosha (sansarga) or both other doshas (sannipata) and mala which are toxic to body are thrown out of the body via rectal route. It is a less tedious procedure than Vamana and hence there is less possibility of complications and it can be carried out with comparative ease.

विरेको मुखपीत गुदमार्गेणान्तः। स्थितस्य दोषस्य निस्सारणं पित्तस्य परमौषधम्।। (A.S.Su.1/39.Indu)

Virechana is the procedure in which the orally administered drug acts on internally situated doshas, specifically on Pitta Dosha and expels them out of the body through anal route.

Importance of Virechana

Vagbhatta says that although Virechana is choice of treatment for Pitta paradhana dosha, even then it is not opposed or contraindicated in kapha pradhana diseases. It is advisable in conditions of sansrishta Kapha and in conditions where kapha reaches Basti sthana.

ETYMOLOGY

Virechana is a napunsaka linga shabda. The word "Virechana" has three components:

विरेचन वि+रिच्+णिच्, ल्युट्-मलादेः निस्सरणम्। (Vachaspatyama 4847)

Vi - Upasarga (prefix)
Ricir - Ric Dhatu (root)
Lut - Pratyaya (suffix) (Malade Nissaranam)
Here (I) "Ricir" - evacuation
(II) "Ric" - Viyojana (separation)
Sansarga (combination)

The word "Rechana" is commonly used in the first sense i.e. Richir = evacuation. As the evacuation is done by both Vamana and Virechana, therefore some times Virechana word is used for both Vamana and Virechana (Ch.K.1/4). But in general Virechana word denotes to evacuation through lower gut by purgation.

The other root word, i.e. "Ric" is also very important to understand the systemic action of Virechana. According to Charaka, the Virechana drugs first get absorbed, then reaches to heart (Dhamani, macro and micro channels of the body) and the place where doshas are accumulated.

DEFINITION

तत्र दोषहरणं अधो भागम् विरेचन संज्ञकं। उभयं वा शरीरमल विरेचनात् विरेचनं संज्ञा लभते।
(Ch.Ka.1/4)

The process of elimination of morbid doshas through Adhobhaga is said to be Virechana. According to Chakrapani, the meaning of Adhobhaga is Guda. Virechana is a broad term which is applied even for Vamana Karma since the expulsion of doshas takes place from either routes.

विपक्वं यदपक्वं वा मलादि द्रवतां नयेत्। रेचयत्यपि तज्ज्ञेयं। (Sh.Sam.Pu.Kh.4/6.)

The process of elimination of Mala either in Pakva or in Apakva avastha but along with excess fluid portions is called as Virechana. In Virechana the Doshas even from the Amashaya are taken to the Pakvashaya and they are removed through Gudamarga.

तत्र दोष हरणं अधोभागम् विरेचन संज्ञकं। उभयं वा शरीरमल विरेचनात् विरेचनसंज्ञकं लभते।
(Ch.Ka.1/4)

As the evacuation of Doshas is done by both Vamana and Virechana, therefore sometimes the word 'Virechana' broadly applies for both.

विरेचनं पित्तहराणाम् (श्रेष्ठं) (Ch.Su.25/50)

Virechana Karma is one of the prime purificatory procedures among Panchakarma, which is a supreme procedure for elimination of Pitta Dosha.

विरेचनं तु सर्वौपक्रमेभ्यः पित्ते प्रधानतमं मन्यते भिषजः।
तद् ध्यादित एवं आमशयम् अनुप्रविश्य केवलं वैकारिकं पित्तमूलम् अपकर्षति,
तत्र अवजिते पित्तेऽपि शरीरान्तर्गताः पित्त विकारः प्रशान्तिम् आपद्यते, यथाऽग्नौ
व्यपोढे केवलम् अग्नि गृहं शीतीभवति तद्वत्। (Ch.Su.20/16)

Virechana is prime modality of treatment for Pitta dosha nirharana, as Amashaya is Samanya sthana for Pitta and Kapha Dosha which holds good for both. How the fire gets cooled by subsiding the fire which had caught the building, in the same way by subsiding Amashayagata Pitta, all other Pitta's gets subsided.

पित्ते तु विरेकं, श्लेष्म संसृष्टेवा तत् स्थानगतेव श्लेष्मणीति। (A.S.Su. 27)

The vitiation of Kevala Pitta, Pitta associated with Kapha and through Pittasthana Gata Kapha, Virechana is the choice of treatment to be followed.

It is also advocated as a part of Ritucharya in Sharad Ritu.

Virechana is not as complicated as Vamana, because of the expulsion of Dosha in normal route.

बुद्धेः प्रसादं बलम् इंन्द्रियाणां धातु स्थिरत्वं बलम् अग्निदीप्तिम्।
चिरात् च पाकं वयसः करोति विरेचनं सम्यग् उपास्यमानम्॥
यथा औदकानाम् उदकेऽपनीते चरस्थिराणां भवति प्रणाशः।
पिते हृते त एव उपद्रवाणां पित्तात्मकानां भवति प्रणाशः॥ (Su.Chi 33/27-28)

By the process of Virechana Karma, it helps in improving the intellectual clarity, strengthens all sense organs, provide stability to Dhatu, Bala, causes Agni dipti and delays ageing process. By removal of water how all dependents of water gets destroyed, in the same way by removal of vitiated Pitta all the diseases caused due to Pitta gets destroyed.

Shodhana is the only means by which the Dosha Dushya SamMurcchana can be broken. This is the reason why the disease gets a radical cure by the administration of Shodhana.

Synonyms

प्रस्कन्दन च स्नेहात्प्रस्कंदन जन्तुः त्रिरात्रौपरतः पिबेत्। (Ch.Su. 13/81)

Rechanam, Praskandanam

Detailed description of Virechana is present in all the Ayurvedic texts. The references of various aspects of Virechana in Ayurvedic classics are listed below.

Text	*Reference*
Charaka Samhita	Sutrasthan Chap.-1, 2, 4, 15, Chikitsasthana Kalpasthana - Chap. 7th to 12th, Siddhisthana-Chap. 1, 2, 6
Sushruta Samhita	Sutrasthana- Chap 39, 41, 44, Chikitsasthana-33, 34 Kalpasthana.
Ashtanga Sangraha	Sutrasthana-Chapter 27
Ashtanga Hridaya	Sutrasthana-Chap. 18, Kalpasthana Chap. 3
Sharangdhara Samhita	Purvakhanda -Chapter 4, Uttarakhanda- Chapter 4
Chakradatta	Chapter-71
Bhava Prakash	Purvakhanda

UTILITY OF VIRECHANA KARMA

Virechana can specifically act on the following Dosha Dushya and Srotasa:

- ❑ **Dosha**: Pitta, Pitta Sthanagata Alpa Kapha, Kapha Sthanagata Bahu Pitta Pittavritta Vata, Sannipata of doshas.
- ❑ **Dushya**: Rasa, Rakta, Mansa, Asthi, Majja, Shukra
- ❑ **Srotasa**: Rasavaha, Raktavaha, Mansavaha, Asthivaha Majjavaha, Shukravaha

1. Indication of Virechana in Different Doshas

केवले पित्ते विरेचनमाचरेत्। स्तोकेन श्लेष्मणा संसृष्टे पित्ते विरेचनमेव। तथा पित्तस्थान गते श्लेष्माणि प्रभूतपित्ते विरेचनमेव। कफस्थागते वा प्रभूत पित्त इति। (Indu on A.S.Su. 27/4)

- Virechana is a specific treatment for Pitta dosha. "Virechanam Pittaharanam (Ch.Su.25/40)

शरीरजानां दोषाणां .... विरेको .... धृतं .... ॥ (A.H.Su. 1/25)

- Virechana is even a treatment for Pitta Sansargaja Doshas, Kapha sanshrishta doshas and also for Pitta sthanagata Kapha.

पित्तं तु विरेकं; श्लेष्म संसृष्टे वातस्थान गते वा श्लेष्माणि इति (विरेक)॥ (A.H.Su. 27)

- Similarly, Virechana is even beneficial for Vata dosha, which is evident from Vatopakrama that :

  वातस्योपक्रमः स्नेहः स्वेदः सशोधनं मृदुः॥ (A.H.Su. 13/1)
- Here mridu Sanshodhana refers to Virechana karma.
- Where Rakta is the pradhana dosha i.e. Kushtha, Visarpa, Raktapitta, Gudapaka.
- Pitta-Kaphaja conditions like Adhoga Amlapitta.
- Pitta invading the site of Kapha.
- Vayu located in Pakvashaya. (Ch.Chi. 28/190)
- If Vayu in association with Pitta, pervades the entire body.(Ch.Chi. 28/190)
- Acharya Bhela has mentioned Virechana in 'sannipata' condition also.

  Chakrapani does not includes Niruha and Shiro virechana under the term Virechana but Gangadhara says that dosha nirharana from any route of the body can be taken as Virechana. Hence Niruha, Shirovirechana should also be considered as Virechana. Hence Virechana is beneficial in tridosha states.

2. Indication of Virechana as Vyadhi Prtyanika Chikitsa

- Pitta Sthana gata Vyadhi like Shvasa.
- Diseases having deep seated pathology like Unmada, Apasmara.
- Diseases involving multiple doshas and dushyas requiring Tikshna Shodhana like Gara visha, Krimi koshtha, Prameha etc.
- Diseases in which Margavrodha as a treatment is indicated like Urdwa Raktapitta and Chhardi.
- In which Anulomana of Vayu is required like Udavarta, Udara roga, Yoni Vyapada.

3. As both Dosha and Vyadhi Pratyanika Chikitsa

- Diseases dominated by Pitta like Kamla, Pandu.
- In diseases like Grahani where aggravated Pitta itself hampers Agni.
- Disease caused by Aama like Visuchika. In Ashtanga sangraha Shodhana (virechana) has been mentioned for the treatment of Sama dosha and Sama dushya.

CLASSIFICATION OF VIRECHANA

1. According to Sharangadhara

Sharangadhara has classified as per the gradation of Virechana which are dependant on action, potency of drug, onset, consistency of excretory product.

i. Anulomana

कृत्वा पाकं मलानां यद्भित्वा बन्धमधो नयेत्। तच्चानुलोमनं ज्ञेयं यथा प्रोक्ता हरीतकी।

(Sh.Sam.Pu.Kh.4)

The process which does the digestion of malas and breaks its compactness and later expels out through adhobhaga is known as Anulomana e.g. Haritaki.

ii. Sransana

पक्तव्यं यदपक्त्वैव श्लिष्टं कोष्ठे मलादिकम्। नयत्यधः स्त्रंसनं तद्यथा स्यात्कृतामलकः।

(Sh.Sam.Pu.Kh.4)

The process which expels half digested and sticky malas without prior digestion is known as Sransana e.g. Kritamalaka.

iii. Bhedana

मलादिकमबद्धं च बद्धं वा पिण्डितं मलैः। भित्वाधः पातयति तद्भेदनं कुटकी यथा।।

(Sh.Sam.Pu.Kh.4)

The drug which breaks abaddha, baddha and pindita malas and eliminates through anus are called as Bhedana e.g. Katuki.

iv. Rechana

विपक्वं यदपक्वं वा मलादि द्रवतां नयेत्। रेचयत्यपि तज्ज्ञेयं रेचन त्रिवृता यथा। (Sh.Sam.Pu.Kh.4/6)

The process which expels both digested and undigested malas after making them watery, through Gudamarga is known as Rechana e.g. Trivrit.

Anulomana and Sransana are the mild types of Virechana, whereas Bhedana and Rechana are of moderate type. Acharya Charaka also described about Bhedaneeya, Virechanopaga and Anulomana, which suggests types of Virechana.

2. According to Guna of Aushadhi

i. Ruksha virechana

Drugs used are of Ruksha guna in form of churna, vati. Administered in Snigdha sharira.

ii. Snigdha virechana

Drugs used are in form of sneha, aasava, aarishtas and administered in ruksha sharira.

3. According to Intensity of Aushadhi

i. Tikshna

Drugs are strong purgatives. Administered in Bahudoshavastha, e.g. Snuhiksheera.

ii. Madhya

Drugs like Aragvadha for Madhyadosha.

iii. Mridu

Mild purgatives for Alpadosha.

INDICATIONS AND CONTRAINDICATIONS OF VIRECHANA KARMA

Prior to subjecting the patient to any therapy, it is necessary to examine whether the patient is fit for proposed therapy or not. Following are the indications and contraindications for Virechana karma.

Indications

विशेषस्तु कुष्ठ ज्वर मेह उर्ध्वरक्तपित्त भगन्दर उदर अर्शो ब्रध्न प्लीह गुल्मार्बुद गलगण्ड ग्रन्थि विसूचिकालसक मूत्राघात क्रिमिकोष्ठ विसर्प पाण्डुरोग शिरः पार्श्व शूल उदावर्त नेत्रास्यदाह हृद्रोग व्यङ्ग नीलिका नेत्रनासिका आस्यस्रवण हलीमक श्वास कास कामला अपच्यपस्मार उन्माद वातरक्त योनिरेतोदोष तैमिर्यारोचकाविपाक च्छर्दि श्वयथूदर विस्फोटकादयः पित्तव्याधयो विशेषेण महारोगाध्यायोक्ताश्च; एतेषु हि विरेचनं प्रधानमित्युक्तं अग्रपशमेऽग्रिगृहवत्। (Ch.Si.2/13)

Kushtha, Jvara, Meha, Urdhva Raktapitta, Bhagandara, Udara, Arsha, Bradhna, Pleeha, Gulma, Arbuda, Galaganda, Granthi, Visuchika, Alasaka, Mutraghata, Krimikoshtha, Visarpa, Panduroga, Shirahshula,Parshvashula, Udavarta, Netradaha, Aasyadaha, Hridroga, Vyanga, Neelika, Netrasrava, Nasika srava, Asya srava, Halimaka, Shvasa, Kasa, Kamala, Apachi, Apasmara, Unmada, Vatarakta, Yoni Dosha, Reto Dosha, Timira, Arochaka, Avipaka, Chhardi, Shvayathu, Udara, Visphota etc.

1. Dosha
   - Utklishta Pitta, Kapha Sansrishta Pitta, Pittasthanagata alpa Kapha, Kaphasthanagata Kapha Pitta.
   - Pitta Avritta Vata, Kapha Avritta Vata.
   - Charaka advices that Tiryakgata Dosha should be taken back to Koshtha, gradually by proper acts and after that elimination should be carried out. This denotes that Virechana is the treatment of choice in Tiryakgata Dosha as seen in Kushtha.
2. Dushya

   For Rasa, Rakta etc. Vikaras Virechana Karma is described in direct or indirect way.
3. In Svastha.
4. Purvakarma for Rasayana and Vajikarana.
5. Virechana is indicated in disorders like, Gulma – Vatadhikya, Kamala – Paittika, Gara – Tridoshaja, Unmada – Tridoshaja, Kushtha – Tridoshaja etc.

From the above references it becomes clear that Virechana karma has a specific action in various conditions of all three Doshas. It is a procedure of choice for healthy as well as diseased person.

Virechana Yogya Indication

Virechana Yogya	*Ch.*	*Su.*	*A.S.*	*A.H.*	*K.S.*	*Sha.S.*	*Y.R.*
Pitta Pradhana Vyadhi							
Jvara	+	+	+	+	+	+	+
Pandu	+	+	-	-	-	+	+
Kamala	+	-	-	+	-	-	-
Halimaka	+	-	+	+	-	-	-
Netradaha	+	+	-	-	-	-	-
Aasyadaha	+	+	-	-	-	-	-
Paittika vyadhi	+	+	+	-	-	-	-
Vata Pradhana Vyadhi							

Contd...

Contd...

Virechana Yogya	*Ch.*	*Su.*	*A.S.*	*A.H.*	*K.S.*	*Sha.S.*	*Y.R.*
Pakvashaya Ruja	-	+	+	+	-	-	-
Shirashula	+	-	+	-	-	-	-
Parshvaruja	+	-	-	-	-	-	-
Gulma	+	+	+	+	-	+	+
Vatarakta	+	+	+	+	-	+	+
Kapha Pradhana Vyadhi							
Prameha	+	+	-	-	-	+	+
Netrasrava	+	-	-	-	-	+	+
Asyasrava	+	-	-	-	-	+	+
Nasasrava	+	-	-	-	-	+	+
Shvasa	+	-	-	-	-	-	-
Shotha	+	+	-	-	-	+	+
Tridoshaja Vyadhi							
Kushtha	+	+	-	-	+	+	+
Visarpa	+	+	-	-	-	-	-
Hridroga	+	+	-	-	-	+	+
Rakta Pradhana Vyadhi							
Pleeha	+	+	+	+	-	+	-
Vyanga	+	-	+	+	-	-	-
Nilika	+	-	-	-	-	-	-
Visphotaka	+	+	+	+	+	+	-
Manasa Roga							
Unmada	+	-	-	-	-	-	-
Apasmara	+	+	-	-	-	-	-
Stri Roga							
Yonidosha	+	+	+	+	-	+	+
Shalya Kriya Sadhya							
Vyadhi							
Arbuda	+	+	-	-	-	-	-
Bhagandara	+	+	+	-	-	+	+
Arsha	+	+	+	+	-	+	+
Vidradhi	-	+	+	+	-	+	+
Granthi	+	+	-	-	-	+	+
Galaganda	+	-	-	-	-	-	-
Bradhna	+	-	-	-	-	-	-
Dushtavrana	-	+	+	+	-	-	+
Vriddhi	-	+	-	-	-	-	-
Apachi	+	-	-	-	-	-	-
Shalakya Vyadhi							

Contd...

Contd...

Virechana Yogya	*Ch.*	*Su.*	*A.S.*	*A.H.*	*K.S.*	*Sha.S.*	*Y.R.*
Timira	+	+	+	+	-	-	-
Abhishyanda	-	+	+	+	-	-	-
Kacha	-	+	+	+	-	-	-
Akshipaka	-	+	+	-	-	-	-
Annavaha Srotasa							
Krimi koshtha	+	+	+	+	-	+	+
Garavisha	-	+	-	+	-	+	+
Visuchika	+	+	-	-	-	+	+
Alasaka	+	+	-	-	-	-	-
Udara	+	-	+	+	-	+	+
Arochaka	+	+	-	-	-	+	+
Avipaka	+	+	-	-	-	+	+
Vibandha	-	+	+	+	-	-	-
Marga Bheda							
Urdhva Raktapitta	+	+	+	+	-	-	-
Udavarta	+	-	+	-	-	-	-
Chhardi	+	+	+	+	-	+	+
Others							
Retodosha	+	-	+	+	-	-	-
Mutraghata	+	+	+	+	-	+	+
Shashtrakshata	-	+	-	-	-	-	-
Ksharagni-dagdha	-	+	+	-	-	-	-

Reason for indication

1. Pitta pradhana vyadhi's are indicated since Virechana is best in these diseases (Ch.Su. 25/40) eg: Pandu, Kamala.
2. Rakta pradoshaja vyadhi: Since there is specific indication of Virechana in these diseases. eg: Kushtha, Visarpa, Raktapitta, Gudapaka (Ch.Su.24/18).
3. Diseases where there is extreme need to eliminate doshas i.e. Bahudoshavastha, such as in Gara visha, Krimi koshtha and Udavarta.
4. Diseases having Viloma gati of doshas, like Urdhvaga Raktapitta and Chhardi etc, Virechana is indicated to reverse the gati of the disease.
5. Diseases in which there will be excessive vitiation of doshas and also having tridosha prakopa and also those diseases requiring Ubhayabhaga shodhana like Kushtha, Virechana is indicated.
6. Those diseases where Pitta has main role in pathogenesis: e.g. Hridroga- Sadhaka Pitta, Jvara- Pachaka Pitta, Kamala- Ranjaka Pitta etc.

Contraindications

अविरेच्यास्तु सुभग क्षतगुद मुक्तनाल अधोंभागरक्तपित्त विलङ्घित दुर्बलेन्द्रिय
अल्पाग्नि निरूढ कामादिव्यग्र अजीर्णि नवज्वरी मदात्ययिताध्मात शल्यार्दिताभिहत
अति स्निग्ध रूक्ष दारुणकोष्ठाः क्षतादयश्च गर्भिण्यन्ताः॥ (Ch.Si..2/11).

Subhaga, kshata guda, muktanala, adhoga raktapitta, vilanghita, durbalendriya, alpagni, nirudha, kamadi vyagra, navajwari, madatyaya, adhmata (adhmana), atisnigdha, atiruksha, daruna koshtha, garbhini, etc.

Virechana Ayogya	*Ch.*	*Su.*	*A.S.*	*A.H.*	*K.S.*	*Sha.S.*	*Y.R.*
Langhita	+	-	+	-	-	-	-
Durbala	+	-	-	-	+	-	-
Durbalendriya	+	-	-	-	-	-	-
Upavasita	+	-	-	-	-	-	-
Subhaga	+	-	-	-	-	-	-
Alpagni	+	+	+	+	-	+	+
Abhighata	+	-	-	-	+	-	-
Kshatkshina	+	+	+	-	-	+	+
Shranta	+	+	-	-	+	+	+
Pipasita	+	+	-	-	+	+	+
Karma Bharadhvahata	+	+	-	-	-	-	-
Vriddha	+	-	-	-	-	+	+
Bala	+	+	+	-	+	-	-
Atikrisha	+	-	+	-	+	+	-
Atisthula	+	+	+	-	+	+	-
Daruna koshtha	+	-	+	+	-	-	-
Kshama	+	-	-	-	-	-	-
Garbhini	+	+	-	-	-	-	-
Bhakta	+	+	-	-	-	+	-
Rikta Koshtha	-	-	-	-	+	-	-
Sukumar	-	-	-	-	+	-	-
Navaprasuta	-	+	-	-	-	+	+
Some Other Conditions							
Ratri Jagarana	-	-	+	-	-	-	-
Anupasnigdha	-	-	-	-	+	-	-
Atisnigdha	+	+	-	+	-	+	+
Atiruksha	+	-	-	-	-	+	+
Bhayoptapta	-	+	-	-	-	+	+

Contd...

Contd...

Virechana Ayogya	*Ch.*	*Su.*	*A.S.*	*A.H.*	*K.S.*	*Sha.S.*	*Y.R.*
Chintaprasakta	+	-	-	-	-	+	+
Maithunaprasakta	+	-	-	-	-	-	-
Adhyayanaprasakta	+	-	-	-	-	-	-
Vyayamaprasaka	+	+	+	+	-	+	+
Shalyardita	+	-	+	+	-	-	-
Kamadi Vyagra	+	+	-	-	-	-	-
Nirudha	+	-	-	-	-	-	-
Samavastha							
Nava Pratishyaya	-	+	-	-	-	-	-
Nava Jvara	+	+	+	+	-	+	+
Diseases of Rectum							
Kshataguda	+	+	+	-	-	-	-
Muktanala	+	-	+	-	-	-	-
Other Diseases							
Madatyaya	+	+	+	-	-	+	+
Adhmana	+	+	+	-	-	-	-
Talushosha	-	-	-	-	+	-	-
Urustambha	-	-	-	-	+	-	-
Ardita	-	-	-	-	+	-	-
Hanugraha	-	-	-	-	+	-	-
Hridroga	-	-	-	-	+	-	-
Kevala Vataroga	-	-	-	-	+	-	-
Rajayakshma	-	-	+	-	-	-	-
Shosha	-	-	-	-	+	-	-
Marga Virodhi Vyadhi							
Adhoga Raktapitta	+	+	+	+	-	-	-
Atisara	-	-	-	+	+	-	-

Reasons for Contraindication

Contraindication	*Reason for contraindication*
सुभग (Ulceration in anal region)	सुभगस्य सुकुमारोक्तो दोषः स्यात् (Leads to Dosha's caused in Sukumaras mentioned in Avaamya like bleeding per rectum, pain in precordial region etc.)
क्षतगुद (Injury to anal region)	क्षते गुदे प्राणोपरोधकरीं रुजां जनयेत् (Gives rise to severe pain in the anal region)

Contd...

Contd...

Contraindication	*Reason for contraindication*
मुक्तनाल (Anal in continence)	मुक्तनालमतिप्रवृत्या हन्यात् (There are chances of Atipravritti of Dosha's)
अधोभाग रक्तपित (Sponataneous bleeding from rectal route and urethrae route)	अधोभागरक्तपित्तिनं तद्वत् (May worsen the condition)
विलङ्घित, दुर्बलेन्द्रिय, अल्पाग्नि, निरूढा (The person who had undergone Langhana, Niruha and who is debilitated and has Alpagni	औषधवेगं न सहेरन् (Cannot tolerate the strain caused due to action of Virechana dravyas)
कामादिव्यग्रमनस (Usually active in sexual behaviours	न प्रवर्तते कृच्छ्रेण वा प्रवर्तमानमयोगदोषान् कुर्यात्(Chances of Ayoga doshas is observed)
अजीर्ण (Indigestion)	आमदोष : (Formation of Amadosha's)
नवज्वरि (Fever of recent origin)	अविपक्वान् दोषान् न निर्हरेद् वातमेव च कोपयेत् (because of unripened state of Dosha's there are chances of complication)
मदात्ययि (Alcoholic)	मद्यक्षीणे देहे वायुः प्राणोपरोधं कुर्यात् (body is weakened in alcoholics. Virechana karma is likely to predispose provocation of vata.)
आध्मात (Distension of abdomen)	अधमतो वा पुरीषकोष्ठे निचितो वायुर्विसर्पन सहसाऽऽनाहं तीव्रतरं मरणं वा जनयेत् (Administration of Virechana may further cause aggravation of disease)
शल्यार्दिताभिहतयो (Traumatic injury)	क्षते वायुराश्रितो जीवितं हिंस्यात् (Further aggravation of Vata)
अतिस्निग्ध (Over oleation)	अतियोगभयं भवेत् (Chances of Atiyoga are seen)
रूक्ष (Excessive dryness in the body)	(Vitiation of Vata)
दारुणकोष्ठ (Habitual constipated)	विरेचनोद्धतादोष हृच्छूल पर्वभेदाहङ्गमर्दच्छर्दि मूर्च्छाक्लमाञ्जन यित्वा प्राणान् हन्युः (Can lead to Ayoga, precordial pain, joint pain, distension of abdomen, body ache, vomiting etc.)

CLASSIFICATION OF THE VIRECHANA DRAVYA, GENERAL PROPERTIES OF VIRECHANA DRAVYA

Classification of Virechana dravya can be done with various viewpoints as follows:

I. Based on the Origin and Utilized Part

1. Animal origin: Ksheera, Mastu, Takra, Mutra (A.S.Su.14/3)
2. Plant origin:

Part used	*Charaka (Ch.Su.1/77-85)*	*Sushruta (Su.Su. 39/4)*	*Vagbhatta (A.S. Su. 14)*
Mula (Mulini)	Hastidanti Shyamatrivritta Shweta, Saptala Danti Gavakshi, Visanika Avartaki Dravanti	Snuka Shyamatrivritta, Raktamula, Danti, Gavakshi, Swarnakshiri, Dravanti, Chitraka, Kusha, Kasa, Kinhi	Shaliparni, Prishnaparni Kantakari, Gokshura, Vartaki Punarnava, Vastuka, Salavriksha
Phala (Phalini)	Shankhini, Vidanga, Aanupklitaka, (Madhuyashti) Prakirya, (Latakaranja) Abhaya, Antahakotarpushpi, Kampillaka, Aragawadha, Udkirya	Puga, Eranda Haritaki Amalaki, Bibhitaka, Nilini, Chaturangula, Kampillaka Kashmari, Puga Parushaka, Vidanga, Draksha, Nili, Yashtimadhu, Putikaranja	Triphala, Pilu, Eranda, Priyala, Badara, Kuvala, Karkandhu
Kshira	Snuhiksheera Arkaksheera		
Tvacha	Putika Tilvaka Krishnagadha	Saptacchada, Jyotishmati, Kampillaka, Ramyaka, Patala, Patola	Saptaparna, Jyotishmati Kampillaka, Lodhra, Mahanimba

II. According to the Intensity of Action

a. **Mridu:** These are the dravyas which causes mild actions when given in low dosage.
Indication: In alpa dosha, in unknown type of koshtha, previously who have taken Shodhana even then who have ample amounts of doshas and in mridu koshtha.
E.g. : Draksha, Payas, Ushnambu, Eranda taila (Sh.Ut.4/13,14)

b. **Madhyama:** Drugs which are madhyama in their guna and karma.
Indication: In madhyama koshtha, madhyama roga and bala (Ch.Ka.12/55)
E.g. : Trivrit, Katuki, Rajavriksha (Sh.Sam.Ut.4/13-14)

c. **Tikshna:** Drugs which are having tikshna guna and karma and which cause numerous motions by eliminating doshas in major quantity, even then doesn't produce glani in payu and hridaya pradesha or antarashaya are called Tikshna Virechana (Ch. Ka.12/51-52)
Indication: Krura koshtha , Balayukta purushas.
E.g. Snukpaya, Hemakshiri, Dantiphala (Sh.Sam.Ut.4/14)

III. According to their Safety of Action

1. **Sukha Virechana:** Drugs which leads to Samyak Virechana without any complication. Indicated in Madhya koshtha, e.g. Trivrit.
2. **Mridu Virechana:** Drugs which are mild in nature and useful in mridu koshtha. Indicated in Mridu koshtha, e.g. Chaturangula.
3. **Tikshna Virechana:** Drugs which cause drastic purgation. Indicated in Krura koshtha e.g. Snuhi paya.

IV. According to Kalpana

Certain kalpanas of virechana dravyas are prepared for the purpose of easy intake, to enhance or to alter the potency and to preserve for longer duration. Kalpana is procedure of mixing and processing Virechaka drug along with other edible substances which increase or decrease its potency. According to Sushruta: Ghrita yoga, Taila yoga, Ksheera yoga, Madya yoga, Mutra yoga, Mansarasa yoga, Bhakshyanna yoga, Avaleha yoga. Apart from these, some other kalpanas include: Asava, Aristha, Varti, Panaka, Shadava, Seedhu, Yavagu, Modaka, Dadhi etc.

V. Based on Dosha :

कषायमधुरैः पित्ते विरेकः, कटुकैः कफे। स्निग्धोष्णलवणैर्वायौ ....॥ (A.H.Su. 18/35)

Vata : Snigdha, Ushna, Lavana
Pitta : Kashaya, Madhura
Kapha : Katu

VI. According to Acharya Sushruta

अरूणाभं त्रिवृतमूलं श्रेष्ठं........सुधापय पयसूवक्तं इति प्रधान्य संग्रहः॥ (Su.Su.44/1,2)

1. Mula virechana- Arunabha trivrit mula
2. Twak virechana- Tilvaka
3. Phala virechana - Haritaki
4. Taila virechana - Eranda taila
5. Svarasa virechana - Karavellaka
6. Paya virechana - Shudha paya (Su.Su.44/3,4).

VII. According to Prakriti

Prakriti	*Virechana drugs*
Vata	Snigdha, Ushna, Lavanayukta aushadhi
Pitta	Kashaya and Madhura rasa aushadhi
Kapha	Katu rasa aushadhi

VIII. According to Dosha

Dosha	*Drugs*
Vata	Trivrit+Saindhava+Shunti churna along with kanji and mansa rasa
Pitta	Trivrit churna+Draksha Kvatha
Kapha	Triphala Kvatha, Gomutra, Trikatu

IX. According to Ritu

Sharangadhara and Bhava mishra have mentioned some of the drugs and their preparations.

Ritu	*Drugs*	*Anupana*
Varsha	Trivrit, Kutaja beeja, Pippali, Shunthi, Draksha, Swarasa,	Kshaudra
Sharada	Trivrit, Duralabha, Musta, Sharkara, Chandana	Draksha Kvatha with Yashtimadhu
Hemanta	Trivrit, Chitraka, Patha, Jivaka, Sarala, Vacha, Hemakshiri	Ushnambu
Shishira	Trivrit, Pippali, Shunthi, Saindhava,	Madhu
Vasanta	Shyama (Sariva)	
Greeshma	Trivrit	Sharkara
Sarvaritu	Trivrit, Hapusha, Danti, Saptala, Katuki, Swarnaksheeri	Bhavana with Gomutra

X. According to Qualities

1. **Snigdha:** Charaka and Sushruta have coined the word Snigdha and Ruksha Virechana. The Virechana given by using snigdha dravyas is known as snigdha Virechana. It is contraindicated in those patients who have been given much of Aabhyantar snehana. (Su.Chi 33/41). Drugs used are - Eranda, Tilvaka, Aragvadha,
2. **Ruksha Virechana:** The Virechana given by using ruksha dravyas, is known as Ruksha Virechana. It is indicated in those patients who have snigdha sharira and having doshotklesha avastha after Snehapana. Drugs used are - Haritaki, Danti, and Katuki.

Virechana Agrya Dravya

Mridu Virechana	Aragwadha
Tikshna Virechana	Snuhi
Sukha Virechana	Trivrit
Bhedana and Anulomana	Amlavetasa
Anulomana	Hingu
Sransana	Yaavashuka

Among all the Virechana Drugs following drugs have been placed at top most position in their respective cadres. (Su.Su.44/1-2)

Mula Virechana	Shyama Trivrit
Phala Virechana	Haritaki
Twak Virechana	Tilvaka
Swarasa Virechana	Karvellaka
Dugdha Virechana	Snuhi

GENERAL PROPERTIES OF VIRECHANA DRAVYA (CH.KA. 1)

1. Ushna
2. Tikshna
3. Sukshma
4. Vyavayi
5. Vikashi
6. Adohobhaga prabhava

Panchabhautikatwa of Drugs

Virechana drugs possess the Prabhava as adhobhagahara, by which it can be inferred that there is a dominance of Prithvi and Jala mahabhuta.

सलिल पृथिव्यात्मकत्वाद् अधोभाग प्रभावाच्च औषधस्याधः प्रवर्त्तते। (Ch.Ka.1/5)

Even the drugs having the dominance of these two mahabhuta may not have Virechaka property,but it is due to the Prabhava, that the Virechana action is appreciated.

Appearance of Virechana Aushadha

विरेचनानि सात्म्य अबीभत्स अदुर्दर्शन सुगन्धीनीति गम्यते। (Su.Chi.33/7.Dalhana)

Virechana dravya's should be accoustomed to patient, good to observe and should have good smell.

GENERAL KNOWLEDGE OF SINGLE VIRECHANA DRAVYA

1. Trivrit (Fig. 5.1)

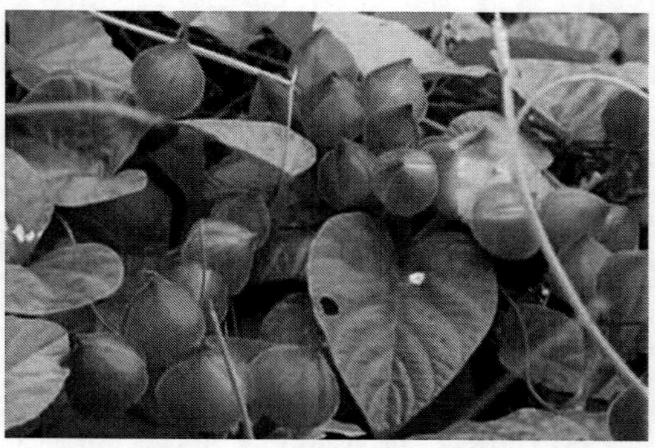

Fig. 5.1: Trivrit

Latin Name	:	*Opuculina turpethum*
Family	:	Convolvulaceae
Synonyms	:	त्रिभण्डी त्रिवृता चैव श्यामा कूटरणा च सा। सर्वानुभूतिः सुवहा शब्दैः पर्यायवाचकैः॥ (Ch.Ka.7/4)

Tribhandi, Trivrita, Shyama, Kutarana, Sarvanubhuti and Suvaha are the synonyms of Trivrit.

Guna Karma

कषाय मधुरा रूक्षा विपाके कटुका च सा। कफपित्तप्रशमनी रौक्ष्याच्चानिलकोपनी॥ (Ch.Ka.7/5)

Rasa	:	Kashaya, Madhura
Guna	:	Laghu, Ruksha, Tikshana
Veerya	:	Ushna
Vipaka	:	Katu
Doshaghnata	:	Pitta Kaphahara
Chemical composition	:	Root contains an active principle glycosideresin named as turpethin, responsible for purgation.

Collection and Preservation

गुणवत्यां तयोर्भूमौ जातं मूलं समुद्धरेत्। उपोष्य प्रयतः शुक्ले शुक्लवासाः समाहितः॥
गम्भीरानुगतं श्लक्ष्णमतिर्यग्विसृतं च यत्। तद्विपाटयोद्धरेद्गर्भं त्वचं शुष्कां निधापयेत्॥ (Ch.Ka.7/10-11)

The roots should be collected from the herb, grown in good soil and place.
Should be collected in Shukla Paksha
Person going to collect should do fasting and wear white garments.
The root that has penetrated deep, which is smooth and has not spread sideways should be gathered. It should be split and pith inside should be removed and the bark should be dried and preserved.

2. Katuki (Fig. 5.2)

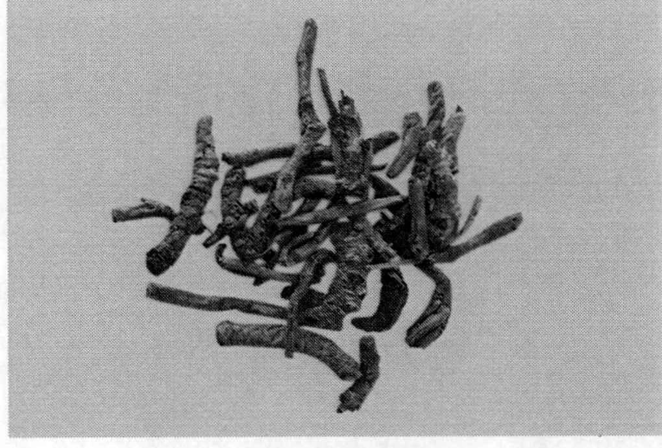

Fig. 5.2: Katuki

Botanical Name	:	*Picrorhiza kurroa*
Family	:	Scrophularaceae
Synonyms	:	कट्वी तु कटुका तिक्ता कृष्णभेदा कटम्भरा। अशोका मत्स्यसकला चक्राङ्गी शकुलादनी।। मत्स्यपित्त काण्डरूहा कटुरोहिणी। (Bha.Pra.Haritakyadi varga)

Katvi, Katuka, Tiktaa, Krishnabheda, Katambhara, Ashoka, Matsyasakala, Chakrangi, Shakuladani, Matsyapitta, Kandaruha, Katurohini.

Guna Karma

कट्वी तु कटुका पाके तिक्त रूक्षा हिमा लघुः। भेदिनी दीपनी हृद्या कफपित्तज्वरपहा।
प्रमेह श्वास कासास्त्र दाह कुष्ठ क्रिमिप्रणुत्।। (Bha.Pra.haritakyadivarga)

Rasa	:	Tikta
Guna	:	Ruksha, Laghu
Vipaka	:	Katu
Veerya	:	Sheeta
Doshaghnata	:	Kapha Pittahara
Chemical Composition	:	Root contain Cathartic acid which is responsible for purgation

3. Haritaki (Fig. 5.3)

Latin name	:	*Terminalia chebula*
Synonyms	:	हरीतक्यभया पथ्या कायस्था पूतना ऽमृता। हैमवत्य व्यथा चापि चेतकी श्रेयसी शिवा।। वयस्था विजया चापि जीवन्ती रोहिणीतिच।। (Bha.Pra.haritakyadivarga)

Haritaki, Abhaya, Pathya, Kayastha, Putana, Amrita, Haimavati, Chetaki, Shreyasi, Shiva, Vayastha, Vijaya, Jeevanti, Rohini.

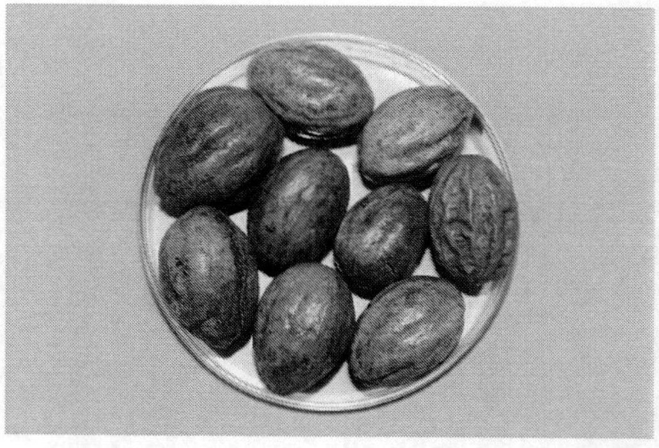

Fig. 5.3: Haritaki

Guna Karma

हरीतकी पञ्चरसाऽलवणा तुवरा परम्। रूक्षोष्णा दीपनी मेध्या स्वादुपाका रसायनी॥
चक्षुष्या लघुरायुष्या बृहणी चानुलोमिनी। (Bha.Pra.haritakyadivarga)

Rasa	:	Pancha rasa, Kashaya Pradhana
Guna	:	Laghu, Ruksha
Veerya	:	Ushna
Vipaka	:	Madhura
Doshaghnata	:	Vatakaphahara
Chemical Composition	:	Myrobalan contains Tannic acid, Gallic acid and Resin.

4. Aragvadha (Fig. 5.4)

Botanical name	:	*Cassia fistula*
Family	:	Leguminosae
Synonym	:	आरग्वधः आरग्वधो राजवृक्षः शम्पाकश्चतुरङ्गुलः। प्रग्रहः कृतमालश्च कर्णिकारोऽवघातकः॥ (Ch.Ka.8/3)

Aragvadha, Rajavriksha, Shampaka, Chaturangula, Pragraha, Kritamala, Karnika, Avaghataka.

Guna Karma

ज्वर हृद्रोग वातासृगुदावर्तादि रोगेषु। राजवृक्षोऽधिकं पथ्यो मृदुर्मधुरशीतलः॥ (Ch.Ka.8/4)

Rasa	:	Madhura
Guna	:	Guru, Mridu, Snigdha
Veerya	:	Sheeta
Vipaka	:	Madhura
Doshaghnata	:	Vata Kaphahara
Chemical Composition	:	Aqueous extract of fruit pulp has significant purgative action, due to the presence of Anthraquinone rhein.

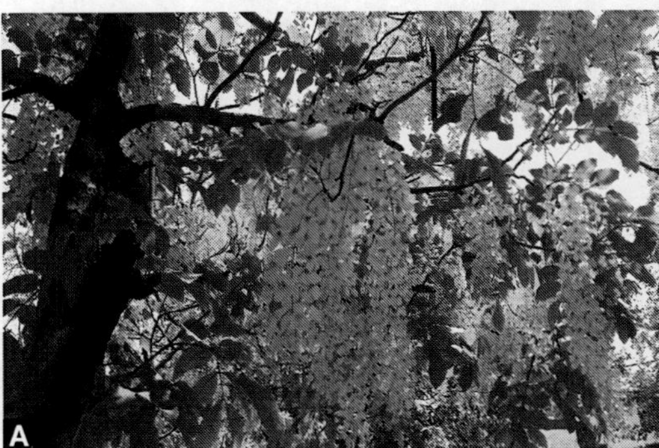
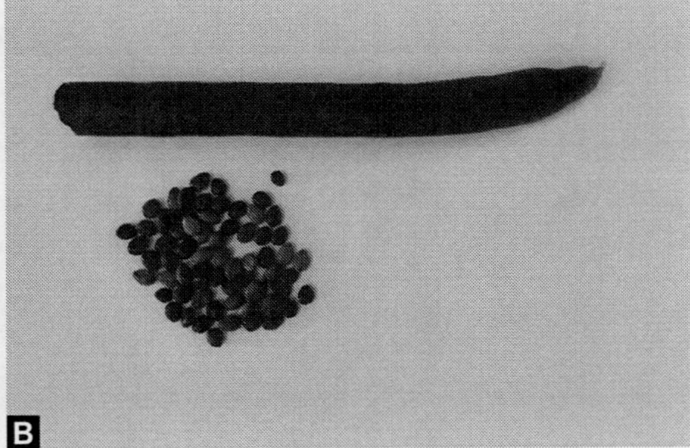

Figs 5.4A and B: Aragvadha

Collection and Preservation

फलकाले फलं तस्य ग्राह्यपरिणतं च यत्। तेषां गुणवतांभारं सिकता सुनिधापयेत्।।
सप्तरात्रा त्तसमुद्धत्य शोषयेदातपे भिषव्। ततोमज्जानमुद्धय शुचौभाण्डेनिधापयेत्।। (Ch.Ka.9/6-7)

- Fruits should be collected in fruiting season.
- Fruits which are heavy and rich in pulp should be collected and preserved in sand.
- After 7 days fruits should be dried in sunlight and pulp should be taken out and preserved.

5. Eranda (Fig. 5.5)

Botanical name	:	*Ricinus communis*
Family	:	Euphorbiaceae
Synonyms	:	एरण्ड आमण्डश्वित्रो गन्धर्वहस्तकः। पञ्चाङ्गुलो वर्धमानो दीर्घदण्डो व्यडम्बकः।। (Bha.Pra)

Eranda, Aamanda, Chitra, Gandharvahasta, Panchangula, Vardhamana, Dheergadanda, Vyadambaka.

Guna Karma

Rasa	:	Madhura, Katu, Anurasa Kashaya
Guna	:	Tikshna
Virya	:	Ushna
Vipaka	:	Madhura
Karma	:	Dipana, Sroto Vishodhanam
Doshaghnata	:	Vata Kaphahara

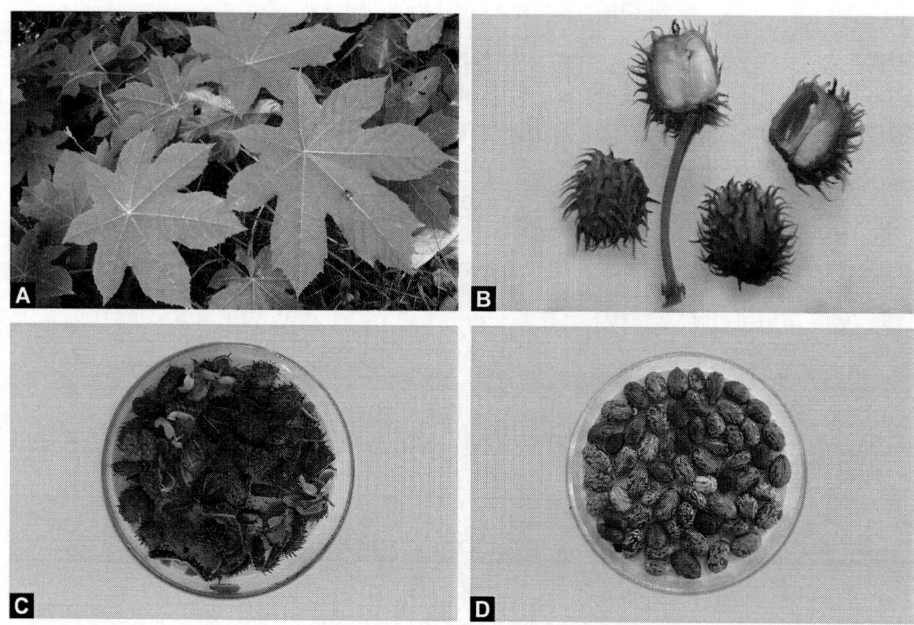

Figs 5.5A to D: (A) Erand Patra, (B) Erand phala fresh, (C) Erand Phala dry, (D) Erand beej

6. Jaipala (Fig. 5.6)

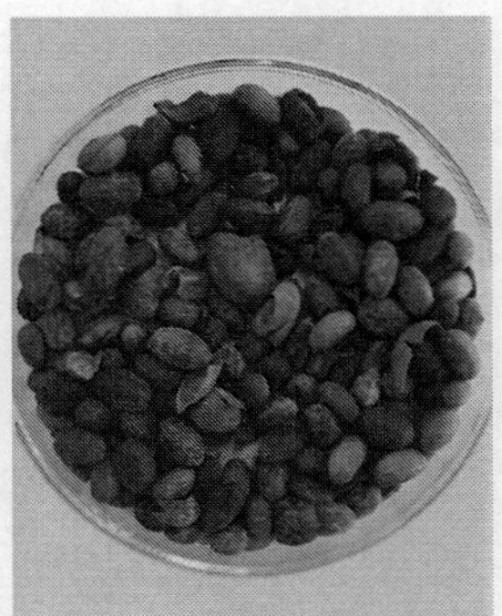
Fig 5.6: Jaipal

Botanical name	:	*Croton tiglium*
Family	:	Euphorbiaceae
Synonyms	:	Danti bija, Tintidiphala

Guna Karma

Rasa	:	Katu
Guna	:	Guru, Snigdha, Tikshna
Veerya	:	Ushna
Vipaka	:	Katu
Karma	:	Kapha-Vatahara, Deepana, Jalodarahara
Doshaghnata	:	Kapha Vatahara

Chemical Composition

Seeds contain tiglic acid, Crotonic or quartendic acid and Croton oil. Crotonic acid is the active principle of croton oil.

VIRECHANOPAGA DRAVYA

द्राक्षा काश्मर्य परूषकाभयामलक बिभीतककुबल बदर कर्कन्धु पीलूनीति दशेमानि विरेचनोपगानि भवन्ति। (Ch.Su.4/13)

S.N.	*Dravya*	*Botanical name*
1.	Draksha (Fig. 5.7)	*Vitis vinifera*
2.	Kashmarya (Fig. 5.8)	*Gmelina arborea*
3.	Parushaka (Fig. 5.9)	*Grewia asiatica*
4.	Abhaya (Fig. 5.10)	*Terminalia chebula*
5.	Amalaka (Fig. 5.11)	*Emblica officinalis*
6.	Bibhitaka (Fig. 5.12)	*Terminalia belerica*
7.	Kuvala (Fig. 5.13)	*Zizyphus sativa*
8.	Badara (Fig. 5.14)	*Zizyphus jujuba*
9.	Karkandhu (Fig. 5.15)	*Zizyphus numularia*
10.	Peelu (Fig. 5.16)	*Salvodara persica*

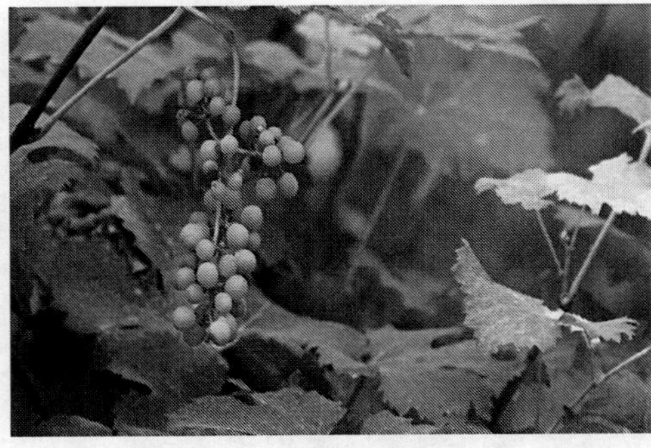
Fig. 5.7: Draksha

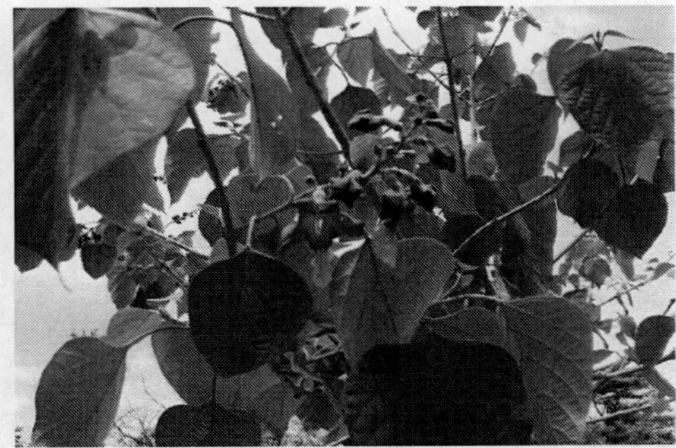
Fig. 5.8: Kashmarya

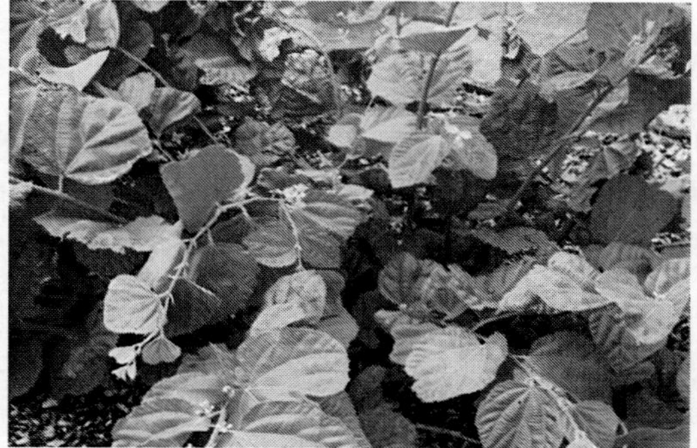

Fig. 5.9: Parushaka

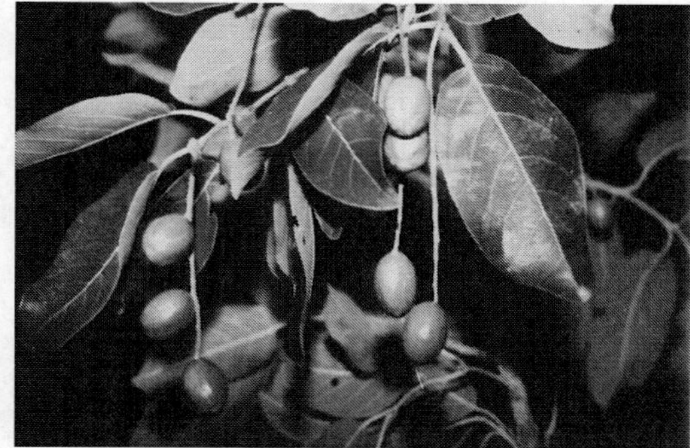

Fig. 5.10: Abhaya

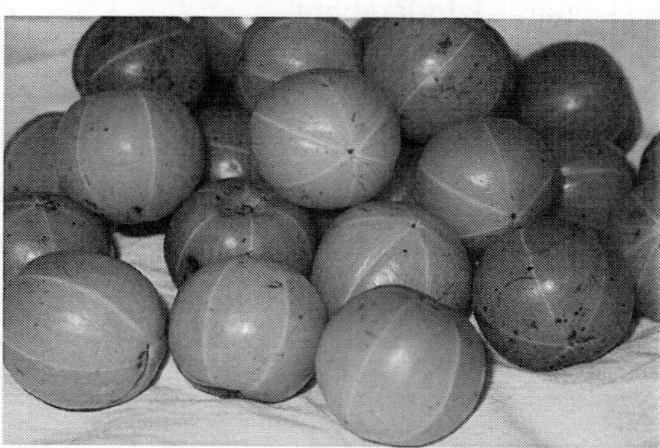

Fig. 5.11: Amalaka

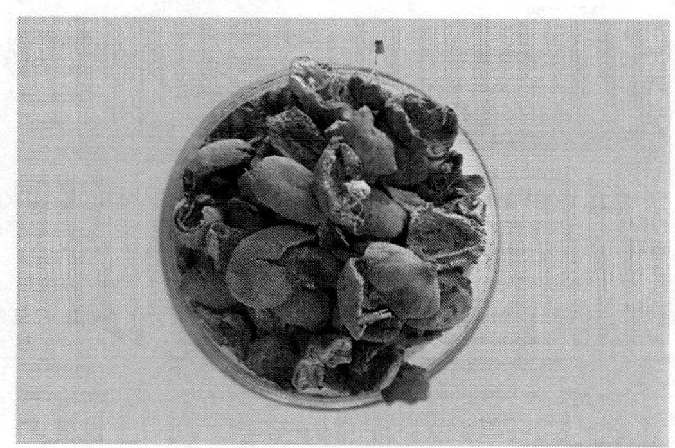

Fig. 5.12: Bibhitaka

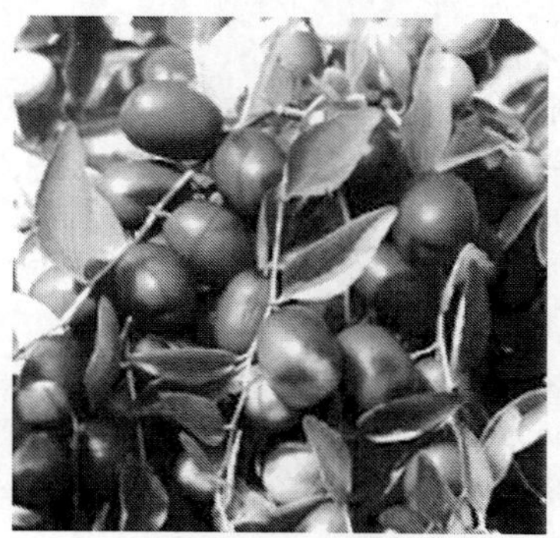

Fig. 5.13: Kuvala

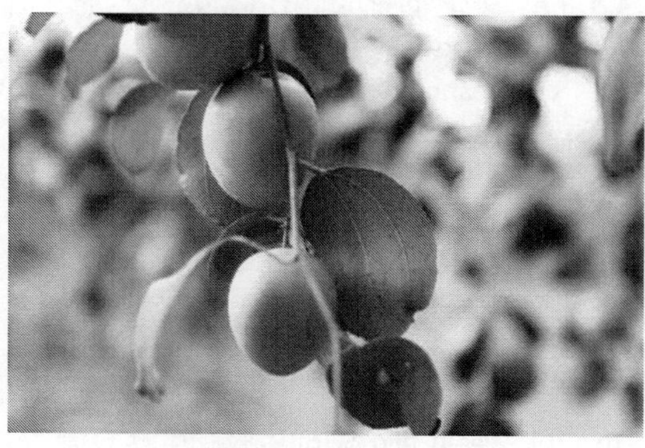

Fig. 5.14: Badara

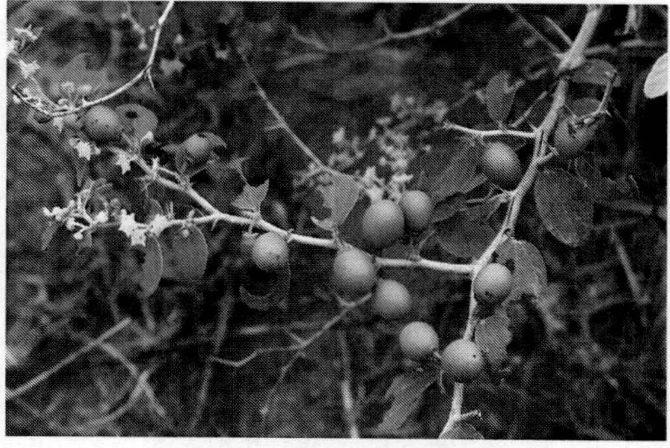

Fig. 5.15: Karkandhu

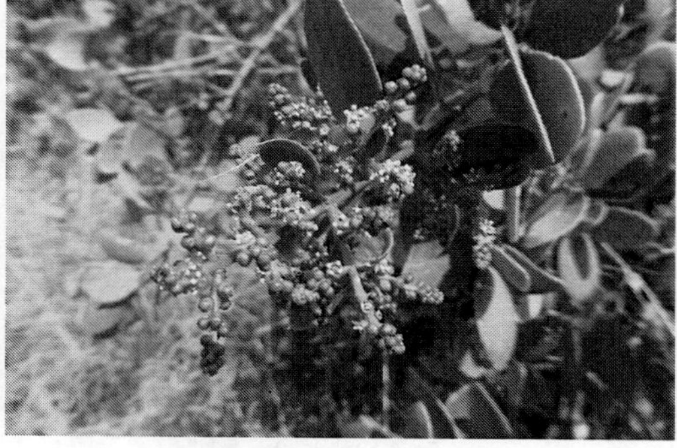

Fig. 5.16: Peelu

VIRECHANA KARMA VIDHI

The main procedure can be classified as:

1. Purva karma 2. Pradhana karma 3. Pashchata karma.

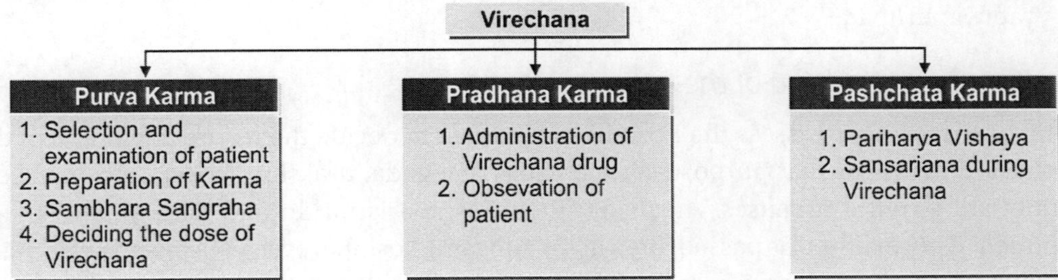

Purva karma

It includes:

a. Sambhara Sangraha

In Sutrasthana-15, Acharya Charaka has given the description of some drugs necessary to manage the complications, which may occur during main procedure and also certain necessary equipments which helps to handle the emergency. Drugs necessary for deepana, pachana such as trikatu, panchakola etc have to be collected and sufficient quantities of Sneha dravya required for Abhyantara Snehapana have to be collected as well. Certain Virechaka drugs like Trivrit, Eranda taila, Aragwadha, Icchabhedi rasa, Jalodarari rasa, Abhayadi modaka have to be stored. Certain Virechanopaga drugs like Draksha, Triphala, Parushaka etc should also be collected. To combat certain complications like Atiyoga, medicines like Kutaja ghana vati, Karpura rasa, Jatiphaladi churna, Sanjeevani vati, Bilwadi churna, Piccha basti ingredients have to be stored.

b. Atura Pariksha

Proper examination of the patient is pre-requisite for carrying out Virechana. Bala of Roga and Rogi should be assessed to achieve proper Shodhana. The following important factors should be considered before administration of Virechana:

- ❑ Factors to be considered for Virechana:

  प्रसमीक्ष्य दोष भेषज देशकाल बल शरीराहार सात्म्य सत्व प्रकृति वयसां सामवस्थान्तराणि विकारांश्च.............॥ (Ch.Su.15/17)

  One should consider Dosha, Bheshaja, Desha, Kala, Bala, Shareera, Ahara, Satmya, Satva, Prakriti, Vaya and Samavastha before administration of Virechana.

- ❑ Examination of the patient for Yogya and Ayogya.
- ❑ Nature of Koshhta and Virechana:

  तत्र मृदौ मात्रा मृद्वी, तीक्ष्णा क्रूरे, मध्ये मध्या कर्तव्येति। (Su.Chi 33/21)

Acharya Sushruta mentions to give Mridu Aushadha for the person having Mridu Koshtha, Tikshna aushadha for the person having Krura Koshtha and Madhyama for Madhyama Koshtha.

- ❑ Deciding the type of Sneha and Virechana yoga by considering Vyadhyanukulata and Vyadhyanurupata.

Identification of Koshtha of the Patient

It is highly necessary to assess the Koshtha of a patient to decide the nature and matra of the Virechaka dravya. For that purpose certain drugs like guda, draksha, ksheera etc, in excess quantity are given, if it causes Virechana; then Koshtha is mridu and bahu pittavastha is confirmed. If normal stool is passed, then it is madhyama koshtha, even with tikshna Virechaka medicines if Virechana occurs occasionally, then Krura koshtha is confirmed.

c. Atura Siddhata

अवान्तस्य हि सम्यग्विरिक्तस्यापि सतोऽधः स्रस्तः श्लेष्मा ग्रहणीं छादयति,
गौरवमापदयति, प्रवाहिकां व जनयति॥ (Su.Chi 33/19)

Prior to Virechana therapy the following should be completed.

1. Snehana
2. Svedana
3. Vamana : Prior to Virechana, Vamana is necessary, otherwise, the Kapha dosha may cause Avarana over Grahani resulting in Mandagni, Gaurava, Aruchi, Pravahika (Sh.Sam. Ut.4/J, Vangasena, Hemadri, Su.Chi.33/14). Niruha basti should be administered prior to Virechana in case of Vatolbana state. In A.S.Su.27/27 it is clearly mentioned not to administer Vamana prior to Virechana in Krura koshtha.
4. Sansarjana Krama
5. Snehana and Svedana

d. Deepana and Pachana Karma before Virechana

निराम देहस्य द्रि भेषजानि तुल्यानि अमृतोपमानि। (Yoga Shataka)

The medicine will act in the body like an Amrita (nectar) when there is Niramavastha. Thus it is very necessary to attain such a state before administration of Virechana drug to get its maximum benefit. Deepana and Pachana drugs help to achieve such state. The outcome of the medicine which has administered in Ama state is compared to the extraction of juice from Amaphala (unriped fruit) A.H.Su.13/28 which is impossible to get.

Charaka mentions in Siddhisthana (6/14) that if Virechana drug is administered in Ajeernavastha it will cause Glani and Vibandha. To enhance the Agni and to digest the Ama, so as to facilitate easy digestion of Sneha and also to get Samyak Snigdha lakshana, Deepana and Pachana should be carried out with drugs like Chitrakadi vati, Trikatu churna and Agnitundi vati till the appearance of Nirama lakshanas for 3 or 5 days.

e. Snehana

It is an essential part in Panchakarma treatment, which helps in dislodging the harmful substances from the body tissues. One which produces snigdhata in the body is known as Snehana. According to Dalhana, doshas which are lodged in Shakhas are made to move towards Koshtha, by means of Snehana and Svedana.

Importance of Snehana as a Purva karma is mentioned in Ch.Si. 6/11, that as the toya (water) from snigdha patra (oleated bowl) glides easily, in the same way, the doshas from the oleated body get separate easily. Without proper Snehana and Svedana, if one performs Sanshodhana, then the body will be destroyed just like a dried stick (A.H.Su.18/59, Su.Chi.33/45).

1. **Dose of the Snehana** depends upon capacity of the Agni to digest it. In texts three types of matra (doses) of Sneha are mentioned (A.H.Su.16/17). These are Hrasva, Madhyama and Uttama matra. Arunadatta while commenting on above reference mentions about Hrasiyasi matra which is said to be a test dose and can be given in the dose of 2 tola usually after assessing Doshadi to know the nature of Agni. The dose of Snehapana in an increasing order for the whole schedule was first mentioned by Kalyanakaraka (6th A.D.).

   स्वयं नरस्त्रेहन तत्परो घृतं तिलोद्भवम् वा क्रमवर्द्धितं पिबेत।
   त्रिपच्चसप्ताहमिह प्रयत्रतः ततस्तु सात्म्यं प्रभवेन्निषेवितम्॥
   क्रियत्प्रमाणं परिणामेति तद्घृतं तु पीत्तं दिवसस्य मध्यताः।
   मदक्लम ग्लानि विदाह मूर्च्छामात्यरोचकाभावत एव शोभनम्। (Kalyanakaraka 22/7)

   Later Vangasena (9th A.D.) has also repeated the same dose schedule that seems to be more practical.

   त्रिकर्षार्द्धकर्षेण वृद्धिः .... । स्नेह मात्रा यथायोगं सप्ताहन्तु कनीयसी।

   Vangasena (Snehapanadhikara)

2. **Kala:** The Snehapana which is administered for Shodhana purpose should be at the time where the diet taken on the previous night should be digested Virechana Karma completely and there should be Anna Abhilasha (desire for food) (A.H.Su.16/18). This time is exactly early in the morning, around 6-7 a.m. If this time is passed, then the administered Sneha will be unable to perform provocation of the doshas and gets digested (Hemadri on above reference).

3. **Duration of Snehapana:**

   मृदुकोष्ठः त्रिरात्रेण स्त्रिह्यात्यच्छोपसेवया। स्त्रिह्यति क्रूरकोष्ठस्तु सप्तरात्रेण मानवः।

   It suggests the occurrence of Samyaka Snigdha lakshana on 3rd day, 5th day and 7th day in Mridu, Madhya and Krura koshtha respectively.

4. **Observation during snehapana:** Observe for samyaka, snigdha lakshana depending on the Koshtha (either 3rd, 5th or 7th day). If within 7 days samyaka snigdha lakshana do not appear then after a gap of few days again Snehapana should be started in an increasing order (Chakrapani on Ch.Si. 1). One should avoid sneha vibhransha, otherwise complications may appear. (Ch.Su.13/75). After the signs and symptoms of samyaka snigdha lakshana are obtained prior to Virechana karma, 3 days gap should be given as per the reference :

स्नेहात् प्रस्कन्दनं जन्तुः त्रिरात्रोपरतः पिबेत्। (Ch.Su.13/80)

Abhyanga and Svedana should be carried out during the gap of these 3 days. Sarvanga abhyanga in all 7 postures should be done followed - by Svedana karma.

f. Diet and Regimen

During Snehapana, drava, ushna, anabhishyandi ahara should be consumed. Ushnodaka is mandatory, one should follow brahmacharya (avoidence of sexual indulgence) and avoid vyayama (exercise), krodha (anger), shoka (grief), hima and atapa (excessive cold and hot atmosphere), pravata (exposure of early morning air), yana (excessive riding on vehicle), adhwabhashya, atyasana sthiti (sitting in a single posture for long duration), dhuma and raja (dust and smoke) also should be avoided (A.H.Su.16/25-27).

Management in Vishrama Kala

स्निग्धद्रवोष्णधन्वोत्थरसभुक् कुर्याद्विरेकं ....। (A.H.Su.16/36)

रसैस्तथा जाङ्गलजैः सयूषैः स्निग्धैः कफावृद्धिकरैर्विरिच्यः। (Ch.Si.1/9)

In 3 days of Vishrama Kala Sarvanga Abyanga and Svedana should be done.

Diet used should be Snigdha, Drava, Ushna, Jangala Mansa Rasa, Yusha and which does not increase Kapha.

Diet on the day before Virechana :

स्निग्ध स्विन्नो विरेच्यस्तु पेयामात्रोषितः सुखम्। (Ch.Ka. 7/12)

अथातुरं श्वो विरेचनं पाययिताऽस्मीति पूर्वाह्णे लघु भोजयेत्, फलाम्लमुष्णोदकं चैनमनुपायेत्। (Su.Chi.33/20)

According to Charaka, after Abhyanga and Sveda, Peya should be administered on the previous day of Virechana whereas Sushruta mentions Laghu Bhojana, Amla Phala along with Ushna jala prayoga.

In certain cases like Mandagni and Krura Koshtha, Snehapana is performed with the kshara, lavana added Sneha to obtain Deeptagni and Vata-Kaphahara state and then virechana should be administered. (A.H.Su. 18/52)

Manasopachara is necessary to get some confidence while performing procedure. (Ch.Su.15/17).

Reason behind 3 Days Gap Prior to Virechana Karma

श्लेष्मोत्तरश्छर्दयति ह्यदुःखं विरिच्यते मन्दकफस्तु सम्यक् अधः कफेऽल्पे वमनं विचरयेद् विरेचनं वृद्धकफे तथोर्ध्वम्।। (Ch.Si.1/9)

Since Snehapana increases Kapha in the body, there will be aggravation of Kapha dosha.Thus to attain Manda Kapha avastha, 3 days of gap is adviced. Snehapana should be carried out after the Shleshma in the body decreases (Ch.Chi.3/164-165). If soon after Snehapana, Virechana is performed, then there may be occurrence of Grahani, Pravahika, Gaurava, since Kapha masks the Grahani and it may even cause Vamana instead of causing Virechana because there is Kaphotkleshavastha. Hence Virechanaushadhi is administered after passing of Shleshmakala.

श्लेष्मकाले गते ज्ञात्वा कोष्ठं सम्यक् विरेचयेत्।। (A.H.Su. 18/33)

Even the Virechanaushadhi requires pachana unlike that of Vamanaushadhi, which is said (A.H.Su.18/47) as **'अपक्वं वमनं दोषान् पच्यमानं विरेचनम्'** suggests the occurrence of Virechana in Pachyamanavastha.

Main Precautions During Virechana

- Kaphakara diet should be avoided.
- If Kapha becomes more than normal, then Virechana drug may produce Vamana (Ch. Si.1/9).
- During Virechana Karma, Amashaya should be empty in contrast to Vamana.
- In Natisnigdha shareera, Snigdha Virechana is indicated and for Snehotklishta Shareera Ruksha Virechana is indicated.
- In certain cases like Mandagni and Krura Koshtha, Snehapana is performed with the kshara, lavana added Sneha to obtain Deeptagni and Vata-Kaphahara state and then virechana should be administered (A.H.Su.18/52).

Management on Morning of Virechana Day

अर्थेनं पुनरेव स्नेह स्वेदाभ्याम् उपपाद्यान् अनुपहममनसम् अभिसमीक्ष्य सुखोषितं सुप्रजीर्णभक्तं कृत होम बलि मङ्गल जप प्रायश्चित्तम् इष्टे तिथि नक्षत्रकरण मुहूर्ते ब्राह्मणान् स्वस्ति वाचयित्वा त्रिवृत्कल्कम् अक्षमात्रं यथार्हालोडनप्रतिविनीतं पाययेत् प्रसमीक्ष्य दोष भेषज देश काल बल शरीरा आहार सात्म्य सत्त्व प्रकृति वय सामवस्थान्तराणि विकारांश्च। (Ch.Su.15/19)

On the day of Virechana karma, patient should be subjected to Bahya snehana and Svedana karma. Patient should be assessed for Sujeerna Anna Lakshana. After offering prayers patient should be administered one Aksha Matra of Trivrit.

Matra Vinishchaya (Dose Determination)

In general, Charaka says while explaining matra of Virechana-aushadhi as :

यावद्धि यस्य संशोधनं पीतं वैकारिक दोष हरणयोपपद्यते .... मात्रा प्रमाणं वेदितव्यं भवति। (Ch.Su.15/10)

The medicine which results in removal of vaikarika doshas, without causing Atiyoga, Ayoga or any other complications is said to be the proper matra for Shodhana. The drug selected should have the following properties:

1. The potency of the drug should be such that in Alpa matra it should act to produce maha vega.
2. Should have the capacity to eliminate Bahudosha.
3. Having laghu paka, good taste, preenana, vyadhinashana property and natiglanikara.
4. Having proper gandha,varna and rasa (Ch.Si.6/1S-16)

One should consider the following 5 points just before the administration of Virechanaushadhi. They are:

1. Nutritional state of patient: Properly nourished or malnourshied.
2. History of prevoius Panchakarma procedures.

3. State of Dosha Vikriti.
4. Constitution of patient: Sthula (obese) or Krisha (thin).
5. State of Koshtha (A.H.Su.18/50,51)

If Koshtha is not properly determined, alpa and mridu medicines should be given. To decide the exact matra, one should have the knowledge of agni and koshtha of the patient.

Dose of the Virechanaushadhi: (Sha.S.Ut.4/16-17, Vangasena)

Kalpana	*Hina for Mridu Koshtha*	*Madhyama for Madhyama koshtha*	*Uttama for Krura koshtha*
Kvatha	2 tola	4 tola	8 tola
Kalka, Churna, Modaka	1 tola	2 tola	4 tola
Svarasa (half of kvatha)	1 tola	2 tola	4 tola
Ushnodaka	2 tola	4 tola	8 tola

Dose of Virechanaushadhi According to Koshtha (According to Vangasena)

Mridu koshtha - 1 tola
Madhyama koshtha - 2 tola
Krura koshtha - 4 tola

Conditions	*Matra (Dose)*
I. Young age, afflicted with visha having Good strength, in skin diseases	Uttama
2. Madhyama balayukta vyadhi with Madhyama bala	Madhyama
3. Alpa dosha with alpa bala	Laghu (Bh.Si. 1/5-12)

Pradhana Karma (Method of Virechana Karma)

Pradhana karma starts with administration of virechana dravyas till the stoppage of virechana vegas. It is as follows :

a. Virechana yoga sevana.
b. Atura paricharya and Nirikshana.
c. Vega nirnaya.
d. Observation of Samyak yoga, Ayoga and Atiyoga Lakshanas.
e. Virechana Vyapat and Pratikara.

Virechana Yoga Sevana

अथैन पुनरेव स्नेह स्वेदाभ्यामुपपाद्यानुपहतमनसम् अभिसमीक्ष्य सुखोषितं
सुप्रजीर्णभक्तं कृत होम बलि मङ्गल जप प्रायश्चित्तमिष्टे तिथि नक्षत्र करण मुहूर्ते
ब्राह्मणान् स्वस्तिवाचयित्वा त्रिवृत्कल्कम् अक्षमात्रं यथार्हालोडनप्रतिविनीतंपाययेत् ....॥ (Ch.Su.15/17)

i. Virechana aushadha is administered after achieving Samyak Snehana and Svedana Lakshanas.
ii. While the patient is cheerful, slept well and has fully digested his previous meal (Suprajirnabhakta).

iii. Virechana is performed in empty stomach after performing Homa, Bali, Mangala and Japa on the auspicious day after doing Swastivachana by Brahmana.

Time of Administration

अथापरेऽहनि विगत श्लेष्म धातुम् आतुरोपक्रमणीयाद् अवेक्ष्यातुरमथास्मै औषधमात्रां पातुं प्रयच्छेत्।
(Su.Chi.33/20)

श्लेष्मकाले गते ज्ञात्वा कोष्ठं सम्यग्विरेचयेत्।। (A.H.Su.18/33)

Sushruta says in the morning after Vigata shleshma dhatu i.e. when the person is devoid of Praseka, Virechana Aushadha should be administered. Whereas, Vagbhatta mentions to administer after Shleshma Kala.

Sushruta says in the morning after Vigata shleshma dhatu i.e. when the person is devoid of Praseka, Virechana Aushadha should be administered. Whereas, Vagbhatta says it should be administered after Shleshma Kala. Ideally virechana aushadha should be administered between 9 am to 10 am for best results.

Vihara after the Administration of Aushadha

विरेचन पीतवास्तु न वेगान् धारयेद् बुधः। निवातशायी शीताम्बु न स्पृशेन्न प्रवाहयेत्।। (Su.Chi.33/22)

After the intake of the medicine person should not do Vegadharana, stay in the room in which there is no direct entry of air, shouldn't touch the cold water and not pressurise during defecation.

Atura Paricharya and Nirikshana

After administration of the Virechana Aushadha, the vaidya must observe for the manifestation of Jeerna and Ajeerna Aushada lakshana, Hrit Dosha and Vyapat Lakshanas.

Aushadha Jeernaajeerna Lakshana

अनुलोमोऽनिलः स्वास्थ्यं क्षुत्तृष्णोर्जो मनस्विता। लघुत्वमिन्द्रियोद्गारशुद्धि जीर्णौषधाकृतिः।। (Ch.Si. 6/26)

- ❑ Vatanulomana
- ❑ Svasthya
- ❑ Kshut
- ❑ Pipasa
- ❑ Mana prasannata
- ❑ Indriya prasannata
- ❑ Shuddha udgara

Ajeernaushadha Lakshana

क्लमो दाहोऽङ्गसदनं भ्रमो मूर्च्छा शिरोरुजा। अरतिर्बलहानिश्च सावशेषौषधाकृतिः।। (Ch.Si.6/27)

- ❑ Daurbalya
- ❑ Daha
- ❑ Angasada
- ❑ Bhrama
- ❑ Murccha
- ❑ Shiroruja
- ❑ Arati
- ❑ Balahani

In case of Ajeernaushadha lakshanas, the Virechana drugs should not be given immediately, as the drug may produce severe purgation i.e. Atiyoga.

Hrita Dosha Lakshana

ऊर्ध्वं कफानुगे पित्ते विट्पत्तेऽनुकफे त्वधः। हृतदोषं वदेत् कार्श्यदौर्बल्ये चेत् सलाघवे।। (Ch.Si. 6/20)

The Lakshanas like passing of Vit, Pitta and Kapha in order, Daurbalya, Laghuta; and Karshya are indicative of Hrithadosha lakshana. These are also indicative of completion of Virechana.

उत्थाने अल्पे दिने तस्मिन्भुक्त्वाऽन्येद्युः पुनः पिबेत्। अदृढ स्नेहकोष्ठस्तु पिबेदूर्ध्वं दशाहतः।।(A.H.Su.18/36)

1. If Aushadhi Jirna Lakshanas are available, but Hritadosha Lakshanas are not found then Virechana Yoga should be administered again on next day. Even then, if Virechana does not occur then Snehana and Svedana should be done again and thereafter Virechana drug should be administered after 10 days.
2. If virechana persists even after manifestation of Hrit dosha lakshanas then vamana should be performed.

.... अप्रवृत्तौ तु पाययेत्। उष्णाम्बु स्वेदस्य पाणितापेन चोदरम्।। (A.H.Su.18/35)

3. If the number of Virechana Vegas are less or occur slow then, ushna jalapana should be administered followed by Svedana over Udara pradesh a by rubbing the hands of patient and placing over the Udara.

Vega Vinirnaya

जघन्यमध्यप्रवरे तु वेगा............................। दशैव ते द्वित्रिगुणा विरेके प्रस्थस्तथा द्वित्रिचतुर्गुणश्च।
द्वित्रान् सविट्कानपनीय वेगान्मेयं विरेके ....।। (Ch.Si.1/13-14)

For the purpose of observation of Pravara, Madhyama and Avara shuddhi, Chakrapani has given four types of criteria i.e. Laingiki, Antiki, Vaigiki and Maniki, but importance should be given to Laingiki shuddhi. For Vega vinirnaya, the physician have to leave the first two-three malayukta Vegas, then counting should be done till kaphantam. Virechana Vega vinirnaya is shown in the following table:

S.N.	*Vega vishaya*	*Pravara shuddhi*	*Madhyama shuddhi*	*Avara shuddhi*
01.	Vega	30 Vega	20 Vega	10 Vega
02	Maniki	4 Prastha	3 Prastha	2 Prastha
03.	Antaki	Kaphanta	Kaphanta	Kaphanta
04.	Laingiki	Samyak Virechana Lakshanas		

OBSERVATION OF SAMYAK YOGA, AYOGA AND ATIYOGA LAKSHANAS

Samyak Lakshana of Virechana Karma

स्त्रोतोविशुद्धीन्द्रियसम्प्रसादौ लघुत्वमूर्जोऽग्निरनामयत्वम्। प्राप्तिश्च विटपित्त कफानिलानां सम्यग्विरिक्तस्य भवेत्क्रमेण।।
(Ch.Si.1/17)

गतेषु दोषेषु कफान्वितेषु नाभ्या लघुत्वे मनसश्च तुष्टौ। गतेऽनिले चाप्यनुलोमभावं सम्यग्विरिक्तं मनुजं व्यवस्येत्।। (Su.Chi.33/26)

Srotovishuddhi	Purification of body channels
Indriya prasada	Clarity of all sense organs
Laghuta	Lightness of the body
Agnideepti	Increase of Digestive strength
Anamayatwa	Remission from disorder
Kramat Vit, Pitta, Kapha and Vata Nissarana	Expulsion of stools, Pitta, Kapha and Vata in sequence
Vatanulomana	Downward movement of vata
Absence of Ayoga, Atiyoga lakshanas	Absence of inadequate and excessive features

Samayaka Shuddhi Lakshana

Lakshana	*Ch.Si.1/7*	*Su.Chi.33/25*	*A.H.Su.18/39*
1. Srotovishuddhi	+	-	-
2. Indriya samprasada	+	+	-
3. Laghutwa	+	+	-
4. Agnivriddhi	+	+	-
5. Anamayatwa	+	+	-
6. Kramat Vata Pitta Kapha Anila Shuddhi	+	+	-
7. Vatanulomana	-	+	-
8. Absence of ayoga lakshana	-	-	+

One should consider finally the Laingiki and Antiki criteria to assess Samyak Virikta lakshana. According to Charaka, Anila shuddhi is mentioned which means that Vata, Pitta and Kapha have been completely eliminated. After elimination of Pitta from large intestine, mucus which is covering it will also be eliminated. Mucus protects the intestinal wall from excoriations. Hence passage of mucus indicates expulsion of Kapha dosha. In case if further Virechana is carried out then the intestinal wall containing capillaries rupture resulting in Jivadana, which is one among Virechana vyapat (complication).

Importance of Assessment Criteria

Laingiki and Antiki criterias are the indicators to stop the Virechana karma.

Maniki and Vaigiki criterias are helpful to assess expulsion of doshas from the body which may be further taken as a criteria to decide Sansarjana krama. Sansarjana krama corrects the body physiology starting from Agni upto homeostasis of all the physiological processes.

Virechana Ayoga

स्यात् श्लेष्मपित्तानिल सम्प्रकोपः सादस्तथाऽग्नेर गुरुता प्रतिश्याय।।
तन्द्रा तथाच्छर्दिररोचकश्च वातानुलोम्यं न च दुर्विरिक्ते।। (Ch.Si.1/18)

हृत्कुक्ष्यशुद्धिः परिदाह कण्डू विण्मूत्र सङ्गश्च न सद्विरिक्ते। (Su.Chi.33/24)

हृत्कुक्ष्यशुद्धिररुचिरुत्क्लेशः श्लेष्मपित्तयोः। कण्डूर्विदाहः पिटिकाः पीनसो वातविड्ग्रहः॥ (A.H.Su.18/38)

Kapha prakopa	Vitiation of kapha
Pitta prakopa	Vitiation of pitta
Vata prakopa	Vitiation of vata
Agnimandya	Decrease in digestive strength
Gaurava	Heaviness of the body
Pratishyaya	Running nose
Tandra	Drowsiness
Chhardi	Vomiting
Aruchi	Lack of taste
Vata pratilomata	Opposite course of vata
Daha	Burning sensation
Hridaya ashuddhi	Dsicomfort in chest region
Kukshi ashuddhi	Discomfort in abdomen
Kandu	Itching
Vitsanga	Constipation
Mutrasanga	Retention of urine
Pidaka	Skin eruptions

Asamyak Lakshana

Ayoga Lakshana of Virechana Karma (Ch.Si. 1/18; Su. Chi. 33/24; A.H.Su.18/38-39)

Lakshana	*Ch.*	*Su.*	*Va.*
Kapha prakopaka	+	+	+
Pitta prakopaka	+	+	+
Vata prakopaka	+	-	-
Agnimandya	+	+	-
Gaurava	+	+	-
Pratishyaya	+	-	+
Tandra	+	-	-
Chhardi	+	-	-
Aruchi	+	+	+
Vata pratilomana	+	-	Vatagraha
Daha	-	+	+
Hridaya Ashuddhi	-	+	+
Kukshi Ashuddhi	-	+	+

Contd...

Contd...

Lakshana	*Ch.*	*Su.*	*Va.*
Kandu	-	+	+
Vita Sanga	+	+	+
Mutrasanga	-	+	-
Pidika	-	-	+

Atiyoga Lakshanas of Virechana

कफास्त्रपित्त क्षयजानिलोत्थाः सुप्त्यङ्गमर्द क्लम वेपनाद्याः॥ निद्राबलाभाव तमःप्रवेशाः सोन्मादहिक्काश्च विरेचितेऽति। (Ch.Si. 1/29)

मूर्च्छागुदभ्रंशकफातियोगाः शूलोद्गमश्चातिविरिक्तलिङ्गम्॥ (Su.Chi. 33/24)

विट्पित्तकफवातेषु निःसृतेषु क्रमात्स्रवेत्। निःश्लेष्मपित्तमुदकं श्वेतं कृष्णं सलोहितम्॥
मांसधावनतुल्यं वा मेदः खण्डाभमेव वा। गुदनिःसरणं तृष्णा भ्रमो नेत्रप्रवेशनम्॥
भवन्त्यतिविरिक्तस्य......................॥ (A.H.Su.18/40-42)

Kapha kshaya	Depletion of Kapha Dosha
Pitta kshaya	Depletion of Pitta Dosha
Vata kshaya	Depletion of Vata Dosha
Supti	Numbness
Angamarda	Body ache
Klama	Tiredness
Vepathu	Tremors
Nidra	Feeling of sleep
Dourbalya	Debility
Tamapravesha	Darkness in font of eyes
Unmada	Obsession
Hikka	Hiccup

Atiyoga Lakshana of Virechana Karma

Lakshana	*Ch*	*Su.*	*Va.*
Kapha kshaya vikara	+	+	-
Pitta kshaya vikara	+	-	-
Vata kshaya vikara	+	-	-
Supti	+	-	-
Angamarda	+	-	-
Klama	+	-	-
Vepathu	+	-	-
Nidra	+	-	-

Contd...

Contd...

Lakshana	*Ch*	*Su.*	*Va.*
Balabhava	+	-	-
Tamah pravesha	+	-	-
Unmada	+	-	-
Hikka	+	-	-
Murccha	-	+	-
Gudabransha	-	-	-
Kapha Pitta rahit shveta Udaka nihsarana	-	-	+
Pitta rahit Lohita Udaka nihsarana	-	-	+-
Mansa Dhavana vat Udak srava	-	-	+
Medokhandavat srava	-	-	+
Trishna	-	-	+
Bhrama	-	-	+
Netrapraveshanam	-	-	+
Raktakshayaja vikara	+	-	-

Management of Atiyoga

1. Sprinkling of water on patient's body.
2. Tandulodaka with honey.
3. Kapittha swarasa with honey.
4. Padmakashtha, nagakeshara, rakta chandana with honey.
5. If mala kshaya occurs then Masha soup should be given along with Kulmasha.

DIFFERENCE IN MODE OF ACTION OF VAMANA AND VIRECHANA DRUGS

Virechana drugs after getting digested (Pakva), expel Doshas from Adhobhaga (through anal route), whereas Vamana drugs expel Doshas from Urdhavabhaga (through oral route) without digestion (Apakva).

यात्यधो दोषमादाय पच्यमानं विरेचनम्। गुणोत्कर्षाद् व्रजत्यूर्ध्वमपक्वं वमनं पुनः॥ (Su. Chi. 33/34)
अपक्वं वमनं दोष पच्यमानं विरेचनम् निर्हरेद्। (Ch.Ka.)

Criteria for Best Virechana Drug: The drug taken in morning hours that will digest within the time period of food digestion i.e. three Prahara, is known as best Virechana drug.

PASHCHAT KARMA

This period starts from cessation of Virechana vegas till the patient takes his normal diet. Certain behavioural restriction like "Ashta Mahadosha Varjyakara Vishaya" should be followed. It includes avoidence of: Uchcha bhashana (speak loudly), Ratha kshobha (overriding on vehicle), Atichankramana (excessive walking), Asana (sitting for long duration), Ajeerna bhojana (eating in indigestion), Ahita bhojana, Diwaswapna (sleeping in day time), Maithuna (sexual act) (Ch.Si.12/11).

Apart from these Atyasana (excessive eating), Atisthana (sitting for long duration), Chankramana (walking excessively), Krodha (anger), Shoka (grief), Atapa (exceesive sun exposure), Avashyaya (exposure to dew), Atipravata (exposure to early morning cold air), Viruddha bhojana, Vegasandharana should be avoided (Ch.Su. 15/15).

Sansarjana Krama

To restore and to boost the hampered Agni special dietatic-procedure called Peyadi krama should be followed. According to jejjata, the need of Peyadi krama is told as the doshas being liquified and reaches Amashaya by Shodhana process which hampers Agni.

Duration of Sansarjana Krama: Sansarjana krama is arranged according to the type of shuddhi.

In Pravara shuddhi – 7 days
In Madhyama shuddhi – 5 days
In Avara/jaghanya shuddhi – 3 days.

After Shodhana karma, Agni is enhanced by providing Laghu Ahara just like with the help of anu kashtha, Agni Sandhukshana occurs (Su.Chi.39/5).

Procedures under Sansarjana Krama

पेयां विलेपीमकृतं कृतं च .... प्रधानमध्यावर शुद्धि शुद्धः॥ (Ch.Si.1/11)

Chakrapani commenting on above opines that depending on character of Shuddhi, i.e. in Pravara shuddhi, Peyadi krama should be started for 3 Annakala (Peya, Vilepi, Akrita yusha- 1 kala, Krita yusha- 2 kala, Akrita mansa rasa- 1 annakala and Krita mansa rasa- 2 annakala), for Madhyama shuddhi 2 Annakala is prefered, whereas for jaghanya shuddhi 1 Annakala is mentioned.

Peyadi Sansarjana Krama

Days	*Anna Kala Shuddhi*	*Pravara Shuddhi*	*Madhyama*	*Avara Shuddhi*
1st	Morning Evening	- Peya	- Peya	- Peya
2nd	Morning Evening	Peya Peya	Peya Vilepi	Vilepi Kritakrita Yusha
3rd	Morning Evening	Vilepi Vilepi	Vilepi Akrita Yusha	Kritakrita Mansa Rasa Normal diet
4th	Morning Evening	Vilepi Akrita Yusha	Krita Yusha Akrita Mansa	- -
5th	Morning Evening	Krita Yusha Krita Yusha	Krita Mansa Rasa Normal diet	-
6th	Morning Evening	Akrita Mansa Rasa Krita Mansa Rasa	- -	- -
7th	Morning Evening	Krita Mansa Rasa Normal diet	-	-

Sushruta has mentioned his opinion regarding the Sansarjana krama that- Depending upon the Hrita Dosha Pramana, Ahara vidhi changes. He considers 3 Pramana of dosha harana i.e. 1 prastha, 1/2 adhaka and 1 adhaka which is Avara, Madhyama and Uttama Pramana respectively (Su.Chi.39/6-7)

The food substances which are prescribed for Sansarjana krama includes :

1. Swalpa tandula yavagu
2. Vilepi
3. Sneha and lavana rahita Mudga Yusha (Akrita)
4. Half of quantity of cooked rice with Mudga Yusha.
5. Krita Yusha along with 3/4th quantity of cooked rice.
6. Lava, krishna mriga susanskrita mansarasa is also given.

The above diet in Avara, Madhyama and Pravara shuddhi is 1, 2 and 3 Annakala respectively (Su.Chi.39/8-11).

Sushruta opines Sansarjana krama is decided according to the Bala Vishesha (strength) of patient i.e. if Pravara bala is present then 3 Anna kala, in Madhyama bala 2 Anna kala, in Alpa bala persons 1 Anna kala is mentioned (Su.Chi.39/17-18).

Tarpanadi Krama

Indication

According to Charaka the following criterias are selected for Tarpanadi krama:

1. Alpa shuddhi of Kapha and Pitta
2. In alcoholic patients
3. In Vata Pitta Prakriti individuals (Ch.Si.6/25)
4. Heena shuddhi (Su.Chi.39/13).

According to Acharya Sushruta Peyadi Krama causes Abhishyanda and aggravation of Kapha in above conditions thus it should be replaced by Tarpana krama (Su.Chi.39/13). Hence in the place of Peya-Svaccha Tarpana can be given and Vilepi is replaced by Ghana Tarpana (Chakrapani on Ch.Si.6125).

According to Jejjata, Mudga Yusha and Mansa-rasa are indicated in 1st, 2nd and 3rd Annakala respectively.

Sequence of Rasa used in Sansarjana Krama

According to Charaka, initially Snigdha, Amla, Madhura and Hridya dravyas are used to pacify Vata dosha then Amla and lavana is used to enhance the Agni followed by Madhura and Tikta rasa for Pitta Shamana. Later to pacify Kapha, Kashaya and Katu rasa should be used (Chakrapani on Ch.Si.l2/6-8). According to Sushruta, initially Svadu (Madhura) and Tikta rasa should be given to pacify Vata, Pitta and to increase Agni, later Snigdha, Amla, Lavana and Katu rasa should be given to pacify Vata and Kapha doshas and also to boost Agni.

To pacify Vata Pitta generated due to previous Rasas, Madhura and Tikta rasa is used in next series. Later Kashaya and Katu rasa should be used to pacify Kapha and Pitta situated in upper part (Dalhana on Su.Chi.39/18-19).

Ruksha and Snigdha dravya are used in Vyatyasat Krama (alternatively) and the same is followed in further days. The intention is to gradually enhance Agni and strength by practicing all rasa in these days. It is even appropriate to continue further for few days while taking normal diet.

COMMONLY USED VIRECHANA YOGAS

Various formulations of Virechana Aushadha are available in the market. By considering the Vyadhi and Koshtha, appropriate formulation along with proper dose is to be considered. This will help in achieving Samyak Virechana Lakshana. Following are the few descriptions of various Virechana formulations which are commonly practiced :

1. Taila yoga – Eranda taila, Gandharva Hastyadi taila, Nimbaamrutadi eranda taila
2. Vati yoga – Rechaka Vati, Icchabhedi Rasa
3. Leha yoga – Aragwadha Lehya, Trivrit Lehya
4. Churna yoga – Avipattikara Churna, Trivrit Churna
5. Guda yoga – Manibhadra Guda, Kalyanaka Guda
6. Rasa yoga – Aswakanchuki Rasa, Abhayadi modaka
7. Sneha yoga – Mishraka Sneha

Important Virechana Yogas

1. **Icchabhedi Rasa** (Ref Y.R. 1/342)

   Ingredients :

Shuddha Parada	–	1 Tola
Shuddha Tankana	–	1 Tola
Maricha	–	1 Tola
Shuddha Gandhaka	–	1 Tola
Trivrit	–	2 Tola
Shunthi	–	2 Tola
Jayapala	–	9 Tola
Anupana	–	Sheeta jala

   Indications: Amaja Vikaras, Ajeerna, Udara Roga, Gulma, Kaphaja Vikara, Shukra Dusti and Kushtha.

   Dosage: 250 mg (1-3 tablets)

2. **Ghandharva Hastyadi Taila** (Ref B.R 43/105-108)

   Ingredients

   Eranda Mula
   Shunthi
   Yava
   Java
   Eranda Taila
   Eranda Mula Kalka
   Godugdha

Anupana: Ushna Jala, Triphala Kashaya, Ksheera, Aragwadha Kashaya
Indication– Vidhradi, Gulma, Udavarta, Udara roga, Maha vata rogas.
Dose: 60–80 mL

3. **Aragwadha leha** (Ch.Ka.8/12)
   Ingredients: Argawadha phala majja, Trivrit Churna and Sita
   Indications: Jvara, Vatarakta, Udavarta, Bala, Vriddha, Sukumara.
   Anupana: Ushna jala.
4. **Trivrit Leha** (Ch.Ka.7/23)
   Ingredients: Trivrit Kashaya, Trivrit Kalka and Sita
   Indications: Urdhva Raktapitta, Pakshaghata, Kamala, Vatarakta, Kasa and Shvasa.
   Anupana: Ushna jala.
   Dosage: 50 to 80 g
5. **Mishraka Sneha** (Ref A.H.Chi.14/89-90)
   Ingredients: Pippali, Amalaki, Draksha, Shyama, Eranda taila, Go-ghrita and Ksheera.
   Indication: Vidradhi, Shula, Vataja Vikara
   Anupana: Ushna jala

Dosage in Practice

The below described dosage is ideal for Virechana. The same dose can be changed conveniently while administering in Children.

Dravya	*Mridu Koshtha*	*Madhyama Koshtha*	*Krura Koshtha*
Eranda taila	20 mL	40 mL	60 mL
Rechaka vati	1 tab	2 tab	2–3 tab
Trivrit Kashaya	40–50 mL	60–70 mL	80–100 mL
Manibhadra Guda	20–30 g	40–50 g	60–80 g
Trivrit Leha	40–50 g	60–70 g	80–100 g
Icchabedi Rasa	1 tab	2 tab	2–3 tab

Guidelines to be Followed After Administration

- ❑ Have some fragrance
- ❑ Repeated intake of water accordingly
- ❑ Vega should not be induced or retained
- ❑ Time should be noted
- ❑ Keen observation of contents of Vega should be made
- ❑ Don't wander
- ❑ Don't sleep
- ❑ Relax and take rest.

VYAPADA (COMPLICATIONS) AND THEIR MANAGEMENT

Because of improper selection in the nature of aushadha and dose of aushadha, patient may develop certain complications.

As per Charaka there are 10 Vyapadas as follows (Ch.Si. 6/29)

1. Adhmana (Distension of abdomen)
2. Parikartika (Gripping pain)
3. Parisrava (Discharge from anus)
4. Hridgraha (Cardiac discomfort)
5. Gatragraha (Stiffness of body)
6. Jivadanam (Discharge of blood per rectum)
7. Vibhransha (Improper action of medication)
8. Stambha (Rigidity)
9. Upadrava (Serious complications)
10. Klama (Exhaustion)

Chakrapani has divided this 10 Vyapada in two groups, i.e. Atiyoga and Ayoga.

Atiyoga	*Ayoga*
Parikartika	Adhmana
Jivadanam	Srava
Vibhransha	Hridgraha
Gudabhransha	Gatragraha
Sangya Vibhransha	Kandvadi Vibhramsha
	Upadrava
	Klama

Sushruta has mentioned 15 complications: Adhmana, Jivadana, Parikartika, Parisrava, Angagraha, Vibandha and Hridayopasaranam are common.

Saavashesha aushadatvam, lina Aushadhatvam, Hina-Doshapritatvam, Vamanasyadhogati and Virechanasya Urdhva-gati (movement of Dosha's in opposite direction) are different explanations gati in Sushruta which are included in the causes of complication by Charaka (Su.Chi. 34/3). Ayoga, Atiyoga and Pravahika are also included in above 15 complications.

Causes of Complications

Adhmana

It is caused when Virechana Aushadhi of low dose and low potency is given to the Ruksha patient, in Bahu Dosha condition or in Agnimandya condition.

Signs and Symptoms

Distention of abdomen, pain in back and sides of the chest and head. Obstruction to breath, feces, urine and flatus.

Treatment

Charaka recommends Abhyanga, Svedana (sudation), Varti (suppository). Niruha and Anuvasana Basti (evacuative and unctuous enema) whereas Sushruta has added Deepana and Langhana.

Parikartika

When the strong (Tikshna) Virechana drug is given to the Snigdha patient having Guru, Ama and Mridu Koshtha and is weak and tired. It may cause acute Kartanavat (cutting) pain and patient may pass stools containing blood and mucus. This is known as Parikartika.

Signs and Symptoms

It is characterized by burning sensation in anus, umbilical region, urethra, head and retention of gases and loss of appetite.

Treatment

Patient should be managed by Langhana, Pachana, Rukshana, Ushna drugs. Brihana should be given to weak patient Sheeta Basti, Piccha Basti or Anuvasana Basti should be given for the purpose.

Srava

If mild drug is given to the patient having excess of Dosha and Krura Koshtha, then the drug is unable to remove the Doshas. These doshas gets aggravated leading to the condition of Parisrava.

Signs and Symptoms

Weakness, itching, swelling, skin diseases, heaviness in the body, loss of appetite, anemia.

Treatment

Tikshna Virechana after Snehana, Asava-Arishtas mentioned in Grahani and Arsha chikitsa should be administered after Shodhana. Asthapana Basti administration has been mentioned by Sushruta. (Su.chi.34/17).

Hridgraha

If a patient tries to retain the Vega generated due to Virechana Karma, after taking Virechana drug, then Vata Dosha gets vitiated and reaches Hridaya leading to Hridgraha.

Signs and Symptoms

Hiccup, cough, pain in flanks, unconsciousness, biting of tongue and teeth, excessive salivation, rotation of eye balls.

Treatment

Patient can be managed by Vamana followed by Pachana to remove Shesha dosha. Abhyanga, Svedana with Dhanya and Anuvasana Basti, Tikshna Nasya, Snigdha-amla-Lavanayukta Aushadhi should be administered.

Gatragraha

This can occur because of two reasons. Firstly, after consumption of Virechana aushadha, if a patient does Vega Dharana, then the Kapha gets aggravated leading to Gatragraha. Also, if there is atiyoga of Virechana, then the aggravated vata leads to Gatragraha.

Signs and Symptoms

Angagraha, Sada, pricking pain, twisting and stirring pain.

Treatment

Patient's should be managed by Vatahara Snehana and Svedana.

Jivadanam

If Tikshna drug is given to the Mridu Koshthi patient in Alpa Dosha avastha, then it creates irritation and leads to heavy discharge of blood.

Signs and Symptoms

Excessive thirst, loss of consciousness, delirium, frank blood loss per rectum.

Treatment

Patient should be given Pittahara Chikitsa, Rakta basti, Piccha Basti, Ghrita Manda yukta Anuvasana are to be administered. Nowadays blood transfusion can be given in very acute condition of blood loss.

Vibhransha

Vibhransha refers to 3 types of complications of Virechana Karma viz., Gudabhransha, Sangya Bhransha and Kandvadi Vibhransha. Gudabhransha is a result of Atiyoga of Virechana which usually manifest following the complication of jivadana.

Signs and Symptoms

Prolapse of Anus, Sangyanasha (unconsciousness), Itching etc.

Treatment

In rectal prolapse, it should be replaced by applying astringent medication, Saurastri powder, Udumbara Sara, Lodhra Churna. Along with this Jatyadi Taila should also be used. In Sangyanasha, recitation of Samaveda and peaceful heart touching singing is advised. The treatment of Kandu should be according to Vyadhi.

Stambha

When Sneha Virechana is given to Snigdha patient it causes Doshavarana, resulting in retention of Dosha.

Signs and Symptoms

Vatasanga, Gudastambha, Ksharati alpashaha sashula (patient passes small amount of feces with pain).

Treatment

Langhana, Pachana, Tikshna Basti and Virechana should be given.

Upadrava

When Ruksha Virechana drug is given to Ruksha patient, it vitiates Vata leading to upadrava complication.

Signs and Symptoms

Stambha, Shula and Gatragraha.

Treatment

Snehana, Svedana and other Vatahara line of treatment.

Klama

When Snigdha and Mridu Koshtha patient is given Mridu drug it causes vitiation of Kapha and Pitta and retention of Vata which creates the following signs and symptoms.

Signs and Symptoms

Tandra, Gaurava, Klama, Daurbalya and Angasada.

Treatment

Ullekhana with Kaphapittahara drugs. Langhana, Pachana, Snehana and Tikshna Shodhana should be carried out.

These are 10 Vyapads mentioned by all the Acharyas. Besides these Sushruta has given few more Vyapads and their treatment.

PARIHARYA VISHAYA

सम्यक् विरिक्तं चैनं वमनोक्तेन धूमवर्जेन विधिनोपपाद येदाबलवर्णप्रकृतिलाभात्। (Ch.Su.15/18)

After attaining Samyak Virechana lakshana patient should follow all the regimen said under Vamana except Dhumapana.

VIRECHANA KARMUKATA (MODE OF ACTION)

1. Deepana and Pachana

Due to Ushna and Laghu guna these drugs enhances the Agni and Ama pachana occurs and facilitates the easy digestion of Sneha during Snehapana.

2. Snehapana

स्नेह सारोऽयं पुरुषः। प्राणाश्च स्नेहभूयिष्ठः। (Su. Chi. 31/3)

Sneha is the sarabhaga of purusha and even the life is dependant on it. By virtue of its qualities like Guru, Sheeta, Sara, Snigdha, Manda, Sukshma, Mridu and Drava (A.H.Su.16/l) it performs the function of Snehana, Vishyandana, Mardava and Kledakaraka (Ch.Su.22/11).

Snehana dravyas are having the properties of keeping the particles together and also to bring about adhesion. Human body is made up of infinitesimal and innumerable units known as Parmanus and they are held in proper position by Sneha dravyas.

Snehana dravyas will produce the following properties in the body :

1. Vatashamana ensues.
2. It makes the body smooth, soft and dissolves and disintegrates the vitiated doshas.
3. Mala sanga in the body is removed - (Ch.Si.1/7).
4. Enhances digestive fire in the body.
5. Purifies the Koshtha.
6. Nourish the body.
7. Helps to maintain proper functioning of Indriyas
8. Vyadhi Kshamatwa is enhanced.

The Kledakaraka action enhances the doshas by liquefying morbid doshas. Here the drava quality helps in liquefying the concentrated doshas.

The Vishyandana quality of Sneha causes liquefaction by virtue of its Snigdha, Mridu, Drava, Sara and Sukshma guna. By liquefying the doshas and Dhatus it helps in bringing them to Koshtha from Shakha for their easy expulsion during shodhana process.

Mridu guna helps to soften and loosen the doshas. Liquidity of doshas increases and also causes Shaithilya in various organs. Sara guna causes Anulomana of the doshas. Vivarana karma i.e. dilating the Srotas, thereby entering into Anusrotas is done by Sukshma guna. Administration of Snehapana in Vardhamana krama helps in bringing the doshas from Shakha to Koshtha by Vriddhi, Vishyandana, Paka, Srotomukha vishodhana and by Nigraha of vata (Ch.Su.28/34).

Vriddhikarma is done by Drava guna of Sneha, which helps even for Vilodana of doshas (A.H.Su.1/18 - Hemadri). Vishyandana is vilayana which is due to Snigdha guna, Srotomukha Vishodhana karma is achieved by Sukshma guna of Sneha dravyas (A.H.Su.1/18- Hemadri).

The mode of action is compared to just like a vessel smeared with oil, water slips down from it, without any application of force, so also in the body, the application of oleation therapy the moistened and vitiated doshas will be alleviated easily (Ch.Si.6/11).

Importance of Snehapana

Snehana is beneficial in durbalagni state to enhance it. Hence prior to snehapana shodhana is contraindicated. If we try to remove the doshas from ruksha shareera, then there may be possibility of lodging the dosha due to rukshata in srotas.

Svedana

The qualities of Svedana drugs are Ushna, Tikshna, Sara, Snigdha, Ruksha, Sukshma, Drava, Sthira and Guru (Ch.Su.22/16).

The Actions Obtained by these Gunas includes

स्तम्भ गौरव शीतघ्नं स्वेदनं स्वेदकारकम्।। (Su. Chi. 22/11)

The action of Svedana is performed by Ushna guna, it also helps in pacifying Stambha. By virtue of Tikshna guna Svedana drugs causes Shodhana of doshas and enter the micro-channels of the body, Sara guna helps in Dosha shamana, Ruksha guna causes Shoshana, Vivarana by Sukshma guna, Vilodhana by Drava guna and dharana karma is produced by Sthira guna (A.H.Su.1/18 -Hemadri), The Agneya property of Tikshna and Ushna gunas produce Paka and Srava.

Due to Snehana, Kledana of doshas takes place and Svedana helps in liquefaction of Doshas thereby they are brought to Koshtha. Svedana pacifies Vata and enhances agni.

Mode of action of Svedana

स्नेह क्लिन्नाः कोष्ठगा धातुगा वा स्त्रोतोलीना ये च शाखास्थि संस्थाः दोषाः स्वेदैस्ते द्रवीकृत्य कोष्ठं नीताः सम्यक् शुद्धिभिः निर्ह्रियन्ते। (A.H.Su.17/29)

Klinna doshas which are present either in Koshtha, Dhatu, Srotasa and Shakhas (includes madhyama roga marga) are liquified by Svedana and brought to Koshtha, thereby eliminated through Shodhana karma. In short, Snehana softens doshas and localizes them. Svedana liquifies those doshas due to its Ushna and Tikshna properties and helps in bringing them back into Koshtha for their easy expulsion through Vamana or Virechana.

Importance of Snehana and Svedana

स्नेह स्वेदावनभ्यस्य कुर्यात् संशोधन तु यः। दारु शुष्कमिवानामे शरीरं तस्य दीर्यते।। (A.H.Su.18/59.)

This suggests the administration of Snehana and Svedana before Shodhana therapy and highlight its importance that if Purva karma is not performed, then the body will be destroyed just like the destruction of Shushka daru (dry wood).

स्नेह पूर्व प्रयुक्तेन स्वेदेनावजितेऽनिले। पुरीष मूत्र रेतांसि न सज्जन्ति कथञ्चन।। (Ch. Su. 14/4)

Svedana is administered after Snehana, ultimately brings Vata under control and thereby helps in facilitating the easy elimination of Purisha, Mutra and Retas.

स्नेह स्वेद प्रचलिताः रसैः स्निगधैरुदीरिताः। दोषाः कोष्ठगता जन्तो सुखा हर्तु विशोधनैः।।

(Su. Chi. 34/47)

Snehana and Svedana enhances the doshas by liquefing them and destroying their compactness and helps in bringing them to Koshtha from Shakha so that they can be removed easily.

क्लिष्टं वासो यथोत्क्लेश्य मलः संशोध्यतेऽम्भसा। स्नेह स्वेदैः तथोत्क्लेश्य शोध्यते शोधनैः मलः॥

(Ch. Si. 6/13)

As the dirty cloth will be separated from dirt after it is washed with water, so also in the body after Snehana and Svedana, vitiated doshas will be thrown out of the body of their entirety.

Mode of Action of Drugs used for Virechana

तत्र उष्ण तीक्ष्ण सूक्ष्म व्यवायि विकाशीन्यौषधानि स्ववीर्येण हृदयमुपेत्य।
सलिल पृथित्यात्मकत्वात् अधोभाग प्रभावाच्चौषधस्याधः प्रर्वत्तते॥ (Ch.Ka.1/5)

The drugs that are having Ushna, Tikshna, Sukshma, Vyavayi, Vikasi properties reaches the Hridaya through Svaveerya (Svaprabhava - Chakrapani) and circulates through large and small blood vessels of the body.

Action of Ushna Guna

By virtue of its Agneya property it causes Vishyandana, i.e. 'Vilininam Kurvanti' (Chakrapani). And helps in facilitating movement of morbid doshas towards koshtha.

Tikshna Guna

'Taikshnyat Vicchindanti': Vicchindanti Cchinnam Kurvanti (Chakrapani), i.e. they break up the doshas, from larger to smaller molecules. Dalhana says that this helps in rapid expulsion of doshas.

Sukshma

Sukshma guna due to its Anupravanabhava, i.e.

अणुत्वात् प्रभणभावाच्च, अणुत्वात्–अणुमार्ग संचरित्वम् प्रवणत्वमिह कोष्ठगमनोन्मुखत्वम्।

(Chakrapani on Ch.Ka.1)

It open micro channels and makes the doshas to move towards Koshtha.

Vyavayi

Due to this property, drug spreads quickly throughout the body and starts their action before its digestion.

Vikasi

Vikasi drugs loosens the Dhatu bandhana (Sh.Sam.Pu.Kh.). It creates the Dhatu Shaithilyata (Dalhana). Hence, drugs initiates their action without being digested. From all these Properties of Virechana drugs, doshas are driven to Koshtha. The presence of Prithvi and Ap bhuta in Virechana drug and the Adhobhaga prabhava, the doshas are eliminated out through guda.

It can be summarised that the above mentioned properties of drug reaches Hridaya by Svaveerya and then with the help of the large and small dhamanis it pervades the whole body.

Due to Agneya property, it causes Vishyandana, i.e. oozing of doshas and by Tikshna property causes Vicchandana (disintegration) of doshas.

Mode of Action of Virechana Drugs

Systemic action: Doshas are brought to Koshtha by Snehana and Svedana, from there they are eliminated by Virechana, which suggests its action throughout the body.

Local action: Locally mild inflammation occurs which is transient due to Ushna and Tikshna properties of the Virechana drugs causing irritation of the intestinal mucosa. Hence hyperaemia results due to arteriolar and capillary dilatation and also exudation of protein substances, which helps in dilution of toxins.

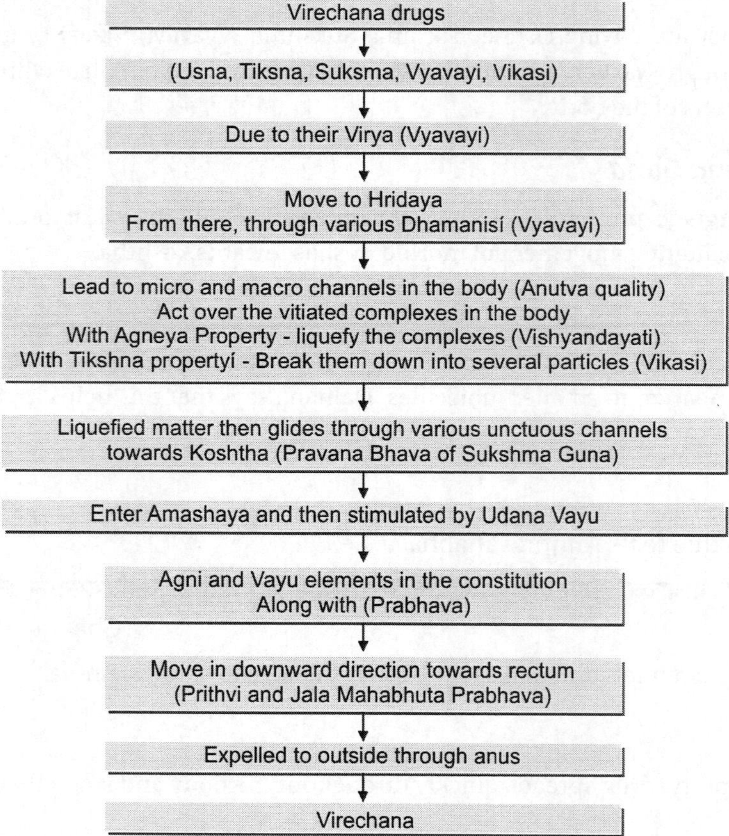

Mode of action of Virechaka Drug According to Pharmacodynamics

Modern View

These are the drugs that promote the evacuation of bowels. Depending on the intensity of action, they are classified into :

1. Laxative or aperient: Which has milder action, and eliminates soft but formed stools.
2. Purgative or cathartic: It has stronger action resulting in more fluid evacuation. Many of the drugs in low doses acts as laxatives and in larger doses as purgatives.

Classification

1. **Bulk forming:** Dietary fibre—bran. Dietary fibre consists of unabsorbable cell wall and other constituents of vegetable food—cellulose, pectins, glycoproteins and other polysaccharides. Bran consists of 40% dietary fibre. It absorbs water in the intestines, swells, increases water content of the faeces, softens it and facilitates colonic transit. Dietary fibre supports bacterial growth in colon which contribute to the faecal mass. Certain dietary fibres like gums, lignins, pectins bind bile acids and promote their excretion in faeces, leads to degradation of cholesterol in liver and then lowering of plasma LDL cholesterol.
   Psyllium (plantago) and Ispaghula: They contain natural colloidal mucilage which forms a gelatinous mass by absorbing water. Methyl cellulose and carboxymethyl cellulose: These are semi-synthetic, colloidal, hydrophilic derivaties of cellulose. Generous amounts of water must be taken with all bulk forming agents.
2. **Stool softener:** Docusates (Dicotyl sodium sulfosuccinate): Is an anionic detergent, which softens the stools by net water accumulation in the intestinal lumen by action on the intestinal mucosa. It emulsifies the colonic contents. By a detergent action, it can disrupt the mucosal barrier and enhance the absorption of many non-absorbable drugs, e.g. liquid paraffin should not be combined with it.
   Lubricant: Liquid paraffin - is a viscous liquid, a mixture of petroleum hydrocarbons. Taken for 2–3 days, it softens stools and is said, it lubricates hard scybala by coating them.
3. **Stimulant purgatives:** They are powerful purgatives and often produce griping. They may irritate the intestinal mucosa and thus stimulate motor activity. The more important mechanism of action is accumulation of water and electrolytes in the lumen by altering absorptive and secretory activity of the mucosal cell. They inhibit Na^+ K^+ ATPase at the basolateral membrane of villous cells- transport of Na^+ and accompanying water into the interstitium is reduced.

   Secretion is enhanced by activation of cAMP in crypt cells and by increased PG synthesis. Larger doses of stimulant purgatives can cause excess purgation, leads to fluid and electrolyte imbalance.

   Anthraquinones: Senna obtained from leaves and pod of certain cassia species. They contain an anthraquinone glycoside called emodins. Glycosides not active as such. Unabsorbed in the small intestine, they are passed to the colon where bacteria liberate the active anthrol form, which either acts locally or is absorbed into circulation. Excreted in bile to act on small intestine. They take 6–7 hours to produce action.

   The active principle is believed to act on the myenteric plexus to increase peristalsis and decrease segmentation. They also inhibit salt and water absorption in the colon. Senna anthraquinone has been found to stimulate PGE_2 production in rat intestine.

   Castor oil: Is one of the oldest purgatives. It is a bland vegetable oil obtained from the seeds of Ricinus communis, has been used on skin as emollient. It mainly contains triglyceride of ricinoleic acid, which was believed to irritate the mucosa and stimulate intestinal contractions.

   The primary action has shown to be decreased intestinal absorption of water and electrolytes and enhanced secretion by a detergent like action on the mucosa.

4. **Osmotic purgatives:** Solutes that are not absorbed in the intestine retain water osmotically and distend the bowel increasing peristalsis indirectly. Magnesium ions release cholecystokinin which may aid purgative action of magnesium salts. All inorganic salts are used as osmotic (saline) purgatives have similar action, e.g. Magnesium sulfate, Magnesium hydroxide, Sodium sulfate, Sodium phosphate, Sodium potassium tartrate Lactulose.

Mechanism of Action

All the purgatives increase the water content of faeces by:

- A hydrophilic or osmotic action, retaining water and electrolytes in the intestinal lumen—increase volume of colonic content and make it easily propelled.
- Acting on intestinal mucosa to decrease net absorption of water and electrolyte, intestinal transit is enhanced indirectly by the fluid bulk.
- Increasing propulsive activity as primary action—allowing less time for absorption of salt and water as a secondary effect.

Certain purgatives do increase motility through an action on the myenteric plexus. Laxatives modify the fluid dynamics of the mucosal cell and may cause fluid accumulation in gut lumen by one or more of following mechanisms.

1. Inhibiting Na^+, K^+, ATPase of villous cells—impairing electrolyte and water absorption.
2. Stimulating adenyl cyclase in crypt cells—increasing water and electrolyte secretion.
3. Enhancing PG synthesis which increases secretion.
4. Structural injury to the absorbing intestinal mucosal cells.

The irritant action of the drug causes inflammation in the small and large intestine and since the mucosa is extensively irritated, secretion rate is enhanced and motility of the intestinal wall usually increases. As a result, large quantities of fluid are propelled by propulsive movements and results in formation of loose stools. The influence of Virechana drugs are even appreciated on nerves, hormones, liver and crypts of Lieberkuhn.

Action on Nerves

Here the defecation centre is irritated in Medulla oblongata. The vagus nerve stimulates pancreas, liver to produce secretions. Bile is secreted due to contraction of gallbladder and also due to irritant vagal stimulation, Brunner's glands are stimulated which secretes mucus. Due to increased peristalsis, sacral and lumbar plexus are irritated, ileocaecal and anal sphincters are relaxed and these secretions are excreted out and is said to be purgation.

Hormonal action causes irritation of liver and pancreas, secretions are increased which adds to further irritation of mucosa. Some other hormones also increase small intestinal secretions like secretin and cholecystokinin. Whenever a segment of large intestine becomes irritated, then mucosa secretes large quantities of water and electrolytes in addition to alkaline mucus. This acts to dilute irritating factors and to cause rapid movement of the faeces towards anus. The mechanism by which marked secretion of watery fluid by crypts of Lieberkuhn occurs is unknown. There is also secretion of chloride ions and bicarbonate ions into the crypts of Lieberkuhn. The secretion of chloride ions causes electrical drag of sodium ions through the membrane. Finally all these cause osmotic movement of water and hence fluidity in the purgation occurs. In diarrhoea, both sodium and potassium are excreted out of the body. The crypts of Lieberkuhn are located at jejunal region of small intestine, cause extreme rate of fluid secretion.

The process of Virechana is regulated and controlled by a special centre situated near Medulla oblongata in the brain. This centre is close to respiratory and vomiting centre. When the Virechana drugs stimulate the purgation centre, indirectly vomiting centre is relaxed. Sacral plexus of the spinal cord also helps in controlling and regulating the act of purgation, and it is also controlled and regulated by local reflex actions. Hence during the act of defecation, the respiration is arrested momentarily, diaphragm is activated and presses transverse colon. Simultaneously, the accessory muscles of the abdomen are also activated and helps in propelling the faecal matter towards anus along with the diaphragm.

Faecal matter, when reaches the intestine, stimulates local nerve plexuses and then enforced peristalsis further helps in expelling contents of intestines towards rectum and finally to anal canal. When these voluntary or involuntary act of defecation starts, finally results in evacuation of bowels.

Elimination of Pitta

Potent stimulus for causing the gallbladder contraction is from cholecystokinin hormone. This causes increased secretion of digestive enzymes from pancreas. The stimulation for this hormone is the presence of fatty food in duodenum. Gallbladder is also stimulated by Acetylcholine secreting nerve fibres from both vagi and intestinal enteric nervous system. Due to the relaxant action of sphincter of Oddi, bile enters into duodenum. This bile containing bile acids, bile pigments, cholesterol, lecithin, water, sodium, potassium bicarbonate ions which are eliminated out can be called as Pitta.

Mechanism of Virechana Karma (Purgation)

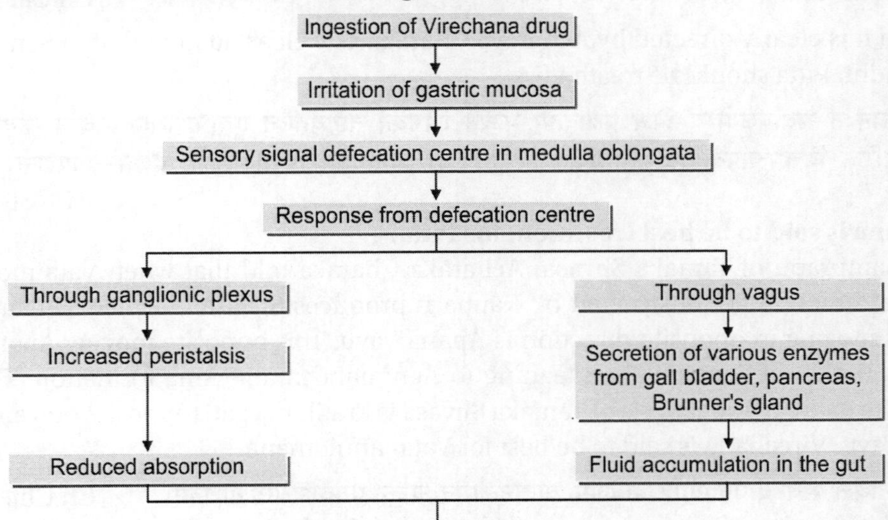

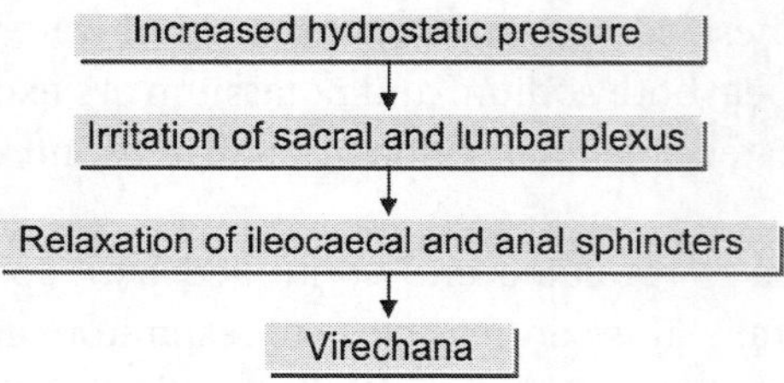

ROLE OF VIRECHANA IN VARIOUS DISEASES

Tamaka Shvasa

वातश्लेष्महरैयुक्तं तमके तु चिरेचनम्। (Ch.Chi. 17/121).

- Here charaka has clearly indicated the Virechana karma in 'Tamaka Shvasa. And he further emphasizes that the Vatanulomana and regular cleaning of the Srotas must be done. The site of origin of Shvasa roga is "Pitta Sthana Samudhbhava." And this Pitta sthana is described by Chakrapani as Adho Amashya. This is the region between the hridaya and nabhi. At this place the main pathology of Shvasa roga takes place and the pre-dominant dosha pitta is present here. And to purify the site of origin Virechana is advocated.
- Harita samhita also quotes the "Navaten Vina Shwase" i.e. Without involvement of Vayu, Shvasa cannot be produced. In Chikitsa sutra, he clearly indicates the use of Snehana, Svedana, and Mridu Virechana is to be done for pacifying Vata. In Tamaka Shvasa there is Predominence of Pitta doshas associated with Vata and Kapha.
- Here it is impotant to mention that intiating dosha of Shvasa is Vata-Kapha but the presenting symptoms in Tamaka Shvasa (like Tamapravesha etc.) appears due to Pitta-Vata. Thus it is Sannipataja Vyadhi.

समवाये हि दोषाणां पूर्व पित्तमुपाचरेत्। ज्वरे चैवातिसारे च सर्वत्रान्यत्र मारूतम्। (Su. Ut.)
संसृष्टे कफपित्ताभ्यां पित्तमादौ विनिर्जयेत। (Ch.Chi 28/188)

And it is clearly directed by Acharaya Charaka as well as Susruta that in Sannipatika Vyadhi, Pitta should be treated first.

विरेचनं तु सर्वोपक्रमेभ्य पित्त प्रधानतम् मन्यते भिषकः तद्धयादित एवामाशयमनुप्रविष्य केवलं वैकारिंक पित्तमूलापकर्षति तत्रावजिते पित्तेऽपि शरीरान्तर्गताः पित्तविकाराः प्रशान्तिमापद्यन्ते।

(Ch.Su. 20/16)

Virechana is said to be best treatment for Pitta.

In the Samprapti of Tamaka Shvasa; Acharaka Charaka told that when Vata moving in opposite direction get obstructed by Kapha it produces Shvasa. Further he clarify that the Vata moving in opposite direction is Apana Vayu. This opposite moving Apana Vayu causes vitiation of Samana Vayu leading to Agnimandya and Ama formation. Thus the root cause in the pathogenesis of Tamaka Shvasa is Pratiloma gati (opposite movement) of Apana Vayu. Virechana is said to be best for Vata- anulomana.

अपानेनावृत्ते सर्व दीपनं ग्राहि भेषजम् वातानुलोमनं यच्च पक्वाशयविशोधनम्। (Ch.Chi.28/243)
ऊर्ध्वगेनावृत्तेऽपाते छर्दिश्वासादयो गदाः स्र्युवाते तत्र वस्त्यादि भोज्यं चैवानुलोमन्। (Ch.Chi.28/209)

Shvasa is one among the symptoms of Udanavrita Apana, here also Acharaya advocate Vatanulomana treatment.

Although Basti is best therapy for Vata but still Mridu Virechana can be used for alleviating Vata as:

वातस्योपक्रमं स्नेह स्वेद संशोधनं मृदु॥ (Vagbhatta)

Basti is best therapy if only Vata is vitiated but when Vata is associated with other doshas, then Mridu Sanshodhana or Mridu virechana (with oilation) is best as:

यद्यनेन सदोषत्वात् कर्मणा न प्रशाम्यति। मृदुभिः स्नेह संयुक्तैः औषधेस्त विशोधयेत्। (Ch.Chi.28/83)

In Tamaka Shvasa there is Sama vayu. For alleviating Vata, and elimination of Ama from body, Virechana is most appropriate. Mridu Virechana not only helps in eliminating Ama from body, but simultaneously it also helps in Vata anulomana. Thus if Vata is associated with Ama, Virechana is most appropriate.

In the conext of Vatika Kasa Acharya give instruction for using Basti in case if Vata is only vitiated and Virechana when Vata is associated with Kapha and Pitta.

बस्तिभिर्बद्धविड्वातं शुष्कोर्ध्व चोर्ध्वभक्तिकैः। घृतैः सपित्तं सकफं जयेत् स्नेहविरेचनैः॥
(Ch.Chi. 12/34)

In Tamaka Shvasa there is obstruction of Vata by Kapha thus there is Kaphavrita Vata and Virechana is mentioned in the treatment of Kaphavrita Vata. Thus it is clear that from the word Virechana Acharya means Adhosanshodhana.

तमकः कफकासे तु स्याच्चेत् पितानुबन्धजः पित्तकासक्रियां तत्र यथावस्थ प्रयोजयेत्॥ (Ch.Chi.18/131)
वाते कफानुबन्धे तु कुर्यात् कफहरीं क्रियाम्। पितानुबन्धयोर्वातकफयोः पितनाशिनीम्॥ (Ch.Chi.18/132)
संसृष्टे कफपित्ताभ्यां पित्तमादौ विनिर्जयेत। (Ch.Chi 28/188)

In the context of Kasa treatment Acharaya Charaka told that if in Kaphaja Kasa, Tamaka Shvasa originated due to Pitta-anubandha then Pittaja Kasa treatment should be followed i.e. Virechana. Further he directed that if Vata is associated with Kapha then Kaphanashaka treatment and if Vata and Kapha both are associated with Pitta dosha then priority should be given to Pittanashaka treatment and best treatment for vitiated Pitta is Virechana.

The patient of Tamaka Shvasa is often weak and in chronic stage, Hridya as the mula of Pranavaha Shrotas is also involved. In this condition Vamana is very difficult and complicated procedure and the Virechana is easily done without threatening the life of the patient.

Pakshaghata

Prior to administration of Shodhana karma, Snehana and Svedana is done. In Pakshaghata the doshas are Shakhagata. Snehana and Svedana will cause Utkleshan and Dravikarana of doshas respectively and by these actions they move from Shakha to Koshtha. These vitiated doshas have to be thrown out of the body through the nearest route (Ch. Ni. 8/39). For this purpose Virechana has been advised because of its wide range of action, i.e., both on Amashaya and Pakvashaya.

In Pakshaghata the main dosha involved is Vata. The natural abode of Vata is Pakvashaya (A.H.Su.12/1). In Pakvashaya gatavata, Virechana is indicated. (Su.Chi. 4/5).

In Pakshaghata, sira snayu vishosha has been described as a symptom. Sira and kandara are the upadhatus of Rakta. Hence in this disease Rakta dhatu involvement is also seen. Pitta being mala of Rakta, its involvement may also occur. Charaka has mentioned Virechana in Raktaja vikara (Ch.Su.24/18) and for Pittaja vikara, Virechana is the treatment of choice.

The adhishthana of Pakshaghata is Indriyayatana (Mastishka). Mastishka is referred as Mustulunga (Ch. Si. 9/101). Dalhana describes the word Mustulunga as Ghritakaram and Mastishka Majja (Su.Sha.10/42, Dal.) He further describes Mastishka Majja as Majja dhara kala and again says that Majja dhara kala and Pitta dhara kala are one and the same. In Pitta dhara kala vikriti, Virechan is the best Shodhan chikitsa. As Majja dhara kala and pitta dhara kala are same, Virechana may also act well in Majja dhara kala vikriti. So, Virechana can be adopted in case of Pakshaghata.

Kaphandubandhit and Pittanubandhit Pakshaghata have been described in Madhava Nidana. This can be compared with Kaphavritta and Pittavritta Vata respectively. In treatment of both these conditions Virechana has been mentioned (Ch. Chi. 28/184,185,189).

In case of Sansargaja dosha, i.e., if Vata is affected by Pitta and Kapha both, then Pitta should be controlled first (Ch. Chi. 28/188) and for controlling Pitta, Virechana is considered to be best. Hence in Doshanubandhit Pakshaghata Virechana can be considered as a treatment.

Vagbhatta has mentioned Mridu Sanshodhana (Virechana) in the general line of treatment of Vata (A.H. Su.13/l), which can also be adopted for Pakshaghata.

Mridu Sanshodhana has been mentioned in treatment of Margavarana. (Ch.Chi.9/25). Hence in Margavaranjanya Pakshaghata Mridu Sanshodhana, i.e., Virechana can be advocated.

Majjavaha sroto dushti takes place in Pakshaghata and in order to combat the morbidity related to Majja, timely Shuddhi has been mentioned (Ch.Su.28/28). So here Virechana can be taken as a Shodhana measure.

In Chikitsasthana 28, Acharaya Charaka told the general line of treatment for Vata vyadhi that after Snehana and Svedana, Virechana should be given as main Shodhana measure. In the patients contraindicated for Virechana, Basti has been mentioned. Hence Virechana is considered to be treatment of choice in Vata vyadhi and so in Pakshaghata.

As described in the virtues of Virechana Karma–

- Srotovishuddhi is done by Virechana. This virtue of Virechana checks the Sanga type of Srotodushti encountered in Pakshaghata.
- Impairment of function of Mana, viz., memory, general intelligence, etc. is seen in Pakshaghata. Virechana is Buddhi Prasadana and checks this impairment.
- Virechana increases the strength of Indriyas and thereby checks the impairment of Indriyas encountered in Pakshaghata.
- Virechan imparts strength to the body and stabilizes all the dhatus. Hence useful in Dhatukshayajanya Pakshaghata. Therefore by all the above statements it can be concluded that virechan is the best Shodhana for Pakshaghata.

VIRECHANA YOGA ACCORDING TO DISEASES

S.No.	Name of Disease	Virechana Yoga	Reference
1.	Jvara	Aragvadha, Trivrita	Ch.Chi. 3/230-233
2.	Vishama Jvara	Ghrita, Dugdha	Ch.Chi. 3/294
3.	Raktapitta	Trivrita, Aragvadha	Ch.Chi. 4/54-57
4.	Gulma	Danti-Haritaki avleha	Ch.Chi. 5/152-160
5.	Kushtha	Trivrita, Danti, Triphala	Ch.Chi. 7/44-46
6.	Unmada	Purana Ghrita	Ch.Chi. 9/68
7.	Shotha	Danti, Trivrita, Eranda sadhita kshira	Ch.Chi. 12/24
8.	Udara roga	Narayan churna Snuhi kshira and ghrita, Eranda taila	Ch.Chi. 13/133,138-140
9.	Grahani	Tikshna Virechana	Ch.Chi. 15/179
10.	Pandu	Tikshna Virechana Danti, Trivrita, Aragvadha, Draksha, Haritaki	Ch.Chi. 16/40, 55-58
11.	Kasa	Trivrita, Tikta Virechana	Ch.Chi. 18/85
12.	Atisara	Haritaki	Ch.Chi. 19/21
13.	Chhardi	Haritaki	Ch.Chi. 20/21
14.	Pittaja Chhardi	Draksha, Trivrita, Vidari, Ikshurasa	Ch.Chi. 20/26
15.	Visarpa	Trivrita, Draksha, Trayamana Triphala, Trivrita Ghrita, Amalaki rasa	Ch.Chi. 21/63-67
16.	Visha (Keeta visha)	Danti, Trivrita	Ch.Chi. 23/203
17.	Madatyaya	Draksha rasa	Ch.Chi. 24/146
18.	Trimarmiya (Udavarta)	Trivrita, Danti, Phalavarti Snuhi kshira, Mulani and Phalini drugs	Ch.Chi. 26/18
19.	Trimarmiya (Aanaha)	Eranda taila	Ch.Chi. 26/29
	Trimarmiya (Mutrakricchra)	Dugdha	Ch.Chi. 26/49
	Trimarmiya (Hridaya roga)	Draksha, Phalasa, Katuki etc.	Ch.Chi. 26/90
20.	Vata vyadhi	Sneha Virechana	Ch.Chi. 28/83
21.	Vatarakta	Kumari swarasa, Triphala Kvatha, Draksha rasa	Ch.Chi. 29/62-68
22.	Vatrakta (Margavrodha-janya, Medovridhi, Kaphvridhi)	Gomutra, Arishta etc.	Ch.Chi. 29/157

Herbs used for Virechana

Operculina Terpethum

Having Anthraquinone glycoside also known as emodin. Unabsorbed in the small intestine, they are passed to the colon where bacteria liberates the active anthrol form, which either act locally or absorbed into circulation and excreted in bile to act on small intestine. The active principle is believed to work on myenteric plexus to increase peristalsis and decrease segmentation.

Water extract of the plant causes mild to moderate relaxation of the isolated guinea-pig ileum and also counteracts Acetylcholine.

Cassia Fistula

Cassia fistula's laxative actions come from a group of well documented compounds called anthraquinones that are found in all Cassia and Senna plants in varying degrees.

Its main property being that of a mild laxative suitable for children and pregnant women.

It is also a purgative due to the wax aloin and a tonic (Satyavati and Sharma, 1989) and has been reported to treat many other intestinal disorders like healing ulcers (Biswas et aI., 1973; Kirtikar and Basu, 1975).

The plant has a high therapeutic value and it exerts an antipyretic and analgesic effect (Patel et al., 1965). Besides, it has been found to exhibit anti-inflammatory and hypoglycaemic activity (Datta and Kumar, 1985).

Terminalia Chebula

- Shows antibacterial and antifungal properties which help in preventing bacterial overgrowth in gut. It has potent action against *E.coli* and *H.pylori*.
- Having anti-allergic action prevent mast cell degranulation and release of histamine.
- It has anti-oxidant effect because it is found to inhibit the lipid peroxidation and reduce the production of Anion superoxide.
- Act as Prokinetic drug and found to be very effective in Diabetic Nephropathy.

Castor Oil

- It is one of oldest purgatives.
- It mainly contains triglyceride of ricinoleic acid which is polar long chain fatty acid.
- It is hydrolysed in the ileum by lipase to ricinoleic acid and glycerol.
- It is believed to irritate the mucosa and stimulate intestinal contractions.
- The primary action is supposed to be decreased intestinal absorption of water and electrolyte and enhanced secretion by a detergent like action on mucosa.

CHAPTER 6

Basti Karma

INTRODUCTION

The urinary bladder of cow, buffalo, sheep was used as pressure pump in olden days to administer the medicinal matter into colon through rectum, urinary bladder or uterus by adjusting a wooden or metal nozel to it. Hence the process is named as Basti. It is a process by which the medicated oil or decoction is administered into the Pakvashaya or Garbhashaya or Mutrashaya with the help of Basti Yantra is known as Basti. Basti therapy is considered as Chikitsardha among all the therapeutic measures used in ayurvedic medicine and some physicians accept it as complete therapeutic measures because Basti has a vast field of action.

"Basti Vataharanam Shreshtham" basti is said to be best therapy to treat all Vata Vyadhis. It not only cures Vatika disorders but it also becomes helpful in Dosha Sansarga and Sannipata, Kaphaja and Pittaja disorder, Shakhashrita and Koshthashrita diseases by combination of different types of Basti Dravya.

ETYMOLOGY

The word Basti is derived from the root 'Vas' by adding 'Tich' Pratyaya and it belongs to masculine gender. According to Vachaspatyam

Meanings of the root ' Vas':

'वसु निवासे' means to reside, to stay, to dwell.

'वस आच्छादने' means to cover, to coat.

'वस् स्नेहाच्छादन प्रहरणेषु' means coating of Sneha for the elimination.

'बस्त गन्ध अर्दने' Here 'गन्ध' denotes bad smell hence it refers to 'Mala' and the verb 'अर्द्धने' is derived from 'अर्दगतौ याचने च' denotes the movement (in the colon) and to beg (drawing of waste material in the colon from all over the body).

'वस् वासने सुरभिकरणे'

Means to produce the effect of pleasant smell.

बस्ते आवृणोति मूत्रम्। वसुंदकतिच्।

Here it denotes an organ which covers the urine.

नाभिस्थोधोभागे मूत्राधारे स्थाने।

It denotes an organ situated below the umbilicus which holds the urine.

औषध दानार्थे द्रव्यभेदे।

It denotes an instrument used for the administration of the medicine. From the above forgoing descriptions, the following two conclusions can be drawn:

1. Basti denotes Karma where the drugs administered (औषधदानार्थे) through the rectal canal stay for certain period in the body (निवासे). Then produce the coating of the Sneha in the body (स्नेहाच्छादन) and draws out the waste substances from all over the body into the colon and eliminates them out of the body by producing movements in the colon resulting into pleasant (beneficial) effect (सुरभिकरण).
2. Basti denotes an organ which is receipted or reservoir of urine, i.e. 'urinary bladder' as it is basically a organ having soft and elastic nature. It was used as an instrument for the administration of the drugs with a constant pressure.

DEFINITION OF BASTI

बस्तिना दीयते इति बस्ति। (A.H.Su.19/1)
बस्तिभिदीयते यस्मात् तस्माद् बस्तिरिति स्मृतः। (Vangasena, Bha.Pra, Sha.Sam.)
बस्तिनादीयते बस्तिं वा पूर्वमन्वेयतो बस्तिः। (A.S.Su.28/2)

The procedure in which animal bladder is used to administer medicine is known as Basti.

IMPORTANCE OF BASTI AS ARDHA CHIKITSA

आपादतलमूर्धस्थान् दोषान् पक्वाशय स्थितः। वीर्येण बस्तिरादत्ते स्वस्थो अर्को भूरसानिव॥ (Ch.Si.7/64)

Basti introduced into the Pakvashaya acts upon the whole body and on every system of the body, from head to toe and draws out the impurities by its potency similar to the sun which evaporates the water from the earth by its heat.

यथा कुसुंभादि युतात् तोयाद्रांग हरेत् पटः। तथा द्रविकृताद् देहाद् बस्तिर्निर्हरेत् मलान्॥ (A.H.Su.19)

As the cloth absorbs the dye from water mixed with kusumba plant, in the same way Basti eliminates the malas from the body which have undergone liquefaction due to snehana and Svedana.

नाभिप्रदेशं कटि पार्श्व कुक्षिंगत्वा शकृद्दोषचयं विलोडयं। संस्नेह्य कायं सपुरीष दोषः सम्यक् सुखेनैति च यः स बस्ति। (Ch.Si.1/40)

The Basti dravya which is administered, churna and collects the accumulated doshas and Shakrit from nabhi, kati, parshwa and kukshi pradesha causes snehana to the body and expels out the doshas.

शाखागतः कोष्ठगताश्चः रोगा मर्मोर्ध्व सर्वावयवअङ्गजाच। ये सन्ति तेषां न हि कश्चिदन्यो वायोः परं जन्मनि हेतुरस्ति॥
विण्मूत्र पितादि मलाशयानां विक्षेप सङ्घातकरः स यस्मात्। तस्याति वृद्धस्य शमाय नान्यद् बस्तिं विना भेषजमस्ति किञ्चित्॥
तस्मात् चिकित्सार्धमिति ब्रुवन्ति सर्वाचिकित्सामपि बस्तिमेके। (Ch.Si.1/38-39)

All acharyas have highlighted the importance of Basti chikitsa; some have even gone to the extent of a ascribing it as purna chikitsa (complete treatment).

Acharya Charaka Says

The root cause for disease is Vata dosha which causes diseases in shakhas, koshthas, marma pradesha, Urdhvanga (head and neck), sarva avayava or all parts of the body.

Vata is responsible for dislodgement or combination of vit, mutra, pitta and kapha. Hence to say any malfunction in the body is caused by Vata dosha and Basti is the prime line of treatment for Vata dosha. None of the treatment modalities are as effective as Basti chikitsa for the mitigation of Vata dosha. Hence it is considered as ardha chikitsa and some even say it is Purna chikitsa or complete treatment.

बस्तिर्वाते च पित्ते च कफे रक्ते च शस्यते। संसर्गे सन्निपाते च बस्तिरेव हितः सदा॥ (Su.Chi.35/6)

Sushruta says basti is useful in treatment of vata, pitta and kapha doshas and even in the derangement of rakta dhatu. It is also effective in combination of two doshas or all the three doshas.

Also,

तत्र स्नेहादिनां कर्मणां बस्तिकर्म प्रधान तममाहुराचार्याः। कस्मात्। अनेक कर्म करत्वाद् बस्तः,
इह खलु बस्तिः नानाविध द्रव्य संयोगात् दोषाणाम् संशोधन संशमन सङ्ग्रहाणि करोति।
क्षीण शुक्रम् वाजीकरोति, कृशम् बृंहति, स्थूलं कार्शयति, चक्षुः प्रीणयति, वली पलित उपहन्ति,
वयः स्थापयति। शरीर उपचयं वर्ण बलमारोग्यम् आयुषः। कुरुते परिवृद्धिं च बस्तिः सम्यगुपासितः।
(Su.Chi.35/3-4)

The varied or multifaceted action of Basti can be ascribed to the permutation and combination of the drugs used for preparing Basti dravya.

Hence the functions like shodhana, shamana, sangrahana are brought about by Basti karma. It causes increased libido in ksheena shukra, increases the weight of the krisha person, decreases the weight of sthula person, causes optimal functions of eyes, delays graying and hair fall, delays degenerative changes, imparts optimal functioning of organs, increases strength and life span.

UTILITY OF BASTI KARMA IN HEALTH AND DISEASE

Effects of Basti

स्त्रोतोशुद्धिकरत्व

It purifies all the systems and makes a clear passage upto micro channel level.

भेषजविशेषयोगात्

It acts on various disorders based on the selection of the drug according to disease.

संशमन कर्म–Curative action

निरत्ययत्वात्–Uncomplicated

सर्वावस्थान् विकारान् उपयोगिता

Basti can be administered at any age and at any stage of disorder after proper examination. It can also be given in normal persons.

1. Promotive Aspects

वयस्थापन– Sustains age

सुखायुर्बलाग्निमेधास्वरवर्णकृत्– Provides better life, improves strength, digestive power, voice and complexion.

सर्वार्थकारि– Perform all functions.

दाढर्यवह– Provide firmness or compactness to body.

पुष्टिकर– Produces pushti or provides strength to body.

आशयलघुत्व– Lightness in visceral systems because of the removal of morbid matter from all over the body.

प्रकृतिस्थ– Restores normalcy.

रुचि– Increases taste perception

2. Curative Aspects

- ❑ **'स्तब्धता'**– Relieves stiffness.
- ❑ **'संकुचिताश्च'**– Relieves contractions and adhesions.
- ❑ **'पङ्ग्वो'**– Effective in paralytic conditions.
- ❑ **'भग्न रुग्णा'**– Effective in dislocation and fracture conditions.
- ❑ **'शाखासु चरन्ति वात'**– Effective in those conditions where Vata is aggravated in Shakha/ extremities.
- ❑ **'शूल'**– Relieves pain.
- ❑ **'कुक्षि आमये'**– Effective in disorders of Gastrointestinal tract.
- ❑ **'शाखाकोष्ठगत रोग'**– Effective in diseases of Shakha and Koshtha.
- ❑ **'मर्मोर्ध्वसर्वावयङ्गश्च'**– Effective in the diseases of vital parts, upper extremities and localized or general parts.
- ❑ **'क्षीणेन्द्रिय, कृशनर'**– Beneficial to debilitated and weak persons.
- ❑ **'वलीपलित अपहन्ती'**– Arrests premature old age and the progress of white hair.

3. Preventive Aspects

- ❑ **'विग्रथित पुरीषः'**– Beneficial in constipation.
- ❑ **'स्त्रोतः शुद्धिकरत्वात्'**– Effective to purify various systems of the body.

4. Rejuvinative Aspect

- ❑ **'शुक्रबलप्रदश्च'**– Increases the quantity and quality of semen.
- ❑ **'रक्तादि प्रसाद'**– Effective to restore the normal functions of blood and other dhatus.
- ❑ **'शुक्रमांसबलप्रदा'**– It provides strength by increasing muscle power.
- ❑ **'बाजीकरोति'**– Beneficial in geriatrics.

5. Psychological Aspects

- 'मेधाकृच्च'– Improves intellectual power
- 'मनः प्रसाद'– Provides clarity of mind
- 'बुद्धिन्द्रियसंप्रसाद'– Improves clarity of sense organs
- 'स्वपनानुवृत्ति'– Induces sound sleep
- 'लघुता'– Lightness
- 'हर्ष'– Exhilaration
- 'चक्षुः प्रीणयति'– (Sushruta) Invigorates eyesight
- 'मनः तुष्टि'– (Sushruta) Lightness of mind.

6. Miscellaneous Aspects

- 'स्वस्थानां आतुरानांवृद्धानाचाविरोधिनां'– Basti is non-antagonistic to healthy, diseased and old persons
- 'सर्वैषुऋतुषु यौगिकाः'– Applicable in all seasons
- 'सर्वार्थकारी शिशुवृद्धानां निरव्यय सर्वगदापहश्च'– Basti can be administered in child and older persons too. Because it is free from complications.

BASTI YANTRA

The instrument through which Basti dravya is administered is known as Basti Yantra. It mainly consists of two parts which are as follows:

1. BASTI-PUTAKA
2. BASTI-NETRA

Much importance is given to basti yantra because, slight negligence in selection of proper Putaka and Netra, may lead to Vyapat.

Material used for Basti Putaka

जारद्गवो माहिष हारिणौ वा स्यात् शौकरो बस्तिः अजस्थ वाऽपि।
दृढः तनुः नष्ट सिरो विगन्धः कषायरक्त सुमृदुः सुशुद्धः। नृणां वयो वीक्ष्य यथानुरूपं नेत्रेषु॥

(Ch.Si. 3/10-11)

Acharyas have insisted the use of Mutrashaya of vriddha go (old ox), mahisha (buffalo), harina (deer), shoukara (pig), aja (goat). The putaka should be dridha (firm), tanu (thin), nashta sira (free from vessels), durgandha rahita (devoid of smell). This Putaka should be made Rakta Varna and Mridu by boiling it in different kashayas. Putaka should be used considering the age of the patient. Putaka should be connected with the appropriate Netra and well tied with strings.

बस्तेः अलाभे प्लवजो गलो वा स्यात् अङ्कपादः सुघनः पटो वा। (Ch.Si.3/12)

If the bladder is not available, throat of a bird, skin of Ankhapada or a very thick cloth can be used.

Basti Putaka Dosha

Structural and functional problems pertaining to Basti Putaka and complications as a result of its uses are listed as follows :

विषम मांसल च्छिन्न स्थूल जालिक वातलाः। स्निग्धः क्लिन्नश्च तानष्टौ बस्तिन् कर्मसु वर्जयेत्॥
गति वैषम्य विस्रत्व स्राव दौर्ग्राह्य निस्रवाः। फेनिल च्युतिः अधार्यत्वं बस्तेः स्यु बस्तिदोषतः॥

(Ch.Si.5/6-7)

S. No.	Nature of problem with Basti Putaka	Complication as a result of its use
1.	विषम (Irregular in shape)	गतिवैषम्य (Does not enter the correct route)
2.	मांसल (Fleshy)	आमगंधता (Raw smell from Putaka)
3.	छिन्नल (Having holes of Putaka which is cut)	स्रावा (Spilling out of medicines)
4.	स्थूल (Thick)	दौर्ग्राह्य दुर्ग्रहता (Difficulty in holding)
5.	जालिक (Presence of veins or small holes)	निस्रवाः (Leaking of medicines)
6.	वातल (Presence of air)	फेनिल (Medicines become frothy)
7.	अतिस्निग्ध (Slimy)	च्युतिः हस्तभ्रंश (May slip out of hand)
8.	अतिक्लिन्न (Putaka which is excessive wet)	अधार्यत्वं बस्तेरिती क्लिन्नत्वाद्धि धारणायोगत्वं बस्तिपुटकस्य (Becomes difficult to hold and hence may slip out of hand)

Basti Netra (Fig. 6.1)

The word meaning of netra refers to 'eye'. In the context of Basti Yantra, netra refers to hollow tube like instrument that which is tied to the Putaka.

नेत्र नलिका (चक्रपाणि)
नेत्रं यन्त्रं (डल्हण)

Netra Dravya

सुवर्ण रूप्य त्रपु ताम्र रीति कांस्य अस्थि शस्त्र द्रुम वेणु दन्तैः।
नलै विषाणौ मणिभिश्च तैस्तैः नेत्राणि कार्याणि सु(त्रि)कर्णिकानि॥ (Ch.Si.3/7)

For the purpose of making basti netra, the Acharyas have insisted using suvarna (gold), raupya (silver), trapu, tamra (copper), riti (brass), kansya (bronze), asthi (bones), druma

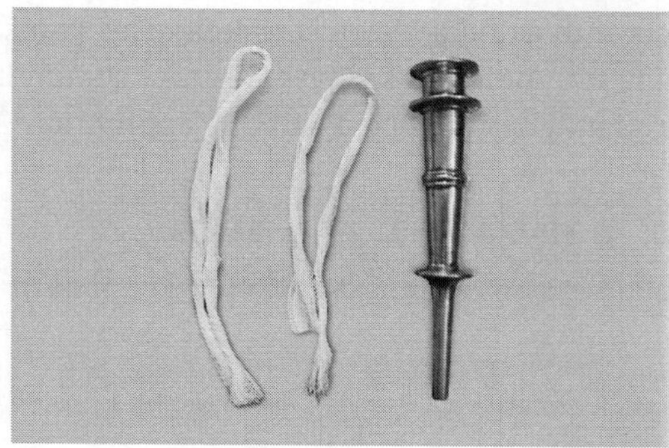

Fig. 6.1: Basti netra

(wood), venu (bamboo), danta (tooth), nala, vishana (horns), mani (beads). There should be 3 karnikas (calyx) for the basti netra.

Specifications of Basti Netra

षड् द्वादश अष्टांगुल संमितानि षड्विंशति द्वादश वर्षजानाम्।
स्युर् मुद्र कर्कंधु सतीन वाहि छिद्राणि वर्त्य अपिहितानि चैव॥
यथावयो अंगुष्ठ कनिष्ठकाभ्यां मूलाग्रयोः स्युः परिणाहवन्ति।
ऋजूनि गोपुच्छ समाकृतानि श्लक्ष्णानि च स्युर् गुडिकामुखानि॥
स्यात् कर्णिकैका अग्रचतुर्थभागे मुलाश्रिते बस्ति निबन्धने द्वे। (Ch.Si.3/8-9)

Basti Netra pramana	*Agrah chidra Pramana (according to Age)*				
	Ch.S. Age and size of opening)	*Su.S. (Age and size of opening)*	*A.S. and A. H. (Age and size of opening)*	*V.S. (Age and size of opening)*	*Sh.S. (Age and size of opening)*
5 Angulas	-	-	Below 1 year Mudgavat	-	-
6 Angulas	1-6 years Mudgavat	Below 1 year Mudgavat	At 1 year Mudgavat	At 6 years Mudgavat	1-6 years Mudgavat
6 ⅓ Angulas	7 years	-	-	-	-
6 ⅔ Angulas	8 years	-	-	-	-
7 Angulas	9 years	-	7 years Mashavat	-	-
7 ⅓ Angulas	10 years	-	-	-	-
7 ⅔ Angulas	11 years	-	-	-	-
8 Angulas	12 years Sushka Sateenavat	8 years Mashavat	12 years Kalayavat	12 years Sushka Sateenavat	6-12 years Kalayavat
8 ½ Angulas	13 years	-	-	-	-
9 Angulas	14 years	-	16 years Klinna kalayavat	-	-
9 ½ Angulas	15 years	-	-	-	-
10 Angulas	16 years	16 years Kalayavat	-	-	-
11 Angulas	18 years	-	-	-	-
11 ½ Angulas	19 years	-	-	-	-
12 Angulas	20 years Karkanduvat (kolasthi)	-	20 years Karkanduvat	20 years Karkanduvat	20 years Karkanduvat
12 Angulas			-	-	-
12 Angulas	Above 25 years Kolasthivat	-	-	-	

Basti Netra Karnikas

Karnikas are the rings over the Basti Netra which help in tying the Putaka and guides the administrator to limit the Netra's entry into the Guda after certain extent. In ayurvedic texts the measure for the first karnika from the tip of the Netra is said to be at 1/4th of the length of given Netra and two other karnikas should be at the base of Netra.

Age	*Distance of Karnika from Agrabhaga*
1 year	1½ Angula
8 year	2 Angula
16 year	3 ½ Angula
25–70 year	3 Angula

Vrana Basti Netra

व्रण नेत्रम् अष्टाङ्गुल मुद्ग वाहिस्त्रोत। (Su.Chi. 35/11)

The Vrana basti Yantra should be 8 angula in length and hole through which the green gram can pass.

Basti Netra Dosha

ह्रस्वं दीर्घं तनु स्थूलं जीर्णं शिथिल बन्धनम्। पार्श्वच्छिद्रं तथा वक्रमष्टौ नेत्राणि वर्जयेत्।।
अप्राप्त्यतिगति क्षोभ कर्षण क्षणन स्रवाः। गुद पीडा गतिर्जिह्वा तेषां दोषाः यथाक्रमम्।। (Ch.Si.5/4-5)

S.No.	*Nature of problem with nozzle*	*Complication as a result of its use*
1.	अतिह्रस्वं (Shorter)	अप्राप्ति (Does not reach Pakvashaya)
2.	अतिदीर्घ (Longer)	अतिगति दूरप्रवेशः (Go behind Pakvashaya)
3.	तनुनेत्र (Thinner in shape)	क्षोभः (Causes irritation)
4.	स्थूलनेत्र (Thicker in shape)	कर्षण (Pressure)
5.	जीर्णनेत्र (Old Netra)	क्षणन (Abrasion)
6.	शिथिल बंधन (Loose binding)	स्राव: (Spilling of medicines)
7.	पार्श्वच्छिद्र (Holes in the sides of Netra)	गुदपीडा (Pain in Guda Pradesha)
8.	वक्रनेत्र (Curved or not straight)	गतिर्जिह्वा कुटिला (Medicines does not enter the correct route because of deviated Netra)

Alternative Basti Yantra

Enema can

The measuring cans attached with the pipe are nowadays used for the administration of niruha Basti. The end of the pipe is attached with catheter of suitable size and it is inserted into the anal canal.

Advantages

- Easily available and easy to administer.
- No need of expertization.
- Chances of complications like Sa-vata Basti is very less.
- By using properly autoclaved instrument even cross infections can be prevented.

Disadvantages

- Dravya should move by gravitational force, no chance for pressing like in Putaka.

Modified Plastic Rubber Bag for Putaka for Niruha

- This Yantra is made from one piece surgical plastic.
- It is transparent and sterilizable and comes with rounded tip for painless insertion.
- Transparent body allows viewing of air in Basti material.

Enema Syringe (Fig. 6.2)

- Nowadays, modified Basti yantras are available in the market. This has a stainless steel body with bronze head or delrin head.
- The disposable Basti tip is screwed to the head.
- This tip has an ideal hole size for Ayurvedic use.
- These are available in the 100 mL/250 mL sizes for Matra Basti and Anuvasana Basti.
- The tips are also available in two sizes: adult and pediatric.

Rubber Catheter

- It can be used in place of Basti Netra.
- Rubber catheter can be used for a single use and then disposed.
- By using rubber catheter one can give high rectal or low rectal enema.
- Different size catheters are available in the market, commonly number 12 size for elders and 8 size for pediatric age group is used.
- Less chance of injury and complications.

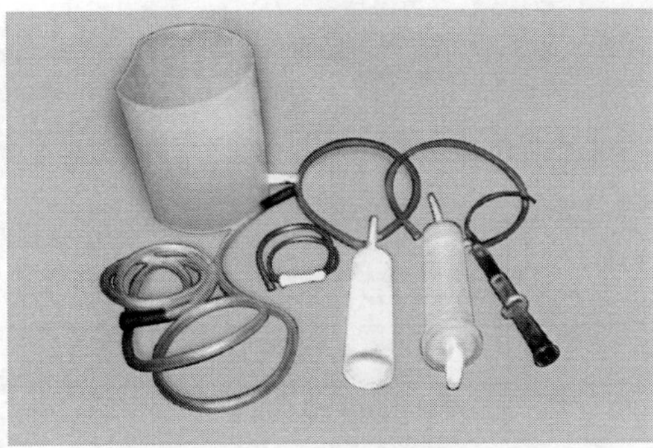

Fig. 6.2: Enema Syringe and pot

CLASSIFICATION OF BASTI

A. Adhishthana Bheda

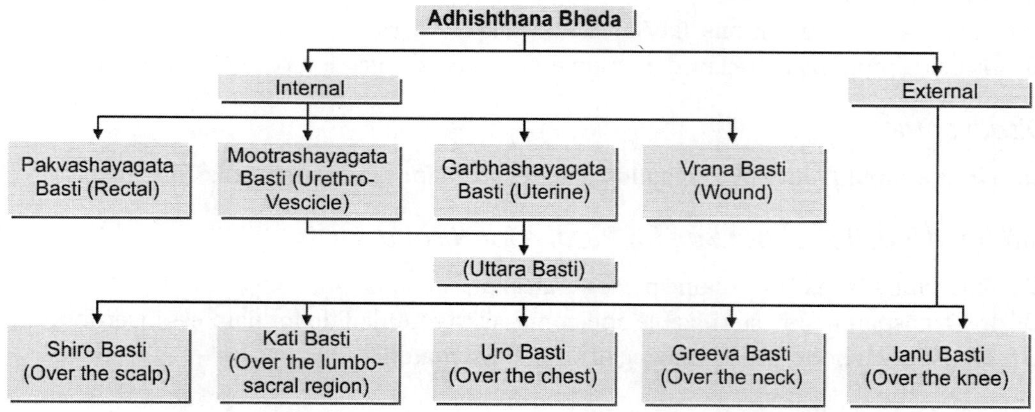

B. तत्र द्विविधो बस्ति नैरूहिकः स्नैहिकश्च।

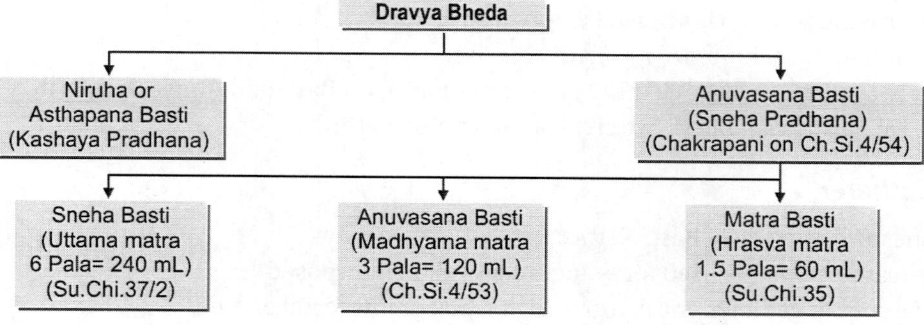

C.

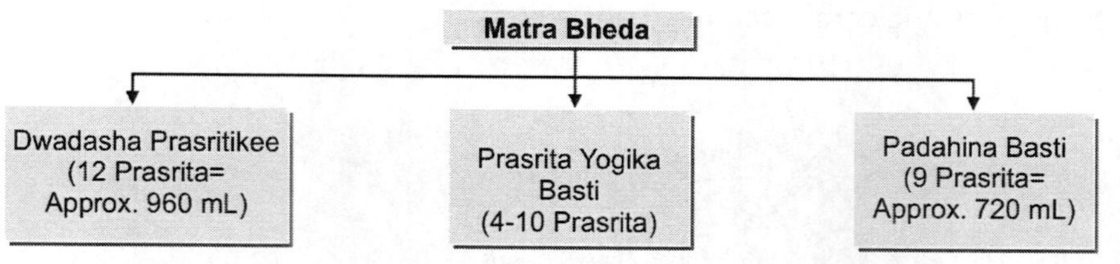

D.

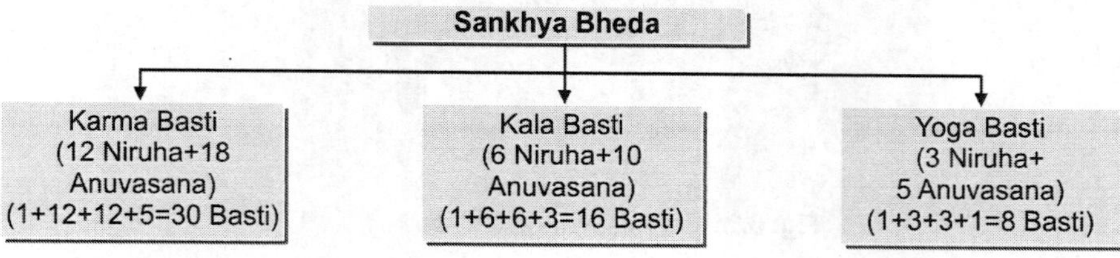

E.

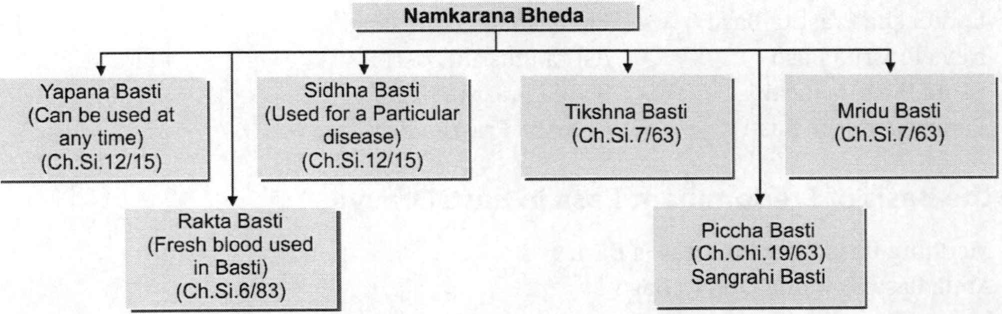

F.

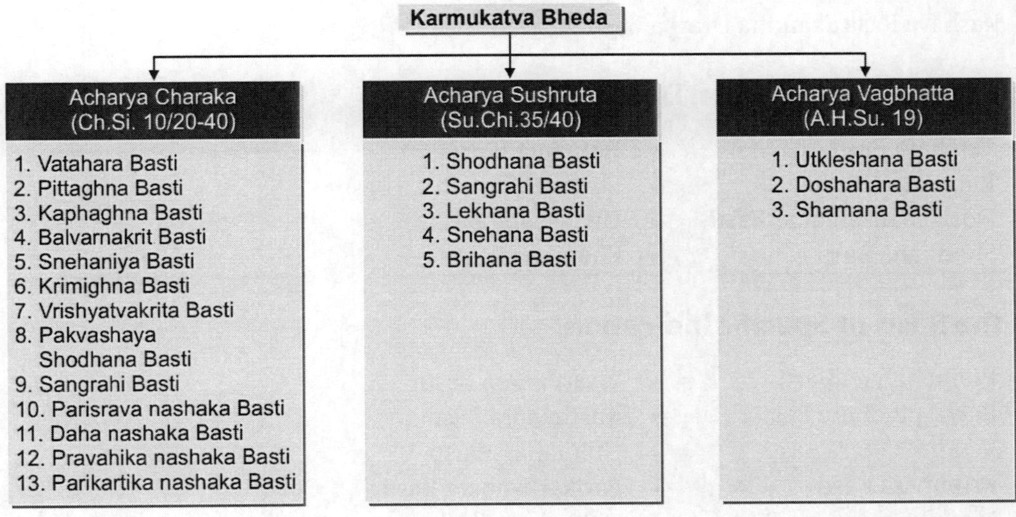

On the Basis of Nature of Basti Dravya

- Mridu Basti
- Madhyama Basti
- Tikshna Basti

On the Basis of Chief Drugs

1. Kshira Basti
2. Mansa Rasa Basti
3. Amla-Kanjika Basti
4. Gomutra Basti
5. Rakta Basti
6. Asavakrita Basti
7. Kshara Basti
8. Dadhi Masha Basti

According to the Dose of Basti

- Dwadasha Prasrita Basti
- Ekadasha Prasrita Basti
- Nava Prasrita Basti
- Ashta Prasrita Basti
- Sapta Prasrita Basti
- Shada Prasrita Basti
- Pancha Prasrita Basti
- Catusha Prasrita Basti

On the Basis of Predominant Rasa in Basti Dravya

- ❑ Madhura Rasa Skandha Dravya Basti
- ❑ Amla Rasa Skandha Dravya Basti
- ❑ Lavana Rasa Skandha Dravya Basti
- ❑ Katu Rasa Skandha Dravya Basti
- ❑ Tikta Rasa Skandha Dravya Basti
- ❑ Kashaya Rasa Skandha Dravya Basti

On the Basis of Action on Dosha and Dushya

- Vatahara Basti
- Pittahara Basti
- Kaphahara Basti
- Shonita Doshahara Basti
- Dosha Sansargahar Basti
- Utkleshana Basti
- Shodhana Basti
- Shamana Basti

On the Basis of Specific Indication

- Pramehahara Basti
- Visarpahara Basti
- Rakta-pittahara Basti
- Kusthahara Basti
- Vata-raktahara Basti
- Gulmahara Basti
- Krimihara Basti
- Parikartikahara Basti
- Mutrakrichhahara Basti
- Dahaghna Basti

CLASSIFICATION OF BASTI ACCORDING TO FIXED SCHEDULE

In our classics, particular format of using Sneha and Niruha Basti has been given. Here, the number of Basti are fixed. These type of Basti can be used as per the disease and the condition of patients. In these types of Basti, only single form of Basti, i.e. either Sneha or Niruha can not be given lonely. These are described as follows -

a. **Karma Basti**- In this schedule, 30 Basti are to be administered.
b. **Kala Basti**- Acharya Charaka opines that Kala Basti includes half the number of Basti to that of Karma Basti. Here, Chakrapani opines that it includes 16 Basti.
c. **Yoga Basti**- This format of Basti includes the group of 8 Basti.

(a) Karma Basti

In this schedule, 30 Basti are to be administered. Out of these 18 are Anuvasana, while remaining, i.e. 12 Basti are Niruha. Initially on the first day, 1 Anuvasana is given which is followed by 12 Niruha and 12 Anuvasana alternatively. Lastly, 5 Anuvasana are to be given.

According to Kashyapa's view, in this schedule of 30 Basti, 24 Basti are Anuvasana, while 6 Basti are Niruha. Initially 5 Anuvasana are to be given then 1 Niruha and 3 Anuvasana are given alternatively, which is followed by 4 Anuvasana at the end.

बाहु .... ते कर्म संज्ञितम्। अत्युदीर्ण बले जाते प्रयोज्यं तद्यथाविधि। (Ka.S.Khi.8/7)

He also mentioned that this schedule can be used in the patients having good strength and Vata predominance. According to Bhela, Karma Basti includes 24 Basti. (Bhe.Si.5/28)

According to Gayadas, Karma Basti can be used when there is a marked vitiation of the Dosha due to the Balavadvigraha.

According to Charaka

1	2	3	4	5	6	7	8	9	10	11	12	13	14	15
A	N	A	N	A	N	A	N	A	N	A	N	A	N	A
16	17	18	19	20	21	22	23	24	25	26	27	28	29	30
N	A	N	A	N	A	N	A	N	A	A	A	A	A	A

According to Kashyapa

1	2	3	4	5	6	7	8	9	10	11	12	13	14	15
A	A	A	A	A	N	A	A	A	N	A	A	A	N	A
16	17	18	19	20	21	22	23	24	25	26	27	28	29	30
A	A	N	A	A	A	N	A	A	A	N	A	A	A	A

Benefits of Karma Basti

अत्युदीर्ण बले जाते प्रयोज्यं तध्याथाविधि॥ (Ka.S.Khi.8/7)

In a person having good Bala one can plan for the Karma Basti.

Indications

गम्भीर अनुगता यस्य क्रमेण अपचिता मलाः। कुपिता वात भूयिष्ठा बस्ति साध्या विशेषतः॥
सम्पन्नस्य सहिष्णोश्च कर्म तस्य परायणम्॥ (Ka.S.Khi.8/28-29)

The person in whom there is gradual accumulation of Doshas and doshas are situated deeply having Vata pradhanata, the diseases are especially Basti Sadhya, the person who is capable of withstanding the treatment of longer duration can be employed with Karma Basti schedule.

(b) Kala Basti

Charaka mentioned that it includes half number of Basti to that of Karma Basti. But Chakrapani clarified that it includes 16 Basti. Day first 1 Anuvasana can be given then afterwards 6 Anuvasana and 6 Niruha given alternatively and at last 3 Anuvasana are to be given.

According to Vagbhatta, it includes 15 Basti.

काल पच्दशैकोऽत्र प्राक् स्नेहोऽन्ते त्रयस्तथा। षट् पच्चवस्त्यन्तरिता...... अत्युदीर्णबले जाते प्रयोज्य मध्यबलान्वये।। (A.H.Su.19/64)

Here Arundatta has clearly mentioned that 1 Anuvasna in the beginning and 3 at the end with 5 Asthapana and 6 Anuvasana on alternate days for 15 consecutive days.

Kashyapa mentioned, 12 Anuvasana and 3 Niruha, 3 Anuvasna in the beginning then 1 Niruha and 3 Anuvasana alternatively and at last 3 Anuvasana are given. He also mentioned that this schedule can be used in the patient having moderate strength and in the disease where along with Vata, Pitta is also vitiated_(Ka.Khi.8/8-9).

पवने पित्तसंसृष्टे विद्यातव्यो विजानता। अल्पत्वात स्नेहबस्तीनां युक्तेर्योगः स लाघवात्। (Ka.S.Khi.8/8-9)

According to Gaydas, it is to be given in the patient where moderate vitiation of doshas due to seasonal changes occurs.

According to Charaka

1	*2*	*3*	*4*	*5*	*6*	*7*	*8*	*9*	*10*	*11*	*12*	*13*	*14*	*15*	*16*
A	N	A	N	A	N	A	N	A	N	A	N	A	A	A	A

According to Kashyapa

1	*2*	*3*	*4*	*5*	*6*	*7*	*8*	*9*	*10*	*11*	*12*	*13*	*14*	*15*
A	A	A	N	A	A	A	N	A	A	A	N	A	A	A

(c) Yoga Basti

Charaka mentioned that it includes 8 Basti out of which 5 are Anuvasana and 3 are Niruha. First day 1 Anuvasana, then 3 Niruha and 3 Anuvasana alternatively and at last 1 Anuvasana should be given. Kashyapa indicates same number of Basti with same Niruha and Anuvasana schedule. According to Kashyapa, due to less use of Sneha it is mild in action. It is used in the patient having Kapha Sansarga along with Vata vitiation. Kashyapa mentioned the Basti course according to their use in pediatric patient. Gayadas mentioned Yoga Basti in mild vitiation of Dosha. It can be given in Svastha Purusha (healthy person) for attainment of Vrishyata.

Note: According to Dalhana, all these Basti schedule, i.e. Karma, Kala and Yoga are for Vata, Pitta and Kapha predominance respectively.

1	*2*	*3*	*4*	*5*	*6*	*7*	*8*
A	N	A	N	A	N	A	A

Indications

अल्पत्वात् स्नेह बस्तिनां युक्तेर्योगः स लाघवम्। प्रयोज्यः कफ संसृष्टे नाति तीव्रबले अनिले।।

(Ka.S.Khi.8/9-10)

Since the number of Sneha Bastis is less and it is laghu, the schedule is known as yoga Basti. The disease in which there is Kapha Sansrishta and Vata is not prabala one should plan for Yoga Basti.

According to Dalhana, the Basti schedule of Karma, Kala and Yoga is as per the predominance of Dosha, i.e. Vata, Pitta and Kapha respectively. Hence, here we can also say that the conditions involving the Vata Dosha are more difficult to cure.

NIRUHA BASTI

Rectal route of administration of medicine predominantly containing Kvatha is called as Niruha. The composition of Niruha basti are honey, saindhava lavana, medicated sneha, kalka and larger quantiy of decoction.

Definition

स दोष निर्हरणात् शरीर नीरोहणाद् वा निरुहः॥ (Su.Chi.35/18)

शरीर आहोरणात् दोष निर्हरणाद् अचिन्त्य प्रभावतया यस्मिन्नूहा सम्भवान् निरुह इति। (A.S.Su.28/6)

निरुहो दोष हरणाद्रोहणाद् अथ वातनोः॥ (Vangasena.Bastiadhikara)

The Basti which causes the removal of aggravated Dosha from the body is known as Niruha. Here, first derivation is on the basis of the pacification of doshas by niruha. In the second derivation, the mode of action of niruha is attributed to 'achintya prabhava'.

Synonyms of Basti

Depending upon the uses, contents, actions the Basti has different synonyms as explained below:

आस्थापनं, निरूह इत्यन् अर्थान्तरं तस्य विकल्पो माधुतैलिकः; तस्य पर्याय शब्दो यापनो, युक्तरथः सिद्धबस्तिर् इति॥ (Su.Chi 35/18)

निरुह, आस्थापन, माधुतैलिक, यापन, सिद्ध।

आस्थापनः

वयः स्थापनाद् आयुः स्थापनाद् वा आस्थापनम्। (Su.Chi.35/18)

तद्वयः स्थापनाद् दोष स्थापनाद् वा आस्थापनम् इत्युच्यते। (A.S.Su.28/6)

आस्थापयेद् वयो देहं यस्माद् आस्थापनः स्मृतः॥ (A.S.Su.28/6)

The Niruha Basti is also called as Asthapana Basti. From above derivations Asthapana means one which stabilizes the youthful age or sustains lifespan by pacifying the vitiated Doshas.

Indications

Niruha Basti is indicated specially in Vata and its disorders, because it eliminates Vata from its root and thus they do not reoccur.

Its other indications are as follows:

विशेषतस्तु सर्वाङ्ग एकांग कुक्षिरोग वात वर्चो मूत्र शुक्र संग बल वर्ण मांस रेतः
क्षयदोष आध्मान अंगसुप्ति कृमिकोष्ट उदावर्त शुद्ध अतिसार पर्वभेद अभिताप
प्लीह गुल्म शूल हृद्रोग भगन्दर उन्माद ज्वर ब्रध्न शिरः कर्ण शूल हृदय पार्श्व

पृष्ट कटिग्रह वेपन अक्षेपक गौरव अतिलाघव रजः क्षयार्त विषमाग्नि स्फिग्जानु जन्गोरु गुल्फ पार्ष्णि प्रपद योनि बाह्वन्गुलि स्तनान्त दन्त नख पर्वास्थि शूल शोष स्तंभ अन्त्रकूज परिकर्तिका अल्पाल्प सशब्द उग्रगन्धो अत्थानादयो वातव्याधयो विशेषेण महारोगाध्यायोक्ताश्च; एतेषु आस्थापनं प्रधानतम् अत्युक्तं वनस्पति मूलच्छेदवत्।। (Ch.Si.2/16)

S.No.	*Asthapya*	*Charaka*	*Sushruta*	*Vagbhatta*
1.	Sarvanga roga	+	+	-
2.	Ekanga roga	+	+	-
3.	Kukshi roga	+	-	+
4.	Vata sanga	+	+	+
5.	Mutra sanga	+	+	+
6.	Mala sanga	+	+	+
7.	Shukra sanga	+	-	-
8.	Bala kshaya	+	-	-
9.	Mansa kshaya	+	-	-
10.	Dosha kshaya	+	-	-
1l.	Shukra kshaya	+	+	-
12.	Adhmana	+	+	+
13.	Anga supti	+	-	-
14.	Krimi koshtha	+	-	-
15.	Udavarta	+	+	-
16.	Shudhhatisara	+	+	+
17.	Parvabheda	+	-	-
18.	Abhitapa	+	-	-
19.	Plihadosha	+	-	-
20.	Gulma	+	+	+
2l.	Shula	+	+	+
22.	Hridroga	+	-	-
23.	Bhagandar	+	-	-
24.	Unmada	+	-	-
25.	Jvara	+	-	+
26.	Bhrama	+	+	-
27.	Shira shula	+	+	+
28.	Karna shula	-	-	-
29.	Hridaya shula	+	-	-
30.	Parshva shula	+	-	-
3l.	Prishtha shula	+	-	-
32.	Kati shula	+	-	-
33.	Kampa	+	-	-

Contd...

Contd...

S.No.	*Asthapya*	*Charaka*	*Sushruta*	*Vagbhatta*
34.	Akshepa	+	+	-
35.	Anga gaurav	+	-	-
36.	Ati laghav	+	-	-
37.	Raja kshaya	+	+	-
38.	Vishamagni	+	-	-
39.	Sphik shula	+	-	-
40.	Janu shula	+	-	-
41.	Jangha shula	+	-	-
42.	Uru shula	+	-	-
43.	Gulma shula	+	-	-
44.	Parshni shula	+	-	-
45.	Prapad shula	+	-	-
46.	Yoni shula	+	+	+
47.	Bahu shula	+	-	-
48.	Anguli shula	+	-	-
49.	Stana shula	+	-	-
50.	Danta shula	+	-	-
51.	Nakha shula	+	-	-
52.	Parva asthi shula	+	-	-
53.	Shosha	+	-	-
54.	Stambha	+	-	-
55.	Antra kunjan	+	-	-
56.	Parikartika	+	-	-
57.	Vata vyadhi	+	+ (Daruna)	
58.	Timira	+	+	-
59.	Pratishyaya	-	+	+
60.	Adhimantha	-	+	-
6l.	Ardita	+	+	
62.	Pakvashayagata shula	+	+	
63.	Sharkara shula	-	+	-
64.	Upadansha		+	
65.	Vatarakta	-	+	+
66.	Arsha	-	+	-
67.	Stanya kshaya	-	+	-
68.	Manyagraha	+	+	-

Contd...

Contd...

S.No.	*Asthapya*	*Charaka*	*Sushruta*	*Vagbhatta*
69.	Hanugraha	+	+	-
70.	Ashmari	-	+	+
71.	Moodhagarbha	-	+	+
72.	Mutrakrichha	-	+	-

Contraindications

क्षीण क्षतानां न विशोधनीयात् न शोषिणां नो भृशं दुर्बलानाम्।
न मूर्च्छितानां न विशोधितानां येषां च दोषेषु निबद्धम् आयुः।। (Ch.Si.1/37)

Niruha Basti is generally contraindicated in persons having Urahkshata (ulcer in lung) who are emaciated, dehydrated due to Shodhana, excessively weak, debilitated and unconscious and where the Dosha is the only matter to withhold the life.
Its other contraindications are as follows:

अनास्थाप्यास्तु अजीर्ण्यतिस्निग्ध पीतस्नेहो उत्क्लिष्ट दोषाल्पाग्नि यानक्लान्त
अतिदुर्बल क्षुत्तृष्णा श्रमार्ता अति कृश भुक्तभक्त पीतोदक वमित विरिक्त कृतनस्य:
कर्मकुद्ध भीतमत्त मूर्च्छित प्रसक्तच्छर्दि निष्टिविका श्वास कास हिक्का बद्ध च्छिद्रो
दकोदरा आध्मान अलसक विसूचिक अमप्रजाताम अतिसार मधुमेह कुष्ठार्त।। (Ch.Si.2/14)

Asthapana Basti Ayogya (Ch.Si.2/14; Su.Chi.35/21; A.H.Su.19/4-6)

S.No.	*Anasthapya*	*Charaka*	*Sushruta*	*Vagbhatta*
1.	Ajirna	+	+	-
2.	Ati snigdha	+	-	+
3.	Pita sneha	+	-	-
4.	Utkleshita dosha	+	-	-
5.	Alpagni	+	+	+
6.	Yan klanta	+	-	-
7.	Ati daurbalya	+	+	-
8.	Kshudharta	+	-	-
9.	Trishnarta	+	-	-
10.	Shramarta	+	-	+
11.	Ati krisha	+		+
12.	Bhukta bhakta	+	-	+
13.	Pitodaka	+	-	-
14.	Vamita	+	-	+
15.	Virikta	+	-	+
16.	Krita nasya karma	+	-	+
17.	Krudhha	+	-	-
18.	Bheeta	+	-	-

Contd...

Contd...

S.No.	*Anasthapya*	*Charaka*	*Sushruta*	*Vagbhatta*
19.	Matta	+	+	-
20.	Murchhita	+	+	-
21.	Prasakta chardi	+	+	+
22.	Prasakta nishthivana	+	-	+
23.	Shvasa prasakta	+	+	+
24.	Kasa prasakta	+	+	+
25.	Hikka prasakta	+	-	+
26.	Baddha gudodara	+	-	+
27.	Chidrodara	+	-	+
28.	Udakodara	+	-	+
29.	Aadhmana	+	-	+
30.	Alasaka	+	-	-
31.	Visuchika	+	-	-
32.	Amadosha	+	-	-
33.	Amatisara	+	-	+
34.	Madhumeha, prameha	+	+	+
35.	Kushtha	+	+	+
36.	Arsha	+	+	+
37.	Pandu	-	+	-
38.	Bhrama	-	+	-
39.	Arochaka	-	+	-
40.	Unmada	-	+	-
41.	Shokagrasta	-	+	-
42.	Sthaulya	-	+	-
43.	Kantha shosha	-	+	-
44.	Kshata kshina	-	+	+
45.	Saptamasa garbhini	-	+	-
46.	Bala, vriddha	-	+	-
47.	Alpa varcha	-	-	+
48.	Gudashotha	-	-	+
49.	Amaprajata	+	-	-
50.	Shopha	-	-	-

Reasons for Contraindication

तत्र अजीर्ण्यतिस्निग्ध पीतस्नेहानां दूष्योदरं मूर्च्छा श्वयथुर्वा स्यात्, उत्क्लिष्ट
दोषा मन्दाग्नेयोर अरोचकस्तीव्रः, यानक्लान्तस्य क्षोभ व्यापन्नो बस्तिराशु देहं

शोषयेत्, अतिदुर्बल क्षुत्तृष्णा श्रमार्तानां पूर्वोक्तो दोषः स्यात् अतिकृशस्य कार्श्यं पुनर्जनयेत् भुक्तभक्त पीतोदकयोर् उत्क्लिश्योर्ध्वम् अधो वा वायुर्बस्तिम् उत्क्षिप्य क्षिप्रं घोरान् विकाराञ्जनयेत्, वमित विरिक्तयोस्तु रूक्षं शरीरं निरूहः क्षतं क्षार इव दहेत् कृत नस्तः कर्मणो विभ्रंशं भृश संरुदध स्रोतसः कुर्याद् क्रुद्ध भीतयोर् बस्तिर् उर्ध्वमुपप्लवेत् मत्त मूर्च्छितयोर् भ्रंश विचलितायां संज्ञायां चित्तोपघाताद् व्याप्त् स्यात् प्रसक्तच्छर्दि निष्ठीविका श्वास कास हिक्कार्तानाम् उर्ध्वीभूतो वायुरुर्ध्व बस्तिं नयेत् बद्ध च्छिद्रो दकोदरा आध्मानार्तानां भृशतरमाध्याप्य बस्तिः प्राणान् हिंस्यात् अलसक विसूचिकऽऽआमप्रजाताम् आतिसारिणाम् आमकृतो दोषः स्यात्, मधुमेह कुष्ठिनोर व्याधिः पुनर्वृद्धिः तस्मादेते न आस्थाप्याः॥ (Ch.Si.2/15)

Condition	*Reason*
Ajeerna, atisnigdha, snehapeeta	Causes udara, murccha, shwayatu
Utklishta dosha	Increases mandagni, aruchi
Yanaklanta	Causes emaciation in the body
Ati durbala, kshut, trishna, shramarta	Causes emaciation in the body
Atikrisha	Causes further emaciation
Bhuktabhakta, peetodaka	Vata getting provoked; throws out enema fluid upward or downwards and produces serious disorders
Vamita, virikta	Burn the dehydrated body as if cauterized with kshara
After nasya karma	Causes impairment of senses and obstruction of the channels
Kruddha, bheeta	Enema will mount very high
Matta, moorchita	Due to derangement of consciousness, there will be complications and injury to the mind
Praskta chardi, nishteeva,	Vata turned into an upward course
Shvasa, kasa, hikka	Will carry the enema fluid upwards
Baddha, chidra, dakodara, adhmanarta	Further increases the distension and may lead to death
Alasaka, visuchika, amaprajata, amaatisara	Causes ama dosha
Madhumeha, kushtha	Further aggravates the disease

a. Dose of Niruha Basti

निरूहमात्रा प्रसृत अर्धम् आध्ये वर्षे ततो अर्ध प्रसृत अभिवृद्धि।
आद्वादशात् स्यात् प्रसृत् अभिवृद्धिर् अष्टादशाद् द्वादशतः परं स्युः॥
आसप्त तेस्त द्विहितं प्रमाणमतः परं षोडशवद् विधेयम्।
निरुहमात्रा प्रसृत प्रमाणा बाले च वृद्धे च मृदुर् विशेषः॥ (Ch.Si.3/31-32)

Charaka has mentioned the detailed dose schedule of Niruha Basti according to the age of the patient.The dose for the child of 1 year is half Prasrita (48 mL), and then half Prasrita increases for the each completed year of the child up to the age of 12 years. The easy formula is half of the age in Prasrita. For example, the dose of 4 years child will be 2 Prasrita and for the 12 years old child it will be 6 Prasrita. After the age of 12 years, the dose of Niruha is to be increased by 1 Prasrita for the each completed year. For instances it will be 7 Prasrita for the age of 13 years, 8 Prasrita for the age of 14 years and so on and it will become maximum, i.e. 12 Prasrita at the age of 18 years. This dose is to be maintained up to the age of 70 years. Thereafter it should be 10 Prasrita, i.e. equal to the dose of 16 years of age.

Age	*Vagbhatta (Dose in Prakuncha)*	*Charaka (Dose in Prasrita)*	*Dose in mL*
1 year	1 Prakuncha	½ Prasrita	48 mL
2 year	2 Prakuncha	1 Prasrita	96 mL
3 year	3 Prakuncha	1 ½ Prasrita	144 mL
4 year	4 Prakuncha	2 Prasrita	196 mL
5 year	5 Prakuncha	2½ Prasrita	244 mL
6 year	6 Prakuncha	3 Prasrita	292 mL
7 year	7 Prakuncha	3½ Prasrita	340 mL
8 year	8 Prakuncha	4 Prasrita	388 mL
9 year	9 Prakuncha	4½ Prasrita	436 mL
10 year	10 Prakuncha	5 Prasrita	484 mL
11 year	11 Prakuncha	5½ Prasrita	532 mL
12 year	12 Prakuncha	6 Prasrita	580 mL

Increase 1 Prasrita from 12 to 18 years

12 year	6 Prasrita	6 Prasrita	580 mL
13 year	7 Prasrita	7 Prasrita	676 mL
14 year	8 Prasrita	8 Prasrita	772 mL
15 year	9 Prasrita	9 Prasrita	868 mL
16 year	10 Prasrita	10 Prasrita	964 mL
17 year	11 Prasrita	11 Prasrita	1060 mL
18 year	12 Prasrita	12 Prasrita	1156 mL

Asthapanopaga Gana

त्रिवृद् बिल्व पिप्पली कुष्ठ सर्षप वचा वत्सक फल शतपुष्पा मधुक मदन फलानीति दशेमानि आस्थापनोपगानि भवन्ति।। (Ch.Su 4/13)

S. No.	*Drug*	*Botanical Name*
1.	Trivrit (Fig. 6.3)	*Operculina turpenthum*
2.	Bilwa (Fig. 6.4)	*Aegle marmelos*
3.	Pippali (Fig. 6.5)	*Piper longum*
4.	Kushtha (Fig. 6.6)	*Saussurea lappa*

Contd...

Contd...

S. No.	*Drug*	*Botanical Name*
5.	Sarshapa (Fig. 6.7)	*Brassica campestris*
6.	Vacha (Fig. 6.8)	*Acorus calamus*
7.	Vatsakaphala (Fig. 6.9)	*Holarrhena antidysentrica*
8.	Shatapushpa (Fig. 6.10)	*Peucedanum graveolens*
9.	Madhuka (Fig. 6.11)	*Glycyrrhiza glabra*
10.	Madanaphala (Fig. 6.12)	*Randia spinosa*

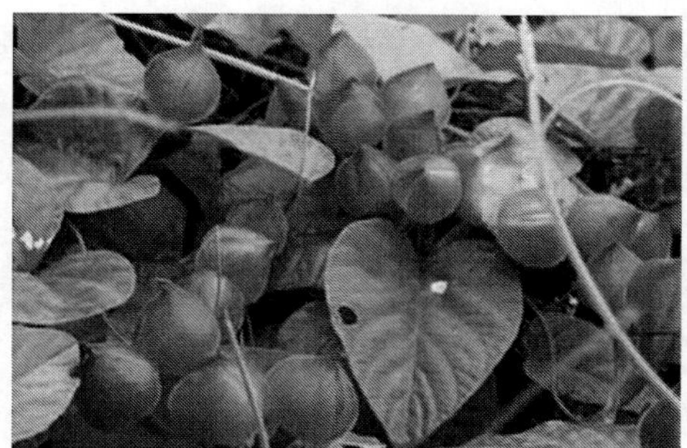

Fig. 6.3: Trivrit

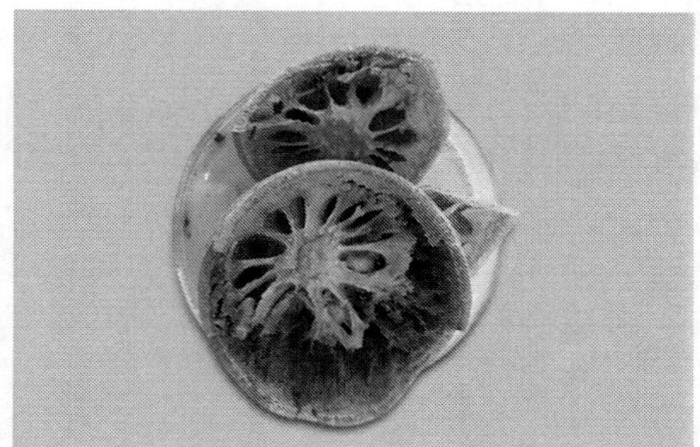

Fig. 6.4: Bilwa

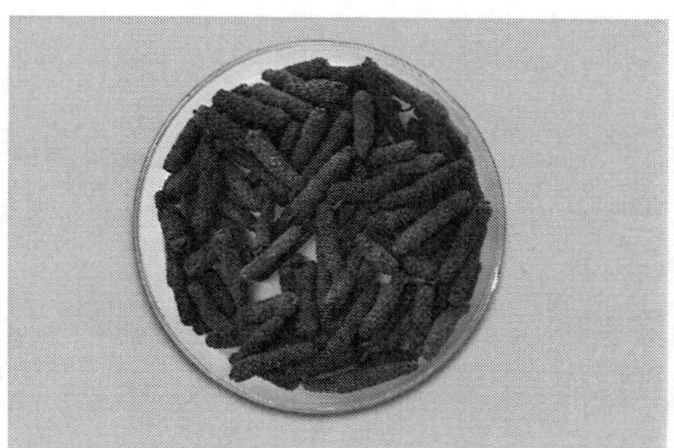

Fig. 6.5: Pippali

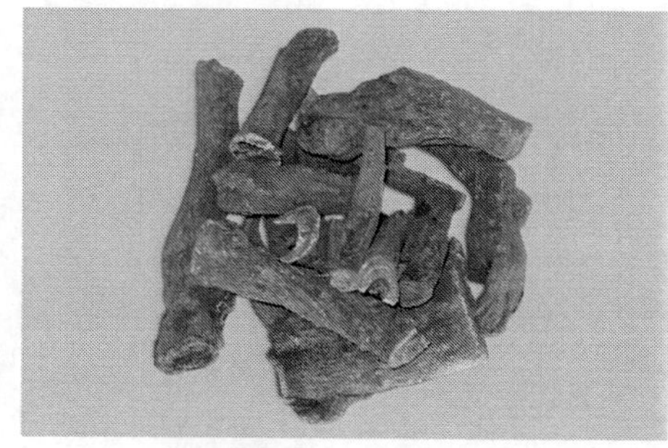

Fig. 6.6: Kushtha

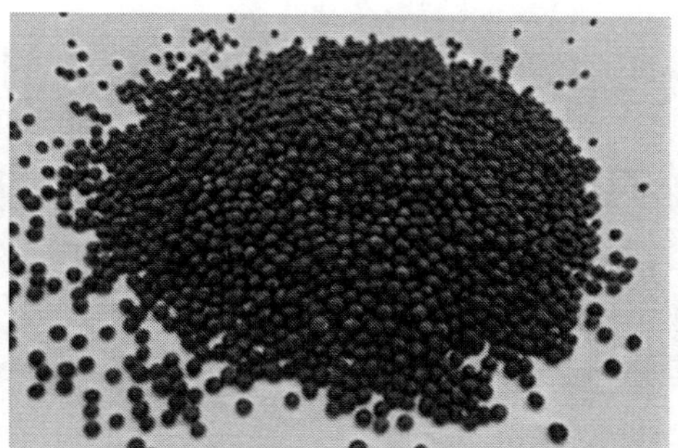

Fig. 6.7: Sarshapa

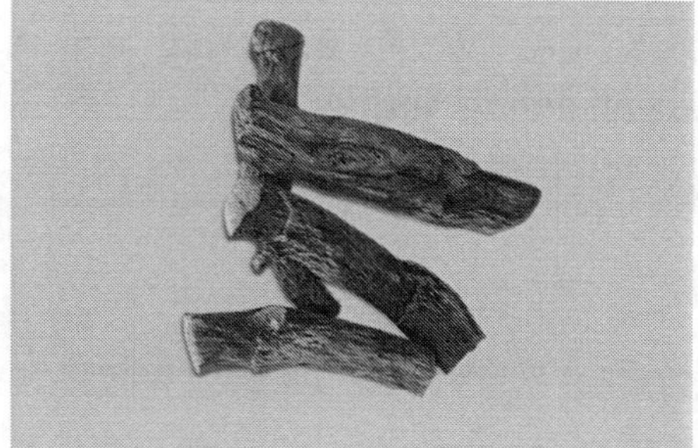

Fig. 6.8: Vacha

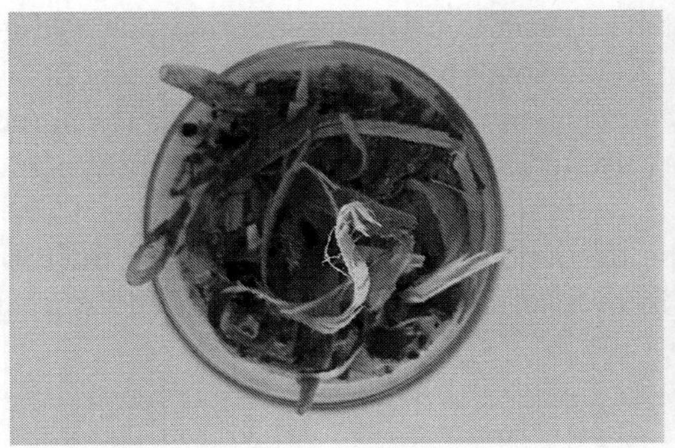

Fig. 6.9: Vatsakaphala

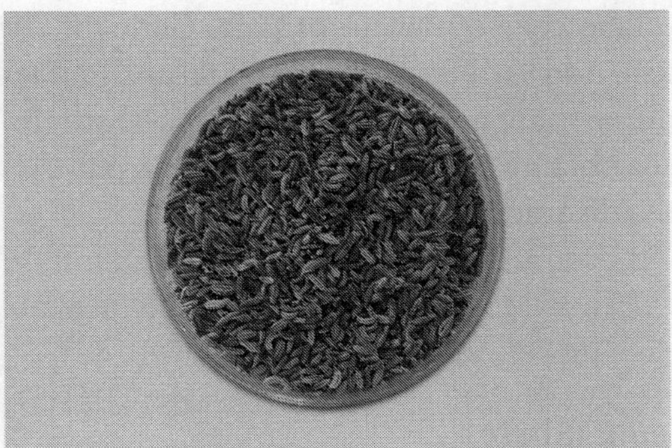

Fig. 6.10: Shatapushpa

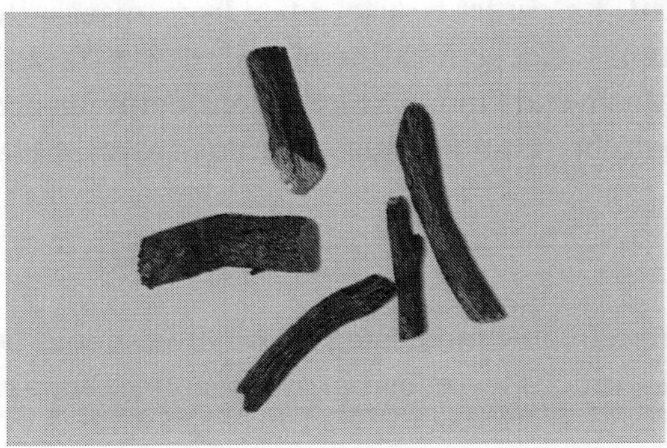

Fig. 6.11: Madhuka

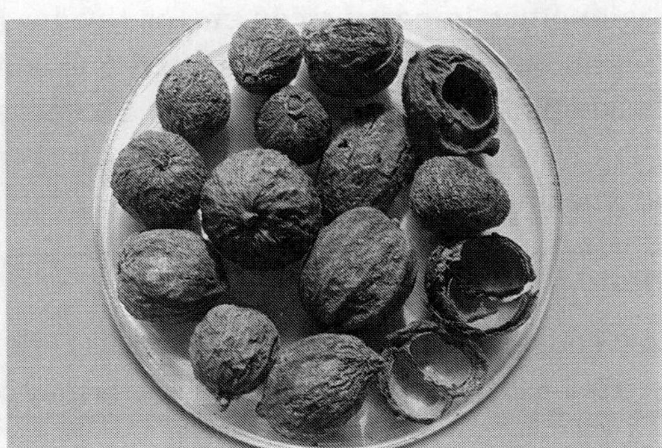

Fig. 6.12: Madanaphala

(b) Composition of Niruha Basti

माक्षिकं लवणं स्नेहं कल्कं क्वाथम् इति क्रमात्। आवपेत निरूहाणाम् एष संयोजने विधिः॥

(A.H.Su.19/45-46)

The preparation of the Basti dravya is a special process in which the order of mixing is unique. Makshika and Lavana are taken first and they are triturated; then the drugs like Sneha, Kalka, Kvatha and Avapa are mixed one by one till the achievement of the homogeneous mixture. Basic idea is to prepare an amalgam by mixing the Makshika and Lavana, then the oil is added and emulsification is achieved by adding the other component into the amalgam. Thus the mixture will become homogeneous.

The main contents of Niruha Basti are Kashaya (decoction), Sneha (oil or ghee), Kalka (paste), Madhu (honey) or Guda (jaggery), Saindhava (rock salt) and Prakshepa Dravya (additional liquids) like milk, cow's urine etc. Their proportion and other details are being described below under separate headings:

Common Kashaya in Niruha

बलां गुडुचिं त्रिफलां स रास्नां द्वे पंचमूले च पलोन्मितानि।
अष्टौ फलानि अर्धतुलां च मांसा च्छागात् पचेद् अप्सु चतुर्थ शेषम्॥ (Ch.Si.3/13)

Take coarse powder of Bala, Guduchi, Triphala, Rasna and Dashamula one pala (48 g) each. Add 8 fruits of Madanaphala and half Tula (2.4 kg) goat's meat and make its decoction by adding water and reducing it to one-fourth by heating on moderate fire. Filter it and the liquid thus obtained is used for Basti. This Kvatha is very useful for providing the relief in most of the Vata disorders.

If even these drugs are not available then the decoction may be prepared from the root of Eranda Mula, which is commonly available in most of the places and is a good drug for relieving Vata and its disorders.

Kalka (Paste)

पूतं यवानि फल बिल्व कुष्ठ वचा शताह्वा घन पिप्पलीनां। (Ch.Si.3/14)

It is another important content of Niruha Basti. Its contents also differ from disease to disease. But Charaka has mentioned one common Kalka comprising of 8 drugs viz. Yavani, Madanaphala, Bilva, Kushtha, Vacha, Shatahva, Musta and Pippali which is commonly termed as Putoyavanyadi kalka. Each of these drugs are to be taken in equal quantity, i.e. one Tola, thus making its total quantity 1 Prasrita.

Sneha (Medicated Oil or Ghee)

Only cooked or boiled (Pakva/Murchita) Sneha preferably medicated oil or ghee should be used in Basti. This is because Ama Sneha may cause mucus secretion from the rectum (Charaka Si. 4: 48).

भागाः कषायस्तु तु पंच, पित्ते स्नेहस्य षष्टः प्रकृतौ स्थिते च।
वाते विवृद्धे तु चतुर्थ भागे, मात्रा निरुहेषु कफे अष्टभागाः॥ (Ch.Si.3/30)

In Baladi Basti, Charaka has mentioned to add 2 Prasrita of Sneha, but in other context, Charaka has mentioned to take Sneha one-fourth part of total quantity of the Basti. In case of Vata, one-sixth in case of Pitta and healthy persons, and one-eighth in case of Kapha.

Madhu (Honey)

The honey is an important content of Niruha Basti. In Dvadasha Prasritaki Basti, according to Sushruta 200 g (2 Prasrita) of honey is to be added. But Ashtanga Hridaya has advised to add 50 g (1 Pala) of jaggery (Ashtanga H.Su.19/40).

Honey contains natural sugars which are quickly absorbed by digestive system and converted into energy. Hence it acts as an instant energizer. As it is hygroscopic, it absorbs excess fluid from tissues thus speeding up the process of healing and aids growth of healing tissue. Honey acts as antibacterial due to its acidic nature and enzymatically produces hydrogen peroxide. Constant use of honey strengthens the white blood corpuscles thereby helps to fight against bacterial and viral disease. Honey is a very good antioxidant which helps in restoring the damaged tissues.

In the present circumstances it is very difficult to get pure honey. In the absence of honey, jaggery can be added without loss of any considerable efficacy of Niruha Basti.

Saindhava (Rock Salt)

In Dvadasha Prasrita (96 Tola) i.e. 1200 mL of Basti, the quantity of rock salt to be added is 1 Karsha i.e. 12 g, thus making it about 1% of salt solution which is very nearer to normal saline, i.e. 0.8%. It is surprising to note that thousands of years earlier the sages of Ayurveda took so much care that the sodium content of Basti should be nearer to normal saline so that the Basti may not disturb the balance of two important electrolytes, i.e. sodium and chloride of the blood.

Saindhava contains 21 essential and 30 accessory minerals. 98% of sodium chloride is present in Saindhava along with traces of potassium. It is useful in regulating acid alkaline balance, maintaining osmosis and activation of ATPase.

Prakshepa Dravya (Additional Substances)

In addition to the above mentioned contents of Basti, some other liquids like milk and urine are also added to make it mild (Mridu) or strong (Tikshna) respectively and they are termed as Prakshepa Dravya. Other such dravyas are curd, juice of sour fruits etc. It may be added up to 2 Prasrita (200 g) in Dvadasha Prasritaki Basti and in that case the decoction is to be added in the quantity of 4 Prasrita (400 g).

General Matra

Dravya	*Pramana In Prasrita*	*%*
Madhu	2 Prasrita	16.67
Sneha	3 Prasrita	25
Kalka	1 Prasrita	8.33
Kvatha	4 Prasrita	33.33
Avapa	2 Prasrita	16.67
Total	12 Prasrita	100%

Dravya	*12 Prasrita In mL*	*Uttama*	*Madhyama*	*Avara*
Madhu	192	160	128	96
Sneha	288	240	192	144
Kalka	96	80	64	48
Kvatha	384	320	256	192
Avapa	192	160	128	96
Total	1152	960	768	576

Preparation of Niruha Basti

दत्वाऽऽदौ सैन्धवस्य अक्षं मधुनः प्रसृत द्वयम्। पात्रे तालेन मथ्नीयात् तद्वत् स्नेहं शनैः शनैः॥
सम्यक् सुमथिते दद्यात् फल कल्क मतः परम्। ततो यथो चितान् कल्कान् भागैः स्वैः श्लक्षण पेषितान्॥
गम्भीरे भाजने अन्यस्मिन् मथ्नीयात्तं खजेन च। यथा वा साधु मन्येत न सान्द्रो न तनुः समः॥
रस क्षीर आम्ल मूत्राणां दोष अवस्थाम् अवेक्ष्य तु॥ कषाय प्रसृतान् पञ्च सूपूतां स्तत्र दापयेत्॥

(Su.Chi.38/33-36)

- First 1 Aksha (12 g) Saindhava and 2 Prasrita Madhu should be taken in an utensil and should be churned with palm (तालेन).
- While churning Sneha should be added little by little followed by kalka of Madanaphala.
- The mixture is taken in deep utensil and other kalka pounded finely in respective parts should be added and churned with churning stick (खज).
- It should be Sama (medium), neither thick nor thin.
- Meat juice, milk, sour and urine should be added in quantity according to condition of Doshas.
- Finally filtered (सुपूत) decoction in quantity of 5 Prasrita should be added.

पूर्वं हि दध्यात् मधु सैन्धवं तु स्नेहं विनिर्गथ्यं ततोऽनु कल्कं।
विमथ्य संयोज्य पुनर्द्रवैस्तं बस्तौ निदध्यान् मथितं खजेन॥ (Ch.Si. 3/23)

All the ingredients of the Niruha Basti are not water soluble. So a special sequence and method of their mixing is to be followed to make a good homogenous mixture. For this purpose first honey and salt are put in the kalva and mixed well with the pestle. Then Sneha is added to it and mixed well. Thereafter the Kalka is added and again mixed well.

At the end all the liquid ingredients like Kvatha and other (Prakshepa) liquids are added and churned well to make the homogeneous mixture. The mixture is kept on hot water bath to warm it to the body temperature and then it is filled in the enema can just before its administration to the patient.

Samyak Sanyojana of Basti

कल्क स्नेह कषायाणाम् अविवेकाद् भिषग्वरैः। बस्तेः सुकल्पना प्रोक्ता तस्य दानं यथार्थकृत्॥
(Su.Chi 38/32)

When kalka, sneha and Kvatha (are mixed well and as such) can not be distinguished this is said by eminent physicians as the ideal preparation of Basti and the application of which is fruitful.

नाति स्निग्धं न वा रूक्षं नातितीक्ष्णं न वा मृदु नातितीक्ष्णं न वा मृदु नाति अच्छ
सान्द्र न ऊना अतिमात्रं ना पटु न अति च। लवणं तद्वदम्लं च। (A.H.Su.19/42)

The proper Niruha Basti should neither contain too much of Sneha nor should it be too dry. It should neither be very strong nor very mild; neither too diluted nor too strong; neither it should be excess in quantity nor in very little dose and neither should it contain excessive of salt and sour (Amla) drugs nor their little quantity.

न धावति औषध पाणिं न तिष्ठति अवलिप्य च। न करोति च सीमन्त स निरूहः सुयोजितः॥ (डल्हण)

A well prepared Basti Dravya should not run quickly out of the palm nor should stick or remain steady on the palm. It should be uniform mixture without separation of its contents.

(c) Diet

सुनिरूढं ततो जन्तु स्नातवन्तं तु भोजयेत्। पित्तश्लेष्म अनिल अविष्टं क्षीर यूष रसैः क्रमात्॥
सर्वं वा जाङ्गल रसैर् भोजयेद् अविकारिभिः। त्रिभाग हीनम् अर्धं वा हीनमात्रम् अथापि वा॥
यथाग्नि दोषं मात्रेयं भोजनस्य विधीयते। अनन्तरं ततो युञ्ज्यातथास्वं स्नेहबस्तिनां॥ (Su.Chi 38/11-14)

After evacuation of Niruha Basti based on the involvement of doshas the diet should be planned.

In Pitta pradhanata - Ksheera pradhana ahara
In Kapha pradhanata - Yusha and
In Vata pradhanata - Mansa rasa should be given.

(d) Basti Pranidana Vidhi (Method of Basti Administration)

The procedure of administration of Basti can be divided into 3 stages which are as follows:

a. Purva Karma
b. Pradhana Karma
c. Pashchat Karma

a. Purva Karma

1. **Selection of the patient:** Before the administration of the Basti one should ensure whether the patient is fit for Basti or not.
2. **Examination of the patient:**

   समीक्ष्य दोष औषध देश काल सात्म्य अग्नि सत्वादि वयो बलानि।
   बस्तिः प्रयुक्तो नियतं गुणाय स्यात् सर्व कर्मानि च सिद्धिमन्ति।। (Ch.Si. 3/6)

   Charaka opines that the Basti should be prepared and administered only after examining the factors like Dosha, Aushadha, Desha, Kala, Satmya, Agni, Satva, Vaya and Bala, etc. It will give definite results bringing about the success of the enema and achieving all its objects.
3. **Preparation of the Basti:** Preparation of Basti dravya has been dealt in detail previously.
4. **Preparation of the patient:**

   तैलाक्त गात्रं कृत मूत्र विट्कं नाति क्षुधार्तं शयने मनुष्यम्। (Ch.Si.3/18.19)

   After passing feces, urine and flatus, the patient on empty stomach should be prepared with Abhyanga and Svedana. However, the patient should not be very hungry.

b. Pradhana Karma

1. **The couch/bed for Basti:**

   ना अति उच्छ्रितं ना अपि अति नीचपादं सपादपीठं शयनं प्रसस्तम्।
   प्रधान मृदु आस्तरण उपपन्नं प्राक् शीर्षकं शुक्लपट्ट उत्तरीयम्।। (Ch.Si.3/33)

   The height of the Basti bed should neither be too high nor be too low and it should have foot rest and provision of slightly lowering the head portion of the bed. It should be well spreaded and prepared with a good soft quilt. The patient should lie on it with his head towards east and cover himself with a white sheet.
2. **Time of administration of Basti:**

   अथ अनुवासितम् आस्थापयेत् स्वभ्यक्त स्विन्न शरीरम् उत्सृष्ट बहिर्वेगम् वाते
   शुचौ वेश्मनि मध्याह्ने प्रततायां।। (Su.Chi.38/3)

Basti should be administered in the afternoon (Madhyahna) after the digestion of previous meal and when the person is not feeling hungry.

3. **Filling the Basti dravya to the Putaka:** (Su.Chi.38/3)
4. **Basti Pranidana:**
   - Position of the patient
   - Introduction of the Basti Netra into the Guda
   - Basti Peedana
   - Observations.

Position of the Patient (Fig. 6.13)

समेऽथ वेषन्नत शीर्षके वा नात्युच्छ्रिते स्वास्तरण अपपन्ने।
सव्येन पार्श्वेन सुखं शयानं कृत्वर्जुदेहं स्वभुजो अपधानं।
सन्कोच्य सव्येतरं अस्य सक्थि वामं प्रसार्य प्रणये तस्तम्।। (Ch.Si.3/18-19)

The patient is asked to lie down comfortably on his left side and to keep his head on his arms in the form of pillow while keeping the body straight and relaxed. Then the patient is asked to flex his right leg over his fully extended left leg.

वामाश्रये हि ग्रहणीगुदे च तत् पार्श्वं संस्थस्य सुखोपलब्धि। (Ch.Si.3/24-25)

As Grahani and Guda are situated on the left side of the body, the enema will be taken well by the person who is lying on his left side; and as the folds and valves of the rectum get straightened out, it is said that the Basti should be administered to the patient while he is lying on his left side. This position allows the flow of solution by gravity into the sigmoid colon and rectum.

This position is the most appropriate position for giving enema because the anatomical characteristics of the colon, do not try to force it, but pull it back slightly if any resistance is felt.

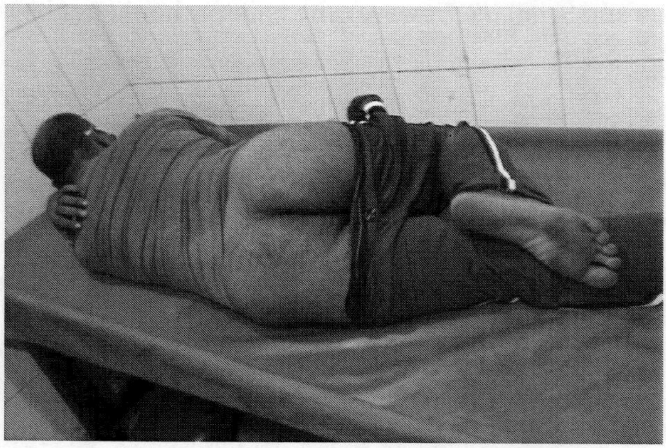

Fig. 6.13: Position of the Patient

Introduction of Basti Netra

स्निग्धे गुदे नेत्रचतुर्थ भागं स्निग्धं शनैरुज्वनु पृष्टवंशम्।
अकम्पन अवेपन लाघवादीन् पाण्योर् गुणाश्चापि विदर्शस्थतमं॥ (Ch.Si.3/19)

Thereafter, the anus and the enema nozzle are lubricated with oil. After removing the air bubble, one-fourth of enema nozzle is introduced in the anus slowly and rightly following the curves of the spinal column without shaking or trembling.

Basti Peedana

प्रपीडय च एकग्रग्रहणेन दत्तं नेत्रं शनैर एव ततो अपकर्षयेत्॥ (Ch.Si. 3/18-19)

With a single act of compression on the receptacle, inject the contents and then he should gradually withdraw the nozzle of the tube from the anus.

बस्तिं सव्ये करे कृत्वा दक्षिणेन अवपीडयेत् एकेन एव अवपीडेन न द्रुतं न विलम्बितम्।
ततो नेत्रम् अपनीय त्रिंशन्मात्राः पीडन कालाद् उपेक्ष्यात् उत्तिष्ठेति आतुरं ब्रूयात्॥ (Su.Chi.38/3-4)

One should squeeze with right hand, while holding the bladder with left hand, neither too fast nor too slow and completely in 1 pressing. The amount of time taken for sqeezing should be 30 matra kala and then ask the patient to get up.

विड्वातवेगो यदि च अर्धदत्ते निष्कृष्य मुक्ते प्रणयेद् शेषम्॥ (Ch.Si.3/25)

If in the middle of the administration of the Basti the patient feels the urge to pass the flatus or feces then the enema nozzle should be withdrawn and the patient is allowed to pass the urge. Thereafter the remaining liquid of the Basti is administered.

Position after Basti Administration

उत्तान देहस्य कृत अपधानः स्याद् वीर्यम् आप्नोति तथाऽस्य देयम्॥ (Ch.Si. 3/26)

After administration of the Niruha basti, patient is allowed to lie on his back comfortably on the bed with his body in raised position by means of a pillow in such a way that the Virya (active principle) of the Basti may spread throughout the body.

उत्तानो दत्तमात्रे तु निरुहे तन्मना भवेत्। कृत अपधानः संजात वेगश्च उत्कटकः सृजेत्॥ (A.H.Su.19/46)

On getting the urge for defecation, one should sit for defecation in squatting position (Utkataka).

Observations

Obseravtions should be done for:

- ❑ Basti Pratyagamana
- ❑ Samyak, Atiyoga or Ayoga Lakshana
- ❑ Vyapad if any.

Basti Pratyagamana

आगतौ परमः कालो मुहुर्तो मृत्यवेपरम्। तत्र अनुलोमिकं स्नेह क्षार मूत्र अम्ल कल्पितं।
त्वरितं स्निग्ध तीक्ष्ण उष्णं बस्तिम् अन्य प्रपीडयेत्। विदध्यात् फलवर्तिं वा स्वेदनो त्रासनादि च॥

(A.H.Su.19/47-48)

The Niruha basti must come out with in a Muhurta (within 48 min) otherwise it may end up in some complications. In case of delay in its evacuation, Sneha Virechana or Basti prepared from Snigdha, Ushna and Tikshna drugs like Sneha, Kshara, Mutra, Amla, etc. or Phala Varti should be given. Svedana and inducing of fear are also advised for this purpose.

स्वयमेव निवृत्ते तु द्वितीयो बस्तिरिष्यते। तृतीयोऽपि चतुर्थोऽपि यावद्वा सुनिरुढता।। (A.H.Su.19/49)

In case Niruha basti comes out automatically in time, then second, third or fourth Niruha basti can be given on the consequent days till the symptoms of proper Niruha appear.

Samyak Yoga Lakshana

प्रसृष्ट विण्मूत्र समीरणत्वं रुच्यग्निवृद्धयाशय लाघवानि।
रोग उपशांतिः प्रकृतिस्थता च बलं च तत् स्यात् सुनिरूढ लिंगम्।। (Ch.Si.1/41)

- Prasrishta Vit - Evacuation of bowel without any discomforts
- Prasrishta mutra - Evacuation of urine without discomfort
- Ruchi in Ahara - Taste in the food
- Agni vriddhi - Increase in the Agni, good appetite
- Ashaya lagahva - Lightness of body
- Rogopashamana - Recovery from disease
- Prakriti sthita - Restoration of normal health
- Bala - Increase in the strength.

Ayoga Lakshana

स्याद् रुक् शिरोहृद् गुदबस्ति लिंगे शोफः प्रतिश्याय विकर्तिके च।
हृल्लासिका मारूत मूत्रसंग श्वासे न सम्यक् च निरूहिके स्युः।। (Ch.Si. 1/42)

If Niruha Basti is not given properly the following symptoms are observed :

- Ruk - Pain in head, cardiac region, and region, urinary bladder and genital organ
- Shopha - Swelling
- Pratishyaya - Rhinitis
- Parikartika - Cutting pain in the anal region
- Hrillasa - Nausea
- Maruta sanga - Obstruction of flatus
- Mutra sanga - Retention of urine
- Shvasa - Difficulty in breathing.

Ati Yoga Lakshana

लिंग यदेवति विरेचितस्य भवेत् तदेवाति निरूहितस्य। (Ch.Si. 1/43)
कफास्रपित्त क्षयज अनिलोत्थाः सुप्ति अङ्गमर्द क्लम वेपनाद्याः।
निद्रा बल आभाव तमःप्रवेशाः स उन्माद हिक्काश्च विरेचितेऽति।। (Cha.Si.1/19-20)

- Anga supti - Numbness all over body
- Angamarda - Pain all over body
- Klama - Exhaustion
- Kampa - Shivering
- Nidranasha - Loss of sleep
- Daurbalya - Feeling of weakness
- Tama pravesha - Darkness in front of eyes
- Unmada - Irrelevent behavior
- Hikka - Hiccup.

Pashchat Karma

योगे तु भोजयेत्। कोष्णेन वारिणा स्नातं तनु धन्वरसो ओदानं। विकारो ये निरुढस्य भवन्ति प्रचलैर्मलैः॥
ते सुखोष्ण अम्बुसिक्तस्य यान्ति भुक्तवतः शमम्॥ (A.H.Su.19/50-51)

After proper evacuation of Niruha basti patient is allowed to take warm water bath and diet comprising of Shali variety of rice mixed with soup of meat or pulses. After the administration of Niruha basti, Mala will get dislodged and starts moving which inturn may lead to disease. Ushnajala Snana and diet is prescribed as per the Dosha avastha so that it will get pacified.

भोज्यं पुनर् व्याधिम् अवेक्ष्यं तद्वत् प्रकल्पयेद् यूष पयो रसाध्यैः।
सर्वेषु विध्याद् विधिमेतम आध्यं वक्ष्यामि वस्तिनत् उत्तरीयान्॥ (Ch. Si 1/34)

The diet should be prescribed according to the disease and condition of the patient comprising of soup of pulse, milk and meat soup. When the meal is digested on the same day evening after consuming light diet, the patient may be given Anuvasana Basti to provide him strength.

Niruha Basti Vyapad

नातियोगौ क्लम आध्माने हिक्का हृत्प्राप्तिं उर्ध्वता। प्रवाहिकाशिरो अंगार्ति परिकर्तःपरिस्रावः
द्वादश व्यापदो बस्तेर् असम्यग्योग संभव॥ (Ch.Si.7/5)

1. Ayoga	2. Atiyoga
3. Klama	4. Adhmana
5. Hikka	6. Hritprapti
7. Urdhvata	8. Pravahika
9. Shiroruk	10. Angarti
11. Parikarta	12. Parisrava

1. अयोग (Absence of Any Action)

Nidana

गुरुकोष्ठ प्रायः अनिल रुक्ष वात अल्बणे अपि। शीत अल्प लवण स्नेह द्रवमत्रो घनो अपि वा॥

The Basti which is Sheeta, Alpa lavana and Sneha Yukta concentrated given to a person who is having Krura Koshtha, Vata vriddhi and Ruksha shareera will lead to ayoga.

Samprapti

दोषं दुर्बलत्वादनिर्हरन्।

Being less potent in nature, this Basti cause the Utkleshana of Dosha but will become unable to eliminate them.

Lakshana

गुरुकोष्ठत्वं वातमूत्रशकृत ग्रहम्। नाभिबस्तिरूं दाहं हृल्लेपं श्वयथु गुदे।
गण्डु गण्डानि वैवर्ण्यं अरुचिं वह्निमार्दवं।।

It causes heaviness in the koshtha pradesha, obstruction to the movement of vata, mutra, pureesha, pain in nabhi and basti region, burning sensation, feeling of cold cloth covered over the hridaya pradesha, edema in guda, itching in the ganda pradesha, discoloration of skin and anorexia.

Chikitsa

उष्ण प्रमथ्या पान, स्वेदाः फलवर्ति, कालं ज्ञात्वा शस्तं विरेचनम्।। बिल्वमूलादि तीक्ष्ण बस्ति।

Prayoga of Ushna pramathya given in Atisara chikitsa, Svedana, phalavarti prayoga. Based on the requirement Virechana is advised. Prayoga of Basti prepared out of Bilwa mula, Trivrit, Devadaru, Yava, Kola, Kulattha Kvatha or Suradi dravya yukta and Gomutra Basti are advised.

2. अतियोग *(Over Action)*

Nidana

स्निग्ध स्विन्ने अति तीक्ष्ण उष्णो मृदुकोष्ठ अतियुज्यते।

Administration of Ati teekshna and Ushna basti in person having Mridu koshtha after doing Abhyanga and Sveda leads to Atiyoga.

Lakshana

तस्य लिंगं चिकित्सा च शोधनाभ्यां समा भवेत्।

Lakshanas are similar to that of Atiyoga of Vamana and Virechana.

Chikitsa

चिकित्सां च शोधनाभ्यां समा भवेत्। पृश्निपर्णि स्थिरां पद्मं काश्मर्यं मधुकं बलां।

The chikitsa is similar to that of vamana and virechana. Prishnaparnyadi Basti mixed with Ghrita is advised in Daha caused due to Atiyoga.

3. क्लम *(Mental Fatigue)*

Nidana

आमशेषे निरुहेण मृदुना दोष ईरितः।

By giving Mridu niruha Basti in the person who is having Ama shesha or Ama left over in the body.

Samprapti

मार्ग रूणद्धि वातस्य हन्त्याग्निं मूर्च्छयत्यपि।।

By this there will be Prakopa of Pitta and Kapha. The aggravated Pitta and Kapha causes obstruction to the movement of Vata. This causes Agnimandya.

Lakshana

क्लम विदाहं हृत्शूल मोहवेष्टनं गौरवम्।

The lakshana's like klama, vidaha, hritshula, moha, vishtana, gaurava are produced.

Chikitsa

कुर्यात् स्वेदैर् विरुक्षैस्तं पाचनैश्च अपि उपचारेत्। पिप्पली कतृष्ण उशीर दारू मूर्वा शृतं जलम्। पिबेत् सौवर्चल न्मिश्रं दीपनं हृद् विशोधनं।। वचा नागरं शटि एला दधिमण्डेन मूर्च्छिताः।। प्रेया प्रसन्नय वा स्युर् अरिष्टेन आसवेन वा।।

Agnideepanartha Kvatha prepared out of pippali, etc. drugs mixed with lavana should be given. Prasanna, Asava, Arishta proyoga should be done. Gomutra Basti is advised. Svedana and Virukshana measures should be carried out.

4. आध्मान *(Flatulence)*

Nidana

अल्पवीर्यौ महादोषे रुक्षे क्रूराशये कृतः।

The Alpa veerya Basti given to person having mahadosha, ruksha, kruraKoshtha.

Samprapti

बस्तिर् दोषावृतो रुद्धमार्गो रुन्ध्यात् समीरणाम्। स विमार्गोऽनिलः कुर्याद्...

Basti will get Avarita by Dosha leading to Dosha prakopa and Vimarga gamana of Vata.

Lakshana

आध्मानं मर्म पीडनम्। विदाहं गुरुकोष्ठस्य मुष्कंदकवंक्षणवेदना रुणद्धि हृदयं शूलेरितश्चेतश्च धावति।

It causes Adhmana, Marma peeda, Vidaha, heaviness in Koshtha, Mushka, Vankshana pradesha. Because of Shula Vriddhi there is Hridaya avarodha.

Chikitsa

श्यामाफलादि सिद्ध अनुवासन बस्ति, गुदवर्ति प्रयोग, दशमूलगोमूत्र सिद्ध निरुहबस्त प्रयोग।

Shyamaphaladi siddha taila Anuvasana, Guda varti, Dashamoola and Gomutra siddha niruha basti is administered in Admana Vyapat.

5. हिक्का *(Hiccup)*

Nidana

मृदुकोष्ठ अबल बस्तिर् अति तीक्ष्णो अति निर्हरन्।

Administration of teekshna Basti in Mridu Koshtha, Durbala person.

Samprapti

This cause the Ati Nirharana of doshas leading to Hikka.

Lakshana

कुर्यात् हिक्कां..........।

Chikitsa

हिक्काघ्नं बृंहणं चिकित्सा, धूम लेह रस क्षीरोदकस्वेदाश्चान्न च वातनुत्।

Brihana chikitsa is advised in Hikka. Bala sthiradi varga siddha taila anuvasana is advised. Vatanashaka Dhuma, leha, mansarasa, Ksheera, Sveda are advised.

6. हृत्प्राप्ति (Medication Reaching Hridaya)

Nidana

अतितीक्ष्णः सवातो वा न सम्यक् प्रपीडितो............

Administration of Ati-teekshna Basti, Savata Basti, not samyak prapeedana of Basti Putaka leads to hritprapti

Lakshana

घट्टयेद हृदयं............।

The Basti administered like this causes pressure over the Hridaya pradesha.

Chikitsa

स आम्ल लवण स्कंध करीर बदर फलै सिद्ध निरुह बस्ति, वातघ्न द्रव्य सिद्धअनुवासन बस्ति।

Amla and Lavana skandha dravya like karira, badara phala siddha niruha basti should be administered and also anuvasna basti prepared by using vataghna oils should be used.

7. उदावर्त (Medicines reaching the Urdhva bhaga of shareera)

Nidana

वात मूत्र पुरीषाणां दत्तै वैगान्निगृण्हतः। अति वा पीडितो...........।

Doing Vegavarodha of Vata, Mutra, Pureesha after giving Niruha, giving Basti by applying mild pressure over Putaka.

Lakshana

बस्तिमुखेनांदकयाति वेगवान्। मूर्च्छा विकार तस्यादौ दृष्टवा.............।

Because of this, the Basti dravya may come out through the Mukha. The patient may also suffer from Murccha.

Chikitsa

शीताम्बु मुखम्। सिंचेत् पार्श्वोदरं च अधः प्रमृज्याद्वी जयेच्च तम्।
वस्त्र पाणि ग्रहैः कण्ठं रुन्ध्यान्न प्रियते तथा। प्राणोदान निरोधाद्धि प्रसिद्धतरमार्हवान्।
अपनः पवनो बस्तिं तमश्चेव अपकर्षयति। शिरःस्थे नावन धूमं प्रच्छाद्यं सर्षपै शिरः।

If patient gets Murccha, then first Sheeta ambu sechana over the face. Mardana should be carried out over Parshwa and udara. The hair should be pulled upwards. He should be feared by telling names of Gaja, etc. (animals).

Throat should be covered by hand or cloth and slight pressure should be given. By this Apana Vayu will move down normally. After this patient should be given kramuka jala for drinking.

If the Basti gets strucked in Pakvashaya, then Bilwadi panchamula Basti should be given. If the medicine reaches Shiras, Navana, Dhuma, lepa of Sarshapa should be applied.

8. प्रवाहिका (Dysentry)

Nidana

स्निग्धे स्विन्ने महादोषे बस्तिर्मृदु अल्पभेषजः।

Administration of mridu basti or alpa matra basti in a person in whom samyak snehana and svedana is done, having Mahadoshas.

Samprapti

उत्क्लिश्य अल्पं हरेत्दोषं जनयेच्च प्रवाहिका।

In such condition, the Basti dravya causes Utkleshana of the Doshas and eliminates only small amount of doshas leading to Pravahika.

Lakshana

स बस्ति पायु शोफ जंघा उरु सदन वा। निरूह मारुतो जन्तुर् अभीक्ष्णं संप्रवाहते॥

The Basti given in this condition causes swelling in Payu, Guda pradesha and sadana in Jangha and Uru pradesha. The Apana vata will not move properly and patient passes stools with lot of difficulty.

Chikitsa

स्वेद अभ्यंग निरुहांच्च शोधनीया अनुलोमिकान्। विदध्यात् लंघयित्वा तु वृत्तिं कुर्याद् विरिक्तवत्॥

Svedana, Abhyanga should be done followed by Basti prepared out of Shodhana and anulomana drugs should be administered. After this dietary regimen said after Virechana should be followed.

9. शिरोर्ति (Headache)

Nidana

दुर्बले क्रुरकोष्ठच तीव्रदोषे तनुमृदुः। शीत अल्प च आवृतो दोषैर् बस्तिस्तद् विहतोऽनिलः।

Administration of Tanu, mridu veerya, sheetala, alpa matra Basti to the person who is durbala and having krura koshtha, mahadosha.

Samprapti

मार्गैर् गात्राणि सन्धावान् उर्ध्व मूर्ध्नि विहन्यते॥ ग्रीवा मन्ये च गृण्हाति...............................।

The Basti administered in such condition will get enclosed by doshas and obstructs the movement of Vata. Because of this the Basti dravya spreads.

Lakshana

शिरःकण्ठंदकभिनस्ति च। बाधीर्यं कर्णनादं पीनसं नेत्र विभ्रमम्॥

It leads to symptoms such as stiffness in Greeva and Manya, bhedana in Shira and Kantha, deafness, tinnitus, coryza, agitation of eyes.

Chikitsa

कुर्याद् अभ्यंजनं तैल लवणेन यथाविधि। युंजात् प्रधमनैर् नस्यैर् धुमैरस्य विरेचयेत्।
तीक्ष्णअनुलोमिकेन अथ स्निग्धं भुक्ते अनुवासयेत्।

Abhyanga should be done with Lavana taila. Pradhamana nasya and dhumapana should be carried out to achieve shirovirechana. After food Teekshna and Vatanulomaka dravya Saadhita Anuvasana Basti is given.

10. अंगर्ति (Malaise)

Nidana

स्नेह स्वेदैर् अनापाद्य गुरु स्तीक्ष्णो अतिमात्रतया। बस्ति प्रयुज्यते.............।

Guru, Tikshna, Atimatra Basti given to a person who had not undergone Samyak Sneha and Sveda ends up in Angarati complication.

Samprapti

सोऽति मात्रं प्रवर्तयेत्। स्तब्ध अदावृत कोष्ठस्य वायुः संप्रतिहन्यते।

There is Ati pravartana of Dosha. Because of ati dosha nirharana, there is stabdhata and udavarṭa in amashaya. There is also obstruction to movement of Vata.

Lakshana

अंगरुजा गात्रवेष्टन निस्तोद भेद स्फुरण जृम्भनैः।

The person ends up with Anga ruja (pain all over the body), pricking and throbboing type of pain, cramps, numbness and yawning.

Chikitsa

तैल लवणाक्त अभ्यंग, उष्ण जल सिंचन, यव कोल कुलत्थ पंचमूल सिद्ध निरूह प्रयोग,
यष्टिमधु अथवा बिल्व तैल अनुवासन प्रयोग।

Abhyanga should be carried out with lavana taila, Ushna jala Sinchana. After this Niruha Basti should be given with Yava, kola, kulattha panchamula siddha Kvatha.

11. परिकर्त *(Fissure in Ano)*

Nidana

मृदु कोष्ठ अल्प दोषस्य रुक्ष तीक्ष्णो अतिमात्रवान्।

Ruksha, teekshna, Atimatra Basti given in mridu koshtha, alpa dosha person is the cause for Parikartika complication.

Samprapti

बस्तिर् दोषान् निरस्य अशु जनयेत् परिकर्तियाम्।

Basti given in such condition will cause the sudden nirharana of Doshas leading to Parikartika.

Lakshana

त्रिकवंक्षणबस्तिनां तोदं नाभेरधो रुजम्। विबंध अल्पाल्पं उत्थानं...........॥

The person suffers from pricking type of pain in lumbar, groin and bladder region, pain below the nabhi region, constipation along with evacuation of little amount of Mala, etc.

Chikitsa

स्वादुशीत औषध, क्षीरबस्ति, व्यक्ताम्ल मृदुभोजिनः।

Basti with Madhura-sheeta dravya, ksheera Basti prepared out of Sarjarasa, Yashtimadhu, Jingini, Rasanjana kalka, Madhura-Amla rasa pradana diet should be given.

12. परिस्राव

Nidana

पित्तरोगे अम्ल उष्णो वा तीक्ष्णो वा लवणोऽथवा।

The Amla, ushna, teekshna, lavana yukta Basti given in person suffering from pittaja vyadhi is the cause for Parisrava Vyapat.

Samprapti

बस्तिर् लिखति पायु तुः क्षिणोति विदहत्यपि।

Basti causes scraping and ulceration in Guda pradesha and daha in Guda region.

Lakshana

स विदग्धः स्रवत्य अस्त्रंपित्तं च अनेक वर्णवत्। सार्यते बहुवेगेन मोहं गच्छति चासकृत्॥

The person also suffers from srava of the blood of various colors; the person may also end up in Murccha.

Chikitsa

पिच्छा बस्ति, रक्तपित्त अतिसारघ्नि क्रिया प्रशस्यते॥

Piccha basti prepared out of shalmali pushpa vrunta, aja dugdha or vatankura + aja dugdha. Madhura gana sadhita sheetala kvatha sechana over guda, raktapitta and atisara nashaka chikitsa should be done.

Acharya Sushruta has Mentioned 76 Basti Vyapat

Table showing various types of basti vyapat	
Pranidhana Dosha (6)- Defects of insertion of Basti nozzle	1. Vichalita—Excessive shaking 2. Vivartita—Breaking just after entry 3. Parshva peedanam—Pressed in sides 4. Atyukshiptam—Too high 5. Avasannam—Too low 6. Tiryak prakshiptam —Obliquely inserted
Netra dosha (11)- Defects of Basti Netra	1. Atisthula—Too thick 2. Karkasha—Hard 3. Avanatarn—Depressed 4. Anu bhinnarn—Slightly cracked 5. Sannikrishta Karnika—Too near Karnika 6. Viprakrushta Karnika—Far away Kamika 7. Sukshma Chhidra—Opening small 8. Atichidra—Too large opening 9. Ati deergha—Too long 10. Ati hrasva—Too short 11. Asrirna—Angular
Basti dosha (5)	1. Bahalata—Muscular attachment 2. Alpata—Small 3. Sacchidrata—Porosity 4. Prasteernata—Having fibrous attachment 5. Durbaddha—Improperly fixed
Peedana dosha (4) Defects of Pressing	1. Ati peedita—Excessive pressing 2. Shithila peedita—Loosely pressing 3. Bhuryo avapeedita—Pressing again and again 4. Kala atikrama—Too delayed pressing
Dravya dosha (11)- Defects of drug	1. Aamata—Uncooked 2. Heenata—Deficient dose 3. Atimaatrata—Excessive dose 4. Ati sheetata 5. Atyushnata 6. Atiteekshnata 7. Atimriduta 8. Atisnigdhata 9. Atirukshata 10. Atisandrata 11. Atidravata

Contd...

Contd...

Shayya dosha (7)- Defects of posture	1. Avak sheersha—Head low 2. Ucha—sheersha—Head high 3. Nyubhjah deha—Facing downwards knee chest 4. Uttana deha—Upwards 5. Sankuchita deha—Flexed limbs 6. Sthitha—Sitting 7. Dakshina paarshva Shayina—Lying in right side
Aatura nimitta (15)- Su.Chi. 39/25-37	1. Krudyataha 2. Aayasyataha 3. Shochato 4. Maithuna 5. Divasvapna 6. Sambashanat 7. Yana 8. Chirasana 9. Atichankramana 10. Sheeta toya 11. Vatapa 12. Viruddha 13. Adhyashana 14. Asatmya Bhojana 15. Anatmavanta
Vaidyaatura nimitta(8) Sneha basti retention	1. Tridosairavruta 2. Ashnabhibhoota 3. Malavyamishra 4. Duranupravishta 5. Asvinnasya- without svedana 6. Anushno 7. Alpabhukatavato 8. Alpa basti
Vaidya Nimitta (9)	1. Ayoga 2. Adhmana 3. Parikartika 4. Parisrava 5. Pravahika 6. Hridayopasaranam 7. Angapragraha 8. Atiyoga 9. Jivadana

Commonly Encountered Complications of Niruha Basti

- ❑ Pain in abdomen
- ❑ Fullness of abdomen
- ❑ Debility
- ❑ Restlessness
- ❑ Burning sensation in abdomen
- ❑ Longer retention time
- ❑ Headache

- ❑ Parikartika
- ❑ Atisara

Pariharya Vishaya and Kala

अत्यासन स्थान वचांसि यानं स्वप्नं दिवा मैथुन वेगरोधान्।
शीतोपचार् आतप शोक रोगांस्त्यजेद् अकाल अहित भोजनं च॥ (Ch.Si.1/54)

1. Atyasana	-	Excessive sitting
2. Atisthana	-	Standing for long time
3. Vacharnsi	-	Excessive talking
4. Yana	-	Travelling
5. Divasvapna	-	Day sleeping
6. Maithuna	-	Sexual intercourse
7. Vegavarodha	-	Suppression of natural urges
8. Shitopachara	-	Indulgence in cold things
9. Atapa	-	Sunlight
10. Shoka	-	Worrying
11. Rosha	-	Anger
12. Akala Bhojana	-	Untimely food
13. Ahita Bhojana	-	Unwholesome food

कालस्तु बस्त्यादिषु याति यावांस्तावान् भवेत् द्विः परिहारकालः। (Ch. Si.1/54)

One should follow the restrictions and diet, double the duration taken for the treatment. Number of days Basti administered × 2 = Basti Parihara kala in days. It is also called as dviguna parihara kala.

Reason Behind Administering Niruha Basti on Empty Stomach

जीर्णनस्याशये दोषाः पुंसः प्रव्यक्तिमागताः। निःशेषाः सुखमायान्ति भोजनेनाप्रपीडिताः॥
नवाऽऽस्थापनविक्षिप्तमग्नमग्निः प्रधावति। तस्मात्स्थापनंदेयं निराहाराय जानता॥ (Su.Chi.38/21-22)

When Niruha basti is administered to a patient whose previous meal is digested, it leads to complete evacuation of vitiated Doshas, as they are not being disturbed by the food present in Amashaya and Pakvashaya.

On administration of niruha basti, Jatharagni gets influenced and does not digest the food properly, therefore the food is not digested properly leading to formation of Ama rasa which further results in aggravation of disease or formation of new diseases. Therefore, it is advised to administer Niruha basti to a person who is empty stomach.

न तु भुक्तवतो देयमास्थापनम् इति स्थितिः।
विसूचिकां वा जनयेच्छर्दिम् वाऽपि सुदारुणाम्॥
कोपयेत् सर्वदोषान् वा तस्मात् दद्याताभोजिने। (Su. Chi. 38/40)

If Asthapana basti is given after foods, it causes the person to suffer from Visuchika and Daruna cchardi, also it leads to vitiation of all the three dosha's. Therefore, asthapana basti shall be given only on empty stomach.

ANUVASANA BASTI

The basti administered predominantly containing sneha which does not harm even if retained for 24 hours and can be administered daily is called as Anuvasana basti.

On the basis of the dose of Sneha used, Sushruta has described three types-viz. Sneha Basti, Anuvasana Basti and Matra Basti. It is very useful for the weak and emaciated persons due to excessive indulgence in walking, exercise, weight lifting, alcohol intake and sex, Vata disorders and fracture. It provides happiness, nourishment and strength, and helps in proper bowel movement. It is Brimhana and cures Vata disorders.

Etymological Derivation

अनुवासन – न. अनु+वास– सौरभ्येल्युटा।
अनुवसति, अनुवासरंदीयतेवा॥ (Vachaspatyam)
अनुवासनः अनुवासनअपिनदुष्यत्यनुविसंवादीयतइतिअनुवासन॥ (Su.Chi.35/18)
अनुवासनंयथाहौँषधसिद्धः स्नेहानार्थः स्नेहः स्नेहविधौसचतुर्धाभिहितः। (A.S.Su.28/7)

The anuvasana word is derived from the root word 'vaasa' with prefix 'anu'. The Basti which is administered every day is called Anuvasana. In second and third derivation, according to dosha vitiation or according to disease the administration of specific sneha is called anuvasana.

Definition

अनुवसन्नपि न दुष्यत्यनुदिवसं वा दीयत इत्यनुवासनः। (Su.Chi.35/18)

The Basti which remains inside the body for a day without causing any harm or Basti which can be administered every day is called Anuvasana.

The word Anuvasana is used in योगरुढार्थ because Anuvasana is a type of Sneha Basti. The word Anuvasana implies Sneha Basti and its types.

Classification of Anuvasana Basti

Based on Matra it is of three types:

षट्पली तु भवेच्छ्रेष्टा मध्यमा त्रिपली भवेत्। कनीयस्यध्यर्धपला त्रिधा मात्राऽनुवासने इति॥ (Su.Chi.37/4)

1. Uttama	6 pala	240 mL
2. Madhyama	3 pala	120 mL
3. Avara	1½ pala	60 mL

Contraindication of Anuvasana

य एवानुस्थाप्यास्तुएवाननुवास्याः स्युः विशेषतस्त्वभुक्तभक्त नवज्वर पाण्डुरोग कामला
प्रमेहार्शः प्रतिश्यायारोचक मन्दाग्निदुर्बल प्लीहकफोदरोरुस्तम्भ वर्चोभेद विष
गरपीत पित्तकफाभिष्यन्द गुरुकोष्ट श्लीपदगलगण्डापचि क्रिमिकोष्टिनः॥ (Ch.Si.2/17)

Anuvasana Basti is also contraindicated in all such conditions where Asthapana is contraindicated.

It is particularly contraindicated on empty stomach, anorexia, impaired digestion, diarrhea, hard bowel, intestinal worms, spleen disorders, Kaphaja Udara Roga, Abhishyanda of Pitta and Kapha, slow or acute poisoning, corrhyza, recent fever, anemia, jaundice, polyuria, piles, Urustambha, elephantiasis, goiter, lymphadenitis and weak patients.

कुष्ठ प्रमेहादिषु मेदुरेषुनरेषुयेचापिविशोधनीयाः। (Ch.Si. 1/36)
उदरि चप्रमेहिच कुष्ठि स्थूलश्चमानवः। अवश्यंस्थपनीयास्तेनानुवास्याः कथंचन॥ (Su.Chi.35/22)

It is specifically contraindicated in Kushta (chronic skin diseases), obesity and polyuria, because Anuvasana Basti may further deteriorate the condition. However in these conditions, if necessary then Niruha may be given.

Both Anuvasana and Niruha are contraindicated in the conditions of indigestion, thirst, anorexia, fear, grief, unconsciousness, psychic disorders (Unmada), cough, dyspnea and tuberculosis (Sharangadara ut.6: 7).

Reasons for Contraindications

- The Sneha of Anuvasana taken in empty stomach may go upwards due to lack of obstruction in the channels.
- In conditions of recent fever, anemia, jaundice and polyuria, if Anuvasana is given then it may provoke Dosha leading to Udara.
- It causes abdominal distension by doing Abhishyanda of piles.
- In anorexia it may further impair the desire for food.
- In weak person and impaired digestion, it may further impair the digestion.
- In corrhyza and splenomegaly, the Anuvasana may further aggravate the conditions by provoking the Dosha.
- Therefore in these conditions, Anuvasana should not be given.

Indications of Anuvasana

यएवास्थाप्यास्तएवानुवास्याः विशेषस्तु रूक्ष तीक्ष्णाग्नयः केवलवातरोगांतश्चः
एतेषुहिअनुवासनंप्रधानतमित्युक्तं मूलेद्रमप्रसेकवत्। (Ch.Si.2/19)

The Anuvasana is also indicated in the condition where Niruha is indicated. It is specifically indicated in the persons who are having dryness in their body, excessive appetite and suffering from the pure disorders of Vata. In these conditions, Anuvasana is the first choice and is like pouring of water at the root of the plant.

रूक्षनित्यस्तुदीप्ताग्निर्व्यायामिमारुतामयि। वन्क्षणश्रोण्युदवृत्तवाताश्चाहार्दिनेदिने।
एषांचाशुजरांस्नेहोयात्याम्बुसिकतासिव। अतोअन्येषां त्र्याहात्प्रायः स्नेहंपचतिपावकः॥ (Ch.Si. 5/46-47)
रूक्षाय बहुवाताय स्नेहबस्ति दिने दिने। दध्यात्वैध्यस्ततोऽन्येषामग्याबाधाभयात्र्यहात्॥ (Su.Chi.37/79)

Anuvasana can be given daily to the persons having good digestion, doing exercise daily, suffering from Vata disorders involving groin and buttocks, Udavarta or whose routine diet constitutes mainly Ruksha (unctuous) type of food articles.

In other than these diseases Anuvasana is given at the interval of 3 days because Agni takes 3 days to assimilate it properly.

Dose Fixation of Anuvasana Basti According to Age

निरूहपादांशसमेनतैलेनाम्लानिलघ्नौधसाधितेन। (Ch.Si.3/28)
यथावयोनिरुहाणांयामात्राः परिकिर्तिताः। पादावकृष्टास्ताः कार्याः स्नेहबस्तिषुदेहिनां॥ (Su.Chi.37/4)

The detailed dose schedule according to Niruha has been mentioned and the dose of the Anuvasana is calculated accordingly. The dose of Anuvasana should be taken as one-fourth of the dose of Niruha mentioned for that particular age.

Anuvasana Basti is further divided into three types depending on its dose viz. Sneha Basti, Anuvasana Basti and Matra Basti.

षट्पलीतु भवेच्छ्रष्टात्रिपलि मध्यमः भवेत्। कनीयस्यार्धपलिकात्रिधामात्राऽनुवासने॥ (Su.Chi.37/4 teeka)

Sneha Basti

The dose of Sneha Basti is one-fourth of the Niruha. In case of maximum dose i.e. Dvadasha Prasrita it comes out to be 3 Prasrita, i.e. Shat Pala or 24 Tola. According to other texts it is the Uttama Matra (optimal dose).

Anuvasana Basti

The dose of the Anuvasana is half of the dose of Sneha Basti as mentioned for that particular age. In case of maximum dose, i.e. Dvadasha Prasrita, it comes out be 1 Prasrita, i.e. 3 Pala or 12 Tola. According to other texts it is the Madhyama Matra (medium dose).

Matra Basti

Matra basti is a type of sneha basti. It is termed so because the dose of sneha used in it is very less compared to the dose of sneha basti. The term "matra", gives various meanings in different context such as measurement, quantity, size, duration, number, degree, movement, unit of time. In the present context the term matra gives the meaning for the unit of measurement, i.e. for the quantity of basti dravya.

कर्म व्यायाम भाराध्वया (पा) नस्त्रीकर्षितेषुच। दुर्बले वातभग्ने च मात्राबस्तिःस सदामतः।
यथेष्टाहाराचेष्टस्य सर्वकालंनिरत्ययः। ह्रस्वायाः स्नेह मात्राया मात्राबस्तिः समोभवेत्॥ (Ch.Si.5/52-53)

The dose of Matra Basti is half of the dose of Anuvasana or one- fourth of Sneha Basti "as mentioned above. In case of maximum dose, i.e. Dvadasha Prasrita it comes out to be 0.75 Prasrita, i.e. 1 Pala or 6 Tola (75 g). According to other texts it is the Hina Matra (minimum dose). During the administration of Matra Basti there is no restriction of diet and regime.

It can be given at any time in all the seasons and is harmless. It promotes strength, causes easy elimination of feces and urine, and cures Vata disorders.

Contents and Method of Preparation of Anuvasana Basti

Anuvasanopaga Dravyas

रास्नासुरदारूबिल्वमदनशतपुष्पावृश्चीरपुनर्नवाश्चदंश्ट्राग्निमन्थश्योनाक इति दशेमान्यनुवासनोपगानि भवन्ति॥
(Ch.Su.4/13)

S. No.	*Drug*	*Botanical Name*
1.	Rasna (Fig. 6.14)	*Pluchea lanceolata*
2.	Suradaru (Fig. 6.15)	*Cedrus deodara*
3.	Bilwa	*Aegle marmelos*
4.	Madana	*Randia dumetorum*
5.	Shatapushpa	*Peucedanum graveolens*
6.	Vrishchira (Fig. 6.16)	*Boerhavia diffusa (shweta)*
7.	Punarnava (Fig. 6.17)	*Boerhavia diffusa (rakta)*
8.	Shvadanshtra (Fig. 6.18)	*Tribulus terrestris*
9.	Agnimantha (Fig. 6.19)	*Premna mucronata*
10.	Shyonaka (Fig. 6.20)	*Oroxylum indicum*

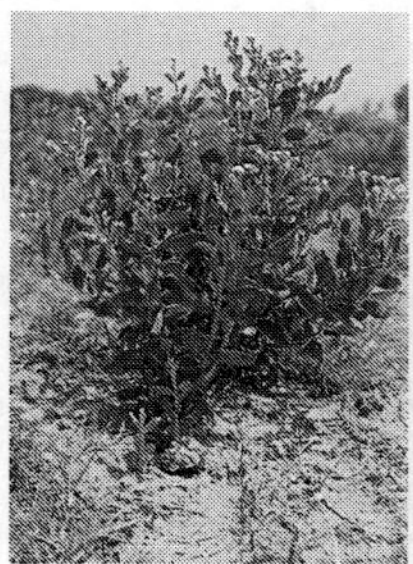

Fig. 6.14: Rasna

Fig. 6.15: Suradaru

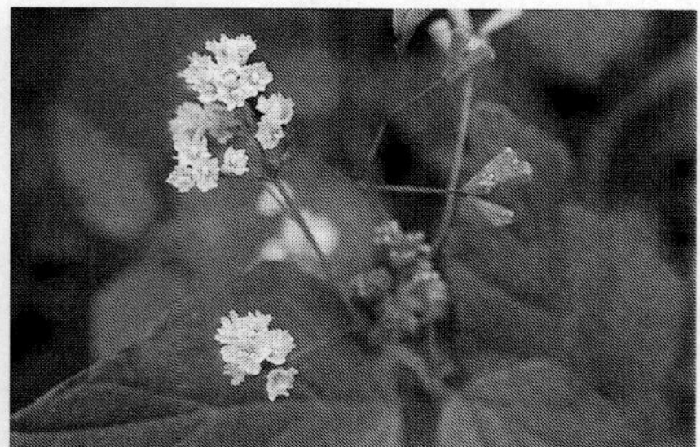

Fig. 6.16: Vrishchira

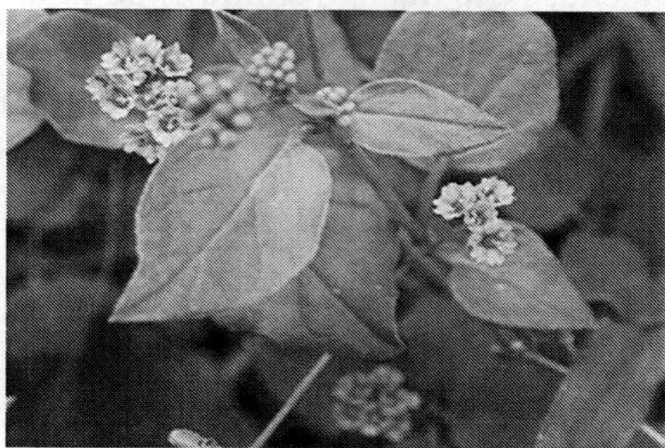

Fig. 6.17: Punarnava

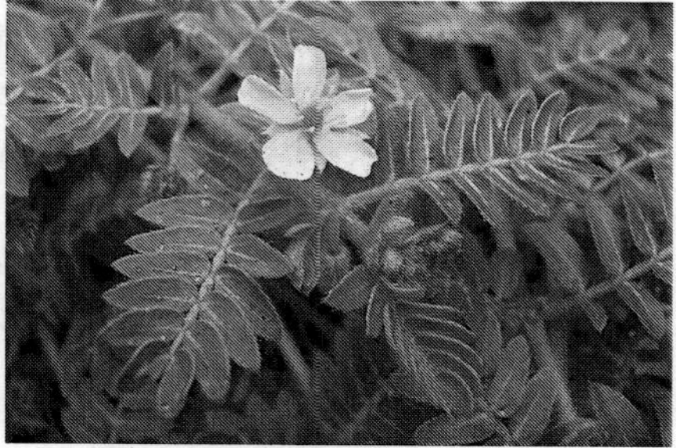

Fig. 6.18: Shvadanshtra

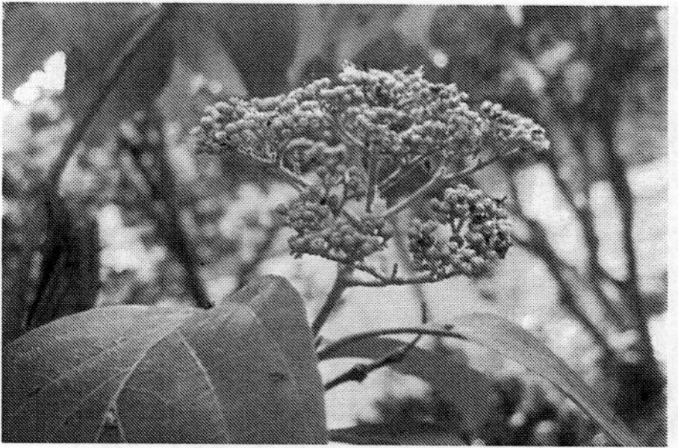

Fig. 6.19: Agnimantha

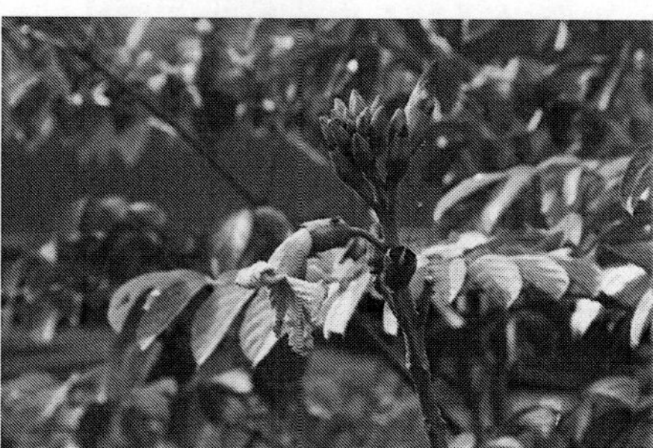

Fig. 6.20: Shyonaka

Prakshepaka Dravyas

सतुसैंधवचूर्णेनशताह्वेनचयोजितः। देयाः सुखोष्णश्चतथानिरेतिसहसासुखं॥ (Su.Chi.37/63)

Saindhava and Shatahva may be added to the oil of Anuvasana because they facilitate its proper and better return.

शताह्वा सैन्धवाभ्यां च देयं स्नेहे च चूर्णकम्। तन्मात्रोत्तममध्यान्ता षट्चतुर्द्वयमाषकैः॥ (Sha.Ut.5/21)

The quantity of powder of Shatahva and Saindhava to be added to Sneha is:

Uttama	-	6 Masha
Madhyama	-	4 Masha
Avara	-	2 Masha

Diet

जीर्णान्नमथ साहाह्ने स्नेहे प्रत्यागते पुनः। लध्वन्न भोजयेत् कामं दीप्ताग्निस्तु नरोयदि।
प्रातरूष्णोदकं देयं धान्यनागर साधितं। तेनास्य दीप्यते वह्निर् भक्ताकांक्षा च जायते॥ (Su.Chi.37/68-69)

After Anuvasana the patient should be given warm water to drink whenever he feels thirsty and in meals light wholesome food should be given. If the patient is having good digestive power then on the same day evening light diet may be given after returning the Basti. In the next morning the warm water or water prepared with Dhaniya and Shunthi should be given. It improves the digestion and appetite of the patient.

युक्तस्नेहं द्रवोष्णं चल घुपथ्योपसेवनं। भुक्तवान् मात्राया भोज्यमनुवास्यर त्र्यहांत्र्यहात्॥ (Ch.Si.4/42)

The next Anuvasana can be given on the third day.

Relation of Food with Anuvasana Basti

न च अभुक्तवतः स्नेहः प्राणिधेयः कथणचनः। शुद्धत्वाच्छून्य कोष्ठस्य स्नेह ऊर्ध्व समुत्पतेत्॥
सदा अनुवासयेच्चापि भोजयित्वाऽऽर्द्रपाणिनम्। ज्वरं विदग्ध भुक्तस्य कुर्यात् स्नेहः प्रयोजितः॥
(Su.Chi.37/53-54)

Sneha Basti should never be given without taking food because in empty Koshtha, the Sneha may go upwards. So always Anuvasana should be given immediately after taking meal (Ardra Paninam) because the Anuvasana Basti given during the digestion period of meal causes fever.

नरस्ततोनिश्यनुवासनार्होनात्याशितः स्यादनुवासनियाः॥ (Ch.Si.1/22)

At the same time care should be taken that the patient should not take excessive quantity of food.

नचातिस्निग्धमशनंभोजयित्वाऽनुवासयेत्। मदंमुर्च्छाचजनयेद् द्विधा स्नेहः प्रयोजिताः॥
रूक्षं भुक्तवतोहि अन्नं बलवर्णम् चहापयेत्। युक्तस्नेहोमतोजन्तुंभोजयित्वाऽनुवासयेत्॥
(Su.Chi.37/55-56)

Meal should not contain excess of fatty substances as the unctuous substances given through both routes, i.e. oral and rectal may cause fainting and unconsciousness. But at the same time if only ununctuous (Ruksha) foods are given then it may be harmful for strength and complexion. So the meal must contain little quantity of fatty substances.

यूष क्षीररसैस्तस्माध्यथाव्याधिसमीक्ष्या। यथोचितात् पादहीनंभोजयित्वाऽनुवासयेत्।। (Su.Chi.37/57)

For this purpose, vegetable or meat soup, milk or other food articles suitable according to the condition of the disease may be given in one-fourth quantity of the usual diet and then Anuvasana is to be given.

Time of Anuvasana

शीते वसन्ते चदिवाऽनुवास्योरात्रौशरद्ग्रीष्मघनागमेषु। तानेव दोषान् परिक्षताये स्नेहस्य पाने परिकीर्तिताः प्राक्।। (Ch.Si.1/22-23)

In winter and spring seasons, Anuvasana is given in day while in the summer, rainy and autumn seasons it may be given in the night with due care to prevent untoward effect of the oleation therapy.

अह्निस्थानस्थितेदोषेवह्नौच अन्नरसान्विते। स्फुटस्त्रोतोमुखेदेहेस्नेहौजः परिसर्पिति।। (Su.Chi.37/48)

Anuvasana is given in day, because at that time the Dosha remain in normal condition at their own place and Agni is also active in digestion and the Srotas also remains open, so the Virya of Anuvasana given in day spreads all over the body.

रात्रौबस्तिंनदध्यात्तुदोषोत्क्लेशोहिरात्रिजः। स्नेहवीर्ययुतः कुर्यादाध्मानंगौरवंज्वरं।। (Su.Chi.37/37)

Generally, Anuvasana should not be given in night because Virya of Sneha by exciting Dosha may cause distension and heaviness in abdomen and fever.

पित्तेऽधिकेकफे क्षीणेरूक्षेवातरूगार्दिते। नरेरात्रौतुदातव्यंकालेचोष्णोऽनुवासनं।।
उष्णोपित्ताधिकेवाऽपिदिवादाहादयोगदाः। सम्भवन्तियतस्तस्मात्प्रदोषेयोजयेद्भिषक्।। (Su.Chi.37/49-50)

But in condition of excessive Pitta and diminished Kapha along with it, if patient is Ruksha then it should be given in night also. In summer and excessive Pitta, if it is given in day then it may cause burning sensation.

Anuvasana and Virechana

संसृष्टभक्तं नवमेऽह्निसर्पिस्तं पाययेताप्यनुवासयेद्वा। (Ch.Si.1/20)

After Sansarjana Krama on ninth day of Virechana the patient either is to be given a potion of ghee or Anuvasana.

पक्षाद्विरेको वान्तस्यततश्चापिनिरूहणं। सध्योनिरूढोऽनुवास्यः सप्तरात्राद्विरेचितः।। (Su.Chi.36/51)
विरेचनात् सप्तरात्रेगतेजातबलायवै। कृतन्नायानुवास्साय सम्यग्देयोऽनुवासनः।। (Su.Chi.37/3)

According to Sushruta after Virechana, Anuvasana should be given after a gap of at least 7 days. But after Niruha, Anuvasana can be given on the same day.

Administration of Anuvasana Basti

Purva Karma

a. Time of administration

शीते वसन्ते च दिवा रात्रौ केचित्ततोऽन्यदा।

During cold season and Vasanta it should be given during day and in other seasons during night.

b. Preparation of the patient

अभ्यक्तस्नातमुचितात्पादहीनं हितं लघु। अस्निग्धरूक्षमशितं सानुपानं द्रवादि च॥
कृतचङ्क्रमणं मुक्तविण्मूत्रं शयने सुखे। नात्युच्छ्रिते न चोच्छीर्षे संविष्ट वामपार्श्वत:॥
सङ्कोच्य दक्षिणं सक्थि प्रसार्य च ततोऽपरम्॥ (A.H.Su.19/21-24)

One should be given Abhyanga and sveda followed with warm water bath and then patient is advised to take food less by one-fourth of the usual quantity (Padaheena); suitable light, neither with more of fats nor very dry followed by an after drink of appropriate liquid.

Next he should walk for some time, eliminate feces, urine and lie on a comfortable cot neither too high nor too low, on his left side, folding his right thigh and extending the other (left thigh).

Pradhana Karma

अथास्य नेत्रं प्रणयेत्स्निग्धे स्निग्धमुखं गुदे। उच्छवास्य बस्तेर्वदने बद्धे हस्तमकम्पयन्॥
पृष्ठवंशं प्रति ततो नातिद्रुतविलम्बितम्। नातिवेगं न वा मन्दं सकृदेव प्रपीडयेत्॥
सावशेषं च कुर्वीत वायु: शेषे हि तिष्ठति॥ (A.H.Su.19/25-26)

Enema nozzle should be pushed into rectum after lubricating nozzle and Guda and removing the air from the bladder. Bladder should be pressed without shaking the hands in the direction of the vertebral column, neither too fast nor too slow, neither with great force nor with low force but in one attempt.

Small quantity of liquid should be allowed to remain in the bag to prevent the entering of air.

Pashchat Karma

तत्रप्रणिहितस्नेहेउत्तानोवाक्शतंभवेत्। प्रसारितैः सर्वगात्रैस्तथावीर्यंविसर्पाति॥
ताडयेत्तलयोरेनंत्रिंस्त्रिन् वारांछनैः शनैः। स्फिचोश्चैततः शय्यांत्रिन्वारानुत्क्षिपेत्ततः।
एवंप्राणिहितेबस्तौमन्दायासौऽथमन्दवाक्। स्वास्तीर्णेशयनेकाममासीताचारिकेरतः॥
(Su.Chi.37/58-62)

When the administration is over, buttocks of the patient are patted with palms for three times and is advised to relax in supine position.

The foot end of the table is raised to little extent for 3 times and then pillow is kept under the head of the patient and soles of the patient are gently rubbed.

In this relaxed position patient should wait for 100 Matra (time taken to count upto 100), to let the Veerya of the Basti spreads all over the body.

The patient may be allowed to take rest on the comfortable bed. He should neither talk loudly nor indulge in anger.

योज्यः शीघ्रं निवृत्तेऽन्यः स्नेहोऽतिष्ठन्नकार्यकृत्। दीप्ताग्नि त्वागतस्नेहं साह्णे भोजयेल्लघु॥
(A.H.Su.19/29)

If the Sneha comes out quickly another enema should be administered immediately because Sneha which does not retain inside will not serve the purpose. If the person has good digestive fire and administered Sneha comes out, light food can be given in the evening.

Pratyagamana Kala (Period of Retention of Anuvasana)

निवृत्तिकालः परमस्त्रयो यामास्ततः परम्। अहोरात्रमुपेक्षेत, परतः फलवर्तिभिः।
तीक्ष्णैर्वा बस्तिभिः कुर्याद्यत्रं स्नेहनिवृत्तये।। (A.H.Su.19/30-31)

The maximum time of retention of Sneha is 3 Yama; after that, can be awaited for 1 day.

Later on, attempt should be made to remove it by force with the help of Phala Varti (suppository) and by administering Teekshna Basti.

यस्यनोपद्रवं कुर्यात् स्नेहबस्तिर् अनिःसृतः। सर्वोऽल्पो वा ऽऽवृतो रौक्ष्यादुपेक्ष्यः स विजानता।।
(Ch.Si.4/41)

However, if it is retained even up to 24 hours and it does not harm the body and in some Ruksha purusha if the Sneha does not return, in that condition if it does not cause any complication, then it should be ignored.

Properties of Warm Water

स्नेहाजीर्णंजरयतिश्लेष्माणंतद्भिनत्तिच। मारुतस्यानुलोम्यंचकुर्यदुष्णोदकंनृणां।।
वमने च विरेको च निरुहेसानुवासने। स्मादुष्णोदकंयंवातश्लेष्मोपशान्तये।। (Ch.Si.4/44-45)

The warm water digests the remaining unctuous substances, breaks down the Shleshma and regulates the peristaltic movements. So after administration of emesis, purgation, evacuative or unctuous enema, warm water should be given.

Samyak Yoga (Symptoms of Proper Anuvasana)

प्रत्येत्यसक्तं सशकृच्च तैलंरक्तादिबुद्धिन्द्रिय संप्रसादो। स्वप्रानुवृत्तिर्लघुताबलम् च सृष्टाश्च वेगाः स्वनुवासितेस्युः।। (Ch.Si.1/44)

The symptoms of proper Anuvasana are:

- ☐ Returning of feces and oil separately without sticking with each other
- ☐ Clarity of senses, intellect and Raktadi Dhatu
- ☐ Feeling of lightness
- ☐ Increase of strength
- ☐ Regulation of excretory urges and
- ☐ Proper sleep

सानिलः सपुरीषश्च स्नेहः प्रत्येतियस्यतु। ओष चोषौ विना शीघ्रं ससम्यगनुवासितः।। (Su.Chi.37/67)

- ☐ There should not be any discomfort or burning sensation.

Ayoga (Symptoms of Improper Anuvasana)

अधःशरीरोदरबाहुपृष्ठपार्श्वेषु रुग्रूक्षखरं चगात्रं। ग्रहाश्चविण्मुत्रसमीरणानासम्यगेतान्यनुवासितस्य।।
(Ch.Si 1/45)

- ☐ Pain in the lower part of the body, abdomen, arms, back and sides
- ☐ Dryness and roughness of the body
- ☐ Retention of feces, flatus and urine

Ati Yoga (Symptoms of Excessive Anuvasana)

हृल्लास मोह क्लम साद मूर्च्छा विकर्तिता चात्यानुवासितस्य॥ (Ch.Si.1/46)

- Nausea
- Stupor
- Fatigue
- Exhaustion
- Fainting
- Griping pain.

Complications of Anuvasana (Vyapad and its management)

वातपित्तकफात्यन्नपुरीषैरावृतस्य च। अभुक्ते च प्रणीतस्य स्नेहबस्तेः षडापदः॥ (Ch.Si.4/25)
स्नेहबस्तौ मरुत्पित्त कफाऽत्याऽऽशनविडावृते। अभुक्ते शूनपाय्याऽऽमदत्तेऽष्टौ व्यापदः स्मृतः॥(A.S.Ka.7/2)

S. No.	*Charaka*	*Vagbhatta*
1.	Vatavrita sneha	Vatavrita
2.	Pittavrita sneha	Pittavrita
3.	Kaphavrita sneha	Kaphavrita
4.	Annavrita sneha	Atyashanavrita
5.	Purishavrita sneha	Vidavrita
6.	Abhuktabhakta pranita sneha	Abhukta
7.	—	Shunapayu
8.	—	Amadatta

Vatavritta Sneha

Nidana

Sheeta and alpa basti in the condition of Vatadhika avastha.

Lakshana

Angamarda, Jvara, Adhmana, Sheeta, Stambha, Urupeedana, Parshvaruk.

Chikitsa

रास्नादि तीक्ष्णबस्ति, रास्नादिसिद्ध तैल अनुवासनबस्ति

Pittavritta Sneha

Nidana

Administration of Atyushna basti in Pittadhika avastha.

Lakshana

Daha, Raga, Trishna, Moha, Tamaka, Jvara

Chikitsa

Basti with Svadu-tikta dravyas.

Kaphavritta Sneha

Nidana

Mridu Basti in Kaphadhika avastha.

Lakshana

Tandra, Sheeta Jvara, Alasya, Praseka, Aruchi, Gaurava, Murccha, Glani

Chikitsa

Teekshna Basti (Kashaya, Katu, Teekshna, Ushna having Sura and Mutra)

Annavritta Sneha

Nidana

Guru Basti after Atibhojana.

Lakshana

Chhardi, Murccha, Aruchi, Glani, Shula, Nidra, Angamarda, Amalinga, Daha

Chikitsa

Pachana with Katu and Lavana churna and Kvatha, Mridu Virechana, Amahara Kriya.

Purishavritta Sneha

Nidana

Alpa bala Basti in Mala Sanchaya.

Lakshana

Sanga of Vit Mutra Anila Arati, Guruta, Adhmana, Hritgraha

Chikitsa

Sneha, Sveda, Varti, Shyamabilwadi Siddha Niruha and Anuvasana Basti.

Abhukta Pranita Sneha

Nidana

Atipeedita Basti in Abhukta Avastha (empty stomach), Shunapayu (empty bowel)

Lakshana

It goes up very high and from there may reach the throat and may come out from the upper orifice of the body.

Chikitsa

Niruha basti prepared with gomutra, Krishna nishotha kvatha added with kalka of yava and kulattha followed by anuvasana basti with taila siddha by same medicines is given. When sneha is coming out of throat, cold water must be sprinkled on the face of the patient and tikshna virechana and/or Vamana nashaka chikitsa should be given.

Commonly Encountered Complications of Sneha Basti

- ❑ Agnimandya
- ❑ Atisara
- ❑ Udarashula
- ❑ Burning sensation in abdomen
- ❑ Jvara
- ❑ Heaviness of body.

Commonly Practiced Anuvasana Basti

❑ Dhanvantara taila	-	Vata kapha hara , apana vishesha
❑ Sahacharadi taila	-	Neurological, varicose veins
❑ Pippalyadi taila	-	Non bleeding piles, atisara, pravahika
❑ Ksheerabala taila	-	Vata pitta shamana, infertility
❑ Balaguduchyadi taila	-	Vatarakta
❑ Murivenna	-	Anal fissures
❑ Lakshadi taila and ptg	-	Osteoporosis
❑ Mahanarayana taila	-	Vata pittahara, osteoporosis
❑ Panchatikta ghrita	-	Sandishoola, kushta
❑ Sukumara ghrita	-	Vitsanga, anaha
❑ Kalyanaka ghrita	-	Manovyadhi, arthavakshaya, kushta
❑ Varunadi ghrita	-	Sthaulya, mutrakrichra, udararoga
❑ Shatavaryadi ghrita	-	Mutrakricchra, mutra dosha.

MODE OF ACTION

नाभिप्रदेशं कटिपार्श्वकुक्षिं गत्वा शकृद् दोषचयं विलोडय संस्नेह्य कायं स पुरीष
दोषः सम्यक् सुखेनैति च यः स बस्तिः॥ (Ch.Si.1/40-41)

The basti when administered does the churning of Doshas situated in Nabhi pradesha, Kati, Parshva, etc. and expels it from the body.

विश्वक् स्थितं दोषचयं निरस्य सर्वान् विकारान् शमयेत् निरुह। (Ch.Si.1/28)

Through the systemic action Basti is capable of removing the Doshas from whole of the body. Though Basti is given in the Pakvashaya its active ingredients, i.e. "Virya of the Basti" spreads in the entire body as stated by Sushruta.

''मूलं गुदं शरीरस्य सिरास्तत्र प्रतिष्ठिताः। सर्वं शरीरं पुष्णन्ति मूर्धानं यावदाश्रिताः''॥ (पराशरे)

Parashara had highlighted the importance of Guda, by saying that Guda is Mula for all the Siras in the body. Hence the nourishment of the Guda by administration of Basti causes nourishment of entire Shareera.

पक्वाशयाद् बस्ति वीर्यं स्वैर्देर् इहम् उपसर्पति। (Su.Chi.35/25)

This Basti virya is also capable of removing the morbid Doshas from the body.

Considering these References

The mode of action can be stated as below:

Absorption of Basti

First sodium ion in Saindhava actively absorb from colon. High concentration of sodium ion facilitates sugar influx. Increase sodium ion in mucosal membrane generate osmotic gradient. Water follows this osmotic gradients thus passive absorption of water take place. Free fatty acid is easily absorbed by passive diffusion in the colon. From above description, it can be understood that how Saindhava, Madhu, Sneha and Kvatha is absorb from the colon along with the Sneha (lipids) and Kvatha. Lipid and water soluble portion is also absorbed from the colon. According to modern pharmacokinetics, it is also proved that rectal drug administration might exceed the oral value due to partial avoidance of hepatic pass metabolism.

Importance of Basti Dravya

Saindhava

This Lavana is considered best among all the Lavana described in Samhita. It plays an important role to initiate the absorption of Basti as discussed earlier.

Madhu

Main role of Madhu is to increase the retention time of Basti by counteract the irritative property of Saindhava. The retention time of irritative substances in rectum may be favoured by making solution as nearly isotonic as possible by using colloidal fluid such as starch water as diluents.

Sneha

By using Sneha the fat soluble portion of the drug easily absorbed from the colon. Lipids and lipid soluble substances can easily enter the cell. In this way Sneha helps the Basti dravya to reach at cellular level.

Kvatha

It is used to get water soluble part of Kvatha dravya. Instead of Kvatha as a drava, dravya like Kshira, Gomutra, Amla, Kanji, Prasanna, Mansarasa, etc. are also used or for the preparation of Kvatha itself.

Avapa Dravya

They are used sometimes in order to make the Basti either Tikshna or Mridu and to affect the particular Dosha.

Action of Basti Dravyas

Saindhava

Because of its:

- Sukshma Guna- It reaches up to the micro channels of the body.
- Tikshna Guna- It breaks down the morbid Mala and Dosha Sanghata.
- Snigdha Guna- Liquifies the Doshas.
- It becomes helpful for the elimination of Basti due to its irritant property.
- It reduces the Pichhila, Bahula and Kashaya properties of Madhu.
- In excess quantity, it can cause Daha and Atisara. Absence or less quantity of Saindhava is responsible for Ayoga. (A.H.19/42).

Madhu

If any drug is administered with appropriate vehicle it can absorbed and assimilated by the body very quickly. Madhu is made of various substances and considered best among the vehicles. (Ch.Su.27/249). It forms the homogenous mixture with the Saindhava. Madhu has predigested sugar and it is easy to digest and rapidly absorbed and assimilated by the body. In this way it energizes body in very short period. Charaka said that Basti dravya containing excess of Madhu when administered to the person makes him extremely virile. (Ch.Si.12/28)

Sneha

Sneha dravya reduces Vata dushti, soften body micro channels (Srotas), destroy the compact Mala and removes the obstruction in the channels. (Ch.Si.1/7). Owing the Snigdha Guna it produces unctuousness in the body, intern helps for easy eliminations of dosha and Mala. Sneha increases the permeability of cell membrane and become helpful in the elimination of dosha and Mala. Because of its Guru-Snigdha Guna it liquefies the Dosha and break down the compact Mala. Apart from this function it also protects the mucous membrane from the untoward effect of irritating drugs in the Basti Dravya.

Kalka, Kvatha and Avapa Dravya

Kalka and Kvatha dravya are the main constituents of the Basti dravya.

- They serve the function of Utkleshana or Doshaharana or Shamana depending upon it's contents and selected accordingly
- They are selected on the basis of Dosha, Dushya and Srotsa so their main action is Samprapti Vighatana of Roga
- Avapa dravya is also used for elimination of particular Dosha.

Some Facts Regarding Basti

There is no therapy equivalent to Basti because:

- It evacuates impurity quickly and easily
- It is free from untoward effect
- It does Asthapana/Santarpana quickly according to the purpose based upon the drugs used in it.

Acharya Charaka quotes that Basti introduced in the colon acts upon the whole body and on every system. Thus, drawing out the impurities by its potency like sun evaporates the liquid from the earth by its heat (Ch.Si.7/65).

Describing the action of Niruha Basti, Acharya Charaka opines that as cloth take away the dye from the water mixed with Kusumbha (plant), in the same way Niruha Basti eliminates excrements from the liquefied body. Only one type of Basti that is either Niruha or Anuvasana should not be used continuously. If Anuvasana is applied continuously than it aggravates morbid matter and reduces the Agni. If Niruha Basti is used continuously then it causes provocation of Vata.

Thus, Niruaha after Anuvasana or vice versa are very much important to restore the body normalcy and to pacify the disease.

- It acts as both Sanshodhana and Samshamana therapy (Su.Chi.35/3).
- It provides immediate strength, hence it is supreme line of treatment particularly in children and aged person (Ch.Si.11/36).
- It cleanses the body immediately with ease and also produces the affect of both Santarpana and Apatarpana immediately by using respective drug (Ch.Si.10/5).
- There is no treatment equivalent to Basti in the protection of Marma and in the management of their affliction which are considered as vital parts in the body (Ch.Si.9/7).
- It can be used in almost all the disease by using specific drugs indicated in that disease condition (Ch.Si.10/4; Su.Chi. 38/111).

Systematic Action of Basti

पक्वाशयाद्बस्तिवीर्यं खैर्देहमनुसर्पति। वृक्षमूले निषिक्तानामपां वीर्यमिव द्रुमम्।। (Su.Chi.35/25)

The Virya of Basti administered through the Basti into the Pakvashaya reaches the whole body through the channels (Srotasa) as the active principles in the water when poured at the root of the tree reaches the whole plant.

Eliminative or Purificative Action of Basti

Basti administered into Pakvashaya draws the Dosha and Mala from all over the body from the foot to the head by the virtue of its Virya, just as the sun situated in the sky draws the moisture from the earth by its heat. (Ch.Si.7/64)

Action of Basti on Vayu

Vayu is considered to be the main controller of the body. Now if Vayu alone or in combination with other Dosha gets vitiated, then Basti by the way of evacuation or elimination normalizes the path of Vayu along with Pitta, Kapha and fecal matter.

Importance of Basti Over Vamana and Virechana

Vamana and Virechana are contraindicated in old person, children and in weak patient. Because they have not gained sufficient strength of Dhatu or their strength is diminished respectively.

Inspite of doing proper elimination, Virechana may produce uneasiness, belching, nausea and abdominal pain due to the use or ingestion of pungent, Kshara and Ushna drugs.

After administration of Basti dravya, a keen observation should be done so as to evaluate the proper function of Basti.

MEDICATION BY RECTAL ROUTE

Rectal Administration

Substances may be introduced into the rectum for exciting evacuation or for medication, which later may be intended for effect in three different locations:

1. For effects on the contents of the colon for which the term “endocolonic” might be suggested to differentiate it from
2. Effect to be exerted on the tissue of the colon, for which the term “encolonic” might be a suitable designation
3. For administration by the way rectal medication intended for systemic action for which the term “diacolonic” might be employed. Before one resorts to rectal administration it is a good rule to make a digital examination of the rectum. Rectum distended with fecal matter should be cleaned out by an evacuant enema before it is given the task of receiving medication. Rectal injections also known as enemas clysters or lavements may be large or small.

Importance of Rectal Administration of Drug

1. When it is desired to spare the stomach and intestine from the action of the drug or to protect the drug from the action of the digestive ferments
2. With children who will not take disagreeable tasting medicaments, or with the insane, who refuse to swallow, rectal administration may become an important recourse
3. Such a bitter substance as strychnine can best be given to children in suppository form provided this method of administration is carried out gently, skilfully and tactfully.

Enemas

Rectal injections also known as enemas, clysters or lavements, may be “large” or “small”. An enema of less than half a liter might be considered a small enema and of more than half a liter is a large enema.

1. When a rectal enema is given by means of a syringe with a short tip, it is deposited just within the sphincter of the anus, a portion of the rectum that is normally very intolerant of sudden distension. It is indeed this irritability which is responsible for the prompt evacuation of any fecal matter that arrives in this part of the bowel. For this reason, even a small quantity of fluid when given rapidly tends to cause evacuation
2. When, on the other hand, the enema is administered very slowly, it suppresses evacuation reflex and reaches to the upper part of the colon which is not only more retentive but also more absorptive than the rectum

3. After the drug once passes the anal sphincter will pass easily up to the sigmoid and descending colon, across and down to the cecum regardless of the position of the body of the patient. Cool large enemas are believed to excite the gallbladder for contraction and are advocated in the treatment of catarrhal jaundice. Irritation of the colon is a long established form of treatment for the various types of jaundice.

Research View

Researches have demonstrated that within a period of three or twelve minutes after the instillation of various solutions high into the rectum a flow of bile was obtained from the duodenal tube that would continue for eighteen to sixty minutes without any interruption. Hence, the introduction of various solutions into the upper part of the rectum produces drainage into the duodenum of bile that comes directly from the liver and without contraction of the gallbladder.

Evacuant Enemas

These types of enemas are used to secure evacuation. Depending on the dose of Basti it can be employed either merely emptying of feces or for cleansing of the bowel. Here if rectum is merely to be emptied of feces then 0.5 liter enema is to be given rapidly. While on the other hand, if colon flushing is required than approximately 1 liter of warm water is slowly introduced to the patient in lateral or in sims' position. Evacuant enema can be repeated every three hour or four hours until the ultimate aim is achieved, here care should be taken that colon should not be overdistended.

Oil Enemas

Though oil enemas are essentially evacuant enemas, they are given with the technique of the retention enema because they are to be retained for many hours usually overnight.

Indications

1. To soften feces, in constipation characterized by the formation of hard scybalous and in that due to partial obstruction of the colon
2. For evacuant action, in so-called spastic constipation, in pelvirectal constipation and in any other form of constipation and in which oral administration of cathartics is contraindicated by gastric disturbance
3. For soothing action, in excessive irritability of the colon and rectum, in colitis and in proctitis
4. It has been suggested that oil enemas might inhibit absorption of toxic products. That the oil has the power of removing substances soluble in it, is shown by the fact that it is passed out as dark yellow or olive green color with offensive odor. There is no definite knowledge, however, of the degree to which this property might be of clinical value.

Precautions

1. The oil must be pure and free from rancidity. This is more important than that it come from a certain source. (Thus poppy seed oil, oil of sesame or cotton seed oil, when pure is just as good for this purpose as olive oil)
2. The oil should be placed in a basin of hot water until it has acquired blood heat (100° F)
3. The oil enema is given at bedtime, unless it produces discomfort and interferes with sleep. In such case it may be taken early in the morning, and the patient may lie in bed for three or four hours afterward
4. The patient should understand that unless the oil remains in the intestine for several hours at least satisfactory results cannot be expected. The total quantity to be injected depends, therefore, on the patient's ability to retain it
5. This is so variable that no definite quantity can be stated. The principle to be followed is to gradually increase the amount injected at successive times until a satisfactory amount can be introduced and retained.

Retention Enemas

Technique

It is well to precede a retention enema by a cleansing enema, so as to unload the lower part of the bowel of fecal matter that may be contained in it, thereby lessening distension and favoring retention.

1. The smaller in bulk the enema, the better it is retained
2. Still, to be retained, it must also be quite devoid of irritating properties
3. The retention of an irritative substance may be favoured by making its solution as nearly isotonic as possible, and by using colloidal fluid such as starch water as dilutents
4. If the fluid is introduced very slowly and steadily, the rectum does not become as readily aware of the distension and retains a quantity of fluid that would otherwise be expelled
5. Giving the enema at body temperature favors retention, as extremes of temperature excite peristalsis
6. The patient should assume the recumbent position for at least an hour after the injection, and should be instructed to resist any liking to evacuation as much as possible.

Nutrient Enemas

The attempt has been made to maintain nutrition by rectal feeding when it is impossible or undesirable to introduce food into the stomach, or when it cannot be retained. But the colon has hardly any digestive power and it absorptive capacity even for a water soluble substance of large molecular size is very poor and nil for fat.

Precautions

1. Not more than three nutrient enemas should be given in the twenty four hours, at about 8 hour intervals. The amount should at first not exceed 150 cc. to be gradually increased to 300 when given as ordinary enemas, though when given by proctoclysis the quantity may reach 1 liter.
2. After each administration the patient should keep as quite as possible for at least two hours and suppress any desire to evacuate the bowel.

3. In point of fact patients who need nutrient enemas should be kept in bed continuously; at rest in bed lessen the consumption of calories by at least 25 percent
4. A daily cleansing enema is advisable. This should precede the nutrient enema by about an hour.

Medicated Enemas

Medicated enemas are given by the technique of retention enemas. They may be employed as previously stated for endocolonic, encolonic or diacolonic action. Oil may be used as a vehicle for diacolonic administration of oil soluble volatile bodies.

Basti is not Merely Enema

After discussing both Basti and enema, it can be concluded that Basti is not merely the enema one, rather it is a highly complex. Sophisticated and systemic therapy having wider range of therapeutic actions and indication. It has been considered as prime treatment modality for Vata Dosha. Innumerable Basti can be formulated using various drugs in different proportions for various diseases and for different patients. Specific rules and regulations are indicated for the administration of Basti which must be followed to obtain the desirable result. On contrary to this, enema is simply used for evacuation of colon and in some instances for rehydration and administration of medicine.

KNOWLEDGE OF DIFFERENT TYPES OF BASTI

1. Madhutailaika Basti

यस्मान् मधु च तैलं च प्राधान्येन प्रदीयते। माधुतैलिक इत्येवं भिषग्भिर् बस्तिर् उच्यते॥

(Su.Chi.38/114)

The basti mainly contains Madhu and Taila in equal proportion. Hence this basti is named as madhutailika basti.

Paryayas of Madhutailika basti are:

Yuktaratha Basti: Madhutailika basti can be used at any time, even while-travelling. Hence it is called as Yuktaratha Basti. (According to Vangasena if Pippali and Madanaphala are added, it is called as Yuktaratha basti.)

Yapana Basti- यापनस्तु बस्तयः सर्व काले देयाः। (Ch.Si.12/15)

It is also called as Yapana basti because it can be used anytime.

Siddha Basti: As it is useful for curing many diseases it is called as Siddha basti.

Doshahara Basti: As it eliminates vitiated doshas it is known as doshahara basti and is also termed as auspicious.

Snigdha Basti: This word denotes the predominant oily nature and the prolonged usage like that of Matra basti (should not be confused with Anuvasana).

Importance

नृपाणां तम् समानानां तथा सुमहताम अपि। नारीणां सुकुमाराणां शिशुस्थ विरयोरपि।
दोषनिर्हरणार्थाय बलवर्णोदयाय च। समासेन उपदेक्ष्यामि विधानं मातुतैलिकं॥

यान स्त्री भोज्य पानेषु नियमश्चात्र नोच्यते। फलं च विपुलं दृष्टं व्यापदां च अपि संभवः॥
योज्यस्तवः सुखेनै च निरुहक्रम मिच्छता। यदेच्छति तदैवैष प्रयोक्तव्यो विपश्चिता॥ (Su.Chi.38/96-99)

- ❑ There are no much restrictions told after administration of this basti like Yana, Maithuna and in terms of Annapana
- ❑ It can be administered in Sarvakala
- ❑ It is a Mridu basti and hence there is less chance for complications
- ❑ It is very beneficial in raja, sukumara, stree, shishu etc and can be administered in above said persons without any restrictions
- ❑ It is very much useful in improving bala and Varna
- ❑ It can be administered without previous shodhana.

Indications of Madhutailika Basti

सुखिनाम् अल्पदोषाणां नित्यं स्निग्धाश्चये नराः। मृदु कोष्ठाश्च ये तेषां विधेया माधुतैलिकाः॥
(Su.Chi.38/117)

It is administered in the person who leads luxurious life who is having mild increase in doshas, the person who is Sukumara, the person who is accustomed to daily usage of snigdha substances and in the person who is having Mridu Koshtha.

मधुतैलं चतुःप्रसृतं शतपुष्प अर्धपलं सैन्धव अर्ध अक्ष युक्तो बस्तिर् दीपनो बृंहणो बल वर्णकरो निरुपद्रवो वृष्यतमो रसायनः क्रिमि कुष्ठो उदावर्त गुल्म अर्शे ब्रध्न प्लीह मेहहरः॥ (Ch.Si. 12/18(13)
मधु तैले समे कर्षः सैंधवाद् द्विपिचुर् मिसिः। एरण्ड मूल क्वाथेन निरुहो माधु तैलिकः।
रसायनं प्रमेहार्शः कृमि गुल्म आंत्र वृद्धिनुत्। सयष्टिमधुकश्चैव चक्षुस्यो रक्तपित्तजित्॥
(A.H.Ka 4/27-28)

Material and Doses

Drug	*Dose*		
	Uttam	Madhyam	Avara
Madhu	175 g	150 g	100 g
Til oil	175 g	150 g	100 g
Eranda Kvatha	350 mL	300 mL	200 mL
Shatapushpa	24 g	24 g	12 g
Madanaphala	12 g	12 g	6 g
Saindhava Lavana	12 g	12 g	6 g

Indications

Krimi, Kushtha, Udavarta, Gulma, Arsha, Bradhna (inguinal swelling), Pleeha and Meha (obstinate urinary disorder including diabetes).

Benefits

Deepana, Brihana, Balavarnakara, Nirupadrava, Vrushya and Rasayana.

Erandamuladi Niruha Basti

Erandamuladi niruha basti is mentioned in Charaka samhita and it contains 35 drugs. It is one of the important kaphahara basti. There are 22 ushna veerya and 7 sheeta veerya drugs. 9 drugs are having katu vipaka and 20 drugs are having madhura vipaka and also kapha-vata shamaka are 10 in number. Most of the drugs are having Laghu, Ruksha Gunas and Katu, Tikta and Kashaya rasa and as avapa dravya, Gomutra is also mentioned.

एरण्डमूलं त्रिपलं पलाषं ह्रस्वानि मूलानि च यानि पंच। रास्न अश्वगन्ध अतिबला गुडूची पुनर्नव आरग्वध देवदारू।
भागाः पलाशां मदनाष्टयुक्ता जलद्विकंसे क्वथिथेऽष्तशेषे।। पेष्याः शतह्वा हपुषा प्रियंगु सपिप्पलीकं मधुकं बला च।
रसाञ्जनं वत्सकबीज मुस्तं भागाक्षमात्रं लवणांशयुक्तम्। समाक्षिक तैलयुतः समूत्रो बस्तिर्नृणां दीपनलेखनीयः।। जंघ अरुपादं त्रिकपृष्ठशूलं कफावृत्ति मारुतनिग्रहं च।। विट् मूत्र वात ग्रहणं सशूलंभ् आध्मान् अश्मरी शर्करे च।
आनाह अर्शो गृहणी प्रदोषान् एरण्डबस्ति शमयेत् प्रयुक्त।। (Ch.Si. 3/38-42)

Ingredients	*Dosage*	*Ingredients*	*Dosage*
Makshika	200 mL	Sneha	200 mL
Saindhava lavana	15 g	Kvatha	300 mL
Kalka	30 g	Gomutra	100 mL

Indications

Pain and heaviness of jangha, pada, trika, prishcha, vibandha (retention of urine, feces and flatus), adhmana, ashmari, anaha, arsha, grahani, vatakapha diseases and also in peripheral vascular disorders.

Benefits

Lekhana, Dipana.

Yapana Basti

आयुषो यापनं दीर्घकालानुवर्तनम् कुर्वन्तीति यापनाबस्त्यः।। (Chakrapani)

These are important sets of basti mentioned in Charaka samhita siddhisthana. Both Anuvasana and niruha yapanas have been mentioned in Charaka samhita. The basti which sustains, support and maintain the life and promotes longevity is called as Yapana basti. It refers to:

- Sustaining the life (Su.Ni.1/12)
- Nourishment of the tissues (Su.Su.14/15)
- Alleviation of the disease (Su.Chi.6/13)
- Supporting and maintaining the life (Ch.Su.18/19)
- Reserving the homeostasis in the body constituents (Ch.Vi.1/14 Chakrapani)
- Checking of ageing process and enhancing the deprived tissues. (Su.Su.14/3 Dalhana)

Importance of Yapana Basti

इत्येते बस्तयः स्नेहश्चोक्ता यापन संज्ञिताः। स्वस्थानाम् आतुराणां च वृद्धानां च अविरोधिनां।
अतिव्यवाय शिलानां शुक्रमांस बलप्रदः। सर्वरोग प्रशमनाः सर्वेष्वृतुषु यौगिकाः॥
नारीणाम् प्रजातानां नराणां चाप्यपत्यदाः। उभयार्थ करो दृष्टा स्नेहबस्तिनिरुहयोः॥ (Ch.Si.12/49-50)

- ❑ It performs both the functions viz. shodhana and Snehana (Ch.Si.12/22) which is done by niruha and sneha basti respectively
- ❑ It is indicated in Svastha, Atura and Vriddha pointing towards its preventive, curative and promotive nature
- ❑ It can be administered in all the seasons at all time and in all the age groups (Ch.Si.12/21)
- ❑ No necessity of administration of sneha basti in between and initially (A.Sa.Ka.5/26)
- ❑ No necessity of prior Vamana and Virechana. (Dalhana)

Ingredients	*Dosage*	*Ingredients*	*Dosage*
Makshika	200 mL	Kalka	30 g
Saindhava lavana	15 g	Kvatha	300 mL
Sneha	200 mL	Mansarasa	100 mL

Indication

Specially indicated in:

- ❑ Shukrakshaya
- ❑ Mansakshaya
- ❑ Balakshaya
- ❑ Indriyakshaya
- ❑ Person indulging in excessive coitus (Ativyavaya)
- ❑ Vandyatwa
- ❑ Klaibya.

Benefits

Deepana, Brihana, Balavarnakara, Nirupadrava, Vrishya and Rasayana

Mustadi Yapana Basti

मुस्तोशीर बलारग्वध रास्नामंजिष्ठकटुरोहिणी। त्रायमाणपुनर्नव विभितक गुडुचि स्थिरादि पंचमूलानि॥
पलिकानि खण्डशः कृप्तानि अष्टौ च मदनफलानि प्रक्षाल्य जलाढके परिक्वाथ
पादशेष रसाह क्षीराद् द्विप्रस्थ संयुक्तः पुनः शृतः क्षीरावशेषः पाद जाङ्गल नसतुल्य
मधुघृतः शतकुसुमा मधुक कुटजफल रसांजन प्रियङ्गु कल्किकृतः ससैंधव सुखोष्णो
बस्तिः शुक्रमांस बलजननः क्षतक्षीण कास गुल्म शूल विषमज्वर ब्रध्न कुण्डल
उदावर्त कुक्षिशूल मूत्रकृच्छ् असृग् रजो विसर्प प्रवाहिक शिरोरूजा जानु जंघागृहा
अश्मरी उन्माद अर्शः प्रमेह आध्मान वातरक्त पित्तश्लेष्म व्याधिहरं सध्यो बलजननो रसायनश्चेति॥
(Ch.Si.12/16-1)

Ingredients	*Dosage*
Makshika	200 mL
Saindhava lavana	15 g
Sneha	200 mL
Kalka	30 g
Kvatha (Kshira kashaya)	300 mL
Mansarasa	100 mL

Kvatha in this basti is prepared with Musta, Ushira, etc. dravya mentioned upto laghupanchmula along with 8 Madanphala. Kalka dravya used are yashtimadhu, kutaja, shatahva, rasanjana and priyangu.

Benefits

Imparts strength to Shukra and Mansa dhatu, increases bala and rasayana.

Indications

Kshatakshina, Kasa, Gulma, Shula, Vishamjvara, Bastikundala, Udavarta, Mutrakrichra, Kukshishula, Raktaja roga, Visarpa, Pravahika, Shirahshula, Janu/jangha graha, Ashmari, Unmada, Arsha, Prameha, Vatarakta, Pitta kaphaja disease.

Ksheera Basti

There are many bastis in which ksheera is used as Avapa dravya or Kashaya dravya in the form of Ksheerapaka. All these bastis are popularly considered as ksheera bastis. Few examples for Ksheera basti are Pancha prasritika basti, Ksheera Vaitarana, Manjishthadi Ksheera basti, Yashtimadhu Ksheera basti, etc.

Milk is an emulsion or colloid of butterfat globules within a water- based fluid that contains dissolved carbhohydrates and protein aggregates with minerals. One of the important factors about the milk is that it contains calcium; it can be absorbed without the help of Vitamin D, under the influence of lactose in the distal small intestine via the paracellular route. This promotes the absorption of calcium and provides simultaneous intake of phosphorous that is essential for bone deposition. Hence Ksheera bastis have a wide and effective applicability in Asthivaha sroto Vikaras.

Ksheera bastis act as Brihana shodhana basti. Ksheera basti can be prepared with varied Ksheerapaka for better effect in varied conditions based on Yukti.

Manjishthadi Ksheera Basti

Ingredients	*Dosage*
Makshika	200 mL
Saindhava lavana	15 g
Sneha (Yashti taila, tiktaka ghrita)	200 mL
Kalka (guduchi, yashti kalka)	30 g
Kvatha (Manjishthadi Ksheerapaka)	300 mL
Gomutra	100 mL

Piccha Basti

Piccha basti is indicated in jeerna atisara avastha and jeerna grahani by charaka and Vagbhatta. Piccha basti acts as grahi (bowel binding), and contains dipana and pachana drugs. Piccha basti is explained as one of the treatment in Arsha roga. Piccha basti cures excess bowel movements and duodenal disorders.

It is also mentioned in Chakradatta, Su.Chi- 38/85-86, Vangasena (Atisarachikitsa)

बदरि एरावति शेलु शाल्मलि धन्वन अंकुराः। क्षीरसिद्धाः क्षौद्रयुक्ताः सास्त्राः पिच्छिल संज्ञिताः।
वाराह माहिष औरभ्र बैड लैणेय कौकुटम्। सध्यस्कम् असृगाजं वा देयं पिच्छिलबस्तिषु॥
कृत अनुवासनस्यास्य कृत संसर्जनस्य च। वर्तते यध्य अतीसारः पिच्छाबस्तिरतः परम्॥
परिवेष्टय कुशैराद्रैर आवृन्तानि शाल्मलेः। कृष्णमृत्तिकया ऽऽलिप्य स्वेदयेद् गोमयाग्निना॥
सुशुष्कां मृतिकां इनात्वा तानि वृन्तानि शाल्मलेः। शृते प्यसि मृद्गीयादापोटथ्यो उलूखले ततः॥
पिण्डं मृष्टिसमं प्रस्थे तत् पूतं तैलसर्पिषोः। स्नेहितं मात्रया युक्तं कल्केन मधुकस्य च॥
बस्तिम् अभ्यक्तगात्राय दध्यात् प्रत्यागते ततः। स्नात्वा भुञ्जीत पयसा जाङ्गलानां रसेन वा।
पित्तातिसार ज्वर शोथ गुल्म जीर्णातिसार ग्रहणीप्रदोषान्। जयत्ययं शीघ्रम् अतिप्रवृद्धान् विरेचन आस्थापनयोश्च बस्तिः॥ (Ch.Chi.19/63-68)

Ingredients	*Dosage*	*Ingredients*	*Dosage*
Makshika	200 mL	Kalka	30 gm
Saindhava lavana	15 g	Kvatha	350 mL
Sneha	200 mL		

Indications

Pittaja Atisara, Jvara, gulma, shotha, jeernatisara, grahani, gudabhransha and raktasrava.

Special Indication

In vatashleshma vibandha (obstruction), in excessive atisara due to kapha or when associated with pain. Here the patient should be given piccha basti prepared with the paste of pippali, bilva, kushta, shatavari and vacha added with salt.

Benefits

It acts as evacuative and sustaining and overcomes the advanced stage of the above diseases. It stabilizes the functions of dosha, dhatu and mala.

Panchatikta Basti

Panchatikta basti contains the group of bitter drugs. Most of these drugs have proven to have antioxidant and anti inflammatory properties along with immunomodulatory and immunostimulatory effect.

पटोल निम्ब भूनिम्ब रास्ना सप्तच्छद अम्भसः। चत्वारः प्रसृता एको घृतात् सर्षप कल्कितः॥
निरूहः पञ्चतिक्तोऽयं मेह अभिष्यन्द कुष्ठनुत्॥ (Ch.Si.8/8)

Ingredients

Ingredients	*Dosage*
Ghrita	1 prasrita
Kalka	1/6th of 1 pala
Kashaya	4 prasruta

Note: The quantity of sarshapa kalka is not mentioned here in the above yoga because it is to be determined according to the general rule (in 12 prasrita of liquid for niruha, 2 pala of the kalka is to be added is general rule. Thus in the above mentioned recipe which has 5 prasrita of liquid the paste should be 1/12th of 5 prasrita, (1/6th of 1 pala).

Sarshapa in more quantity leads to pitta prakopa and leads to excessive and burning micturation in prameha patients. Hence, care should be taken to avoid adverse effect.

Indications

Meha, Abhisyanda and Kushtha

Benefits

As it contains all the tikta dravyas it is very beneficial in the diseases like meha and kushtha

Vaitarana Basti

According to Garuda purana, Vaitarana is the name of the river which a person is supposed to cross during death in his astronomical kingdom. This vasti is so powerful in a sense that it can bring back life of a person who is about to cross the vaitarana river.

पल शुक्ति कर्ष कुडव अम्ली गुड सिन्धुजन्म गोमूत्रैः। ईषतैलयुतो अयं बस्ति शूल आनाह आमवातहरः॥
वैतरणः क्षारबस्ति भुक्ते चापि प्रदियते॥ (C.D.73/32)

Ingredients

Ingredients	*Quantity*	*Quantity in g*
Amlika kalka	1 pala	50 g
Guda (Jaggery)	1 sukti	25 g
Saindhava lavana	1 karsha	15 g
Gomutra	1 kudava	200 mL
Taila	Not specified	50 mL (usually)
Total	350 mL	

Indications

Shula, anaha and amavata.

Lekhana Basti

त्रिफलाक्वाथ गोमूत्र क्षौद्र क्षार समायुताः। ऊषकादि प्रतिवापा बस्तयो लेखनास्मृता॥

(Su.Chi 38/82)

Ingredients

Dravyam	*Quantity*	*Quantity in G as in classics*	*Quantity generally practiced*
Makshika	4 pala	200 mL	200 mL
Saindhava lavana	1 Aksha	12 g	12 g
Triphala kashaya	8 pala	400 mL	300 mL
Go mutra	3 pala	150 mL	100 mL
Kshara	3 karsha	36 g	5 g
Katu taila	6 pala	300 mL	100 mL
Ushakadi prativapa	2 pala	100 g	45 g

Indications

Lekhana, hyperlipidaemia and obesity.

Note: Ushakadigana contains a lot of mineral drugs, so it is not used in practice. The other kalka dravyas are commonly used. For drava-dravya instead of dhanyamla, kulattha kashaya can also be used. It is better to do Anuvasana basti on the same day to avoid inflammatory colitis.

Kshara Basti

सैन्धवाक्ष समादाय शताह्वाक्ष तथैवच। गोमूत्रस्य पलानि अष्टौ अम्लिकाया पलद्वयम्।।
गुडस्य द्वैपले चैव सर्वमालोडय यत्नतः। वस्त्रपूतम् सुखोष्णम् च बस्तिम् दध्यात् विचक्षणः।।
शूलम् संग आनाह मूत्रकृच्छ्रं च दारुणम्। क्रिमि उदावर्त गुल्मादिनाम् साध्यो हन्यात् निषेवितः।।

(C.D. 73/29-31)

Ingredients

Ingredients	*Quantity*	*Quantity in g*
Saindhava lavana	1 aksha	12 g
Shatapushpa	1 aksha	12 g
Gomutra	8 pala	400 mL
Guda	2 pala	100 g
Amlika	2 pala	100 g

Indications

Shula, Vibandha, Anaha, Mutrakrichra, Daruna, Krimi, Udavarta and Vata disease.

Krimihara Basti

विडङ्ग त्रिफला शिग्रु फल मुस्ताखुणिजात्। कषायात् प्रसृताः पञ्चतैलाद् एको विमथ्यतान्।।
विडङ्ग पिप्पली कल्को निरुहः क्रिमिनाशनः।। (Ch.Si.8/9-10)

Ingredients

Drug	Quantity
Tila taila	1 prasrita
Kalka-vidanga and pippali	As per condition
Kashaya	5 prasrita

Kashaya dravya: Vidanga, haritaki, vibhitaki, amalaki, shigru, madanaphala , musta and akhukarni (danti).

Indication

Krimi nashartha.

Ardhamatrika Basti

According to Vangasena and Chakradatta Ardhamatrika basti stands superior among all basti karmas because it has many advantages like:

न च स्नेहो न च स्वेदः परिहार विधिर् न च। आत्रेय अनुमतो ह्येषं सर्वरोग निवारणः।।
पक्ष्मघ्नश्च शूलघ्नश्च क्रिमिघ्नश्च विशेषतः। शुक्रसञ्जनो ह्येष वातशोणितनाशनः।।
बल वर्णकरो वृष्यो बस्तिः पुंसवनः परः।। (C.D.Niruhadikara)

- It can be administered without any preparatory measures, i.e. snehana and Svedana and it is not essential to follow the post procedure regime, i.e. pashchat karma (CD)
- It can be administered to sukumara, aged, women and to those who have fear about basti karma
- Its action is must faster than other bastis
- It can be administered in any dosha predominance and in sannipataja conditions
- It arrests the re-occurrence of the diseases
- It can be done daily or on alternate days.

दशमूली कषायेण शताह्वाक्षं प्रयोजयेत्। सैन्धवाक्षच मधुनो द्विपलं द्विपलन्त्था।।
तैलस्य फलमेकन्तु फलस्यैकत्र योजयेत्। अर्धमात्रिकसं वस्तिर्देयों निरुहवत्।।

Ingredients	Dosage
Makshika	2 pala (100 mL)
Saindhava lavana	1 aksha (12 g)
Sneha	2 pala (100 mL)
Kalka	1 karsha (12 g)
Kvatha (dashamula + madana)	4 pala + 1 pala (350 mL)

Indications

Yakshma, Shula, Krimi, Vatarakta and can be used in almost all the diseases.

Benefits

Shukrala, Varnakara, Balakara, Vrishyakara and punsavanakara.

UTTARA BASTI

Uttara Basti is an important Ayurvedic procedure which is defined in Ayurvedic classics very descriptively. It is mentioned for the genito urinary disorders of both, males and females. The procedure was selected as a method of drug administration in case of tubal blockage for the present study. Hence, its elaborative classical description along with interpretation on modern tools is made here.

There are two routes for administration of Basti described in classics, viz. Basti (through anal canal) and Uttara basti (through urogenital tract). The Basti yantra is also used to inject the medicines through urinary and vaginal passage for which the term Uttara basti is given. The Uttara basti deals with both males and females. But the following discussion is carried out taking females in view only, as required here.

Definition

उत्तरबस्तिसञ्ज्ञा उत्तरमार्गदीयमानतया, किंवा श्रेष्ठगुणतया उत्तरबस्तिः। (Chakrapani Ch.Si.9/50)

The administration of drugs through uttara marga and which has Shreshtha Guna.

स निरूहादुत्तरमुत्तरेण वा मार्गेण दीयत इत्युत्तर बस्तिः॥ (A.S.Su.28/11)

Basti which is administered after Niruha Basti and through the Uttara Marga.

गुदादुत्तरेण मार्गेण दीयत इत्युत्तरबस्तिः। (Arunadatta A.H.Su.19/70)

The administration of drugs through route above guda marga.

उत्कृष्टावयवे दानाद्बस्तिरुत्त्रसंज्ञितः। (Vangasena Basti.9)

Administration of drug to utkrishta avayava.

Thus uttara basti may be defined as the route of administration of drugs through vesicular / urethral route in males and vesicular/urethral or genital route in females.

Classification of Uttara Basti

उत्तरबस्तिपिस्नेहोऽनुवासनवत्वशोधनंनिरूहवद्पिकेचिदाहुः॥ (A.S.Su.28/10)

On the basis of form of drug to be administered Uttara Basti may be classified as follows:

Snaihika Uttara Basti

The uttara basti procedure where only sneha dravyas are used is called as snaihika uttara Basti. There is no mentioning of addition of any avapa dravyas in it.

Niruhika Uttara Basti

The uttara basti procedure where only kashaya dravya are used. There is no mentioning of addition of madhu, sneha, kalka, etc. which are being added commonly in Niruha basti.

On the Basis of Route of Administration it is Classified as:

1. Mutrashayagata uttara basti - The administration of drugs through urethral route
2. Yonigata uttara basti - The administration of drugs through vaginal route
3. Garbhashayagata uttara basti - The administration of drugs through uterine route

Male: Mutrashaya (Vesicular/urethral route)
Female: Yoni marga and Garbhashaya (vesicular/urethral or genital route)

Indications

शुक्रं दुष्टं शोणितं चा ङ्गनानां पुष्पोद्रेकं तस्य नाशं च कष्टम्।
मूत्राघातान्मूत्रदोषान् प्रवृद् धान् योनिव्याधिं संस्थितिं चापरायाः॥
शुक्रोत्सेकं शर्करामश्मरीं च शूलं बस्तौ वङ्क्षणे मेहने च।
घोरानन्यान् बस्तिजांश्चापि रोगान् हित्वा मेहानुत्तरो हन्ति बस्तिः॥ (Su.Chi.37/125-126)
बस्तिजेषु विकारेषु योनिविभ्रंशजेषु च। योनिशूलेषु तीव्रेषु योनिव्यापत्स्वसृग्दरे॥
अप्रस्त्रवति मूत्रे च बिन्दुं बिन्दुं स्त्रवत्यपि। विदध्यात् उत्तरं बस्तिं यथास्वौषधसंस्कृतम्॥
(Ch.Si.9/63-64)

Uttara Basti is indicated in the following conditions:

1. Shukradushti
2. Atyartava
3. Rajah Nasha
4. Kashtartava
5. Mutraghata
6. Mutradosha
7. Yoni Vyadhi
8. Obstruction to Apara
9. Shukrotseka
10. Sharkara
11. Ashmari
12. Basti Shula
13. Vankshana Shula
14. Meha Shula

Contraindications

In Males	*In Females*
• Urethral stricture • Bleeding disorders • Carcinoma of the bladder • Carcinoma of penis • Hypo/epispadiasis	**Intrauterine uttara basti** • Hypersensitivity • Carcinoma cervix • Heavy bleeding • Virginity • Vesicovaginal fistula
	Intravaginal uttara basti • Hypersensitivity • Menorrhagia • Rectovaginal fistula

Basti Yantra

It has 2 parts which are as follows:

1. Basti Netra

Synonym: Pushpa Netra

Characteristic of Netra for Male

Material	*Hema (gold), Raupya (silver)*
Length	12 Angula (Charaka and Vagbhatta), 14 Angula (Sushruta)
Structure	Agra (tip)- Jatipushpavruntal Ashvamara
Gopucchasamstitha	It should have a broad base with tapering end so that it resembles Gopuccha and the insertion end should be similar to the buds of Karaveera or Jathikusuma
Cchidra (opening)	Sarshapa Nirgamana
Karnika	2 Karnika One at the base to tie the Putaka and the other at the center from the tip (at 6 angula according to Chakrapani) indicating the length to be inserted.
Length of insertion (Netra pranidana)	Charaka - Length of Medhra Sushruta - 7 angula Ksharapani - 4/5/6/7 Angula

Characteristics in Female

Material	*Hema (gold), Raupya (silver)*
Length	10 Angula
Structure	Agra (tip)- Jatipushpavrunta Ashvamara
Gopucchasamstitha	It should have a broad base with tapering end so that it resembles Gopuccha and the insertion end should be similar to the buds of Karaveera or Jathikusuma
Karnika	2 Karnika one at the base to tie the Putaka and the other at 4 Angulas from the tip indicating the length to be inserted
Cchidra (opening)	Mutra marga- Mudga pramana Yoni marga- Medrasama
Length of insertion (Netra Pranidana)	Mutra marga: Bala (upto 12years) - 1 Angula Stree (reproductive age) - 2 Angula Apatya Marga (Garbhashaya) - 4 Angula

2. Basti Putaka

औरभ्रः शौकरो वाऽपि बस्तिराजश्च पूजितः। तदलाभे प्रयुञ्जीत गलचर्म तु पक्षिणाम्॥ (Su.Chi.37/107)

It should be made of the Basti of small sized animals like goat, sheep, pig, etc. or the leather of birds as the quantity of drug is less. It should be smooth, devoid of siras, processed with Kashaya Dravya, clean and devoid of foul smell.

Method of Administration (for Male)

It is divided in to 3 steps.

(1) Purvakarma

(a) Preparation of the Patient

द्वित्रास्थापनशुद्धेभ्यो विदध्यात् बस्तिमुत्तर। (A.H.Su.19/70)
अथातुरमुपस्निग्धं स्विन्नं प्रशिथिलाशयम्। यवागुं सघृतक्षीरां पीतवन्तं यथाबलम्॥ (Su.Chi.37/107)
स्नातस्य भुक्तभक्तस्य रसेन पयसाऽपिवा। (Ch.Si.9/53)

About 2–3 Niruha Basti are to be given before the administration of Uttara Basti. It is also in practice to give morning Niruha Basti and in the afternoon Uttara Basti. However, it is not clear whether Niruha should be given as Purva karma when Kashaya is taken as medicine for Uttara Basti.

On the day of Uttara Basti, Sthanika abhyanga and Nadi Sveda is to be given to the lower abdomen, thighs and groins and advice to take bath.

In Snaihika Uttara Basti Yavagu added with ghee and milk should be given before the administration of Basti.

(b) Time of Administration

तेन पूर्वाह्ने चोत्तरबस्तिप्रणिधानम्। (Dhalhana Su.Chi.37/109)

Should be administered in the morning time.

(c) Position of the Patient

सृष्टाविण्मूत्रवेगस्य पीठे जानुसमे मृदौ। ऋजौः सुखोपविष्टस्य हृष्टे मेढ्रे...॥ (Ch.Si.9/53)

After voiding the urges of mala and mutra, patient should be seated on a knee high and soft seat in a straight and comfortable position. His phallus should be made erect.

(d) Preparation of Trolly for Uttara Basti

- Uttara basti yantra
- Lithotomy table
- Hole towel
- Cuscus speculum
- Sponge holding forceps
- Xylocaine jelly
- Medicine
- Kelley's pad
- Tray
- Tampoon
- Gauze pieces
- Cleaning agents

(e) Preparation of the Medicine and Fixation of Dose

Preparation of the Medicine

- Take the medicated oil in required quantity in a precleaned container
- Autoclave the oil along with all the required materials
  This description of uttara basti netra suggests the intravesicular/urethral administration of uttara basti. With this basti netra intraurethral administration may not be possible

The following may be taken as Uttara-Basti Netra for Urethral administration.

- Urinary rubber catheter no. 8 or 11

50 cc syringe (glass or dispersible) may be used as Basti Putaka.

Fixation of Dose

वयोबलदेहसत्वसात्म्यादिवशान्निरूप्य वा। (Arunadatta A.H.Su.19/73)

Dose should be fixed considering Vaya, Bala, Satva, Satmya etc.

Sneha :

Charaka	-	Ardhapala (24 mL)
Vagbhatta	-	1 Shukti (24 mL)
Sushruta	-	1 Prakuncha (1 pala) at the age of 25 years
Kashayap:	-	1 Prasrita (96 mL)

(2) Pradhana Karma

........................घृताक्तया। श्लोकयाऽन्विष्य गति यद्यप्रतिहता व्रजेत्।।
ततः शेफः प्रमाणेन पुष्पनेत्रं प्रवेशयेत्। गुदवन्मूत्रमार्गेण प्रणयेदनु सेवनीम्।।
हिंस्यात् अतिगतं बस्तिमूने स्नेहो न गच्छति। सुखं प्रपीडय निष्कम्पं निष्कर्षेन्नेत्रमेव च।। (Ch.Si.9/54-56)

After smearing the ghee, the probe should be inserted into urethra. If the probe can be passed without any obstruction, then the Basti Netra should be introduced according to the length of phallus in the same manner as that of Netra for Guda, i.e. carefully without shaking.

If it enters too far, it hurts and if insufficiently inserted, the medication will not reach the destination. Slowly medicine should be pressed in.

After pressing, without shaking it and without causing discomfort Netra should be withdrawn.

(3) Pashchat Karma

प्रत्यागते द्वितीयं च तृतीयं च प्रदापयेत्। (Ch.Si.9)
ततः प्रत्यागतस्नेहमपराह्णे विचक्षणः। भोजयेत् पयसा मात्रां यूषेणाथ रसेन वा।। (Su.Chi.37/113)

After the medicine has returned, a second and third enema should be given. In the evening considering the Dosha, Ksheera, Yusha or Mansa Rasa has to be taken.

Medhod of Administration (for Female)

It is divided in to 3 steps which are as follows:

1. Purva Karma

(a) Preparation of the Patient

Same that of male.

(b) Time of Administration

स्त्रीणामार्तवकाले तु प्रतिकर्म तदाचरेत्। गर्भासना सुखं स्नेहं तदाऽऽदत्ते ह्यपावृता।। (Ch.Si.9/62)

Ritukala is the apt time for the administration of uttara basti, as during this period the yoni or garbhashaya will be avaranarahita, thus receives the drug easily, i.e. does Snehana easily. However, it can be administered other than ritukala in anrutavapi and atyayika conditions like Asirgdhara, Yonishula, etc.

(c) Position of the Patient

उत्तानायाः शयानायाः सम्यक् सङ्कोच्य सक्थिनी। (Ch.Si.9/67)

Patient should be made to lie down in supine position with well flexed thighs.

2. Pradhana Karma

अथास्याः प्रणयेन्नेत्रमनुवंशगतं सुखम्। (Ch.Si.9/68)
सम्यक् प्रपीडयेत् योनिं दध्यात् सुमृदुपीडितम्।। (Su.Chi.37/115)

Basti netra should be administered gently in the direction of vertebral column. Medicine should be administered into the Yoni by gently pressing the Putaka. Like this 2, 3 or 4 enema should be administered in the course of day and night.

3. Pashchat Karma

Same as that of male. Procedure should be repeated after an interval of 3 days.

Observations

Basti Pratyagamana Kala

बस्तिर्मात्राशतादूर्ध्वं प्रत्यागच्छति अनागच्छति वर्ति पायौ नाले प्रदापयेत्।। (Su.Chi.37/117)

The uttara basti dravya pratyagamana is 100 matrakala. In the absence of uttara basti dravya pratyagamana one may wait and neglect. If it is upadravakari it has to be expelled using teekshna uttara basti.

Chikitsa for Apratyagamana

A. Kashaya of shodhana dravya is used as niruha basti in the dose of 1 and 2 prasrita in mutra and yoni marga respectively.
B. Shodhana dravya siddha phala varti.
C. Probe is inserted in mutramarga and abdomen is pressed forcefully below the umbilicus.
D. Varti of size of mudga, ela, sarshapa should be prepared by triturating aragwadha patra with nirgundi patra swarasa, gomutra and saindhava lavana and dried in shade. This varti is smeared with ghee and inserted into mutamarga with the help of shalaka.
E. Sthula varti of 4 angula prepared out of above said drugs is placed in yoni marga to achieve the returning of sneha.

Complication and its Management

शर्करामधुमिश्रेण शीतेन मधुकाम्बुना।दह्यमाने तदा बस्तौ दद्यात् बस्तिं विचक्षणः॥
क्षीरवृक्षकषायेण पयसा शीतलेन च॥ (Su.Chi.37/123-124)

If Daha is present after the administration of Uttara Basti then

- Sharkara + Madhu mixed in Sheeta Kashaya of Yashti Madhu
- Ksheera Vriksha Sheeta Kashaya + Ksheera for Basti

In practise, complications found can be categorized as:

Immediate : 1. Shock
2. Pain

Late : 1. Peritonitis
2. Infection

- Shock (Neurological): Neurological shock may be due to the forceful insertion of rubber catheter in urethra and in spinchter of urinary bladder or a patient in anxious mood. This condition needs immediate resuscitation or else may be life-threatening.
- Pain (Spasmodic): Pain may be due to the forceful insertion in urethra. It is usually self limiting and if necessary antispasmodics can be given.
- Peritonitis: If the medicine is forcefully pushed it may spill in to peritoneal cavity leading to inflammation there.
- Infection: The source of infection may be either through the improper sterilization of the instrument or medicament or poor aseptic precautions during the procedure. This condition may require a course of antibiotic therapy and a good nursing care.

Uttara Basti Currently in Practice

Mutrashayagata Uttara Basti

Requirements

- ❑ Table for administration
- ❑ Cleaning agents like savlon, betadine etc.
- ❑ Sponge holding forceps and artery forceps
- ❑ Sterile gauze, Surgical towel and towel clips
- ❑ Sterile gloves
- ❑ Anesthetic jelly (Xylocaine 2% - 1 tube)
- ❑ Urinary rubber/disposable catheter No. 6-8
- ❑ Aspiration syringe, 30 mL capacity (disposable)
- ❑ Steel bowl of 30–50 mL capacity
- ❑ Kidney tray - 1
- ❑ Medicated oil, decoction or ksheerapaka selected according to the condition
- ❑ Autoclave facility

Preoperative Procedure

- ❑ All the instruments used during the procedure including the medicine have to be autoclaved and kept ready.

- Patient is examined for the parameters like BP, pulse, temperature, etc. before he is put to table
- Patient must lie down on supine position on the clean table by exposing the part. The hands are flexed and clasped below head
- Wash the genitalia and the surrounding area with savlon by using sponge holding forceps and gauze. Retract the prepuce completely and wash thoroughly the glans penis and then apply Betadine to glans penis
- The physician should wear the gloves after washing hands spread the surgical towel over patient, exposing the penis. Towel clips may be applied
- When once the assistant transfers the autoclaved medicine into steel bowel the medicine is filled into the syringe. Fix the catheter to the nozzle of the syringe, push the oil to the tip of the catheter.

Operative Procedure

- Lubricate the catheter with the Xylocaine jelly. Gently introduce the catheter into the urethra; slowly introduce the catheter into the bladder
- Ensure that the catheter has entered the bladder, and then slowly inject the medicine into the bladder. If more amount of medicine has to be injected clamp the catheter with artery forceps, remove the syringe and then inject the medicine with the same syringe or by another.

Post-operative

- When once the injection of medicine is over remove the catheter and allow the patient to lie down in the same position for 5 to 10 minutes, and then patient may be sent home. Check the tip of the catheter to ensure that there is no bleeding.

Garbhashayagata Uttara Basti

The mode of administration of drugs either in sneha or kashaya form through vagina to uterus as a therapeutic measure is called as garbhashayagata uttara basti.

This description of uttara basti netra suggests the intra vaginal administration of uttara basti. With this basti netra intrauterine administration may not be possible.

The following may be taken as uttara basti netra for intrauterine administration.

- Infant feeding tube (with the tip cut to a length of about 10 cm)
- IV cannula
- Intrauterine insemination cannula
- Urinary rubber catheter no. 11 or 12
- A 100 cc syringe (glass or dispersible) may be as basti putaka.

Preoperative

- Yoni prakshalana should be done with suitable antiseptic lotion/kashaya.
- All the instruments used during the procedure including the medicine have to be autoclaved and kept ready.

- The patient is examined for the parameters like BP, pulse, temperature, etc. before she is put to table.

Operative

- Then the patient is kept in lithotomy position with the part exposed, cleaned and draped.
- The part is covered with the ring towel and only the perineum is exposed.
- Later the lubricated cusco's speculum is slowly inserted to expose the cervix. Cervix and the surrounding areas are cleaned with suitable antiseptic lotions.
- The direction of the uterus can be understood by the insertion of uterine sound which opens the os if it is closed. In case of closed internal os, Hegar dilator may be used.
- The autoclaved dravya is then taken in the basti yantra. The netra (cannula or infant feeding tube) is carefully introduced to the uterus through the cervix (after removing the air bubble) and the dravya is pushed in slowly taking 2 - 3 minutes.

Postoperative

The patient has to lie down for 30 minutes in head low position.

Probable Mode of Action of Uttara Basti

Mode of action of Uttar Basti lies not only in the Pradhana Karma but also in its Purva Karma.

Mode of action of Purva Karma in Uttara Basti

Snehana and Svedana are very important procedures and are used as both, the Pradhana Karma as well as Purva Karma of several Panchakarma procedures. Snehana and Svedana are very efficient and multifaceted procedures, but the current discussion deals with its efficacy as an adjuvant to Uttara Basti only. Though, classics have not specifically emphasized much upon Snehana and Svedana before Uttara Basti, but this approach seems to be genuine and appropriate. Uttara Basti deals mainly with the Apana Vayu, as the nearby situated organs are its seat. Snehana and Svedana prior to Utttara Basti does its Anulomana and thus, Uttara Basti becomes more efficacious. Besides this, chances of any type of complication are also less, if Vatanulomana is done prior to procedure. Other than it, Snehana and Svedana just prior to Uttara Basti relax the abdominal muscles. Good relaxation is very important for Uttar Basti, so that uterus does not get irritated by the instillation of medicine from outside. If it is not relaxed adequately, it may contract at once and may not retain any of the medicine. Snehana and Svedana before Uttara Basti also lessen the pain during and after procedure. Yoni Prakshalana done prior to Uttara Basti with Kvatha of antiseptic property nullifies the possibility of any type of infection as a complication.

Pradhana Karma

Mode of action of Uttara Basti can be understood in two ways:

Local effect of Uttara Basti

Effect of Uttara Basti will depend on various points like method, instrument, drug used, etc. If medicine is put in cervical canal, it may act more on the cervical factors. For the factors like cervical stenosis, a Katu-Ushna Taila based medication can be more useful, while for increasing the secretion of mucous from cervical glands, a nutritive and Madhura - Shita Ghrita based medicine will be more efficacious. In the same way, drug selection for ovulatory and tubal factor will be totally different from each other. On ovary, the effect of drug will be after absorption and then by promoting the Hypothalamic - Pituitary - Ovarian axis, while in tubal block, Uttara Basti acts locally. In ovulation, a drug with Snehana property can be good while for tubal block, a drug with Lekhana Karma will be better. Advantage of intrauterine instillation of oil is proved in modern science also as it is said that approximately 30% of the patients who have normal hysterosalpingography, conceive over the following 6 months and it was thought to be a characteristic of only oil- based contrast medium. Apart from this, Uttara Basti may also stimulate certain receptors in the endometrium leading to correction of all the physiological processes of reproductive system. It may also help in rejuvenation of endometrium. Thus, mode of action of Uttara Basti can be understood in the following ways:

- Intravaginal Uttara Basti helps in removing the infections, if given with antiseptic drugs.
- Intravaginal Uttara Basti may also facilitate the absorption of drug as posterior fornix has a very rich blood supply and it may also act as reservoir of drug.
- Intracervical Uttara Basti with oil based drug helps to remove the cervical stenosis and to restore the function of cervix in conception and helps to treat dysmenorrhoea caused by stenosis.
- Intracervical Uttara Basti with Brihana drugs may stimulate the secretion of cervical mucous leading to ascent of sperms in uterine cavity.
- Intrauterine Uttara Basti with Ghrita based Snehana and Brihana drugs helps in rejuvenation of endometrium, especially where apart from regular ovulation, poor endometrium is causing infertility or scanty menstruation.
- In cases of menorrhagia due to hyperplastic endometrium, intrauterine Uttara Basti with Lekhana Dravyas may help.
- For tubal factor of infertility, a high intrauterine Uttara Basti with Lekhana dravyas acts in two ways. It removes the blockage of tubal lumen by directly acting on obstruction mechanically and restores the normal function of tubal cilia by stimulating it. As endometrial covering is continuous in the tubes too, its scraping and regeneration of also leads to normalization of tubal functions.

Systemic Effect of Uttara Basti After Absorption

It seems that Ayurveda had a clear distinguishing approach between oral and parenteral route of drug administration from the very beginning. Thus, Acharyas have described the administration of drug from almost all the possible route and have considered the Basti (rectal administration) the most efficacious. On the same pattern, Uttara Basti can also act after getting absorbed from rich blood circulation of uterus and posterior fornix. Then, it may act on whole body system and can act as a parenteral route. On ovlulatory factor and certain other gynecological disorders related to Bandhyatva, it may act by stimulating some neuroendocrine pathways after getting absorbed.

Systemic effect of Uttara Basti can also be understood with the help of system biology concept. System biology is the latest concept emerging and getting accepted in modem science. This concept believes in the holistic approach similar to as advocated in Ayurveda from the very beginning. It considers the need of a paradigm shift of modem science from reductionist to holistic. It believes that all the bodily systems and organs are interconnected at molecular level. And any change in any organ on molecular level will certainly change the other. This concept actually is the first step of modern science towards the concept of Mahabhuta and Tridosha. Ayurveda also considers whole the body as one unit on Mahabhuta level. Still, Tridosha and Mahabhuta are something broader, but more abstract than molecule which will be explored in modern science too in coming future. Even then it is clear that whatever the effect Uttara Basti drugs have on the physiology of reproductive system, it will definitely involve the physiological functions and corrections of other systems.

MATRA BASTI

Matra basti is a type of sneha basti. It is termed so because of the dose of sneha used in it is very less compared to the dose of sneha basti. The term' "matra", gives various meanings in different context, such as measurement, quantity, size, duration, number, degree, movement, unit of time. In the present context the term matra gives the meaning for the unit of measurement, i.e. For the quantity of basti dravya.

ह्स्वया स्नेहपानस्य मात्रया योजितः समः। मात्राबस्तिः स्मृतः स्नेहः ....॥ (A.H.19/67)

Acharya Vagbhatta has defined Matra basti as the Basti in which the dose of Sneha is equal to Hrasvamatra of Snehapana.

Indications

कर्म व्यायाम भाराध्वयान स्त्री कर्षितेषु च। दुर्बले वातभग्रे च मात्राबस्तिः सदा मतः॥ (Ch.Si.4/52)

बाल वृद्धाध्वभर स्त्री व्यायामासक्त चिन्तकैः। वातभग्नबलाल्पाग्निनृपेश्वरसुखात्मभिः॥

(A.H.Su.19/67-68)

S. No.	Indications	Ch.	A.H.	A.S.
1.	Karmakarshita	+	-	-
2.	Bharakarshita	+	+	+
3.	Adhvakarshita	+	+	+
4.	Vyayamakarshita	+	+	+
5.	Yanakarshita	+	-	+
6.	Streekarshita	+	+	+
7.	Durbala	+	+	+
8.	Vata Rogi	+	+	+
9.	Bala	-	+	+
10.	Vriddha	-	+	+
11.	Chintatura	-	+	+
12.	Stree	-	-	+

Contd...

Contd...

S. No.	Indications	Ch.	A.H.	A.S.
13.	Nripa	-	+	+
14.	Sukumar	-	-	+
15.	Alpagni	-	+	+
16.	Sukhatma	-	+	-

Contraindications

तथापि तौ नाजीर्णे योज्यौ न च दिवास्वप्नः सेव्यः॥ (A.S.Su.28/8)

Matra basti should not be administered in the persons having Ajirna, and who indulges in Divasvapna.

Time of Administration

सेव्यः सदा च माधुतैलिकवत्। (A.S.Su.28/8)
सर्वकालं निरत्ययः। (Ch.Si.4/53)

Ashtanga Sangraha, emphasizes regular administration of Matra basti and it can be administered at all times and in all the seasons like Madhutailika Basti.

Dose of Matra Basti

According to Vagbhatta, Matra basti is recommended in the dose equal to the dose of Hrasva Snehamatra. The Matra which gets digested in 2 Yama, i.e. 6 hours is called as Hrasva Matra of Snehapana.

According to Chakrapani, the dose of Sneha basti is 6 Pala, dose of Anuvasana Basti is 3 Pala and that of Matra basti is 1 Pala.

Kashyapa prescribed the quantity of Matra basti as 2 palas as Uttamamatra, 1 pala as Madhyama matra and 1 Prakuncha as Hrasva matra. He even stated that half Pala of Sneha can be given in newborn baby; it can be administered without any hesitation and complication.

Composition of Matra Basti

Shatahva and Saindhava lavana can be added with sneha of matra basti in the proportion of 6 g, 4 g and 2 g for maximum, medium, and minimum quantities of Sneha. The therapeutic effect of Basti will be higher by adding this kalkas. It helps in increasing the Vata shamana property of the sneha dravya.

Increment Dosage of Matra Basti

कनीयसी यस्य मात्रा सार्धा पलमात्रन्विता तस्य प्रथममर्धपलोचितं।
ततो वृद्धिरष्टमाषकैरेव नवभिर्दिनैः सार्धपलं स्यात्॥ (Sha.Sam)

Adamalla commentator of Sharangadara Samhita explained the dosage of Matra basti for 9 days in increment order by increasing 6 mL every day. Even Vangasena and Chakradatta has explained the same concept of increment dosage of matra basti.

DAYS	1	2	3	4	5	6	7	8	9
Quantity of Matra Basti in mL	24	30	36	42	48	54	60	66	72

Administration of Matra basti: Same like that of Anuvasana Basti.

Benefits of Matra basti

दोषघ्नो निष्परीहारो बल्यः सृष्टमलः सुखः॥ (A.H.Su.19/67-68)

यथेष्टाहारचेष्टस्य सर्वकालं निरत्ययः। बल्यं सुखोपचर्यं च सुखं सृष्टपुरीषकृत्।

स्नेहमात्राविधानं हि बृंहणं वातरोगनुत्॥ (Ch.Si.4/52-54)

There will not be restrictions for taking any food and one can indulge in any activities, can be given at any time and its free from complications.

Matra basti promotes strength, demands no strict regimen of diet, causes easy elimination of feces and urine, nourishes the body and cures Vata disorders.

Importance of Matra Basti

We can summarize the importance of Matra Basti by considering its advantages by following points:

It can be given to Bala, Vriddha, Sukumara, Stree, and everybody. There are no restrictions of Vihara; even one can perform routine works after administration of Matra Basti. It does not give any complications as other Basti. Even though Matra is less it has widespread action throughout the body. Niruha Basti and Anuvasana Basti can be administered alternatively, but Matra Basti alone can be administered everyday continuously without any complications.

Matra basti has no restrictions as of Asthapana and Anuvasana. Matra basti can be administered any time irrespective of age, day, and time. No such Ahara sevana krama is explained before or after the administration of matra basti. Matra Basti improves Varna and Bala, and is indicated for Bala, Vriddha, and Alpagni persons.

No need of Parihara kala after administration of Matra basti. It acts as Varnya, doshaghna, etc. It can be administered to Durbala Purusha where other Bastis are contraindicated. It eliminates vitiated Doshas along with Mala from the body. It acts as Shodhana, Shamana, Brihana, Vatahara and even Balya. (Ch.Si.4/52-54)

Important Factors

Other than the factors that have to be assessed before administration of the Basti that is told in the classics, one has to observe and consider some other factors in today's context.

Temperature

Temperature is an important factor .The temperature of the Basti Dravya should be maintained from 36 to 40° Celsius which is an optimum temperature. If the Basti is given at more than this temperature then there may be fear of burning of the intestinal mucosa and if the Basti is given in the lesser temperature then the fear of more retention will be there which is not the purpose what we are looking for as far as the Niruha Basti is concerned.

Position of the Patient

वामाश्रये हि ग्रहणी गुदे च तत् पार्श्व संस्थस्य सुख उपलब्धिः।
लीयन्त एवं वलयश्च तस्मात् सव्यं शयानोऽर्हति बस्तिदानम्॥ (Ch.Si.3/24-25)

In the classics, the position that has to be followed is left lateral. Charaka has given explanation that Grahani and Guda are coming in the same direction. Therefore, one has to follow the same position.

Logical thinking says that only in the left lateral position due to the gravitation the drugs may enter into the colon. In the medial side, the middle rectal valve is there which controls the sphincter continence which may get injured when the enema is given in the right lateral position. However, in cases like situs inversus and dextrocardia totalis the administration of the Basti in right lateral position may be considered.

Niruha Prior to Anuvasana Basti

स्नेहबस्तिर् विधेयस्तु न अविशुद्धस्य देहिनः। स्नेह वीर्यं तथा दत्ते च अनुविसर्पति॥ (Su.Chi.37/6)
निरुह शोधितान् मार्गान् सम्यक् स्नेहो अनुगच्छति। अपेत सर्प दोषासु नाडिषु इव वहज्जलम्॥
सर्वदोषहरश्च असौ शरीरस्य च जीवनः। तस्माद् विशुद्धदेहस्य स्नेहबस्तिर् विधियते॥
(Su.Chi.35/19-20)

The Sneha Basti should not be given to unpurified person because for the proper absorption and circulation of active principle (Virya) of the medicated oil in the body, it is necessary that channels should be cleaned by purificatory Basti.

अशुद्धमपि वातेन केवलेन अपि पीडीतम्। अहो रात्रस्य कालेषु सर्वेषु एषु अनुवासयेत्॥ (Su.Chi.37/43)

But in some cases where the patient is suffering from excessive and pure Vata, Anuvasana Basti can be given directly without prior administration of Niruha Basti.

In such condition, Anuvasana Basti can be given at any time even in night where generally it is contraindicated. In such case as well as when the patient is having excessive dryness then first 2 or 3 Anuvasana should be given and when the patient becomes unctuous then Niruha Basti may be given for purification. In such conditions Niruha Basti may be given by adding excessive quantity of the Sneha.

त्रिन् पंच वाऽऽहुश्चतुरो अथ षड्वा वात अधिकानम् अनुवासनीयान्।
स्नेहान् प्रदायाशु भिषग् विदध्यात् स्त्रोतो विशुध्यर्थम् मतो निरुहान्॥ (Ch.Si.1/49)

Also, after giving 5 or 6 Anuvasana Basti continuously or when proper Snehana of the body is achieved by it, then it is necessary to administer Niruha for Shodhana. Niruha Basti and Anuvasana Basti can also be given on the same day. For this purpose Niruha is given in the forenoon and when it returns, the patient is allowed to take his meal.

In the evening when the ingested meal is digested properly, then again the patient is asked to take light meal in little quantity and then Anuvasana Basti is given by using medicated oil from sour and Vatahara drugs.

For Vata disorders, the oil should be prepared with Bilva.
For Pitta disorders with the drugs of Jivaniya group or Yashtimadhu and
For Kapha disorders, it should be prepared with Madanaphala.

स्नेह बस्तिं निरुहं वा न एकमेव अतिशीलयेत्। स्नेहाद् अग्निवधो उत्क्लेशौ निरुहात् पवनात् भयम्॥
तस्मात् निरुढो अनुवास्यो निरुहाश्च अनुवासितः। नैवं पित्त कफ उत्क्लेशौ स्यातां न पवनाद् भयम्॥
(Su.Chi.37/78)

Anuvasana or Niruha basti should not be given alone continuously for a longer period. Because if Anuvasana alone is given for a longer period then the impairment of Agni and nausea occurs. On the other hand Niruha taken continuously for a longer period may lead to the vitiation of Vata. Therefore, Anuvasana should follow the Niruha and Niruha should follow Anuvasana and in that case there will be no fear of vitiation of Vata, Pitta or Kapha.

एकं तथा त्रीन् कफजे विकारे पित्तात्मके पंच तु सप्त वाऽपि।
वाते नवे एकादश वा पुनर्वा बस्तिन् युग्मान् कुशलो विदध्यात्॥ (Ch.Si.1/25)

However, in the Ruksha persons, the Anuvasana can be given in smaller dose for a long time, While in unctuous persons, Niruha can be given in the smaller dose for a long period. In Kapha disorders 1 or 3 Anuvasana, for the Pitta 5 or 7 Anuvasana and for Vata 9 or 11 Anuvasana Basti are advised. Generally, it is advisable to administer Anuvasana in odd numbers.

INDICATION OF BASTI IN DIFFERENT DISEASES ACCORDING TO CHARAKA

S. No.	*Name of the Disease*	*Basti indicated*	*Reference*
1.	Jvara	Patoladi basti, Argavadhadi Niruha Guduchyadi Niruha	Chi.3/240-241
2.	Jvara	Anuvasana basti: Jiventyadi Anuvasana, Patoladi Anuvasana, Chandanadi Anuvasana	Chi. 3/250-253
3.	Punaravartaka Jvara	Yapana basti	Chi.3/339
4.	Gulma	Basti is best treatment	Chi. 5/100
5.	Pittaja Gulma	Kshira basti	Chi. 5/34
6.	Kushtha	Niruha and Anuvasana basti	Chi. 7/46
7.	Vatodara	Dashmula Niruha Eranda taila Anuvasana	Chi. 13/63 Chi. 13/65
8.	Pittodara	Kshirabasti	Chi. 13/68, 71
9.	Baddhodara	Trikshana Niruha with Gomutra	Chi. 13/89
10.	Plihodara	Niruha and Anuvasana basti	Chi. 13/77
11.	Arsha	Piccha basti	Chi. 14/255-229
12.	Atisara (Gudabhransha)	Anuvasana with Dashmula, Bilvadi taila, Satavryadi taila	Chi. 19/49
13.	Raktatisara	Piccha basti	Chi. 19/98,99
14.	Trimarmiya	Niruha and Uttar basti (Muttrakricchra)	Chi. 26/45
15.	Vatavyadhi (Avarana Vata)	Yapana basti	Chi. 26/219
16.	Vatarakta	Basti should be use repeatedly	Chi. 29/41
17.	Yoni vyapada	Uttar basti with Trivrita sneha	Chi. 30/119

CHAPTER 7

Nasya Karma

INTRODUCTION

As discussed earlier, Sanshodhana chikitsa in ayurveda is primarily dependent upon Panchakarma therapies. We have already learnt about various ways to cleanse the Urdhva Bhaga by Vamana, adho bhaga by virechana and to an sarvanga extent vata everywhere by basti. Even then there is still a part of body left which does not get treated completely with these sanshodhana therapies which is above jatru i.e. Uttamanga or Shiras. To cure the diseases occurring in the shiras region medicine is administered through nasal orifices and is known as Nasya Karma.

Ayurveda is such a system of medicine where the importance of both prevention and cure are highlighted. As per Ayurvedic texts, diseases are deep seated at different Dhatu levels. Hence, a procedure should be there to uproot the deep seated disease. The Tridoshas are the main causative factors in the pathogenesis of any disease. Specific management for specific doshas has been elaborated in all Ayurvedic texts e.g. Vamana is done for shodhana of Kapha, virechana for Pitta and Basti for Vata.

The importance of Panchakarma lies in the fact that it helps in uprooting the disease and bringing the vitiated doshas to their original places. The main logic behind the manifestation of any disease in terms of Doshas moving from Koshtha to Shakha and bringing them back to Koshtha is one of the main principles of Panchakarma procedures laid down in the Ayurvedic texts. A skillful vaidya is the one who knows about the Tridosha concept along with Dosha-Dushya Sammurchchhana. The advantage of Panchakarma goes to the fact that it enables to cleanse off the doshas at minute levels. The preference of knowing the manifestation of a disease at every level is of utmost importance in controlling the disease. As Sushruta says:

संचयेऽपहृता दोषाः लभन्ते नोत्तरा गतिः। तेत्तूत्तराषु गतिषु भवन्ति बलवन्तराः॥ (Su.Su.21/36)

Urdhvajatrugata Rogas and their management have a special place in Ayurveda. Shirah being the prime seat of knowledge and also the prime controller of the entire body has been termed as Uttamanga.

ऊर्ध्वजत्रु विकारेषु विशेषान्नस्यमिष्यते। नासा हि शिरसो द्वारम् तेन तद्व्याप्यहन्तिान्। (A.H.Su. 20/2)
नस्तः कर्म च कुर्वीत् शिरोरोगेषु शास्त्रवित्। द्वारं हि शिरसो नासा....... ॥ (Ch.Si. 9/88)

Nasa is considered to be that Indriya, whose functions are not only limited to respiration but is also considered as a pathway for drug administration. In Ayurveda, special procedure called Nasya has been mentioned. The Acharyas have also said-"नासा हि शिरसो द्वारम्", because Nasa is indirectly connected with the brain centers in the head. Perfect balance of oxygen levels in the body can be attained with Nasya Karma, thereby also clearing all the morbid Doshas.

ETYMOLOGY

The word Nasya Karma is composed of two words Nasya and Karma.
Nasya : 'Nas' is substituted for Nasa when it is followed by the suffix 'Yath'.
Nasika + Yath = Nasadeshancha
Nasikaayaihitam – Nasya

नासिकाये हितं तत्र भवोवायत् नासादेशः। (Vachaspatyam)

According to Vachaspatyam the word 'Nastah' means beneficial for the nose.

The word Nasya is derived from 'Nasa' Dhatu which conveys the sense of Gati-motion (Nasa Gatau).

The literal meaning of the word Nasya is being in the nose or the things beneficial to the nose.

According to Shabdakalpadruma

नासिकायायैः हितं इति नस्यः।
नासिकादेयचूर्णादि।
नासाद्वारादेयौषधविशेषा।

DEFINITION

औषधं औषध सिद्धोवास्नेहो नासिकाभ्यां दीयते इति नस्यम्। (Su.Chi. 40/21)

Administration of medicine (drug) or medicated oil through the nose is known as Nasya.

नस्यमिति नासया दीयते इति नस्यम्॥ (Sha.Ut.8/1. Adamalla)

Administration of medicine through the nose is known as Nasya.

नासायां प्राणीयमानौषधं नस्यम्। नावनं नस्तः कर्मेति च संज्ञा लभते॥ (A.S.Su.29)

Administration of medicine through the nasal route is known as Nasya. It is also known as Navana or Nasta Karma.

Synonyms

Shirovirechana **Shirovireka** **Murdha virechana**	Indicates its main function; elimination of morbid Doshas from parts above the clavicle.
Navana **Nasta karma**	Denotes the site of administration and the measures which are beneficial to the nose.

SIGNIFICANCE OF NASYA KARMA

The main aim of Panchakarma is to remove the Doshas through the easiest/nearest route.

द्वारं हि शिरसो नासा तेन तद् व्याप्य हन्ति तान्। (Ch.Si.9/88)

Nasa is said to be the door of the Shiras. Medicine administered through the nose, spreads through the Shiras and helps in the evacuation of Dosha, thereby pacifying the diseases. Nasya Karma is the main line of treatment for diseases above the clavicle and it is the only Shodhana Karma for Urdhvanga. Along with these, Nasya Karma has the following benefits:

- Can be used even in Unconscious patients.
- Promotion of health as a part of Dinacharya.
- Rapid drug absorption via highly vascularised mucosa.
- Avoiding the gastrointestinal tract and first-pass metabolism
- Improved bioavailability
- Lower side effects

CLASSIFICATION OF NASYA

All the Acharyas have classified Nasya in different way but sum total of classification is that all are practically the same. Mainly classified according to its function and on the basis of use of preparation for the Nasya e.g. Churna, Sneha etc. The classification according to Charaka, Sushruta and Vagbhatta in details are as follows:

According to Charaka's Classification of Nasya. It is of five types viz. Navana, Avapida, Dhmapana, Dhuma and Pratimarasa. (Ch.Si.9/89-92)

नावनं चावपीडश्च ध्मापनं धूम एव च। प्रतिमर्शश्च विज्ञेयं नस्तः कर्म तु पञ्चधा। (Ch. Si 9/89-92)

Classification of Nasya

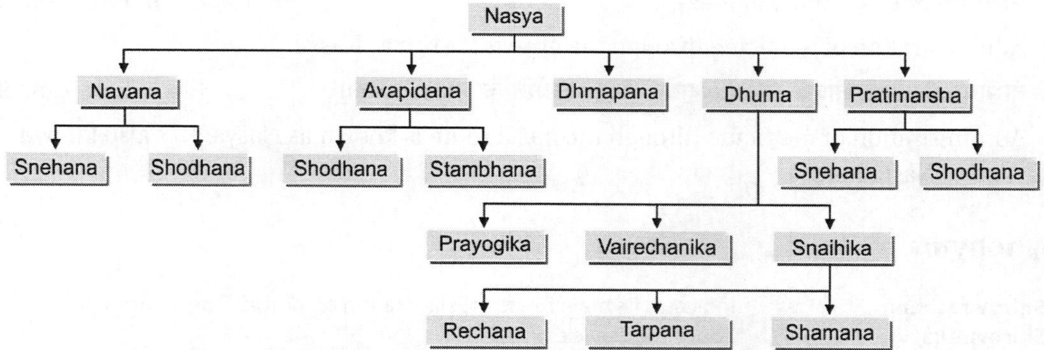

Navana is further divided into Snehana and Shodhana, Avapidana into Shodhana and Stambhana, Dhuma into Prayogika, Vairechanika and Snaihika while Pratimarsha is divided into Snehana and Shodhana.

The above mentioned five types of Nasya are regrouped according to their function into three groups viz. Rechana, Tarpana and Shamana. (Ch.Si. 9/89-92)

Charaka has also mentioned 7 types of Nasya according to parts of the drugs to be used in Nasyakarma viz.- Phala, Patra, Mula, Kanda, Pushpa, Niryasa, Twaka. (Ch.Vi. 8/154)

Classification of Nasya

1. Navana, Avapidana, Dhmapana, Dhuma, Pratimarsha
2. Snehana, Shodhana, Prayogika, Snaihika, Vairechanika
3. Shodhana, Stambhana, Snehana, Virechana.

According to Action of Nasya therapy

- ❑ Rechana, Tarpana, Shamana

On the basis of Parts used in Nasya

- ❑ Phala, Patra, Mula, Kanda, Pushpa, Niryasa, Twaka

Classification of Nasya According to Sushruta

According to Sushruta Nasya is also of 5 types Viz. Nasya, Avapida, Pradhamana, Shirovirechana and Pratimarsha. These 5 types of Nasya are further classified according to their functions into two groups viz. Shirovirechana and Snehana.

तद् द्विविधम् शिरोविरेचनं स्नेहनं च। तद् द्विविधमपि पञ्चधा तद्यथा–नस्यं, शिरोविरेचनं, प्रतिमर्शः अवपीडः प्रधमनं च॥ (Su.Chi 40/21)

Shirovirechana, Avapida and Pradhamana are used for Shirovirechana. i.e. for the elemination of morbid doshas from Shira, Pratimarsha and Nasya type may be used for Snehana. (Su.Chi. 40/21)

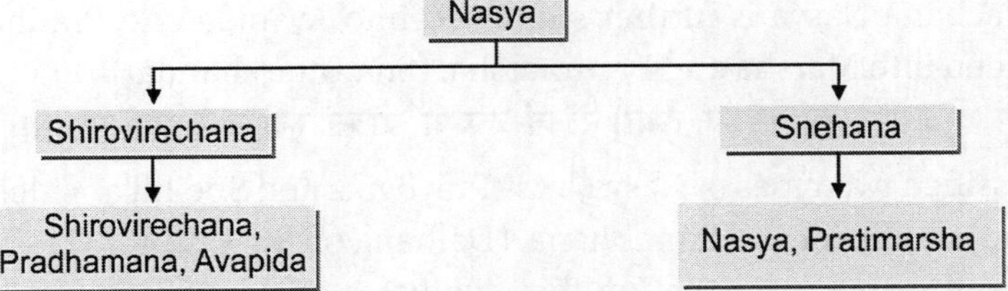

Vagbhatta's Classification of Nasya

Ashtanga Samgraha has mainly classified Nasya according to the functions viz. Virechana, Brihana and Shamana. Snehana and Brihana Nasya have been further subdivided according to the doses into two groups i.e. Marsha and Pratimarsha.

विरेचनं बृहणं शमनं च तिधामपि तत्। (A.H.Su. 20/2)

Avapida nasya may be given for both Virechana and Shamana while Pradhamana Nasya is given only for Shirovirechan.

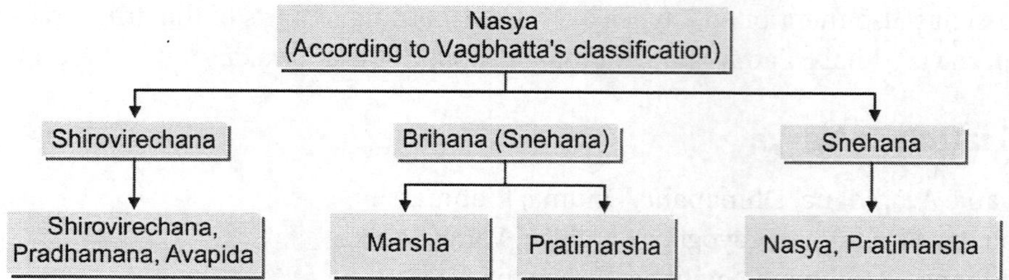

Ashtanga Hridaya has mainly classified Nasya in 3 types viz. Rechana, Brihana and Shamana.

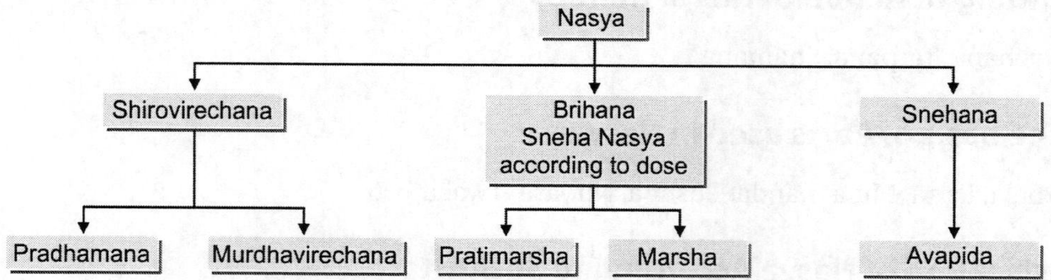

Kashyapa's Classification of Nasya

According to Kashyapa Samhita Nasya has been classified into two groups i.e. Brihana and Karshana. These two types are also known as: Shodhana and Purana Nasya.

बृहणं कर्षणं चैव द्विविधं नस्य कर्म तु। शोधनं पूरणं चैवं द्विविधं नस्यमुच्यते। (Ka.Si.2; Ka.Si.4)

Sharangdhara's Classification of Nasya

Sharangdhara has also classified Nasya according to the functions into two groups viz. Rechana and Snehana. Rechana Nasya is further subdivied into Avapida and Pradhamana. Snehana Nasya is subdivided into Marsha and Pratimarsha. (Sha.Uttarkhanda. 8/2, 11,24)

नस्य भेदो द्विधा प्रोक्तो रेचनं स्नेहनं तथा। रेचनं कर्षणं प्रोक्तं स्नेहनं बृहणं मतम्।।

Bhoja has classified two types of Nasya, viz - Prayogika and Sneihika. Videha has stated two types i.e. Sangyaprabodhaka and Stmabhana. (Dalhana on Su. Chi. 40/31)

It is clear from the above description that two types of classification of Nasya Karma are available in Ayurvedic literature. One is based on the pharmacological actions viz. Rechana, Tarpana etc. and the other is based on the preparation of drug and the method of its application e.g. Dhmapana (Powder is blowed), Avapida (Extracted Juice is used) and Dhuma (inhalation of medicated smoke through nose) etc.

GENERAL DRAVYA USED FOR NASYA

A large-number of drugs have been indicated for nasya karma in Charaka.

(Ch.Su.2/3-5), (Ch.Vi.8/154), (A.H.15/4), (Su.Su.39/6) etc.

अपामार्गस्य बीजानि पिप्पलीर्मरिचानि च। विडङ्गान्यथ शिग्रूणि सर्षपांस् तुंबरूणि च।।

अजाजीं च अजगन्धा च पीलून्येलां हरेणुकाम्। पृथ्वीकां सुरसां श्वेतां कुठेरक फणिज्झकौ।।
शिरीषबीजं लशुनं हरिद्रे लवणद्वयम्। ज्योतिष्मतीं नागरं च दद्यात् शीर्षविरेचने।। (Ch.Su.2/3-5)

Name of the dravya	*Botanical Name*
Apamarga (Fig. 7.1)	*Achyranthes aspera*
Pippali (Fig. 7.2)	*Piper longum*
Maricha (Fig. 7.3)	*Piper nigrum*
Vidanga (Fig. 7.4)	*Embelia ribes*
Shigru (Fig. 7.5)	*Moringa oleifera*
Sarshapa (Fig. 7.6)	*Brassica campestris*
Ajaji (jiraka) (Fig. 7.7)	*Cuminum cyminum*
Tumburu (Fig. 7.8)	*Zanthoxylum alatum*
Ajagandha (Fig. 7.9)	*Gynandropsis gynandra*
Pilu (Fig. 7.10)	*Salvadora persica*
Ela (Fig. 7.11)	*Elettaria cardamomum*
Harenuka (Fig. 7.12)	*Vitex negundo*
Pruthvika (Fig. 7.13)	*Ammomum subulatum*
Surasa (Fig. 7.14)	*Ocimum sanctum*
Shweta (Fig. 7.15)	*Clitoria ternaka*
Phaningaka (Fig. 7.16)	*Riven hypocrateri formis*
Shirisha (Fig. 7.17)	*Albizzia lebbek*
Lashuna (Fig. 7.18)	*Allium sativum*
Haridra (Fig. 7.19)	*Curcuma longa*
Daruharidra (Fig. 7.20)	*Berberis aristata*
Saindhava lavana (Fig. 7.21)	*Sodium chloride*
Jyotishmati (Fig. 7.22)	*Celastrus paniculatus*
Shunthi (Fig. 7.23)	*Zingiber officinalis*

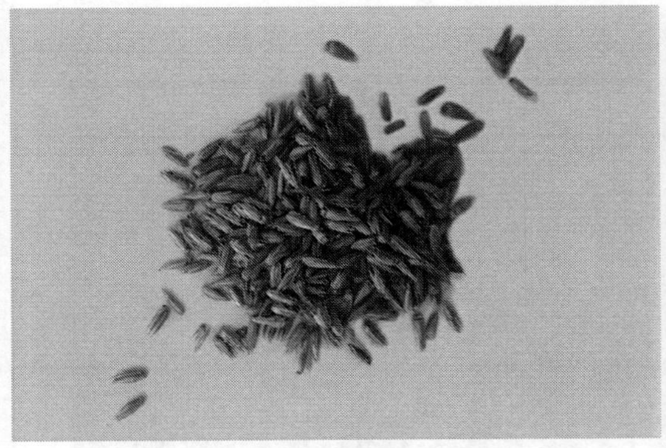

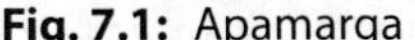

Fig. 7.1: Apamarga

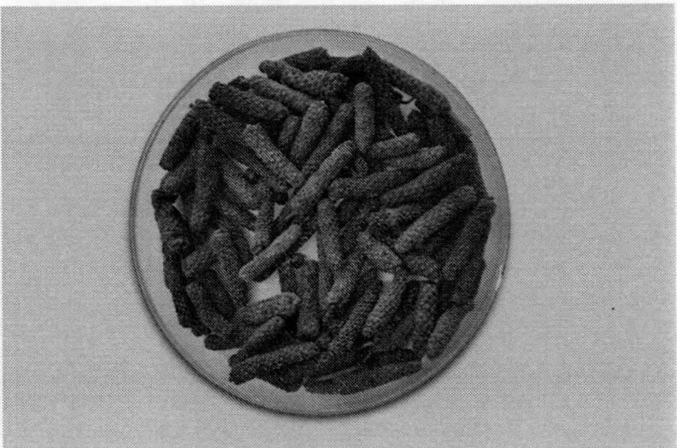

Fig. 7.2: Pippali

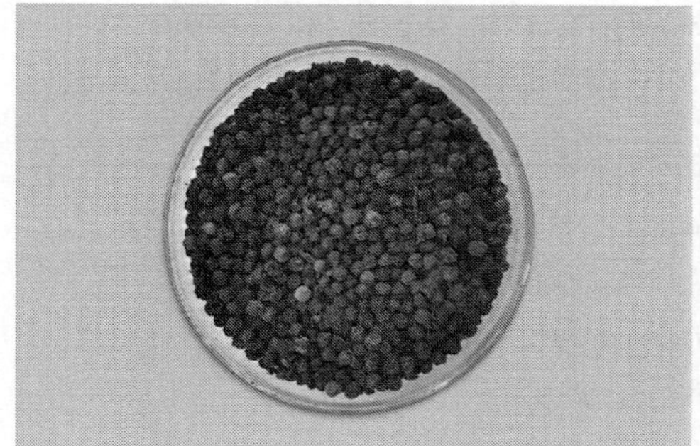

Fig. 7.3: Maricha

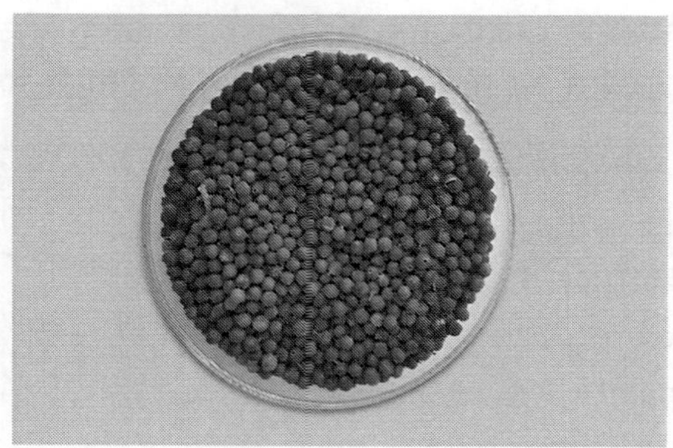

Fig. 7.4: Vidanga

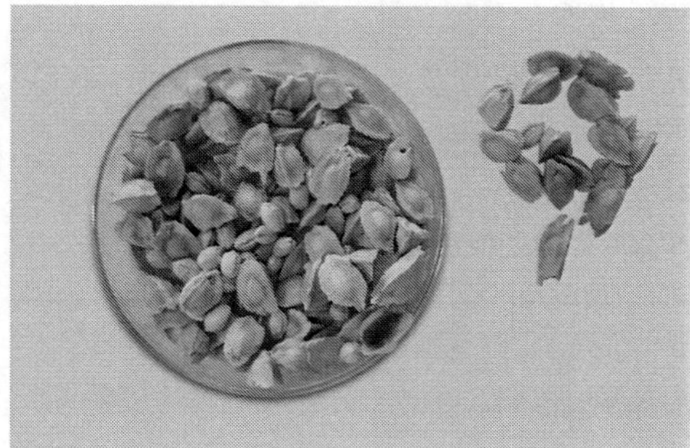

Fig. 7.5: Shigru

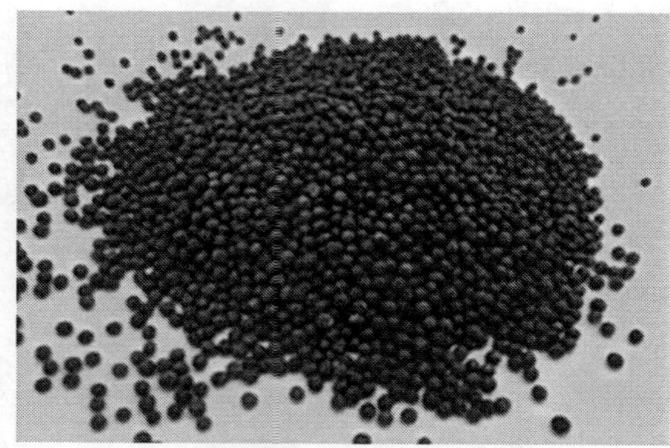

Fig. 7.6: Sarshapa

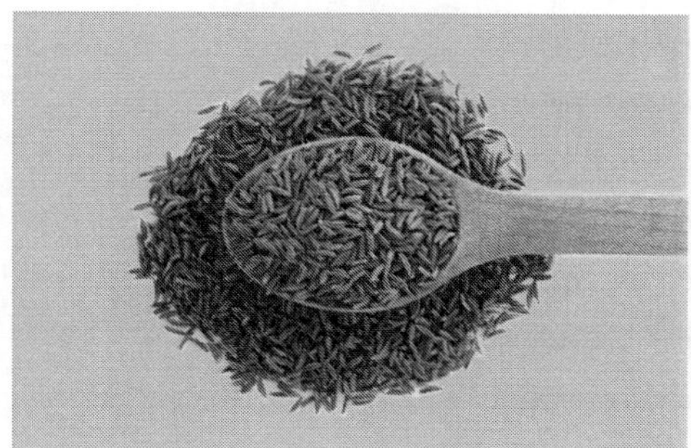

Fig. 7.7: Ajaji (jiraka)

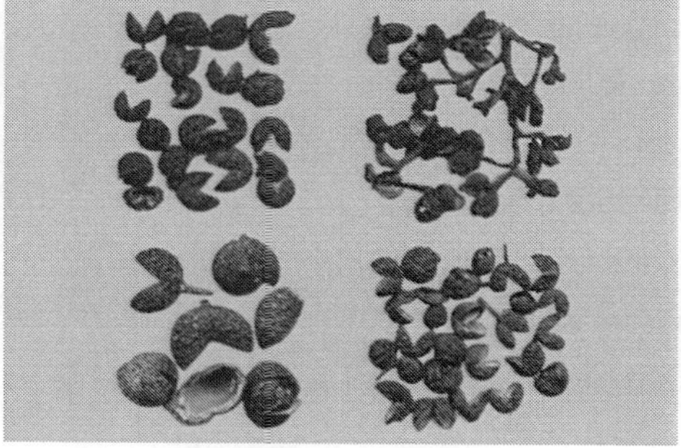

Fig. 7.8: Tumburu

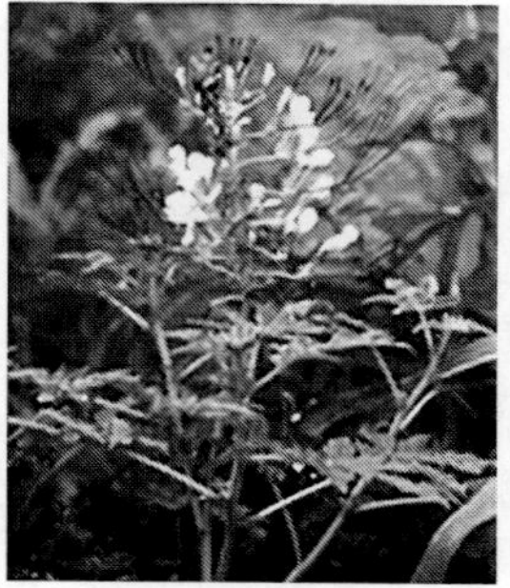

Fig. 7.9: Ajagandha

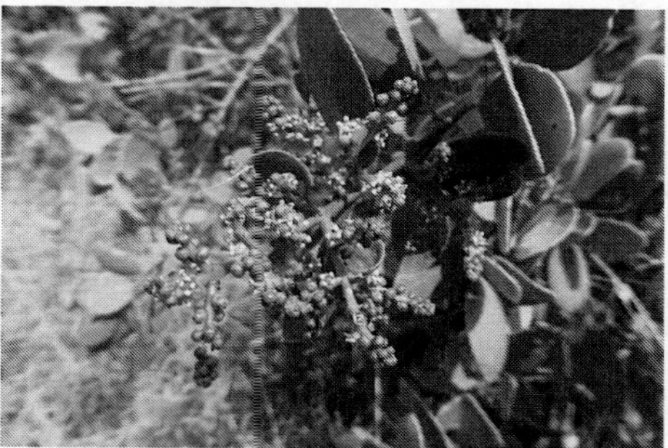

Fig. 7.10: Pilu

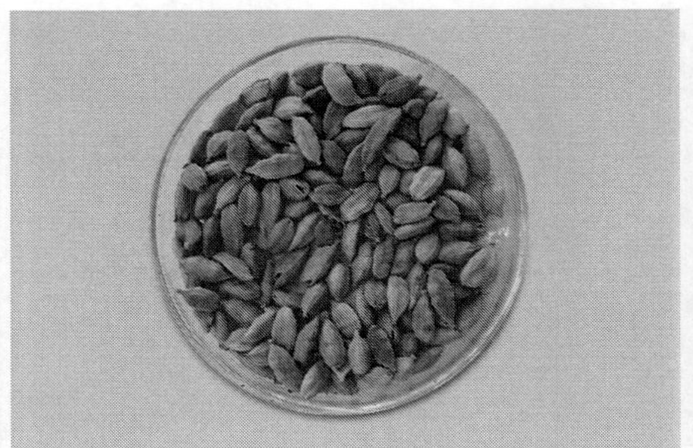
Fig. 7.11: Ela

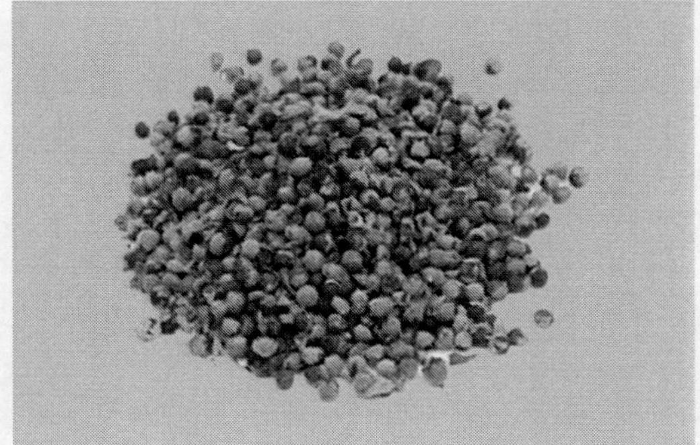
Fig. 7.12: Harenuka

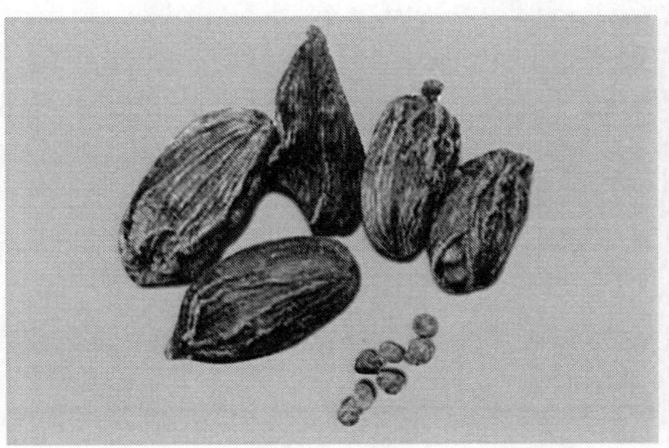
Fig. 7.13: Pruthvika

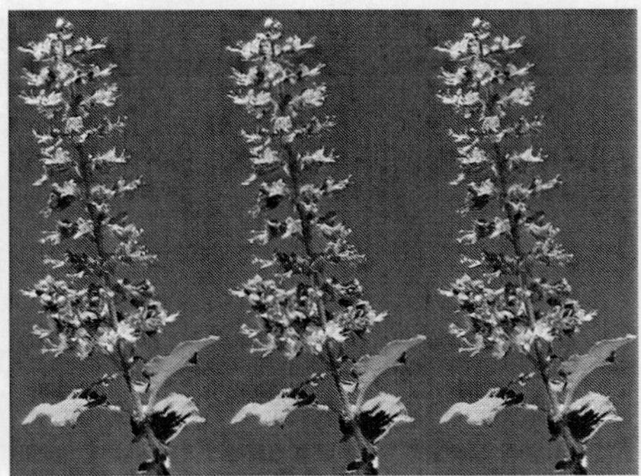
Fig. 7.14: Surasa

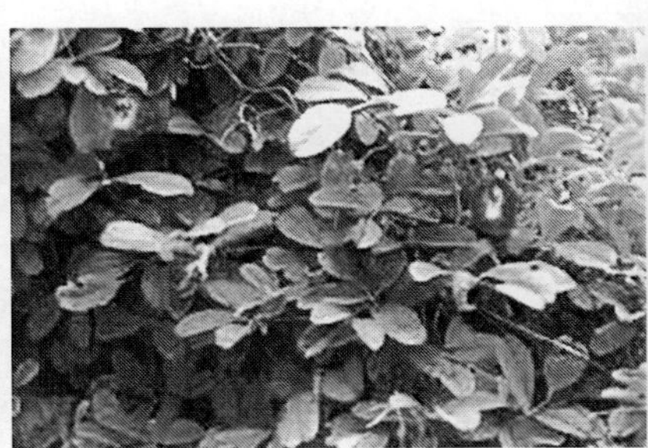
Fig. 7.15: Shweta

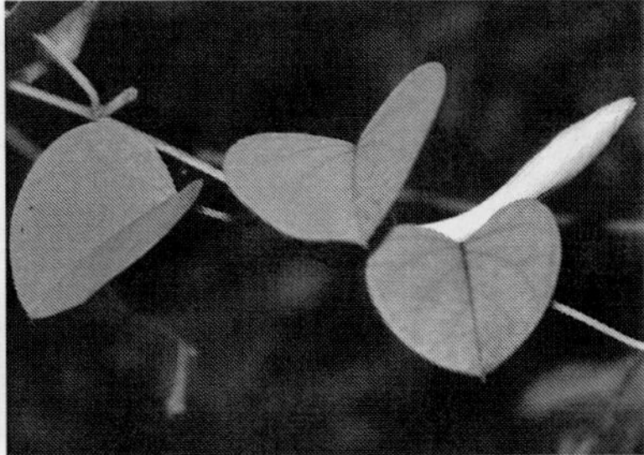
Fig. 7.16: Phanijaka

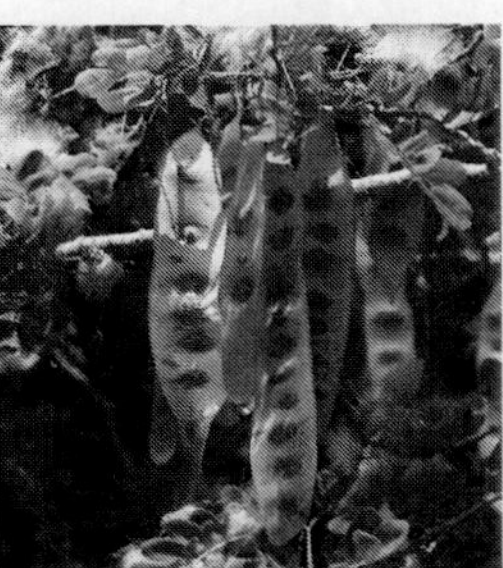
Fig. 7.17: Shirisha

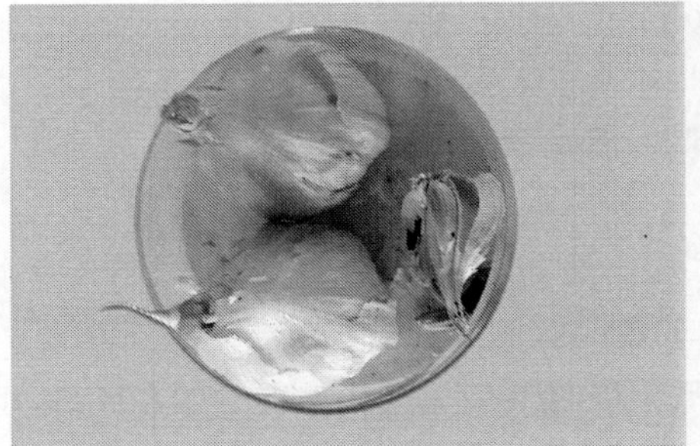
Fig. 7.18: Lashuna

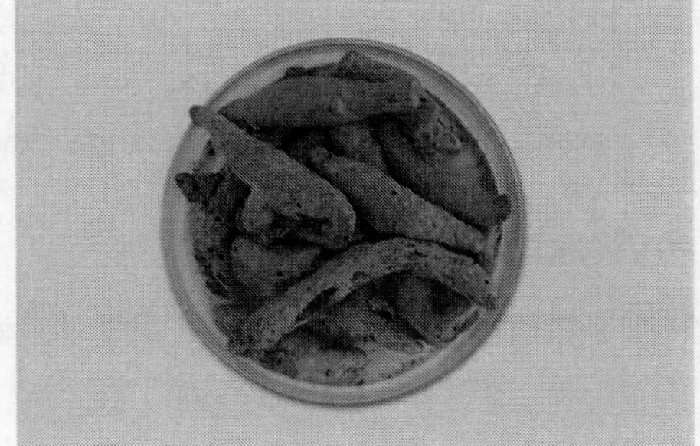
Fig. 7.19: Haridra

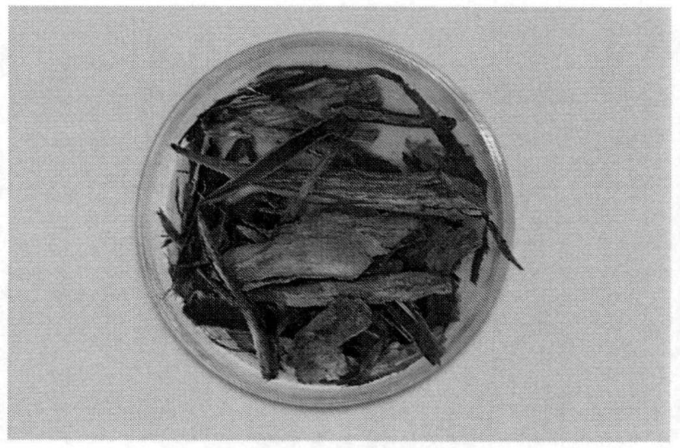

Fig. 7.20: Daruharidra

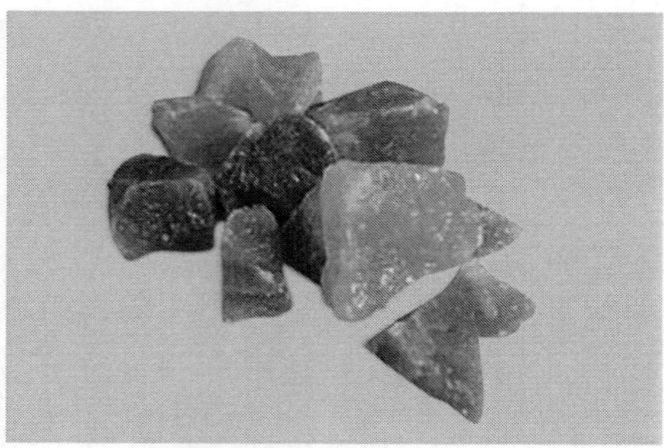

Fig. 7.21: Saindhava lavana

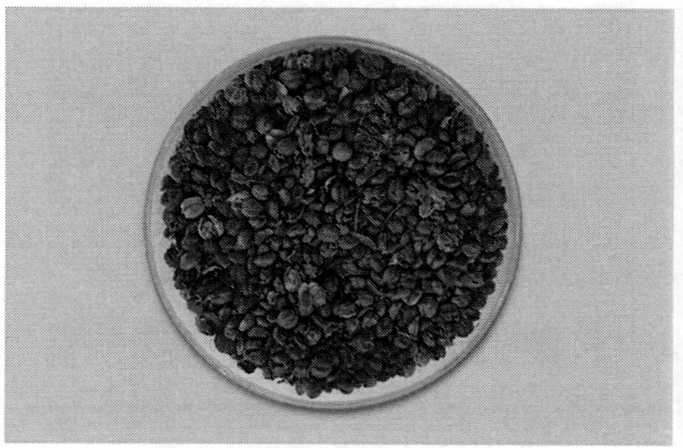

Fig. 7.22: Jyotishmati

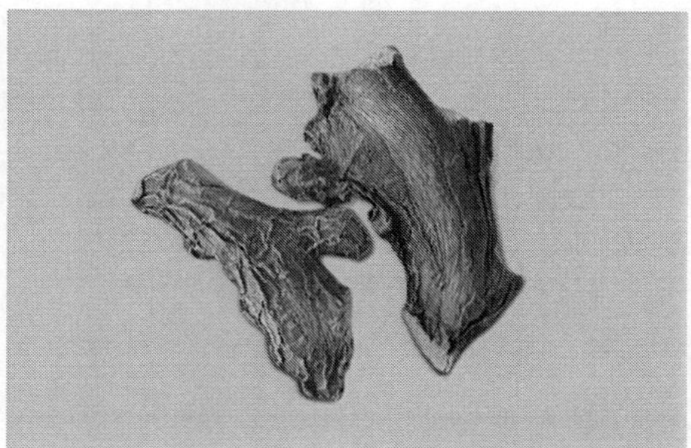

Fig. 7.23: Shunthi

Shirovirechana Dravya according to useful part: (Ch. Vi.8/151)

S.No.	*Useful part*	*Name of the drugs*
1.	Phala (fruit)	Apamarga, Pippali, Maricha, Vidanga, Shigru, Shirisha, Tumburu, Pilu, Ajaji, Ajamoda, Vartaka, Pruthvika, Ela, Harenuka.
2.	Patra (leaves)	Sumukha, Surasa, Kuteraka, Gandeera, Kallamalaka, Parnasa, Kshvaka, Phanijaka, Haridra, Shringavera, Mulaka, Nata, Tarkari, Sarshapa.
3.	Mula (root)	Arka, Alarka, Kushta, Nagadanti, Vacha, Apamarga, shweta, Jyothishmati, Gavakshi, Gandeera, Vakpushpi, Vushika,Ativisha.
4.	Kanda (tuber)	Haridra, Shringavera, Mulaka, Lashuna.
5.	Pushpa (flower)	Lodhra, Madana, Saptaparna, Nimba, Arkapushpa.
6.	Niryasa (resin)	Devadaru, Agaru, Sarala, Shallaki, Jingini, Asana, Hingu.
7.	Twak (bark)	Tejovati, Varanga, Hingu, Shobhanjana, Bruhati, Kantakari.

Shirovirechana Gana

वेल्ला अपामार्ग व्योष दार्वी सुराल बीजं शैरीषं बार्हतं शैग्रव च।
सारो मधुकः सैन्धवं तार्क्ष्यशैलं त्रुटयौ पृथ्वीका शोधयन्तु उत्तमाङ्गम्।। (A.H.Su.15/4)

Vella (vidanga), Apamarga, Vyosha, Darvi, Surala (Sarjarasa); Shirisha beeja, Bruhati Beeja, Shigru Beeja; Madhuka Sara, Saindhava, Tarkshyashaila (Rasanjana), Trutyou (Sukshma and sthula ela),Pruthvika (Hingu).

Shirovirechanopaga Dravya

ज्योतिष्मती क्षवक मरिच पिप्पली विडङ्ग शिग्रु सर्षप अपामार्गतण्डुल श्वेता महाश्वेता
इति दशेमानि शिरोविरेचनोपगानि भवन्ति।। (Ch.Su.4/13)

S. No.	Drug	Bootanical Name
1.	Jyotishmati	*Celastrus paniculatus*
2.	Kshavaka	*Centipada minima*
3.	Maricha	*Piper nigrum*
4.	Pippali	*Piper longum*
5.	Vidanga	*Embelia ribes*
6.	Shigru	*Moringa oleifera*
7.	Sarshapa	*Brassica campestris*
8.	Apamarga	*Achyanthes aspera*
9.	Sweta	*Utonia teraka*
10.	Mahasweta	*Albizzia procera*

INDICATIONS AND CONTRAINDICATIONS

Indications

In general Nasya Karma is useful in the disorders of organs situated above the clavicle. It is particularly indicated in the following conditions:

विशेषतस्तु शिरो दन्त मन्यास्तम्भ गल हनुग्रह पीनस गलशुण्डिक शालूक
शुक्रतिमिर वर्त्मरोग व्यङ्ग उपजिह्विक अर्धावभेदक ग्रीवा स्कन्ध अंसास्य नासिका
कर्णाक्षि मूर्धकपाल शिरोरोगा अर्दित अपतन्त्रक अपतानक गलगण्ड दन्तशूलहर्षचल
अक्षिराजि अर्बुद स्वरभेद वाग्ग्रह गद्गद क्रथनादय ऊर्ध्वजत्रुगताश्च वातादिविकाराः
परिपक्वाश्चः एतेषु शिरोविरेचनं प्रधानतमम् इत्युक्तं।। (Ch.Si.2/22)

Shiro, Danta, Manya Stambha, Galagraha, Hanugraha, Peenasa, Galashundika, Galashaluka, Shukla roga, Timira, Vyanga, Upajihwika, Ardhavabhedaka, Greeva, Ansa, Asaya, Nasika, Kama, Akshi, Murdha, Kapala, Shiroga, Apatantraka, Apatanaka, Galaganda, Danta Shula, Dantaharsha, chala, Akshiraji, Arbuda, Swarabheda, Vakgraha, Gadgada, Krathana, Urdhvajatrugata Vatadi Vikara

Shiro roga	Ardhavabhedaka (migraine), Shirostambha
Netra roga	Akshiraji (congestion of eyes), Shukla roga, Timira (cataract), Vartma roga (disease of eyelid)
Danta Roga	Danta Shula (tooth ache), Dantaharsha (sensitivity), Dantastambha, Dantachala (loose tooth)

Mukha Roga	Upajihwika
Speech disorders	Swarabheda (hoarseness of voice), Vakgraha (difficulty in speech), Gad-gada (spasmodic speech), Krathana
Kantha Roga	Galaganda (goitre), Galagraha, Hanugraha, Galashundika, Galashaluka
Samanya Roga	Greeva (Neck), Amsa (Shoulder), Asya (Oral Cavity), Nasika (Nose), Karna (Ear), Akshi (Eye), Murdha (Head), Kapala Shiroroga, Urdhvajatrugatavata vikara, Vyanga (Moles), Peenasa (Rhinitis)
Other	Arbuda (Tumour), Apatanaka (Contractions), Apatantraka (Convulsions), Manyasthambha (Spasm of neck)

Indications of Nasya

Nasya therapy may be given in all diseases except in the conditions mentioned earlier. The specific indications of Tarpana Nasya, Shodhana Nasya, Shamana Nasya, Shirovirechana, Navana, Avapida, Dhmapana and Dhuma Nasya etc. have already been discussed in the classification of Nasya, but Charaka had described the following general indications where Nasya therapy should be used.

1. Shirostambha
2. Manyastambha
3. Danta Stambha
4. Danta Shula
5. Hanugraha
6. Peenasa
7. Galashundika
8. Galashaluka
9. Shukra Roga
10. Timira
11. Vartmaroga
12. Vyanga
13. Upajihvika
14. Ardhavabhedaka
15. Grivaroga
16. Skandharoga
17. Ansashula
18. Mukharoga
19. Karnashula
20. Nasa Shula
21. Akshishula
22. Shirashula
23. Ardita
24. Apatantraka
25. Apatanaka
26. Galaganda
27. Danta Harsha
28. Danta Chala
29. Raji-Netra Roga
30. Arbuda
31. Svarabheda
32. Vaggraha
33. Gadgadatva
34. Krathana etc.

According to Ashtanga Sangraha if the Nasya is to be given as the part of performing the complete Panchakarma then, it should be given after Bastikama.

Contraindications

Anasyarha	*Charaka*	*Sushruta*	*Vagbhatta*	
1.	Bhuktabhakta	+	+	+
2.	Ajirna	+	+	+
3.	Pita Sneha	+	+	+

Anasyarha	*Charaka*	*Sushruta*	*Vagbhatta*	
4.	Pita Madya	+	+	+
5.	Pita Toya	+	+	+
6.	Snehadi Patukamah	+	-	+
7.	Snatah Shirah	+	-	+
8.	Snatukamah	+	+	+
9.	Kshudharta	+	-	+
10.	Shramarta	+	+	-
11.	Matta	+	-	-
12.	Murcchita	+	-	-
13.	Shastradandahrita	+	-	-
14.	Vyavayaklanta	+	-	-
15.	Vyayamaklanta	+	+	(Shranta)-
16.	Panaklanta	+	-	-
17.	Navajvara Pidita	+	-	-
18.	Shokabhitapta	+	-	-
19.	Virikta	+	-	+
20.	Anuvasita	+	+	+
21.	Garbhini	+	+	+
22.	Navapratishyayarta	+	-	-
23.	Apatarpita	-	+	+
24.	Pitadravah	-	+	+
25.	Trishnarta	+	+	-
26.	Gararta	-	+	+
27.	Kruddha	-	+	-
28.	Bala	-	+	-
29.	Vriddha	-	+	-
30.	Vegavarodhitah	-	+	+
31.	Raktasravita	-	-	+
32.	Sutika	-	-	+
33.	Shvasapidita	-	-	+
34.	Kasapidita	-	-	+

Reasons for Contraindications

Condition	*Reason*
Ajeerni and Bhuktabhakta	Obstructs the Urdhvavahasrotas and causes Kasa, Shvasa, Chhardi, Pratishyaya.

Peetasneha, Madya Toyapaatukama	Causes excessive discharge from Mukha, Nasa and causes Timira and Shiroroga
Shirah snata, Krute cha Snana	Causes Pratishyaya
Kshudharta	Causes Vata Prakopa
Trishnarta	Increases Trishana and causes dryness of mouth
Vyavaya, Vyayama, Pana Klanta	Affects Shira, Skandha, Netra and Uras
NavaJvara, Shokabhitapta	The heat spreading in the vessels in the eyes, will cause Timira and Jvara.
Shastra, Dandahata	Increases pain
Virikta	Indriya Upaghata
Anuvasita	Causes Shirogurutva, Kandu, Krimi Dosha
Garbhini	Causes Garhastambha
Anritu and Durdina	Causes diseases due to cold, Puti nasa Shiroroga

TIME OF ADMINISTRATION OF NASYA

प्रावृट् शरद्वसन्तेतरेष्वात्ययिकेषु रोगेषु नावनं कुर्यात् कृत्रिमगुणोपधानात्:, ग्रीष्मे पूर्वाह्णे, शीते मध्याह्णे, वर्षास्वदुर्दिने चेति। (Ch.Si.2/23)

Pravrit, Sharada, Vasanta Ritu and during emergency it can be given in any season by creating artificial conditions of the required seasons. In Grishma, morning time, in cold season during afternoon and in Varsha Ritu when the sky is free from clouds.

तत्रैत द्विविधमपि अभुक्तवतो अन्नकाले पूर्वाह्णे श्लेष्मरोगिणां, मध्याह्णे पित्तरोगिणां, अपराह्णे वातरोगिणाम्॥ (Su.Chi.40/2)

Both types of Nasya i.e. Snaihika and Vairechanika should be administered during the time of meal in empty stomach.

Doshaja vikara	*Nasya*
Kaphaja	Morning
Pittaja	Afternoon
Vataja	Evening

प्रातः श्लेष्मणि, मध्याह्णे पित्ते, सायंनिशोश्चले। स्वस्थवृत्ते तु पूर्वाग्रह्णे शरत्काले वसन्तयो:॥
शीते मध्यंदिने, ग्रीष्मे सायं वर्षासु सातपे। वाताभिभूते शिरसि हिध्मायाम् अपतानके॥
मन्यास्तम्भे स्वरभ्रंशे सायंप्रातर्दिनेदिने॥ (A.H.Su.20114-15)

श्लेष्म	–	प्रात:काल (Morning)
पित्त	–	मध्याह्ण (Afternoon)
वात	–	सायं (Evening)
स्वस्थ	–	पूर्वाह्ण (Morning) in Sharad and Vasanta Rutu
शीते	–	मध्यन्दिने (Afternoon)
ग्रीष्मे	–	सायं (Evening)
वर्षा	–	आतप (During the presence of sunlight)

Daily morning and evening: Vataprakopa in Shiras, Hikka, Ayama, Apatanaka, Manyastambha and Swarabhramsha.

लालास्त्राव सुप्त प्रलाप दन्तकटकटायन क्रथन कृछ्रोल्मीलन पूतिमुख कर्णनाद
तृष्णार्दिते शिरोरोग श्वास कासोन्निद्रेषु रात्रौ॥ (A.S.Su.29/16)

During Night : Lalasrava, Supti, Pralapa, Dantakatakatayana, Krathana, Krichronmilana, Putimukha, Karnanada, Trishna, Shiroroga, Shvasa and Kasa.

Course of Nasya Karma

Nasya Karma may be given for seven consecutive days. In conditions like Vata Dosha in head, hiccup, torticollis, loss of voice etc. It may be done twice a day (in morning and evening). (A.H.Su. 20/16).

The use of Nasya on 3rd, 5th, 7th and 8th day or till the patient shows the symptoms of Samyak Nasya as stated in Ashtanga Sangraha (A.S. Su. 29/16). Bhoja says that if Nasya is given continuously beyond nine days then it becomes Satmya (adaptable) to patients and if given further, it neither benefits nor harm to the patients.

According to Sushruta, Nasya may be given repeatedly at the interval of 1, 2, 7 and 21 days depending upon the condition of the patient and the diseases he suffer (Su. Chi. 40/42, 43). Charaka has not mentioned specific duration of the Nasya therapy, but suggested to give according to the severity of diseases.

DOSE OF NASYA KARMA

The dose of Nasya is calculated in terms of Bindu pramana. In the context of Nasya, Bindu doesn't mean a drop. It is as follows:

प्रदेशिन्यङ्गुली पर्वद्वयान् मग्र समुद्धृतात्। यावत्पतत्यसौ बिन्दु ....॥ (A.H.Su.20)

The amount of oil that falls, when two phalanges of the index finger is dipped into oil and taken out is termed as Bindu.

S.N.	*Type of Nasya*	*Matra in Bindu Pramana in one nostril*		
		Avara	*Madhyama*	*Uttama*
1.	Shamana Nasya	8	16	32
2.	Shodhana Nasya	4	6	8
3.	Marsha Nasya	6	8	10
4.	Avapida Nasya	4	6	8
5.	Pratimarsha Nasya	2	2	2
6.	Pradhamana	3 Muchyuti (the churna which will come in between index finger and thumb is 1 muchuti).		

Sharangadhara has described the following dosage schedule for Nasyakarma (Sha.Ut.8/9-10).

Nasya Doses	
Tikshnaushadhi	1 Shana (4 masha)
Hingu	1 Yava
Saindhava	1 Masha
Dugdha	8 Shana
Jala (aushada siddha)	3 Karsha
Madhuradravya	1 Karsha

One bindu is equal to 0.5 mL, one yava is 1/6th of shana (0.5 g), one masha-2 g, one karsha is 12 g.

PATHYA-APATHYA

रजोधूम स्नेह आतप मद्य द्रवपान शिरःस्नान अतियान क्रोधादीनि च परिहरेत्। (Su.Chi.40/31)

Pathya	*Apathya*
Laghu Ahara,	Rajo
Sukhoshna Jala	Dhuma
	Sneha
	Atapa
	Madya
	Dravapana
	Shirasnana
	Atiyana
	Krodha
	Divaswapna

ADMINISTRATION OF MARSHA, PRATIMARSHA, AVAPEEDAKA NASYA AND DHUMAPANA ETC.

The procedure of administration of Nasya can be divided into 3 steps :

A. Purva Karma
B. Pradhana Karma
C. Pashchat Karma

Purva Karma

1. Selection of the patient : Before posting a patient for Nasya Karma one should check whether the patient is fit or unfit for the treatment.

2. Examination of the patient: Patient should be examined according to Deshadi factors.
3. Sambhara Sangraha:

i.	Medication for Nasya	-	Q.S
ii.	Oil for Abhyanga	-	Q.S
iii.	Oil and Churna for Talam	-	Q.S
iv.	Cotton pad, gauze, lotus petals to protect eyes during Svedana.		
v.	For Svedana	-	Boiling water, towels or Nadi Svedayantra
vi.	Gokarna yantra	-	2 (for instilling medicine)
vii.	Warm water for Kavala	-	Q.S
viii.	Dhumavarti (Prayogika, Snaihika, Vairechanika)		

4. Preparation of the Patient

स्निग्ध स्विन्न उत्तमाङ्गस्य प्राक्कृतावश्यकस्य च। निवात शयनस्थस्य जत्रूर्ध्वं स्वेदयेत् पुनः॥ (A.H.Su.20/17)

After evacuating the natural urges like urine and feces, the patient is advised to wash the face and mouth with luke warm water. He should be given Abhyanga and Sveda over Uttamanga.

He should be made to lie in a room devoid of breeze and fomentation should be given to parts above his shoulders.

5. Position of the Patient

उत्तानस्य शयानस्य शयने स्वास्तृते सुखम्। प्रलम्बशिरसः किञ्चित् पादोन्नतस्य च॥ (Ch.Si.9/99)
अथ उत्तानर्जुदेहस्य पाणिपादे प्रसारिते। किञ्चिद् उन्नतपादस्य किञ्चिन्मूर्द्धनि नामिते॥
(A.H.Su. 20/18)

The Patient should be made to lie straight in supine position extending his arms and legs, legs should be slightly raised and the head slightly extended up to 45 degree.

Pradhana Karma

नासापुटं विधायैकं पर्यायेण निषेचयेत्। उष्णाम्बुतप्तं भैषज्यं प्रणाडया पिचुनाऽथवा। (A.H.Su.20/19)
नासाम् उन्नाम्य वामेन अंङ्गुष्ठ पर्वणा। हस्तेन दक्षिणेनाथ कुर्यादुभयतः समम्॥
प्रणाडया पिचुना वाऽपि नस्तः स्नेहं यथाविधि॥ (Ch.Si.9/102-103)
वस्त्राच्छादित नेत्राय वामहस्त प्रदेशिन्यग्र उन्नमित नासाग्राय विशुद्धस्त्रोतसि दक्षिणहस्तेन
स्नेहमुष्णाम्बुना प्रतप्तं रजत सुवर्ण ताम्र मणि मृत् पात्र शुक्तिनाम् अन्यतमस्थं
शुक्त्या पिचुना वा सुखोष्णं स्नेहं अद्रुतम् आसिञ्चेदव्य अवच्छिन्नधारं यथा नेत्रे न प्राप्नोति॥
(Su.Chi.40/25)

- After fulfilling all the pre requirements, eyes of the patient are covered with Chaturguna Vastra (four folded cloth).
- The medicament to be administered is placed in a vessel made of Suvarna (gold), Rajata (silver), Tamra (copper), Mrit Patra (small mud vessel) or Shukti (conch shell) and then made luke warm by placing it in a vessel containing hot water.
- Later, tip of patients nose is drawn upward by the Vama Pradeshni (left index finger), and with the Dakshina Hasta (right hand), the lukewarm medicament is instilled into both nostrils using Suktika or Pichu.

- The medicine is administered to both nostrils in an Avichinadhara (a continuous stream), one after the other, keeping one nostril closed while the other is instilled with medicine.
- The patient should remain relaxed during and after the time of administration of Nasya and has to avoid speech, anger, sneezing, laughing and excessive shaking of the head.

Pashchat Karma

दत्ते पादतल स्कन्ध हस्त कर्णादि मर्दयेत्। शनैरूच्छिद्य निष्ठीवेत् पार्श्वयोर् उभयोस्ततः।। (A.H.Su.20120)
आभेषज क्षयादेवं द्वि स्त्रिर्वा नस्यमाचरेत्।। (A.H.Su.20/20)
कृते च स्वेदयेद्धूय आकर्षेश्च पुनः पुनः। तं स्नेहं श्लेष्मणा साकं तथा स्नेहो न तिष्ठति।। (Ch.Si. 9/103)

The following regimen should be followed after the administration of Nasya.

- The Patient should lie in supine position for hundred Matrakalas.
- After administration of Nasya, the regions of ears, forehead, scalp, and cheek, nape of neck, shoulders, palms and sole are massaged.
- The Patient is asked to inhale the medicine with moderate force and to spit it through his mouth turning the head to either side alternatively without rising from the cot.
- Frequent fomentation is given till all the medicament is brought out and care is taken that no portion of the medicament is left behind.
- Depending on the type of Shuddhi, Dhumapana can be advised.
- Kavala with hot water is done to get the mouth and throat cleaned.

Rechana Nasya (Virechana Nasya)

The Rechana Nasya denotes to eliminations of vitiated Doshas from Urdhvajatrugata part of the body. Churns (powder) of the required drug or the Sneha prepared with the Shirovirechana drugs like Apamarga, Pippali, Maricha etc. may be used (Ch.Si.9/96-97). It may also be given with Snehs, Kvatha or Swarasa of Shirovirechana drugs or by dissolving these drugs in Madya, Madhu, Saindhava, Asava, Pitta and Mutra or mixed with the drugs specific for that diseases. (A.S.Su.29/5)

Indications

It is indicated specifically in Kaphaja type of Shiroroga like Stambha, Supti and Guruta of Shira. (Ch.Su.9/13). Sushruta and Vagbhatta have given its other indications as Shleshma. Abhivyapla in Talukantha and Shirokrimi.

Arochaka, Shula, Shirogaurava, Pinasa, Pratishyaya, Urdhvajatrugata Kaphaja Vikara (Su. chi.40/23). Urdhvajatrugata Shopha, Praseka, Vairasya, Arbuda, Dadru and Kotha (A.S. Su. 29/5).

- ❑ Rechana Nasya prepared in Sneha is particularly indicated to the afraid, women, weak and delicate patients.
- ❑ The patients of Galaroga, Sannipataja jvara, Atinidra, Manovikara, Abhishyanda Sarpadansha and Murccha may be given Shirovirechana Nasya with Kalka, Churna and Swarasa also, but if the immediate effects is required, then Churna (powder) should be used. (A.S.Su.29/6).

Tarpana Nasya

Tarpana Nasya of Charaka, Snehana Nasya described by Sushruta and Sharangdhara and Brinhana Nasya mentioned in Ashtanga Sangraha may be considered as the synonyms of each other. The Sneha prepared with Vatapittahara drugs should be used and the drugs of Madhura Skandha (Ch.Vi.8/139) may also be employed (Ch.Si. 9/97). According to Vagbhatta, Sneha prepared with Snigdha and Madhura drugs or with the drugs described useful for that particular disease should be used. Exudations of certain trees, meat soup and blood also may be administered. (A.S. Su. 29/6)

Indications

It is specifically used for Vatika Shiroroga, Dantapata, Keshapata, Damnaka and other Vatapittaja Roga. Sushruta also advised the use of Snehana Nasya for prompting the strength and increasing the vision power. It is also used for curing the Shirahkampa and Ardita. (Ch.Si. 9/94).

Shamana Nasya

As the name indicates, Shamana Nasya is used for the alleviation of Dosha situated in Shirah (head). Shamana Nasya has been described by Charaka and Vagbhatta only. It may be correlated with Snehana and Marsha- Pratimarsha. The Sneha prepared with the beneficial drugs may be used for Shamana Nasya.

Indications

It is used to stop bleeding in Raktapitta. (Ch.Si.9/95). It is also indicated in Akala Valita, Palita and Khalitya, Darunaka, Raktaraji, Vyanga and Nilika. Anutaila Nasya as a measure of Svasthavritta should be administered in Pravrit, Sharada and Vasant Ritu to promote the functions of eyes, ears and nose to prevent Khalitya and Palitya and other diseases like Manyastambha, Shirahshula, Ardita, Hanustambha, Pinasa, Ardhavabhedaka, Shirokampa and sudden onset of other disease which may occur in the Urdhvajatrupradesha.

Avapida Nasya

Definition

Avapeeda Nasya is a type of Nasya in which extracted juice from Kalka is used for instillation.

अवपीडय यत्र कल्कादीनि दीयन्ते इत्यवपीडः। (Ch.Si.9/90.Chakrapani)

Instillation of extracted juice of leaves or paste (Kalka) of required medicine is Avapida Nasya.

For this Kalka of different Shirovirechana drugs can be used like Pippali, Maricha etc.

कल्काद्यैरवपीडस्तु स तीक्ष्णैर्मूर्धरेचनः।

Avapida is from Kalkadi (Kalka, kvatha, Svarasa etc). It is teekshna Murdha Rechana and is a strong purgative to head.

Method

कल्कीकृताद् औषधाद्यः पीडितो निःसृतो रसः। सोऽवपीडः समुद्दिष्टः तीक्ष्णद्रव्यसमुद्भवः।। (Sha.Ut.8112)

Materials Required

1. Drugs in wet form like Patra, Kanda, Kashaya, other Drava Dravyas.
2. KhalvaYantra
3. Clean white cloth
4. Cotton/ clean cloth

Preparation of Medicine

- ❑ Clean drug is taken in a Khalva and triturated well to prepare a Kalka (paste).
- ❑ Prepared Kalka is placed in a clean white cloth and squeezed to get juice.
- ❑ If Kvatha is used then cotton/cloth is dipped in it and then it is squeezed.

Dose	Avara	4 Bindu
	Madhyam	6 Bindu
	Uttama	8 Bindu

Type of Dravya used	*Indications*
Shirovirechana dravya	Abhishyanda (increased Kapha and Medas), Sarpadashta, Visangya (unconscious)
Sharkara, Ikshurasa, Ksheera	Ksheera, Raktapitta
Ghrita, Mansarasa Kalka	Krisha, Durbala, Bheeru, Sukumara, Yoshita

Types of Avapida Nasya

1. Stambhana Nasya: For this type Ikshu rasa, Ksheera etc are used.
2. Shodhana Nasya: In this Shirovirechana dravyas like saindhava, pippali etc are used.

According to Videha– 2 types

1. संज्ञा प्रबोधन : Which arouses consciousness
2. स्तम्भन : Which checks intrinsic haemorrhage

Pradhmana or Dhmapana Nasya

Dhmapana or pradhmana is type of Nasya mainly used for the purpose of Shodhana.

.... प्रध्मानस्य तु। तत् षडङ्गुलया नाडया धमेच्चूर्णं मुखेन तु।। (Ch.Si.91/107)

The powder should be blown by mouth into nostril through a tube of 6 angula length.

Instrument and Method

.... युञ्ज्यात्तं मुखवायुना। षडङ्गुल द्विमुखया नाडया भेषजगर्भया।
स हि भूरितरं दोषं चूर्णत्वादपकर्षति।। (A.H.Su.20/8)

Materials Required

1. Six inches long pipe (or straw)
2. Fine powders of Shirovirechana dravyas, preferably obtained from micro-pulveriser or powder filtered with cotton cloth.

1st Method

- 2-3 pinch of fine powder is filled at the one end of the straw.
- Placing that end at the opening of nostril air is blown from the other end of the straw.

Dose: 3 Muchyuti matra (3 pinch)

2nd Method– According to Videha

शुक्तिप्रमाणं जिघ्रेद्वा बद्धं सूक्ष्मेण वाससा।।

One shukti (24 g) of fine powder is kept in a pottali of thin cloth and then patient is asked to inhale deeply, so that the subtle particles of medicine enter into nostrils.
Benefits– It expels out the Doshas in more quantity.

Indications

चेतोविकारकृमि विषाभिपन्नानां चूर्णं प्रधमेत्। (Su.Chi.40/44)
अत्यन्त उत्कटदोषेषु विसंज्ञषु च दीयते। चूर्णं प्रधमनं धीरैस्तद्धि तीक्ष्णतरं यतः।। (Sha. Ut.8/17)

Those suffering from: Cheto Vikara (mental disorder)
Krimi (worm infestation)
Visha (poisoning)
Utkata Dosha (excessively vitiated Doshas)
Visangya (loss of consciousness)

Dhuma Nasya

Inhalation of medicated smoke/fumes through the Nasal route and exhalation of the same through the mouth is called Dhuma Nasya. There is always a confusion between the two words Dhumapana and Dhuma Nasya. It is cleared by Chakrapani in the context of Nasya states:

तेन प्रायोगिक स्नैहिक वैरेचनिक धूमानां नासादीयमानानाम् इह ग्रहणं, मुखपेयस्तु धूमो न नस्यम्।।
(Ch.Si.9/91.Chakrapani)

Prayogika, Snaihika, Vairechanika Dhuma which are administered through Nasa Should be considered as Dhuma Nasya and those which are administered through mouth is Dhumapana.

Types of Dhuma Nasya

It is of three types:

1. Prayogika
2. Snaihika
3. Vairechanika

1. Prayogika Dhuma

प्रायोगिकी च नित्यपेय धूमवर्ति संज्ञा।

That which is used daily is called Prayogika.

Kala

प्रयोगपाने तस्याष्टौ कालाः संपरिकीर्तिताः। वात श्लेष्म समुत्क्लेशः कालेष्वेषु हि लक्ष्यते।
स्नात्वा भुक्त्वा समुल्लिख्य क्षुत्वा दन्तान्निघृष्य च। नावन अञ्जन निद्रान्ते चात्मवान् धूमपो भवेत्॥
(Ch.Su.5/34)

1. Snatva - Soon after bath
2. Bhuktva - After meals
3. Samullikhya - After vomiting
4. Kshutva - After sneezing
5. Dantanigrushya - Brushing teeth
6. Navana - After putting nasal drop
7. Anjana - After applying collyrium
8. Nidrante - After the end of sleep

2. Snaihika Dhuma

स्नैहिकी स्नेहनकारिका।

Dhuma which causes Snehana is Snaihika Dhuma. It is prepared with drugs of Madhura Gana added with a suitable quantity of Vasa, Ghrita and Madhuchista.

3. Vairechanika Dhuma

This is used for the elimination of Dosha.

श्वेता ज्योतिष्मती चैव हरितालं मनःशिला। गन्धाश्वगुरुपत्राद्या धूमं मूर्धविरेचने॥ (Ch.Su.5/26)

Drugs like Apamarga, Jyotishmati, Haratala, Manashila, Agaru etc are used in Vairechanika Dhuma Nasya.

Type of Dhuma	*Length of Nalika*	*Times of inhalation in a day*
Prayogika	36 Angula	2 times
Snaihika	32 Angula	1 time
Vairechanika	24 Angula	3-4 times

Method of Dhuma Nasya

ऋज्वङ्ग चक्षुस्तच्चेताः सूपविष्टः त्रिपर्ययम्। पिबेच्छिद्रं पिधायैकं धूममात्मवान्॥ (Ch.Su.5/48)

The Person should sit comfortably keeping his body and eyes straight and his mind steady.

Then, patient should inhale through one nostril keeping the other one closed. It is repeated three times.

Smoke inhaled through nostril should be exhaled from the mouth and that which is inhaled through the mouth should also be exhaled from the mouth.

प्रतिलोमं गतो ह्याशु धूमो हिंस्याद्धि चक्षुषी।

This is to be followed because the smoke moving in upward direction may harm the eyes.
Age for Dhuma : 12–70 years

Samyak Dhuma Lakshana

यदा च उरश्च कण्ठश्च शिरश्च लघुतां व्रजेत्। कफश्च तनुतां प्राप्तः सुपीतं धूममादिशेत्॥

(Ch.Su.5/52)

- ❑ Lightness in Ura, Kantha and Shira
- ❑ Tanuta of Kapha

Asamyak Lakshana

अविशुद्धिः स्वरो यस्य कण्ठश्च सकफो भवेत्। स्तिमितोमस्तकश्चैवम् अपीतं धूममादिशेत्॥

(Ch.Su.5/53)

- ❑ Avishuddha Swara
- ❑ Coating of Kapha in Kantha
- ❑ Stimita in Mastaka

Atiyoga Lakshana

तालु मूर्धा च कण्ठश्च शुष्यते परितप्यते। तृष्यते मुहय्ते जन्तू च स्त्रवतेऽधिकम्॥
शिरश्च भ्रमतेऽत्यर्थं मूर्च्छा चास्योपजायते। इन्द्रियाणि उपतप्यंते धूमेऽत्यर्थं निषेविते॥ (Ch.Su.5/54-55)

- ❑ Dryness in Talu, Murdha and Kantha
- ❑ Increased thirst
- ❑ Excessive secretion
- ❑ Murccha
- ❑ Affects Indriyas

Marsha–Pratimarsha Nasya

Marsha and Pratimarsha both consist of introduction of oils through the nostrils. It is well tolerated and is very much convenient procedure. Pratimarsha and Marsha are same in principle, but the main difference between them is of dose. In Pratimarsha Nasya 1-2 drops are given while in Marsha Nasya the dose is 6 to 10 drops.

Pratimarsha Nasya: Pratimarsha Nasya can be given daily and even in all the seasons at morning and evening. It is given by dipping the finger in the required Sneha and then dropping it in the nostrils. The patient should be advised not to sniff the Sneha given in the form of Nasya.

Dose

2 drops morning and evening. The Sneha should at least reach from nose to gullet, but it should not be too much that can produce secretion in gullet (Chakrapani on Ch.Si. 9/117.)

Indications

Pratimarsha can be given in any age, any season and even in Akala. i.e in Varsha and Durdina. It can be given to Bala, Vriddha, Bhiru. Sukumara and weak patients and also to the patients of Kshatakshama, Trishna Pidita, Mukhashosha, Valita and Palita. (A.S. Su. 29/19)

Contraindications

It is contraindicated in Dushta Pratishyaya, Bahudosha and Krimija Shiroroga and also in Madyapi (drunkers -habitual), Badhirya (deafness) and the persons having Utklishta Doshas. (A.H. Su.20/26-28).

It should not be given to them because the Sneha Metre is quite insufficient to eliminate doshas or Kriminasha and already aggravated Doshas may get vitiated further (A.S.Su.29/19). Sushruta and Sharangdhara have described 14 suitable times for Pratimarsha Nasya, while Vagbhatta has mentioned fifteen Kala.

समयाः प्रतिमर्शस्य बुधैः प्रोक्ताश्चतुर्दश। प्रभाते दन्तकाष्ठान्ते गृहान्निर्गमने तथा।।
व्यायामाध्वव्यवायान्ते विण्मूत्रान्तेऽञ्जने कृते। कवलान्ते भोजनान्ते दिवासुप्तोप्यिते तथा।।
वमनान्ते तथा सायं प्रतिमर्श प्रयुज्यते। (Sha.Uttarkhanda-8/41-42)

Time for Pratimarsha

Nasya	*Sushruta*	*Ashtanga*	*Sharangdhara*
1. After leaving the bed in Morning	+	+	+
2. After cleaning the teeth (with Dantadhavana)	+	+	+
3. Before going outside	+	-	+
4. After exercise	+	+	+
5. After sexual intercourse	+	+	+
6. After walking	+	+	+
7. After urination	+	+	+
8. After passing Apanavayu	+	-	-
9. After Kavala	+	+	+
10. After Anjana	+	+	+
11. After meal	+	+	+
12. After sneezing	+	+	+
13. After sleeping in the noon	+	+	+
14. In the evening	+	+	+
15. After vomiting	+	+	+
16. After Shirobhyanga	+	+	+
17. After defaecation	+	+	+
18. After laughing	+	+	+

Difference Between Marsha and Pratimarsha

आशुकृत् चिरकारित्वं गुणोत्कर्षा अपकृष्टता। मर्श च प्रतिमर्श च विशेषो न भवेद्यदि।
को मर्श सपरीहारं सापदं च भजेत्ततः।। (A.H.Su.20/34-35)

Marsha Nasya	Pratimarsha Nasya
Age : 7–80 years	Age: Birth to death
Effect: Ashukari (immediate)	Effect: Chirakari (delayed)

Benefits : More	Benefits : Less
Dose : 6, 8, 10 Bindu	Dose : 2 Bindu
Should follow the regimen strictly	Not essential to follow
More chances of complications	No complications

SAMYAKA YOGA, AYOGA AND ATIYOGA OF NASYA KARMA

After Nasya Karma the symptoms of its Samyaka yoga, Ayoga and Atiyoga should be observed, which are being described here under.

Samyaka Yoga

The symptoms of adequate Nasya according to Charaka, are Urah-shiro-laghava (Feeling of lightness in chest and head). Indriyavishuddhi (sensorial proficiency) and Srotovishuddhi (cleansing of channels) (Ca. Si. 1/51). In addition, Sushruta has described Sukhasvapna-prabodhane (good sleep and awakening), Chitta- Indriyaprasannata (mental and sensorial happiness) and Vikaropashama Nasya Karma (Improvement). Besides these proper respiration and sneezing have been described by Vaghbhatta (A.S.Su. 29/18) as the general symptoms of Samyaka Yoga of Nasya Karma.
It is shown in following table:

Symptoms	*Ch. Si 1/51*	*Su.Chi. 40/32-33*	*A.H.Su 20124*	*Sa.U.K 8/58*	*B.P*	*Ka.*	*Bh*
1. Urah Laghuta	+	-	-	-	+	-	-
2. Shiro Laghuta	+	+	-	-	-	-	-
3. Netra Laghuta	-	+	+	-	+	-	-
4. Gatra Laghuta	-	-	-	+	-	-	-
5. Srotovishuddhi	+	+	-	+	+	+	-
6. Svaravishuddhi	-	+	-	-	-	-	-
7. Vaktravishuddhi	-	+	-	-	-	-	-
8. Indriya prasada	+	+	-	+	+	+	+
9. Netrateja Vriddhi	-	+	-	-	+	-	-
10. Chitta Prasada	-	+	-	+	+	+	+
11. Vikaropashama	-	+	-	+	+	-	+
12. Sukha Svapna Prabodha	-	+	+	-	-	-	-
13. Sukhachchvasa	-	+	-	-	-	-	-
14. Arati	-	-	-	-	-	-	+
15. Medha	-	-	-	-	-	-	+
16. Bala	-	-	-	-	-	-	+

Ayoga

If Nasya is not given in proper way or the dose is less, features of inadequate Nasya arise which are Shirogaurava (heaviness in head), Galopalepa (throat coated with mucous) and Nishthivana (excessive spitting) (Ch.Si.1/52). According to Sushruta-Kandu (Itching in nose). Upadeha (feeling of wetness), Guruta (heaviness), Srotasam Kapha Steve (excess mucous secretion in channels) are the symptoms of Hina Shuddhi (Su.Chi.40/39). Vitiation of Vata, dryness in Indriya and no relief in the symptoms of the diseases (Su.Chi.40/35); dryness in mouth and nose (A.H.Su.20/24) are also the symptoms of Ayoga of Nasyakarma.

Symptoms of Ayoga Nasya

Symptoms	*Ch. Si 1/51*	*Su.Chi. 40/32-33*	*A.H.Su 20/24*	*Sha.U.K 8/58*	*B.P.*	*Ka.*	*Bh.*
1. Shirogaurava and	+	-	-	+	+	+	+
Dehagaurava	+	-	-	-	-	-	+
2. Galopalepa	+	-	-	-	-	-	+
3. Nishthivana	-	+	+	+	+	-	-
4. Kandu	-	-	-	-	-	-	-
5. Kaphapraseka	+	-	+	+	-	-	-
6. Upadeha	+	-	-	+	+	+	-
7. Rukshata	+	-	-	-	-	-	-
8. Vata Vaigunya	-	-	-	-	+	-	-
9. Srototiktste	+	-	-	+	+	+	-
10. Srotasam kaphasrava	-	+	-	-	-	-	-
11. Nasashosha	-	+	-	-	-	-	-
12. Asyashosha	-	+	-	-	-	-	-
13. Akshistabdhata	-	+	-	-	-	-	-
14. Shiroshunyata	-	-	-	-	-	+	-
15. Vyadhi Vridhdhi							

Atiyoga

According to Charaka, the general features of excessive Nasya are, feeling of Arati (unceasiness) and Toda (pricking like pain in the head, eyes, temporal region and ears) (Ch.Si. 1/52). Kapha Srava (Salivation), Shirahshula (headache) and lndriya Vibhrama (confusion) are the other symptoms of Atiyoga of Nasya (Su. Chi. 40/34). Mastulungagama, Vatavriddhi, Indriyavibhrama, Vatavriddhi, and Shiroshunyata (emptiness of head) are also the symptoms of Atiyoga of Shirovirechana.

Symptoms of Atiyoga Nasya

Symptoms	*Cha.Si 1/51*	*Su.Chi. 40/32-33*	*A.H.Su 20/24*	*Sa.U.K 8158*	*B.P*	*Ka.*	*Bh*
1. Shirogaurava	-	+	+	+	+	-	-
2. Shiroshunyata	-	+	-	+	+	-	-
3. Shirovedana	+	-	-	-	-	+	-
4. Netra Vedana	+	-	-	-	-	-	-
5. Shankhavedana	+	-	-	-	-	-	-
6. Suchitodavata Pida	+	-	-	-	-	-	-
7. Indriya Vibhrama	-	+	-	+	+	+	-
8. Mastulungagama	-	+	-	-	-	-	-

Contd...

Contd...

Symptoms	*Cha.Si 1/51*	*Su.Chi. 40/32-33*	*A.H.Su 20/24*	*Sa.U.K 8158*	*B.P*	*Ka.*	*Bh*
9. Snehapurna Srotasa	-	-	-	-	+	-	-
10. Kama Talu Upadeha	-	-	-	-	-	-	-
11. Vata Vriddhi	+	-	-	-	-	+	+
12. Kandu	-	+	-	-	-	-	-
13. Praseka	-	+	+	+	-	-	-
14. Pinasa	-	+	-	-	-	-	-
15. Aruchi	-	-	+	-	-	-	-
16. Deha Daurbalya	-	-	-	-	-	+	-
17. Unmada	-	-	-	-	-	-	+
18. Pitta Vriddhi	-	-	-	-	-	-	+
19. Hridaya Shula	-	-	-	-	-	-	+
20. Suryavarta Roga	-	-	-	-	-	-	+
21. Atripti	-	-	-	-	-	-	+

COMPLICATIONS OF NASYA

तत्र हीन अतिमात्र अतिशीत उष्ण सहसाप्रदाना अतिप्रविलम्बित शिरस उच्छिङ्क्तो
विचलतो अभ्यवहरतो वा प्रतिषिद्ध प्रदानाच्च व्यापदो भवन्ति तृष्ण उद्गारादयो
दोषनिमित्ताः क्षयजाश्च॥ (Su.Chi.40/48)

नस्ये शिरोविरेके च व्यापदो द्विविधा स्मृताः। दोषोत्क्लेशात् क्षयात् च एव विज्ञेयास्ता यथाक्रमम्॥ (Su.Chi.40/49)

निदानः– हीनमात्र, अतिमात्र, अतिशीत, अति उष्णं, अतिप्रविलम्बित शिरस्, उच्छिङ्क्तो, विचलतो, अभ्यवहरतो, प्रतिषिद्ध प्रदान।

If administered like this it will lead to Dosha Utklesha or Dosha Kshayajanya Vyapad like Trishna, Udgara etc.

Management

Doshotklesha Janya - Shamana, Shodhana
Kshaya Janya - Brihana

अजीर्णे भोजने भुक्ते तोये पीते अथ दुर्दिने। प्रतिश्याये नवे स्नाते स्नेहपाने अनुवासने॥
नावनं स्नेहनं रोगान् करोति श्लैष्मिकान् बहून्। तत्र श्लेष्महरः सर्वस्तीक्ष्णोष्णादिर् विधिर्हितः॥ (Ch.Si.9/111-112)

If nasya is given in contraindicated conditions like Ajirna, Bhuktabhakta, Jalapita etc. or in a season or time where nasya is contraindicated e.g. cloudy atmosphere, then there is possibility of production of Kapha Roga like asthma, cough, sinusitis and indigestion etc. In such conditions, the treatment should be done with kapha-nashaka upachara like use of ushna and tikshna aushadha karma.

MODE OF ACTION OF NASYA KARMA

The clear description regarding the mode of action of the Nasya Karma is not available in Ayurvedic classics. According to Charaka, Nasa is the portal (gate way) of Shirah (Ch.Si. 2/22). The drug administered through nose as Nasya reaches to the brain and eliminates only the morbid Doshas responsible for producing the disease. In Ashtanga Sangraha it is explained that Nasa being the door way to Shira, the drug administered through nostrils, reaches Shringataka (a Sira Marma by Nasa Srota and spreads in the Murdha (Brain) taking route of Netra (eye), Shrotra (ear), Kantha (throat), Siramukhas (opening of the vessels) etc. and scratches the morbid Doshas in supraclavicular region and extracts them from the Uttamanga (A.S.29/2).

Sushruta has clarified Shringataka Marma as a Sira Marma formed by the union of Siras (blood vessels) supplying to nose, ear, eye and tongue. It has been further pointed out that injury to this Marma may be fatal immediately (Su. Sha. 6/27). Commentator Indu of Ashtanga Samgraha opined Shringataka as the inner side of middle part of the head i.e. Shiraso Antarmadhyam.

Under the complications of Nasya Karma Sushruta noted that the excessive eliminative nasya may cause Mastulunga (cerebrospinal fluid) to flow out to the nose (Su. Chi. 40/40).

According to all Acharyas Nasa is said to be the portal of Shira. It does not mean that any anatomical channel connects directly to the brain but it might be connected pharmacodynamically through blood vessels or through nervous system (olfactory nerve etc.).

Advantages of Nasal Drug Delivery System

1. Drug degradation is absent.
2. Hepatic first - pass metabolism is absent.
3. Rapid drug absorption.
4. Quick onset of action.
5. The bioavailability of larger drug molecules can be improved by means of absorption enhancer or other approach.
6. Better nasal bioavailability for smaller drug molecules.
7. Drugs which can not be absorbed orally may be delivered to the systemic circulation through nasal drug delivery system.
8. Convenient route when compared with parenteral route for long term therapy.
9. Potential side effects of the drugs on the peripheral system could be minimized.
10. Smaller amount of drug is reqired to produce the desired concentration of drugs in CNS, which can reduce treatment cost.
11. The noninvasiveness of intranasal drug delivery can minimize the pain patients suffer.
12. Intranasal drug delivery may be conducted by patients themselves or other non-professional which could minimize the delay of medical treatment.

Limitations

1. Surface area for absorption is less when compared to Gastrointestinal tract.
2. Once administered the drug can not be removed.
3. Nasal irritation

Mechanism of Drug Absorption given through Nasal route

Passage of drug through the mucus is the first step in the absorption from the nasal cavity. Uncharged as well as small particles easily pass through mucus. However, charged as well as large particles may find it more difficult to cross. Several mechanisms have been proposed but the following two mechanisms have been considered predominantly.

The first mechanism of drug absorption involves an aqueous route of transport (Paracellular route). Paracellular route is slow and passive. In above route there is an inverse log correlation between the molecular weight of water soluble compounds and intranasal absorption. Drugs with a molecular weight greater than 1000 Daltons shows poor bioavailability.

The second mechanism includes transport of drug through a lipoidal route (transcellular process). Transcellular route is responsible for the transport of lipophilic drugs that show a rate dependency on their lipophilicity. Cell membranes may be crossed by drugs by an active transport route via carrier mediated means or transport through the opening of tight junctions.

Factors Influencing Nasal Drug Absorption

The following factors affect drug absorption:

Nasal Physiological Factors

i. Blood flow: Rich supply of blood and a large surface area makes the nasal mucosa an optimal location for drug absorption. Nasal absorption of drugs is influenced by blood flow rate, as it increases the amount of drug that passes through the membrane and hence reaching the general circulation. Kao et al. stated that nasal absorption of dopamine was relatively slow and incomplete probably due to its own vasoconstrictor effect. From above observations, it was concluded that vasoconstriction decreases nasal drug absorption by diminishing the blood flow.

ii. Mucociliary clearance: Mucociliary clearance (MCC) also referred to as Mucociliary apparatus is the self clearing mechanism of the bronchi. Nasal mucus layer defend the respiratory tract by preventing the lungs from foreign substances, pathogens and particles carried by inhaled air. These agents adhere to the mucus layer and transported to the gastrointestinal tract. Above elimination is designated by MCC and it influences significantly the nasal drug absorption. The MCC system has been described as a "conveyer belt" wherein cilia provide the driving force whereas mucus acts as a sticky fluid that collects and disposes foreign particles. Hence MCC efficiency depends on the length, density and beat frequency of cilia as well as the amount and viscoelastic properties of mucus. MCC may be increased by all factors that increase mucus production, decrease mucus viscosity or increased ciliary beat frequency. In physiological conditions, mucus is transported at a rate of 5 mm/min and its transit time in human nasal cavity is reported to be 15–20/mins. The values which are not within the range of these references are abnormal and suggestive of impaired MCC. From the above discussion we can say that the residence time of the drugs in nasal mucosa increased and hence permeation may be enhanced when MCC decreases. When MCC increased permeation rate of drug is decreased.

Enzymatic Degradation

Internasal administration of drugs avoids gastrointestinal and hepatic first pass effect. Drugs may be metabolized in lumen of nasal cavity due to the presence of a broad range of metabolic enzymes in nasal tissues. Some examples of enzyme which may play role in enzymatic degradation of drugs are carboxyl esterase, aldehyde dehydrogenases, epoxide hydrolases, glutathione S transferases and Cytochrome P450 isoenzymes have been found in nasal epithelial cells. The proteolytic enzymes (amino peptidases and proteases) were also found and they play an important role in degradation of calcitonin, insulin and desmopressin. The pharmacokinetic and pharmacodynamic profile of drugs administered through nasal route may be affected by xenobiotic metabolizing enzymes.

Transporters and Efflux Systems

The absorption of drugs into systemic circulation and CNS through nasal route is of great interest. Multidrug resistance transporters have been identified which may be involved in the transportation of hydrophobic and amphiphilic drugs. The apical area of ciliated epithelial cells and sub mucosal vessels of the human olfactory region contain P-gp an efflux transporter which plays an important role in avoiding the influx of drugs from nasal membrane.

Physicochemical Properties of Drugs

Some physicochemical properties of drugs (molecular weight). Lipophilicity, pKa, stability and solubility) can influence nasal absorption.

Molecular Weight, Lipophilicity and pKa

Lipophilic drugs are well absorbed from the nasal cavity, exihibiting pharmacokinetic profiles similar to those obtained after intravenous administration. These drugs are absorbed quickly and efficiently across the nasal membrane via transcellular mechanisms. This observation is true for lipophilic compounds having molecular weight lower than 1 kDa.

The extend of nasal absorption of lipophilic drugs bigger than 1 kDa is significantly reduced. On the other hand, the rate and degree of nasal absorption of polar drugs is low and highly dependent of the molecular weight. Drug absorption is expected to be diminished with decrease lipophilicity because the nasal membrane is lipophilic. Thus we can say that polar drugs may not easily transport across nasal membrane. Whenever lipophilicity is too high, the drug permeation through the wall may be reduced because drug does not dissolve easily in the aqueous environment of nasal cavity.

Stability

Biological, chemical and physical drug stability studies are a major consideration in all process during the development of new drug formulations. The biological stability of nasally administered drugs may reduce due to the metabolism of drugs by defensive enzymatic mechanisms by nasal cavity. To overcome this difficulty a variety of strategies may be followed, mainly through the use of prodrugs and enzymatic inhibitors.

Solubility

For drug absorption, drug dissolution is a pre-requisite because molecularly disperse form of a drug may cross the biomembranes. Therefore the drug must be dissolved in the nasal cavity fluid before absorption. Drug allowed enough contact with the nasal mucosa which may show slow absorption. Drugs with poorly soluble in water may require high doses hence can cause a problem. The problem can be overcome by enhancing drug solubility using various techniques.

Effect of Drug Formulation

Viscosity

Formulation with higher viscosity has a better contact time thus increases the absorption. At the same time, high viscosity enhanced the permeability of drugs. This has been observed during nasal delivery of insulin, acyclovir and metoprolol. Zaki et al. observed that the residence time enhanced as viscosity increased but drug absorption diminished.

pH: The pKa of drug and pH at the absorption site plays important role in absorption of drug through nasal route. Thus the stability can achieve by proper selection of pH of formulation. However, the pH of formulation should be near to human nasal mucosa (5.0-6.5) to prevent the sneezing.

Pharmaceutical Form

Nasal drops are the simplest and the most convenient nasal pharmaceutical dosage form, but the exact amount of drug delivered is not easily quantified and often results in overdose. Moreover, rapid nasal drainage can occur when using this dosage form. Instead of powder sprays solution, suspension sprays are preferred because powder spray may cause nasal mucosa irritation. Nowadays nasal gel has been developed for accurate drug delivery. This increases the nasal absorption by enhancing the drug residence time and diminishing MCC.

Application of Nasal Drug Delivery System

Systemic delivery: The intranasal administration of drugs is an effective way for systemic availability of drugs as compared to oral and intravascular routes. Actually, it seems to present fast and extended drug absorption, and it has been supported by many studies planned to compare intranasal drug delivery against oral and parenteral administration. Examples include analgesics (morphine), cardiovascular drugs as propranolol and carvedilol, hormones such as levonorgestrel, progesterone and insulin, anti-inflammatory agents as indomethacin and ketorolac, and antiviral drugs (acyclovir).

CNS Drug Delivery Through Nasal Route

Intranasal route has promosinng approaches for delivery of drugs to the brain. The delivery of drugs to the CNS from the nasal route may occur via olfactory neuroepithelium. The transport via trigeminal nerve system from the nasal cavity to CNS has also been described. Drug delivery through nasal into CNS has been reported for Alzheimer's disease, brain tumors, epilepsy, pain and sleep disorders.

Scientific Explanation for Probable Mode of Action of Drug Administered Through Intranasal Route

In the 1970s and 1980s there were multiple studies carried out suggesting that intranasal administration may enable substance to directly enter into the brain by pathways involving the olfactory epithelium and olfactory bulb. In 1995, Thorn, et.al. reported the first quantitative study indicating that intranasal administration could deliver large sized molecule into the brain by passing Blood Brain Barrier. A key obstruction for developing effective drugs through oral route is the blockade of drug entrance into the CNS by the BBB. Less than 2% of all small molecule drug and virtually no larger molecule drugs can cross the BBB. Thus intranasal route of drug administration is of great significance that can effectively deliver the drugs directly into CNS.

Multiple recent studies have also suggested that the intranasal drug delivery could produce beneficial effects on human subjects. For example intranasal oxytocin administration, can increase confidence in human subjects (Kosfeld M, et.al. 2005). Insulin given through intranasal route can improve the memory and mood of healthy adults (Benedict C, et.al. 2007). Similarly research studies shows that intranasal delivery of Insulin can improve the memory in Alzimer disease patients without altering blood levels of Insulin or glucose.

There are three likely mechanisms underlying the direct nose -to -brain drug delivery; there could be at least one intracellular transport mediated route and two extracellular transport mediated routes.

1. **Intracellular transport:** The intracellular transport based route is a relatively slow process, taking hours for intranasally administered substances to reach the olfactory bulb. The olfactory neuron in the olfactory epithelium could uptake the molecules by such processess as endocytosis, which could reach the olfactory bulb by axonal transport.
2. **Extracelllular transport:** The two likely extracellular transport based routes could underlies the rapid entrance of drug into the brain, which can occur, within minutes of intranasal drug administration.

   In the first extracellular transport based route intranasally administered substances could first cross the gap between the olfactory neurons in the olfactory epithelium which are subseqently transported into the olfactory bulb.

   In the second extracellular transport based route, intranasally administered substances may be transported along the trigeminal nerve to bypass the BBB. After reaching the olfactory bulb or trigeminal region the substance may enter into other brain region by diffusion which may also be facilitated by " perivascular pump" that is driven by arterial pulsation. In addition intranasally administered drugs may also partially enter into the CNS after the drugs enter into the systemic blood circulation from the nose.

Effect on Neurovascular Function

The lowering of the head, elevation of lower extremities and fomentation of face, seem to have an impact on blood circulation of the head and face. As the efferent vasodilator nerves are spread out on the superficial surface of the face, receive stimulation by fomentation and it may endanger the increased blood flow to the brain, i.e. momentary hyperemia. It has been approximately calculated that 22% of total dilatation of cerebral capillaries, caused by the facial efferent stimulation will lead to 150% blood in flow. It is also possible that the fall of arterial pressure due to vasodilatation may encounter with Cushing's reaction. In which, when the ratio between the CSF pressure and cerebral arterial pressure has reduced, the increased CSF pressure tends to compress the arteries in brain causing a transient ischaemia in the brain. By this, the aroused "ischaemic response" will subsequently raises the arterial pressure (Cushing). This act convince us more of "Slush" created in intracranial space, probably forcing more transfusion of fluids into the brain tissue. Probably this may be the explanation for the benzyl penicilline like drugs, which do not attain a therapeutic level in the brain in normal conditions, found to be effective during the inflammatory conditions of meninges (Gillman and Goodman 1980).

In this ground, we can state that the modus of operandi of Nasya Karma has a definite impact on central neurovascular system and likely to lower the blood brain barrier to enable certain drug absorption in the brain tissue.

Effect at Neuro Endocrinal Level

The peripheral olfactory nerves are chemoreceptor in nature. This olfactory nerves differs from other cranial nerves, excepting optic nerve, in its nature. It is phylogenetically closely related to brain. Rather it should be considered as the fiber tracts of brain itself.

There are adjacent nerves called terminal nerves which run along the olfactory nerves and their functions are unknown.

However, it is known that these nerve are connected with limbic system of the brain including hypothalamus. This limbic system and hypothalamus are having control over endocrine secretions. Moreover, hypothalamus is considered to be responsible for integrating the function of the endocrine system and the nervous system. It is known to have direct nervous connections with the posterior part of pituitary. In addition hypothalamus is indirectly having connections with anterior lobe of pituitary through portal vessels which supplies blood to the gland, having previously ramified in the corpora mammilaria of the hypothalamus in animals is capable of inducing secretion in the anterior pituitary, and it is believed that the products of such hypothalamic stimulation are drained by the portal vessels into the anterior lobe. The experimental stimulation of olfactory nerves caused stimulation in certain cells of hypothalamus and amygdaloid complex, but the nature of the effects is not properly understood. It is understood that just like premitive mammals, man also responds to the language of smell in the environments Abraham and colleagues (1979) in their experimental studies have noticed that more exposure to the smell of the Jasmine flower reduces the activity of mammary gland. If the fragrance could have the effect, it may be acting through impulses traveling via the olfactory pathways influencing hypothalamus which inturn, causes the inhibition effect through the pituitary (Abraham et al 1979).

Effect at Neuro Psychological Levels

The adjacent nerves called terminal nerves which run along the olfactory are connected with limbic system of the brain including hypothalamus (Hamilton 1966). This limbic system is also concerned with behavioural aspect of human beings, besides control over endocrine secretions. Thus, certain drugs administered through nose may have an impact on immediate psychological functions by acting on limbic system through olfactory nerves.

These things certainly supports the recommendation of Nasya mentioned by Ayurveda for mental disorders like Apasmara and Unmada.

Effect on Drug Absorption and Transportation

Keeping the head in lowered position and retention of medicine in nasopharynx help in providing sufficient time for local drug absorption. Any liquid soluble substance has greater chance for passive absorption directly through the cell of lining membrane. On other hand, massage and local fomentation also enhances the drug absorption.

The Later Course of Drug Transversion Can Occur in Two Ways

(i) By systemic circulation (ii) Direct pooling into the intracranial region. This direct transportation can be assumed again in two paths, viz. (a) By vascular path, (b) by lymphatic path. Vascular path transportation is possible through the pooling of nasal venous blood to the facial vein, which naturally occurs. Just of the opposite entrance the inferior ophthalmic veins also pool into the facial vein. Interestingly, both facial and ophthalmic veins have no valves in between. So that, blood may drain on either side, that is to say the blood from facial vein can enter cavernous venous sinus of the brain in reverse direction. Thus, such a pooling of blood from nasal veins to venous sinuses of the brain is more likely in the head lowered position due to gravity. On this lines, the absorption of drug materials into meninges and related parts of intracranial organs, is a worth considering point. Moreover the modern scholars have noted that the infective thrombosis of the facial vein may lead to infection of the meninges easily through this path.

Pooling of blood from paranasal sinuses also possible in the same manner. Vaghbhatt's notation of Shringataka Srotas (anterior cranial fossa) seems to relation with the above explanation.

Drug transportaion by lymphatic path, can reach direct into the CSF as it is known that the archanoid matter sleeve is extended to the submucosal area of the nose along with olfactory nerve. Experiments have shown that the dye injected to arachnoid matter has caused colouration of nasal mucosa within seconds and vice versa also (Hamilton 1971).

Preliminary studies reported from AIIMS Laboratories, clearly showed that steroids enter the CSF rapidly following their administration as a nasal spray. Surprisingly their levels in the CSF was found to be much higher as compared with systemic injections (Anand Kumar et al 1977).

Here it may be worthy to recall Sushruta's caution that the excessive administration of Virechana Nasya (eliminative errhine) may cause oozing of Mastulunga (CSF) into the nose. On this basis, we may say that ancient scholars of Ayurveda were aware of the lymphatic path as direct absorption into the brain from nose.

Importance of Post Nasya Massage

The Ayurvedic texts have recommended light massage on the frontal, temporal, maxillary, mastoid and on Manya region. A comfortable massage on the above region may help to subside the irritation of somatic construction due to heat stimulation.

On the basis of the foregoing observations it can be stated that the procedures, postures and conducts explained for Nasya Karma are of vital importance in drug absorption and transportation. The facts discussed above are also convincing about the definite effect of Nasya karma in the disorders of central nervous system, mental and some endocrinal disturbances also.

INDICATION OF NASYA IN DIFFERENT DISEASES ACCORDING TO CHARAKA

S.N.	*Name of Disease*	*Types of Nasya*	*References*
1.	Jvara	Nasya with Shirovirechaniya dravya Anu taila.	Chi.31254,255
2.	Raktapitta	Nasya with Neelkamala, Gairika and chandana mixed with sugar and water. Durva swarasa, Dhamasa, Palandu swarasa Dadima phoola swarasa, Draksha, Ikshurasa	Chi.4/97-104
3.	Kushtha	Vidanga churna, Vairechanika Nasya	Chi. 7/48,49
4.	Unmada	Nasya with Lashunadi Ghrita	Chi. 9/56-58
5.	Unmada	Purana, Prapurana Ghrita for Nasaya	Chi. 9/65-68
6.	Unmada	Nasya with Shirishadii dravya, Vyoshadi (Trikatu) nasya	Chi. 9/71, 72 Chi. 9/73
7.	Apasmara	Nasya with Gomutra Nasya with Bharangi, Vachadi dravya, Shyamadi Nasya, Nasya with Pipplyadi dravya.	Chi 10/40-45
8.	Hikka-Shvasa	Nasya with Sharkara, Tamalaki, Drakshadi, Nasya with Guda and Sunthi, Lashuna and Palandu, Dugdha and Chandana Nasya	Chi. 17/129-134
9.	Kasa	Kshira, Ghrita Nasya	Chi. 18/142
10.	Visha	Nasya with Shobhanjana, Maricha Churna and Shrisha pushpa swarasa.	Chi. 23/193
11.	Trimarmiya	Rohishadi Nasya in Nasa roga Manashiladi churna	Chi. 26/137 Chi. 26/151-152
12.	Trimarmiya	Lakshadi taila Nasya in Kaphaja Pinasa	Chi. 26/154
13.	Trimarmiya	Agurvadi taila, Rasnadi taila, Mayuradi Ghrita Nasya	Chi. 26/151 174
14.	Trimarmiya	Jivaniya Ghrita Nasya and Avapida Nasya in Pittaja Shiroroga	Chi. 26/176 178
15.	Trimarmiya	Tikshana Nasya in Krimija Shiroroga	Chi. 26/183-85
16.	Vata Vyadhi	Baladi Ghrita manda Nasya	Chi. 26/124
17.	Trimarmiya	Jivaniya Ghrita Nasya in Suryavarta	Si. 9/82-83

CHAPTER 8

Raktamokshana

INTRODUCTION

Raktamokshana is a technical term employed to denote procedure(s) in which vitiated blood from selected areas of the body is expelled out (also called bloodletting) by a specific method. It is fifth karma of Panchakarma. Vitiated Pitta causes vitiation of Rakta due to Ashraya-ashrayi bhava and gets pacified with nirharana of rakta through raktamokshana.

DEFINITION

रक्तस्य मोक्षणं रक्त मोक्षणम्। (Shabda Kalpadrum)

The procedure of letting out impure blood from the body is known as Raktamokshana. Mokshana means liberating emancipating, shedding or causing to flow.

Synonyms of Raktamokshana: Asravisravana, Shonitamokshana, Rakta nirharana, Rakta sravana and Rakta harana.

IMPORTANCE OF RAKTAMOKSHANA

Raktamokshana is the ideal treatment when the Doshas get vitiated by Rakta. Raktamokshana is an important line of management for Rakta Pradoshaja Vikaras.

शीत उष्ण स्निग्ध रूक्षाद्यैरूपक्रान्ताश्च ये गदाः। सम्यक् साध्या न सिध्यन्ति रक्तजांस्तान् विभावयेत्॥

(Ch.Su.24/17)

Raktamokshana is the most important treatment when a disease doesn't get subsided even after being treated with Snigdha, Ruksha, Sheeta or Ushna upakramas.

यानीहोक्तानि कर्माणि विसर्पणां निवृत्तये। एकतस्तानि सर्वाणि रक्तमोक्षणमेकतः॥ (Ch.Chi.21/14)

Among all the treatment principles employed for treatment of Visarpa, Raktamokshana is considered on one side and all other treatments on the other side. This shows the significance of Raktamokshana in Visarpa.

त्वक् दोषा ग्रन्थयः शोफ रोगाः शोणितजाश्चये। रक्तमोक्षण शीलानां न भवन्ति कदाचन॥

(Su. Su. 14/34)

Those who undergo Raktamokshana at the proper time interval will not suffer from disorders like Tvak Dosha, Granthi, Shopha and other Raktaja Vikaras.

One should undergo Raktamokshana in Sharad Ritu as Rakta undergoes vitiation by Kala Svabhava in this Ritu.

तद्विशुद्धं हि रुधिर बल वर्ण सुख आयुषा। युनक्ति प्राणिनं प्राणः शोणितं हि अनुवर्तते।। (Ch.Su.24/4)

The blood which becomes pure by these is responsible for endowment of strength, complexion, happiness and a long life.

सिराव्यधः चिकित्सार्धं शल्यतन्त्रे प्रकीर्तितः। यथा प्रणिहितः सम्यक् बस्तिः कायचिकित्सिते।। (Su.Sha.8/23)

Siravyadha, a type of Raktamokshana is considered as half of the treatment in Shalya Tantra like that of Basti in Kayachikitsa.

The diseases which are not cured by Snehadi kriya or Lepanadi Kriya are cured instantaneously by Siravyadha.

GENERAL PRINCIPLES AND RULES OF RAKTAMOKSHANA

One should know about Rakta and its properties before dealing with Rakta Mokshana.

Nirukti of Rakta

रसंजने, तेन रंजनः राग वर्ण युक्तः रागकृत्व धातुः रक्तम् इत्यर्थो भवति।

रसंजने - Means to stain

रागकृत् - If white cloth is stained with this Rakta, it becomes red colored. Word Raagakrit indicates this.

रक्तेन संयुतं शुक्ल वस्त्रं रक्तवर्णं भवति इत्यतः। रागकृत्व अयं धातुः इति स्पज्टमेव।

Synonyms

रुधिरम्, असृक्, शोणितम्, अस्त्रम्, क्षतजम्, लोहितम्। (Sha.Ka.Dru)

असृक्, शोणितम्, लोहितम्—Indicates red color

क्षतजम् —Indicates any injury/bleeds

Importance of Rakta

देहस्य रुधिरं मूलं रुधिरेणैव धार्यते। तस्माद् यत्नेन संरक्ष्यं रक्तं जीव इति स्थितिः।। (Su. Su. 14/44)

The root of the body is Rakta and the body is sustained verily by blood. As such, Rakta should be protected carefully; as in fact, Rakta is life.

Rakta is also one among the Dasha Pranayatanas. Acharya Sushruta considers Rakta as the fourth Dosha.

शाखा दुष्टे तू रुधिरे रक्तमेव आदितो हरेत्। (Ch.Chi. 12/68)

Rakta plays an important role in spreading diseases from one part to another part of the body by carrying the toxins or Vikrit Doshas. Raktamokshana method of Siravyadha is considered to be supreme as it drains out vitiated Rakta and cures diseases.

Rakta Svarupa

Sarva shareerastha – Resides in whole body

Jeevasya adhara uttama - Important base for life
Snigdha - Unctuous
Guru - Heavy
Chala - Moving
Svadu - Sweet
Vidagdham Pittavat - Vidagdha like Pitta
Sthana of Rakta- Yakrit and Pleeha are the mulasthana of Rakta.
Quantity of Rakta- The quantity of Rakta in the body is 8 Anjali.

Shuddha Rakta Lakshana

तपनेन्द्रिय गोपभं पद्मालक्त सन्निभम्।
गुन्जाफल सवर्ण च विशुद्धं विद्धि शोणितं॥ (Su. Su. 14/44)

S.No.	*Charaka Su.24/22*	*Sushruta Su.14/22*	*Vagbhatta H.Su. 27/1*
1.	Tapaneeya	Indragopa sannibham (the color resembles the insect Indragopa)	Madhura (Sweetish)
2.	Indragopa	Asamhata (Non-coagulant)	Lavana (Saltish)
3.	Padma-Alaktaka Sannibha	Avivarna	Kinchit Sheeta Ushna
4.	Gunja phalavarna (Color of Gunja seeds)		Hema
5.			Avi, Shasha lohita

Panchabhautikatva of Rakta

विस्रता द्रवता रागः स्पन्दनं लघुता तथा।
भुम्यादीनाम् गुणा ह्येते दृश्यन्ते चात्र शोणिते॥ (Su. Su. 14/10)

S.No.	*Sign*	*Causing Mahabhuta*
1.	Visra/ Amagandha	Bhu/ Prithvi
2.	Dravata	Jala/ Aapa
3.	Raga/ Lalima	Teja/ Agni
4.	Spandana	Vayu
5	Laghuta	Aakasha

Rakta Dhatu Karma

1. The Shreshtha Karma of Rakta Dhatu is Jeevana (Sustaining life)
2. Mansa pushti (Nourishing Mansa dhatu)
3. Dhatu purana (Filling the Dhatus)
4. Sparsha gyana (Sensation of touch)
5. Sthairya (Strength)
6. Dhatu pushti (Nourishing Dhatus)

Upadhatus of Rakta

Charaka : Kandara and Sira
Sushruta : Kandara and Sira
Sharangadhara : Raja

Mala of Rakta Dhatu

Charaka and Vagbhatta : Pitta
Sharangadhara : Ranjaka Pitta

Rakta Dushti Nidana

विदाहीन्यान्नपानानि स्निग्धोष्णानि द्रवानि च।
रक्तवाहिनी दुष्यन्ति भजतां चातपानिलौ॥ (Ch. Vi. 5)

Pradushta Madya (vitiated alcohol), Bahu Teekshna Madya, Bahu Ushna Madya, Ati lavana (excessive salt consumption), Ati kshara (excessive alkali), Ati amla (excessive sour), Ati katu (excessive pungent), Kulattha (Dolichos biflorus), Masha (Phaseolus Mungo), Nishpava (Dolichos lablab), Tila Taila (Seasame oil), Pindaalu (Diascoria alata), Mulaka (Raphanus sativus), Harita, Jalaja – Anupa – Prasaha Mansa, Amla Dadhi (Sour curds), Mastu (Supernatant fluid over curds), Sukta, Sura, Sauvira, Viruddha ahara, Upaklinna ahara, Pooti ahara (Stale food), Bhuktava diva prasvapatam (Day sleep after having food), Atyadaana (Excessive heat), Krodha (Excessive anger), Atapa (excessive exposure to Sun rays), Anala, Chhardi vega pratighata (Withholding urge of vomiting), Kale anavasechana (Not doing raktamokshana in Sharad ritu), Shrama (Excessive strain), Abhighata (Injury), Santapa (Excessive grief), Ajeernashana (Indigestion), Adhyashana, Sharat kala svabhavam (naturally in Sharad Kala).

Rakta Dushti Lakshana

Mukhapaka (Stomatitis), Akshiraga (Congestion in eyes), Putighrana (Bad smell in the nose), Asyagandha (Halitosis), Gulma, Upakusha, Visarpa, Raktapitta, Prameelaka, Vidradhi (Abcess), Raktameha, Pradara, Vatashonita, Vaivarnya (Discoloration), Agnisada (Reduced appetite), Pipasa (Excessive thirst), Gurugatrata (heaviness in body), Santapa (Raised body temperature), Atidaurbalya (Excessive weakness), Aruchi (Tastelessness), Shiroruk (Headache), Vidahashcha annapanasya (Burning sensation after consumption of food and beverages), Tikta udgara (bitter belching), Amlodgara (sour belching), Klama (dullness of fatigue), Krodha prachurata (Excessive anger), Buddhe samoha (Loss of orientation), Lavanasyata (saltish taste in mouth), Sveda (Sweating), Shareera daurgandhya (bad smell from body), Mada, Kampa (shivering), Swarakshaya (Feebleness of voice), Tandra (stupor), Ati nidra (Excessive sleep), Tamasacha atidarshanam (Darkness before eyes), Kandu (Itching), Kotha (Various eruptions over body), Pidaka, Kusha, Charmadala, will not get subsided by Sheeta, Ushna, Snigdha, Rukshadi upkaramas.

Doshanusara Rakta Dushti Lakshana

As blood does not aggravate without doshas, signs of aggravation should be known according to respective Dosha lakshanas.

S.N.	*Vata*	*Pitta*	*Kapha*
1.	Phenila	Neela	Gairikodaka pratikasha
2.	Aruna	Peeta	Snigdha
3.	Krishna	Harita	Sheeta
4.	Parusha	Shyava	Bahala
5.	Tanu	Visra	Picchila
6.	Sheeghra Gama	Anishta pipilika, Makshika	Chirasravi
7.	Sheeghra skanda	Askandi	Mansa peshi prabha

In case of Sannipatika Rakta dushti, all the above symptoms will be present and Rakta will appear like Kanji and will have a very bad odor to it.

Samprapti of Raktavaha Sroto Vikara

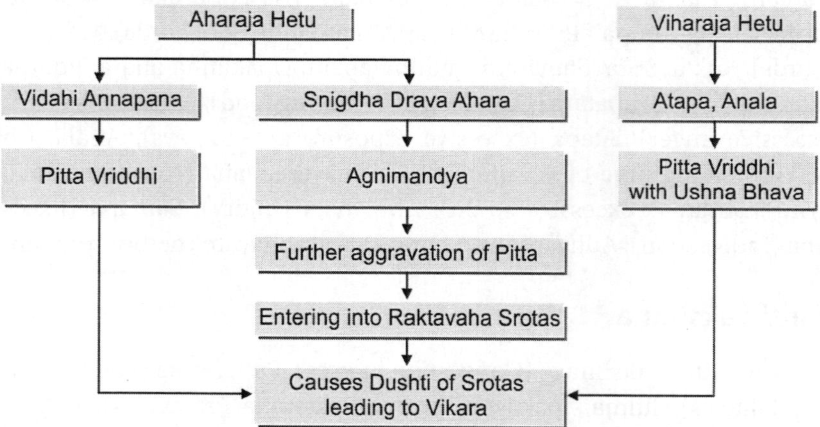

Probable Samprapti of Raktavaha Sroto Vikara

Samprati Ghatakas

Dosha – Samana vata, Vyana vata
Pachaka pitta, Ranjaka pitta,
Kledaka kapha
Dushya – Rasa, Rakta
Ama – Due to Jatharagni and Dhatvagni Mandya
Srotas – Rasavaha, Raktavaha
Sroto dushti prakara – Sanga, Vimargagamana
Udbhava Sthana – Amashaya

Sanchara Sthana – Sarva Shareera
Vyakta Sthana – Sarva Shareera
Roga Marga – Abhyantara and bahya

Raktavaha Sroto Vikaras/ Raktaja Roga

Only Acharya Charaka has explained Raktavaha Sroto vikara under Rakta pradoshaja Vikara. Acharya Vagbhatta has included all these in Rakta vriddhi lakshana whereas Sushruta has explained Sroto viddha Lakshanas.

कुष्ठ वीसर्प पिडका रक्तपित्तम् असृग्दरः। गुद मेढ्र आस्यपाकश्च प्लीह गुल्मोऽथ विद्रधिः॥
नीलिका कामला व्यङ्ग पिप्लवः तिलकालकाः। दद्रुः चर्मदलं श्वित्रं पामा कोठ अस्रमण्डलम्॥

(Ch.Su.28/11-12)

1. Kushtha
2. Visarpa
3. Pidaka
4. Raktapitta
5. Asrigdara
6. Gudapaka
7. Medhrapaka
8. Asyapaka
9. Pleeha
10. Gulma
11. Vidradhi (5 types except Sannipatjanya)
12. Neelika
13. Kamala
14. Vyanga
15. Piplava
16. Tilakalaka
17. Dadru
18. Charmadala
19. Shvitra
20. Pama
21. Asramandala
22. Kotha

Chikitsa Sutra

कुर्यात् शोणित रोगेषु रक्तपित्तं हरीं क्रियाम्। विरेकम् उपवासं च स्रावणं शोणितस्य च॥ (Ch.Su.24/18)

One has to follow the treatment pinciples of Raktapitta, Virechana, Upavasa (fasting) and Rakta sravana (Blood-letting).

Precautions

A. Raktamokshana shall be done in Saumya ritu to prevent any complications arising due to ushna in kala
B. Patient shall undergo Snehana, Svedana and also must be given Yavagu to eat before undergoing Raktomokshana
C. Emergency kit shall be kept ready, to deal with ayoga/ atiyoga etc. if situation arises.

CLASSIFICATION OF RAKTAMOKSHANA

Raktamokshana is of following two types

S. No.	Types	Subtypes	Uses
1.	Ashastra/ Anushastra krita अशस्त्रकृत/अनुशस्त्र	A. Jalauka जलौका	1. Beneficial in Pittaja dushti, gambhira dhatu dushti. 2. It removes the rakta in the area of approx. 1 hasta pramana.
		B. Alabu अलाबु	1. Beneficial in Kaphaja dushti and if the rakta is in avagadhatara state. 2. It removes blood from the area of approx. 12 angula.
		C. Shringa शृङ्ग	1. Beneficial in Vataja dushti and if the rakta is in avagadhatam state. 2. It removes blood from the area of approx. 10 angula.
		D. Ghati घटीयन्त्र	Beneficial in Vataja dushti and where dosha are tvakastha
2.	Shastrakrita शस्त्रकृत	A. Siravyadha सिराव्यधन	1. Beneficial in sarva shareeragata avastha and if the rakta is in avagadhatama state. 2. Choice of treatment in Mahakushtha.
		B. Pracchana प्रच्छान	1. Beneficial in conditions where rakta gets pindibhuta. 2. When rakta is with alpa doshavastha and in kshudra kushtha.

GENERAL CONTRAINDICATIONS AND INDICATIONS

Contraindications

अथ अविस्रत्राव्या:सर्वांग शोफ क्षीणस्य च आम्लभोजन निमित्तः पाण्डुरोगि
अर्श स उदरि शोषि गर्भिणीनां श्वयथवः॥ (Su. Su. 14/24)

बाल स्थविर, रूक्ष क्षतक्षीण भीरु परिश्रान्त मद्यप अध्व स्त्रीकर्शित वमित
विरिक्त आस्थापित अनुवासित जागरित क्लीब कृश गर्भिणीनां कास श्वास शोष
प्रवृद्धज्वर आक्षेपक पक्षाघात उपवास पिपासा मूर्च्छा – प्रपीडितानां च सिरां न विध्येत्॥ (Su. Sha.8/3)

In general, these conditions can be divided as follows for better understanding of the cause behind them being classified as contraindications.

Shodhana	Snehapeeta, Vamita, Virikta, Astapita, Anuvasita
Physiological conditions	Garbhini, Bala, Bhiru, Parishrantha, Upavasa, Pipasa, Jagarita, Krisha
Diseased conditions	Shvasa, Kasa, Shosha, Murchhita, Pravriddha Jvara Akshepaka, Pakshaghata, Sarvanga shopha, Pandu, Ruksha Strikarshita, Madyapana (mada), Kleeda, Arshas (Bleeding piles), Udara (Jalodhara, vatodara, pittodara)

Indications

According to Sushruta

स्राव्या विद्रधयः पञ्च भवेयुः सर्वजादृते। कुज्टानि वायुः सरुजः शोफो यश्च एकदेशजः॥
पालि आमयाः श्लीपदानि विषजुष्टं च शोणितम्। अर्बुदानि विसर्पाश्च ग्रन्थयश्च आदिश्च ते॥
त्रयः त्रयः श्व उपदंशाः स्तनरोग विदारिक। सुषिरो गलशालुकं कण्टकाः कृमिदन्तकः॥
दन्तवेष्टः स उपकुशः शीतादो दन्तपुप्पुटः। पित्त असृक् कफजाश्च औष्टयाः क्षुद्ररोगाश्च भूयशः॥

(Su.Su.25/12-15)

According to Charaka

ततः शोणितजा रोगाः प्रजायन्ते पृथग्विधाः। मुखपाको अक्षिरागष्ठच पूतिघ्राण आस्यगन्धिता॥
गुल्म उपकुश वीसर्प रक्तपित्त प्रमीलकः। विद्रधी रक्तमेहष्ठच प्रदरो वातशोणितम्॥
वैवर्ण्यम् अग्निसादष्ठच पिपासा गुरुगात्रता। सन्तापश्च अतिदौर्बल्यम् अरुचिः शिरश्च रुक्॥
विदाहश्च अन्नपानस्य तिक्त आम्लोद्रिरणं क्लमः। क्रोधप्रचुरता बुद्धेः सम्मोहो लवणास्यता॥
स्वेदः शरीर दौर्गन्ध्यं मदःकम्पः स्वरक्षयः। तन्द्रा अनिद्र अतियोगश्च तमसश्च अतिदर्शनम्॥
कण्ड्वरुः कोठ पिडका कुष्ठ चर्मदल आदयः। विकाराः सर्व एवैते विज्ञेयाः शोणिताश्रयाः॥
शीत उष्ण स्निग्ध रूक्षाद्यैर् उपक्रान्ताष्ठच ये गदाः। सम्यक् साध्या न सिध्यन्ति रक्तजांस्तान् विभावयेत्॥

(Ch.Su.24/11-17)

According to Vagbhatta

.... कुरुते ततः। विसर्पविद्रधिप्लीहगुल्माग्निसदनज्वरान्।
मुखनेत्रीष्ठिरोरोगमदतृड्लवणास्यताः॥ कुष्ठवातास्त्रपित्तास्त्रकट्वम्लोद्रिरणभ्रमान्।
शीतोष्णस्निग्धरूक्षाद्यैरूपक्रान्ताश्च ये गदाः॥ सम्यक्साध्या न सिध्यन्ति ते च रक्तप्रकोपजाः।

(A.H.Su.27/2-4)

In general, these conditions can be divided as follows for better understanding of the cause behind them being classified as indications.

Vaya	16–70 yrs
Ritu	Sharad
Twak vikara	Sarvakushtha and Visarpa
Kshudraroga	Ajagallika, Arunshika, Chippa, Kunakha, Yova-napidikas, Nyaccha, Vyanga, Alaji, Nilika, Padadari, Alasa, Indralupta, Darunaka, Shleepada, Vranashotha
Udara	Pleehodara, Yakrittodara
Vidradhi	All types except sarvaja
Vatavyadhi	Gridhrasi, Avabahuka, Vatashonita, Kroshtukasheersha, Khanja, Pangu, Bahushosha, Vishvachi
Others	Stanaroga, Mutra vriddhi, Parshvashula, Pramehapidakas
Jvara	Tritiyaka and Chaturthaka
Manasa roga	Unmada and Apasmara

Specific Uses of Raktamokshana According to Types

प्रच्छानेन एकदेशस्थं सुप्तं शृङ्ग आदिभिर् हरेत्। ग्रथितं तु जलौकोभिरसृग्व्यापि सिराव्यधैः॥
प्रच्छानं पिण्डिते वा स्यादवगाढे जालौकसः। त्वक्स्थेऽलाबुघटोशृङ्गं सिरैव व्यापकेऽसृजि॥
वातादिधाम् वा शृङ्गजलौकोऽलाबुभिः क्रमात्। (A.S.Su.35/7)
उष्णं सुमधुरं स्निग्धं गवां शृङ्गं प्रकीर्तितम्। तस्माद्वातोपसृष्टे तु हितं तदवसेचने॥
शीताधिवासा मधुरा जलौका वारिसंभवा॥ तस्मात् पित्तोपसृष्टे तु हिता सा त्ववसेचने।
अलाबु कटुकं रूक्षं तीक्ष्णं च परिकीर्तितम्॥ तस्माच्छलेष्मोपसृष्टे तु हितं तदवसेचने॥ (Su.Su.13/5-7)

S. No.	*Type of Raktamokshana*	*Guna*	*Site and type of dushti*	*Doshavastha*	*Area of action*
1	Pracchana	---	Ekadeshasthita Pindita rakta	Tridosha	Localised
2	Siravedha	---	Vyapaka Rakta	Tridoshaja	Sarvadeha
3	Shringa	Ushna, Madhura, Snigdha	Supti (numbness), Tvak	Vataja	Dashangula
4	Jalauka	Sheeta, Madhura	Avaghada (deeply seated)	Pittaja	Hastamatra
5	Alabu	Katu, Ruksha, Teekshna	Supti (numbness) Tvak	Kaphaja	Dwadashangula
6	Ghati	---	Twak	Vataja	Localized

JALAUKAVACHARANA

Sushrutacharya also known as father of Surgery has listed two types of Raktamokshana as already described earlier. Out of these, Jalaukavacharana (bloodletting by Jalauka/Leech) has been renowned for its safest, quick acting nature and less complicating effect. He counts the benefits of Raktamokshana for the Chikitsa purpose that it not only purifies the channels but also let the other parts become free from disease and action is faster than other remedies. (Su. Chi.1/44)

Introduction

According to Charaka, ideal medicine is one which relieves from all kinds of miseries. Drug, not necessarily be given orally. Ayurveda speaks about many modes of healing art, even surgery and Para-surgical techniques. Among the Para-surgical measures, Raktamokshana or bloodletting enjoys a pride place from the dawn of medical history. "The clinician who knows all about the leeches, habitat, and their method of collection, varieties, storage and method of application is successful in treating the diseases amenable to them". Earliest references of bloodletting are found in the basic works of all systems of medicine. The oldest civilization of the world too used this method to bestow health on its subjects from time immemorial. All the major classics of Ayurveda have dealt the topic with minute details.

Since the time of Veda, Ayurveda has much productive materials about Raktavasechana/ Raktamokshana karma as a part of treatment. The method of application of leech for bloodletting is mentioned in Kaushika Sutra (4/26/8) which is a Sutragrantha of Atharvaveda. The awareness of Jalaukavacharana is as old as the Ayurveda.

All Samhita have given detailed description of Raktamokshana and Jalaukavacharana (A. H. Su. 26; A. S. Su. 37; Sha. Sam. Ut. 12). Charaka has enumerated Raktaja Roga and their treatment by Shonitavasechana (Ch. Su. 24; Ch. Chi. 75/2) and various techniques of Raktamokshana are also mentioned (Ch. Chi. 28).

Sushruta has discussed in detail about Raktamokshana and its type. He described special chapter only for Jalaukavacharana (Su. Su. 13), where types of Jalauka, their habitat etc. have been described in details. Jalaukavacharana is claimed to be the best therapy amongst raktamokshana/shalya, because of its safety and high efficacy in the disorders involving the vitiation of blood. It is safely indicated even for the king, rich, old, fearful, weak, women and the people of tender nature.

Jalauka

Etymology

जलमासामायुरिति जलायुकाः, जलमासामोक इति जलौकसः। (Su.Su. 13/9)

The word Jalauka is a compound word with two components Jala + Ayu; i.e. the animals having water as the life. The term Jalauka can be split into Jala + Oka; i.e. water dwelling animals.

Synonyms

Jalauka, Jalaragi, Jalayuki, Jalika, Jalasika, Jalajantuka, Veni, Jalaloka, Jalaukasa, Rakta Payani, Rakta Sandamshika, Jalajivani, Raktapata, Jala Sarpini, Jala Soochi, Jalatanou, Jalaluka.

Definition

For which Jala is Ayu is Jalayuka. That which resides in Jala is Jalauka.

Types of Jalauka

'ता द्वादशः, तासां सविषाःषट्, तावत्य एव निर्विषाः'। (Su.Su. 13/10)

1. Savisha Jalauka

The Savisha Jalauka originates in the decomposed urine and fecal matter of toads and poisonous fishes in ponds of stagnant and turbid water.

General characters of Savisha Jalauka

स्थूलमध्याः परिक्लिष्टाः पृथ्व्यो मन्दविचेष्टिताः। अग्राहिण्योऽल्पपान्यियः सविषाश्च न पूजिताः॥ (Su. Su. 13/18)

Such types of Jalauka are having the following characters according to the Ayurvedic texts:

a. Thick
b. Slow in motion
c. Fatigues quickly
d. Middle part elongated

e. Delay in sucking
f. Not commendable type
g. Sucks little quantity of blood

Individual Features of Savisha Jalauka

1. Krishna

'अञ्जनचूर्णवर्णा पृथुशिराः कृष्णा'। (Su.Su. 13/11)

i. Thick
ii. Black in color.

2. Karbura

'वर्मिमत्स्यवदायता छिन्नोन्नतकुक्षिः कर्बुरा'। (Su.Su. 13/11)

i. Resemble the fish of vermin type.
ii. Ventral surface is convex (Ayata)

3. Alagarda

'रोमशा महापार्श्वा कृष्णमुखी अलगर्दा'। (Su.Su. 13/11)

i. Thick
ii. Hairy
iii. Round at sides
iv. Black at the mouth

4. Indrayudha

'इन्द्रायुधवदूर्ध्वराजिभिष्चितचित्रा इन्द्रायुधा'। (Su. Su. 13/11)

i. Having different colors like rainbow.
ii. Number of linings on the body.

5. Samudrika

'ईषदसितपीतिका विचित्रपुष्पाकृतिचित्रा सामुद्रिका'। (Su. Su. 13/11)

i. Blakish yellow with dotted skin.

6. Gochandana

गोवृज़णवदधोभागे द्विधाभूताकृतिरणुमुखी गोचन्दनेति। (Su. Su. 13/11)

i. Narrow mouth
ii. Marked by bifurcating lines
iii. Bottom (end part) like the scrotal sac on a bull.

Features of Savisha Jalauka Bite

If Savisha Jalauka is applied then a person suffers from following clinical symptoms: (Su. Su. 13/11)

1. Burning
2. Itching
3. Swelling
4. Drowsiness
5. Fever

6. Delirium
7. Unconsciousness
8. Irresistible inclination to scratch the seat of bite.

2. Nirvisha Jalauka

Nirvisha Jalauka originates in decomposed vegetable matter, as the purified stems of the several aquatic plants knwon as Padma, Utpala, Nalina, Kumuda, Pundarika and common zoophytes, which live in clear water.

पद्मोत्पलनलिनकुमुदसौगन्धिककुवलपुण्डरीकशैवालकोथजाता विमलेष्वम्भःसु च निर्विषाः।

(Su.Su. 13/14)

Geographical Distribution

According to Sushruta, the leeches are found in Yavana (Turkesthana, Pandya, Sahya, Pautana etc.)

Habitat

Such leeches swim in sweet scented water, live on, non-poisonous weeds, and lie on the leaves of flowering water plants in spite of on the dark and oozy beds of pools and suck blood from the affected part of a human being without causing any discomfort.

General Characters of Nirvisha Jalauka

Such types of Jalauka are characterized by following points :

1. Strong and large body
2. Ready suckers
3. Greedy for blood

Individual features of Nirvisha Jalauka :

1. Kapila

मनः शिलारञ्जिताभ्यामिव पार्श्वाभ्यां पृष्ठे स्निग्धामुद्ग वर्णा कपिला। (Su. Su. 13/12)

i. Color like Manahshila at the sides
ii. Dorsal surfaces are slimy and colored like Mudga pulse.

2. Pingala

किञ्चिद्रक्ता वृत्तकाया पिङ्गाऽऽशुगा च पिङ्गला। (Su. Su. 13/12)

i. Color – Reddish
ii. Shape – Round
iii. Locomotion – Speedy.

3. Shankumukhi

यकृद्वर्णा शीघ्रपायिनी दीर्घतीक्ष्णमुखी शङ्कुमुखी। (Su. Su. 13/12)

1. Color – blackish red like that of liver.
2. Provided with the greatest swiftness.

4. Mushika

मूषिकाकृतिवर्णाऽनिष्टगन्धा च मूषिका। (Su. Su. 13/12)

1. Color – like the common blind moles
2. Emit a foetid smell from the body

5. Pundarikamukhi

मुद्गवर्णा पुण्डरीकतुल्यवक्त्रा पुण्डरीकमुखी। (Su. Su. 13/12)

1. Color – like Mudga pulse
2. Presence of resemblance of the mouth of the full blown lotus lillies.

6. Savarika

स्निग्धा पद्मपत्रवर्णाऽष्टादशाङ्गुलप्रमाणा सावरिका। (Su.Su. 13/12)

1. Marked with impressions like lotus leaves.
2. Measured eighteen fingers in length.
3. Directed to apply only in the lower animals.

The leaches are further classified according to sex by Acharya Vagbhatta. Those which are delicate, having thin skin, small sized head, the lower body being large are female leeches and the ones with opposite characters along with being semi lunar in look with large front portion are male.

Leech

Kingdom : Animalia
Phylum : Annelida
Class : Clitellata
Subclass : Hirudinea

External Features

Shape and Size

- ❑ Leeches are small, soft, invertebrate vermiform worm like structure.
- ❑ Elongated, dorso-ventrally flattened,
- ❑ Almost cylindrical when contracted and ribbon shaped when extended
- ❑ Length is between 7 and 15 cm, having 6 longitudinal reddish or brown strips.
- ❑ Broadest near the posterior and narrowest near the anterior end
- ❑ Dorsal surface is somewhat convex and ventral surface is more or less plane.
- ❑ Transverse outline is almost oval.
- ❑ Dorsal surface brightly olive green and ventral surface is orange yellow or black and yellow.
- ❑ Black stripe marks on median longitudinal at dorsal side of the body.

Suckers

Hollow muscular organs on each end of the body are known as suckers.

1. Anterior sucker (oral/cephalic sucker): It is comprised of a cup like hollow, preoral chamber and the mouth. It contains three jaws with sharply serrated edges, which are used like circular saws, and on them are about 100 horny teeth used to incise the host. Sucks blood with this end. After sucking inverted Y shaped mark at the site is seen.

2. Posterior sucker (anal sucker): The posterior sucker is mainly used for leverage and is also useful for the purpose of locomotion.

Chemical Constituents of Saliva

Leeches produce a number of important substances which contribute to the special property of the bite, including an anticoagulant, a local vasodilator and local anesthetic, like Hirudin, Hyaluronidas etc. A study has found that high anti-thrombin activity was maintained in starved leech. A medicinal leech is a small "factory" which manufactures a number of biologically active substances, which help in following:

- ❑ Normalization and improvement of capillary circulation.
- ❑ Expressed anti-inflammation effect.
- ❑ Anti stressful and adaptogenic effects.
- ❑ Blood purification effect by expelling out the vitiated blood.
- ❑ Immune stimulation and immune modulating effects.
- ❑ Improvement of an endocellular exchange.
- ❑ Early wound healing effect.
- ❑ Reduces the high blood pressure and blood viscosity.
- ❑ Positive haemopoietic effect.
- ❑ Anesthesia, Anticoagulation, Antibacterial effect.

Leeches are also useful in removing the blood from areas where tissue has been transplanted or reattached.

Availability

Since the time of the Samhitas, Jalaukas have been available in India at the sea-coast regions. As per Sushruta Samhita, Jalaukas were seen in many parts of ancient India.

- ❑ Yavana (Turka sthana)
- ❑ Pandya (South region country - Deccan)
- ❑ Sahya (Tract of land traversed by the Ghat- Mountains)
- ❑ Pautana (Modern time of Mathura) etc. are the places for leech origination.

Purva Karma

Collection of Leech

In Sushruta Samhita, there is a detailed instruction on the subject of application of Jalauka in Sutrasthana (13th chapter). Knowledge from ancient time seen that, the leeches can be caught with a piece of wet leather or fresh meat from ponds, tanks, streaming water and where there are lotuses. For collection of the leeches, the another method, i.e. the fresh meat of dead animals, fish or milk must be applied on the thigh of an animal or the human being himself, may apply on his thigh and keep that part in the water for sometime. Jalauka will attract and will catch the place. Then remove them from the skin of that part with the application of Saindhava (rock salt), all Jalauka will detach and collect them. The best time for collecting leeches is Sharad Ritu (autumn) according to Dalhana.

Preservation of Leeches

After collecting the leeches, they should be kept in a wide and new earthen pot. The pure water of tank with lotus should be filled into that pot. Feed it with leaf of lotus plants (Kamala Nala), Shaivala, and powder of stem of small plants. The grass and leaves of plants must be kept inside water in the pot for the bed. The meat of pig and other animals, which are living in watery and marshy areas, may also to be kept inside the pot. Vriddha Vagbhatta suggests diet for Jalauka like; Sringataka, Kaseruka, Shalaka, Shaivala, Mruhala,Vallura, Mrutsana, Pushkara beeja Churna, sweet-cold clean water etc. Water should be changed on every 3rd day and fresh feeding should be dropped inside the pot. After 7 days the pot itself should be changed. Vagbhatta mentioned that the pot should be changed every five days. Poisonous leeches must be thrown out differentiating from all.

अथ जलौको अवसेक साध्य व्याधितमुपवेश्य संवेश्य वा, विरूक्षस्य चास्य तमवकाशं मृद्गोमयचूर्णैयद्यरुजः स्यात्।
गृहीताश्चताः सर्षपरजनीकल्कोदक प्रदीग्धगात्रीः सलिलसरकमध्ये मुहूर्तस्थिता विगतक्लमा ज्ञात्वा ताभी रोगं ग्राहयेत्॥

(Su.Su. 13/19)

i. Atura siddhata (Preparation of patient)
ii. Jalauka siddhata
iii. Sambhara sangraha

Atura Siddhata (Preparation of Patient)

In Yogya patients the vital data is checked to confirm fitness for the procedure. Part to which Jalaukavacharana is to be carried out is rubbed with mud, cow dung or with gauze is used to dry the affected area. This helps Jalaukas to stick easily.

Jalauka siddhata (Preparation of Jalauka)

A Jalauka of good quality is taken and kept in Rajani and Sarshapa kalkodaka. By this procedure Jalaukas become active and get rid of exhaustion.

Sambhara sangraha (Collection of Required Materials)

Shastra, Shalaka, Pichu, Plotha, Patra, Patta, Saindhava, Taila, Kashaya and Alepana Kalka are to be collected.

Pradhana Karma (Fig. 8.1)

श्लक्ष्णशुक्लार्द्र पिचु प्रोत अवच्छन्नां कृत्वा मुखमपावृणुयात् अगृह्णन्त्यै क्षीरबिन्दुं शोणितबिन्दुं वा दद्यात् शस्त्रपदानि व कुर्वीत; यद्येवमपि न गृह्णयात् तदा अन्यां ग्राहयेत्॥ (Su.Su. 13/19)
यदा च निविशते अश्वखुरवद् आननं कृत्व उन्नम्य च स्कन्धं तदा जानीयाद् गृह्णात्
इति गृह्णन्तिं च आर्द्रवस्त्र अवच्छन्नां कृत्वा धारयेत्॥ (Su.Su. 13/20)

The patient is made to sit or lie in the supine position. The Jalauka is applied on the site which is dried already. The Jalauka bites the skin and suck the blood by itself. If the Jalauka does not suck or bite the skin, a drop of milk or blood is shed on the surface or a mild prick is made. In spite of this if the Jalauka does not suck, another Jalauka is taken for application. As soon as the Jalauka starts sucking the blood, it should be covered with wet white gauze leaving its facial region uncovered. When its face appears like the hoof of a horse and it raises its neck, we can understand that it has started sucking (Fig. 8.2).

दंशे तोद कण्डु प्रादुर्भावैर् जानीयात् शुद्धमियम् आदत्त इति; शुद्धमाददाना अपनयेत्
अथ शोणित गन्धेन न मुञ्चेत मुखम् अस्याः सैन्धव चूर्णेनावकिरेत्। (Su.Su. 13/21)

When the patient gets itching and pain at the site of Jalaukavacharana we can understand that it has started sucking pure blood. Then it should be removed. If the Jalauka does not stop sucking due to its desire for blood, it is removed by sprinkling powdered rock salt or Haridra powder at its mouth region.

If Dushta Rakta is still there, it must be made to flow out by the application of the paste of turmeric, jaggery and honey at the bite spot. This is done because Dushta Rakta is mobilised from its Ashaya, comes near the Dansha Sthana and stagnates there. It may lead to pus formation.

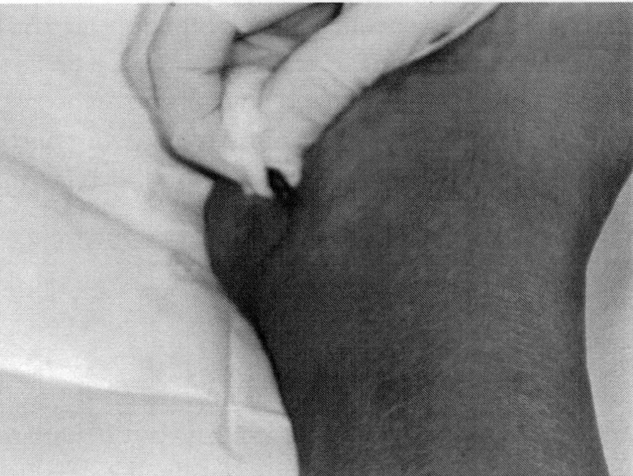

Fig. 8.1: Jalaukavcharana

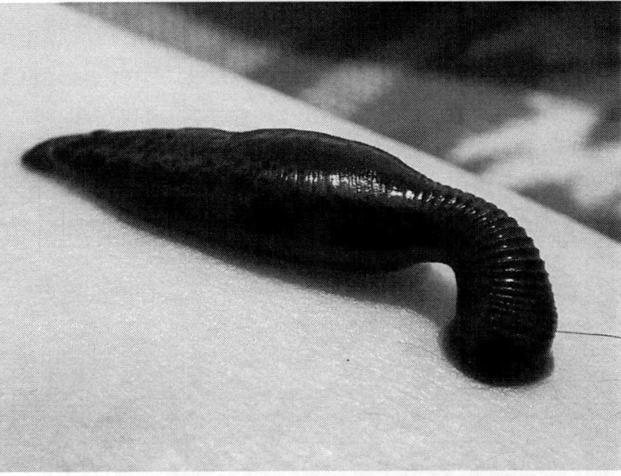

Fig. 8.2: Jalauka procedure (note position of head – horse shoe type)

Pashchat Karma

Management of Patient

शोणितस्य योग अयोगान् अवेक्ष्य शतधौत घृत अभ्यङ्गः , तत् पिचुधारणं वा;
जलौको व्रणान् मधुना अवघट्टयेत् शीताभिर् अद्भिः परिषेचयेद् बध्नीत वा,
कषाय मधुर स्निग्ध शीतैश्च प्रदेहैः प्रदिह्यादिति॥ (Su.Su. 13/23)

After the detachment of Jalauka, the wound caused by the Jalauka is smeared with Shatadhauta Ghrita and tightly bandaged. Also a paste of haridra and Arjuna can be applied instead of Shatadhauta ghrita.

Pashchat Karma for Jalauka after Jalaukavacharana

अथ पतितां तण्डुल कण्डन प्रदिग्ध गात्रीं तैल लवण अभ्यक्त मुखीं वामहस्त
अङ्गुष्ठ अङ्गुलीभ्यां गृहीत पुच्छां दक्षिण हस्त अङ्गुष्ठ अङ्गुलिभ्यां शनैः शनैर्
अनुलोमम् अनुमार्जयेद् आमुखात्, वामयेत् तावद् यावत् सम्यक् वान्त लिङ्गान् इति। (Su.Su. 13/19)

As soon as the Jalauka is freed from sucking, paste of Tandula is to be applied over its body and a mixture of Taila and Saindava Lavana or haridra is smeared on its mouth. Then with the help of the thumb and small finger of the left hand, the tail end of the Jalauka is to be held. The body of the Jalauka is squeezed with the fingers of right hand and pushed gently towards its face. This maneuver will induce vomiting of the sucked blood. This is continued until the signs of proper vomiting in jalauka are found.

सम्यक् वान्ता सलिलसरके न्यस्ता भोक्तु कामा सती चरेत्।
या सीदती न चेष्टते सा दुर्वान्ता, तां पुनः सम्यक् वामयेत्।
दुर्वान्ताया व्याधिर् असाध्य इन्द्रमदो नाम भवति। (Su.Su. 13/22)

After that, the Jalauka is kept in a vessel containing water. If the Jalauka moves in the container actively then it is suggestive of proper emesis. If it is lethargic and settles in the bottom of the vessel emesis should be performed once again. If it still does not vomit the whole blood, it becomes inflicted with a disease called Indramada or Raktamada where that leech should not be used in future for blood-letting.

After proper vomiting, the Jalauka is kept in an earthen pot, containing water. Jalauka once applied should not be reapplied for the next seven days. After proper vomiting, the Jalauka regains activeness and becomes strong. If too much vomiting is induced, it becomes very weak or even may die. If vomiting is improper, it becomes intoxicated or lazy.

They should be transferred from one pot to another pot filled with good mud and the water is changed in order to prevent putrefaction of its saliva. If this is not properly maintained the Jalauka becomes poisonous with such contact.

Complications of Jalaukavcharana and their Management with Ayurveda and Modern medicine

Complications

तत् दंशात् दाह शोफ पाक कण्डू पिटका विसर्प ज्वर मूर्च्छा श्वित्र उत्पत्तिः। (A.S.Su. 25/3)

If Savisha Jalauka is used it will cause Daha, Shopha, Paka, Kandu, Pitaka, Visarpa, Jvara, Murccha and Shwitra.

Treatment

स्रुत असृजः प्रदेहाद्यः ष्टीतैः स्याद् वायुकोपतः। स तोद कण्डूः ष्टोफस्तं सर्पिज़ उज़्णेन सेचयेत्॥

Hinayoga

To achieve Samyak yoga the wound is rubbed (Avagattana) with Madhu.

Atiyoga

Sheetala Jala Parishechana and Rakta Stambhaka drugs are sprinkled. Bleeding may continue for sometime, due to leechs hirudin. Bleeding time will vary depending on location, from a few hours to three days. This is a function of hirudin and other compounds that reduce the surface tension of the blood. Anti-clotting medications also affect the bleeding time.

Applying pressure can reduce bleeding, although blood loss from a single bite is not dangerous. The wound normally itches as it heals, but should not be scratched, as this may complicate healing and introduce other infections. An antihstamine can reduce itching, and applying a cold pack can reduce pain and swelling.

Some people suffer from severe allergic or anaphylactic reactions from leech bites and require urgent medical care. Symptoms include red blotches or an itchy rash over the body, swelling around the lips or eyes, feeling dizzy and difficulty in breathing.

Diet for Patient After Jalaukaavacharana

नाति उष्ण शीतं लघु दीपनीयं रक्ते अपनीते हितम् अन्नपानम्।
तदा शरीरं हि अनवस्थित असृक् अग्निर् विशेषाद् इति रक्षितव्य॥ (A.S.Su.36/21)

After bloodletting, the intake of foods and drinks which are neither too hot nor too cold, light and stimulants of digestion are recommended.

Pathya Apathya

The pathya-apathyas are same as those for any type of Raktamokshana. Exercise, sexual intercourse, cold bath, day sleep, exposure to breeze, food having Kshara, Amla, Katu Rasa and Ṣhoka should be avoided till the body gets normal strength.

Actions and Medicinal uses of Jalauka

Dosha: Pitta Shamaka
Useful in Grathita or Avagadha Sthana.

PRACCHANA

The procedure of incising the skin superficially and thereby accomplishing the bloodletting is known as Pracchana. This procedure is specially indicated to eliminate Pindita Doshas.

A. Purva Karma

Sambhara Sangraha

S. No.	*Requirement*	*Types*
1	Shastras	Mandalagra shastra, Karapatra shastra
2	Rakta pravartaka	Powder of Ela, Kushtha, Devadaru, Tagara, Vayuvidanga, Chitraka, Trikatu, Maricha, Pippali, Haridra, Arka and Naktamala.
3	Ratka skandana	Powder of Lodhra, Priyangu, Madhuka, Patanga, Gairika, Sarja rasa, Rasanjana, Shalmali flowers, Shankha, Shukti, Masha, Yava, Godhuma or the powder of barks of Sita, Sarja, Arjuna, Irimeda, Dhava, Dhanvana.
4	Rakta Sandana	Kakolyadigana (Kakoli, Ksheera Kakoli, Jeevaka, Rishabaka, Mudgaparni, Mashaparni, Meda, Mahamedha, Chinna Ruha, Karkataka Shrungi, Rudhi, Tugaksheeri, Padmaka, Prapaundareeka, Vriddhi, Mridveeka, Jivanthi and Madhuka).
5	Rakta Pachana	Kshoumavastra
6	Dahana	Kshara, Agnikarma Shalakas
7	Others	Collecting vessels, Sheetalaghara, attenders, Vrana Bandhana Dravyas etc.

Preparation of the Patient

No specific purva karmas are needed for carrying out the Pracchana procedure. However, to get the maximum benefit from the procedure, Stanika Snehana and Svedana can be carried out. It is said that doshas gets dissolved by the process of snehana and svedana and thereby easily flow out.

B. Pradhana Karma

गात्रं बध्वो अपरिदृढं रज्ज्वा पट्टेन वा समम्। स्नायु सन्धि अस्थि मर्माणि त्यजन् प्रच्छानम् आचरेत्।
अधो देष्ठा प्रविसृतैः पदैर् उपरि गामिभिः। न गाढ घन तिर्यग्भिर् न पदे पदम् आचरेत्।। (A.S.Su.35/7)
तत्र ऋजु असंकीर्णं सूक्ष्मं समं अनवगाढं अनुत्तानं आशु च। शस्त्रं पातयेत मर्म सिरा स्नायु सन्धीनां च अनुपधाति।। (Su.Su. 14/26)

The affected area should be cleaned well and then ligation (Bandhana) should be made above the site of Pracchana. Sharp instruments like Mandalagra Shastra or Scalpel blade should be taken and the area of Pracchana should be scraped. Pracchana should be avoided in areas such as snayu, sandhi, asthi, marma, sira etc.

Qualities of Pracchana

Riju (straight), Naati uttana (not too superficial), Naati Gambhira (Not too deep), Asankirna (Not very near to another pracchana line), Naati Tiryak (Not oblique)

Conventionally one can use lancet needle or insulin needle for pracchanna.

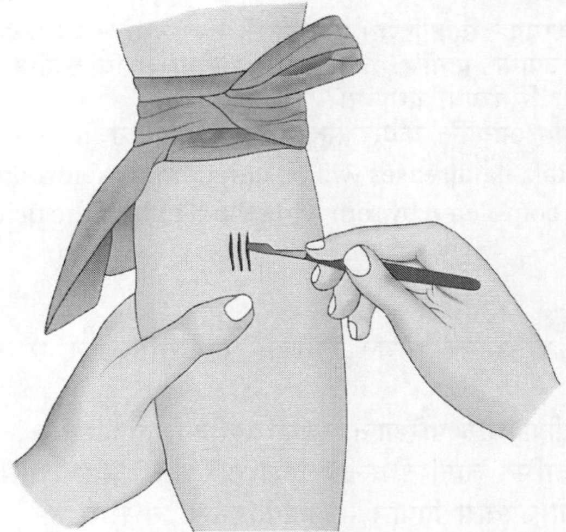

Fig. 8.3: Pracchana karma

C. Pashchat Karma

When the bleeding stops, area of the wound is dressed by applying Jatyadi Ghrita or powder of Yashtimadhu.

Indications

Pindita Rakta. The procedure is also done prior to the application of Shringa, Alabu, or Ghati for the purpose of accomplishing Raktamokshana.

Contraindication

Same as that of general contraindications of Raktamokshana.

SIRAVYADHA

Siravyadha is one of the important methods of Raktamokshana. The surgical procedure of puncturing a vein for therapeutic purpose, after suitable preparation of patient is called as siravyadhana. Raktamokshana, by the method of Siravyadha is preferred in physically strong as well as courageous people.

Importance

सिराव्यध चिकित्सार्ध संपूर्ण वा चिकित्सितं। शल्यतन्त्रे स्मृतो यद्वद्वस्तिः कायचिकित्सते॥ (Su.Sha.8/23)

Siravyadha is considered to be as half the treatment or even a complete treatment in Shalya tantra, just as Basti is considered in Kayachikitsa. The disorders which are not cured by Sneha, Lepa etc. are spontaneously cured by Siravyadha.

Indications

यथा रक्तं अधिष्ठानां विकाराणां विकारिणां। अन्यन्य हि तथा दूष्यं कर्मेदं प्रथमं ततः।। (A.S.Su.36/3)
बहवो हि रक्त अवसेचन उपायाः प्रागभिः हितः तेषाम् अन्येषां च विरेकादीनाम्
उपक्रमाणां तत्साधेष्वामयेजु सिराव्यधः प्रधानम्।
अमुला हि ते समूलाः शोषम् आयान्ति केदार सेतु भेदेन शल्यादय इव।। (A.S.Su.36/2)

By Siravyadhana, all Raktaja diseases will be cured from their roots just like rice and other crops in the field dry out completed by removing the bunds in the field.

Contraindications

सर्वाङ्ग शोफः, क्षीणस्य च आम्ल भोजन निमित्तः पाण्डुरोगि अर्श स उदररि शोषि गर्भिणीनां च श्वयथवः।। (Su.Su. 14/24)
बाल स्थविर रूक्ष क्षत क्षीण भीरु परिश्रान्त मद्यपाध्वस्त्रीकर्शित वमित
विरिक्त आस्थापित अनुवासित जागरित क्लीब कृश गर्भिणीनां कास श्वास शोष
प्रवृद्धज्वराक्षेपक पक्षाघातो उपवास पिपास मूर्च्छाप्रपीडितानां च सिरां न
विध्येत्याचाव्यधाः, व्यध्याश्चादृष्टाः, दृष्टाश्चायन्त्रिताः, यन्त्रिताश्चानुत्थिता इति।। (Su.Sha.8/3)

Bala (Child), Sthavira (Vriddha)	Kshatha Ksheena (emaciated due to injury)
Rooksha (dryness of body)	Kleeba (Impotent)
Bheeru (fearful)	Parishrantha (Tired)
Madhyakarshita (Emaciated due to alcohol)	Adhva (Excessive travelling)
Stree Karshita (Emaciated due to coitus)	Vamita, Virikta, Asthapita, Anuvasita
Ratri jagarana (night awakened)	Kasa, Shvasa, Shosha, Jvara, Akshepa, Pakshaghata, Murccha, Pipasa, Upavasa

Different Sites of Siravedha according to Disease

S. No.	*Disease Name*	*Vedhya Sira Sthana*
1	Padadaha, Padaharsha, Apabahuka, Chippa, Visarpa, Vatakan-taka, Vicharchika, Padadari, Vata Rakta	Two angula above the Kshipra Marma
2	Koshtukashirshaka, Kanja, Pangu	In leg four angula above Gulpha
3	Ghridhrasi	Four angula below or above Janu Sandhi
4	Apachi	Two angula below Indra Basti Marma in legs
5	Galaganda	Uru Mula
6	Pleeha roga	Kurpara Sandhi or sira between littleand index finger or left upper limb

Contd...

Contd...

S. No.	Disease Name	Vedhya Sira Sthana
7	Yakrit roga, Kasa, Shvasa	Kurpara Sandhi or sira between little and index finger of right upper limb
8	Pravahika, Udarashoola	Two angula near Shroni
9	Parikartika, Upadansha, Shukra Dosha	Medhra sthita Sira
10	Muthravriddhi	Posterior side of the Vankshana
11	Jalodara	Four angula lateral and below umbilicus
12	Antravriddhi, Parshvashula	Vein between Parshwa, Kaksha, Stana
13	Bahushosha, Apabahuka	Sira between two ansa

Procedure of Siravyadha

The procedure is carried out in three steps i.e., Purva karma, Pradhana karma and Pashchat karma.

1. Purva Karma

A. Sambhara Sangraha

अथ खल्वप्रवर्तमानेरक्ते एला शीत शिव कुष्ठ तगर पाठा भद्रदारु विडङ्ग चित्रक
त्रिकटुक आगारधूम हरिद्रा अर्काङ्कुर नक्तमाल फलैर् यथा लाभं त्रिभिः श्चतुर्भिः
समस्तैर्वा चूर्णीकृतैत् लवण तैल प्रगाढैर् व्रण मुखम् अवघर्षयेत्, एवं सम्यक् प्रवर्तते। (Su.Su. 14/35)
प्रागेव च उपकल्पयेत् शयन शासन उदकुम्भ वस्त्र पट्टादि।
तथा यथा लाभं च तगर एला शीत शिव कुष्ठ पाठा विडङ्ग भद्रदारु त्रिकटुक
आगारधूम हरिद्र अर्काङ्कुर नक्तमाल चूर्णम् असकृक्स्त्रावणाय।
असृक् स्थापनाय च लोध्र मधुक प्रियङ्गु पत्तङ्ग गैरिक रसाञ्जन शाल्मली शङ्ख यव गोधूम माष चूर्णम्।
वट अश्वत्थ अश्वकर्ण पलाश बिभीतक सर्ज अर्जुन धन्वन धातकी सालसार अरिमेद तिन्दुक त्वगङ्कुर
निर्यास श्रीवेष्टक मृत्कपाल मृणाल अञ्जन चूर्णम्। क्षौम मषी लाक्षा समुद्रफेन चूर्णं वा। (A.S.Su. 36/10)

Sambhara sangraha canbe divided into following sub parts for better understanding of the things required:

Shastras	Vrihimukha Shastra, Kurcha Shastra, Kutharika Shastra, Jalauka, Alabu and Shringa
Rakta pravartaka churnas	Powder of Ela, Kustha, Devadaru, Tagara, Vayuvidanga, Chitraka, Trikatu, Maricha, Pippali, Haridra, Arka and Naktamala
Rakta skandhana churnas	Powder of Lodhra, Priyangu, Madhooka, Patanga, Gairika, Sarja rasa, Rasanjana, Shalmali flowers, Shankha, Shukti, Masha, Yava, Godhuma or the powder of barks of Sita, Sarja, Arjuna, Irimeda
Rakta Sandhana churnas	Kakolyadhigana (Kakoli, Ksheera Karoli, Jeevaka, Rishabaka, Mudgaparni, Mashaparni, Meda, Mahamedha, Guduchi, Karkataka Shrungi, Rudhi, Tugaksheeri, Padmaka, Prapoundareeka, Vrudhi, Mrudveeka, Jeevanthi and Madhuka
Rakta Pachana	Kshoumavastra
Dahana upakarana	Kshara, Agnikarma Shalakas
Others	Collecting vessels, Sheetala aghara, attenders, Vrana Bhandhana Dravyas (Pichu, Plotha etc.)

B. Preparation of the Patient

तत्र स्निग्ध स्विन्नमातुरं यथादोष प्रत्यनीकं द्रवप्रायमन्नं भुक्तवन्तं यवागुं पीतवन्तं वा यथा कालम् उपस्थाप्य आसीनं स्थितं वा प्राणान् अबाधमानो वस्त्र पट्ट चर्मा अन्तर्वल्कल लतानाम् अन्यतमेन यन्त्रयित्वा नातिगाढं नाति शिथिलं शरीर प्रदेशमासाद्यप्राप्तं शस्त्रमादाय सिरां विध्येत्॥ (Su. Sha. 8/6)

Snehapana

The patient is made to undergo Snehapana either with Ghrith/Taila which is selected according to the condition. (Either Sadyo-snehapana or Arohana Snehapana).

Svedana

After Snehana, Svedana is administered. As pitta is dominant in Raktaja disorders Mridu Svedana is given. It is said that, the Doshas are dissolved by the process of Snehana and Svedana, and the liquefied Doshas will pass in to the Siras.

Yavagupana

The physician should ask the patient to perform all the auspicious ceremonies. After determining the strength of the disease and desha of the patient, the physician should give him either Mansarsa of Jangala animals or Yavagu mixed with Snigdha Dravyas (ghee or oil) as a drink. After this, the patient should be allowed to rest comfortably for about a Muhurta (48 minutes).

Kala

Generally the Pitta Dosha gets increased in the Sharada (autumn) season. There will be natural vitiation of Rakta in Sharada ritu because of vitiated pitta. So raktamokshana should be carried out during this season.

Sushruta has further specified that blood-letting should not be performed on a patient in extremely hot or cold weather, neither in one who is too much heated or improperly heated (before the act of bloodletting).

In addition to the above said season, the following are the periods where raktamokshana can be carried out :

1. In rainy season, but when the sky is clear and devoid of clouds.
2. In summer season, but in cool time (i.e., morning and evening).
3. In Hemanta Ritu (autumn), but in the noon.

The above cited periods are suitable for Raktamokshana. Besides these time factor depends on the condition of the disease and state of the patient during which the surgeon has to take his own decision for Raktamokshana. (Su. Sha. 8/19)

2. Pradhana Karma (Fig. 9.3)

The patient should be made to sit comfortably on a stool of the height of the knee, placing his elbows on his knees and the feet together comfortably on the floor and facing the sun.

The site of Siravyadhana should be selected according to the disease. A tight bandage either of moiost cloth, leather or inner bark of the trees should be tied above the site of Siravyadhana. This will help in making the vein prominent and visible for puncture.

Then the physician should raise the vein by tapping on it with his middle finger triggered by the thumb. On finding that the vein is palpable he should hold the Khutarika with his right hand keeping its handle up, place it on the vein in its centre and puncture the vein. At places where the vein is hidden or the skin is thick, pressing with the thumb should be done.

Vyadhana Pramana (Size of puncture): In muscular areas, puncturing should be of the size of Yava (barley grain) and in other areas it should Yava or one Vrihi (rice) using a Vrihimukha Shastra. Veins over the bones should be punctured to the size of Yava using a Kutharika Shastra.

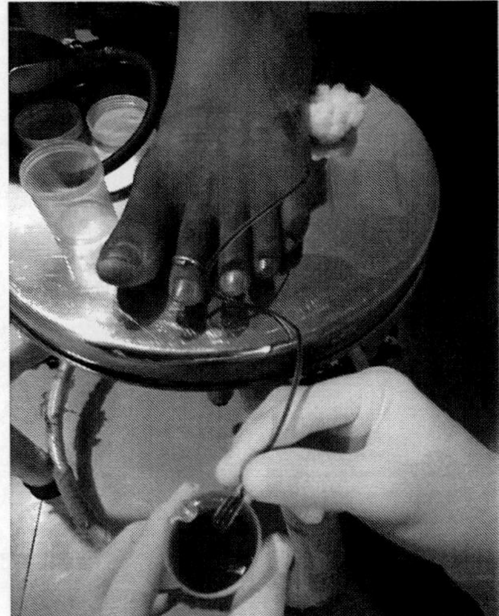

Fig. 8.4: Siravyadha

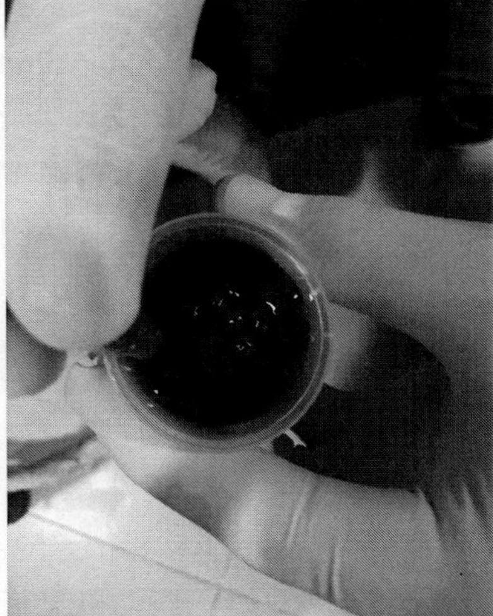

Fig. 8.5: Phenila rakta collected during Siravedha

Amount of Rakta Visravana in Siravyadha

बलिनो बहुदोषस्य वयःस्थस्य शरीरिणः। परं प्रमाणमिच्छन्ति प्रस्थं शोणितमोक्षणे॥ (Su.Sha.8/16)

One Prastha has been advocated as the maximum limit of bloodletting in a strong adult person with excessively vitiated doshas. In this regard Dalhana elaborated that Rakta can be let out in amounts as shown in the table below:

Uttama, Madyama and Hina wise Rakta Visravana Matra

Uttama	1 Prastha	648 mL
Madyama	1/2 Prastha	324 mL
Hina	1 Kudava	196 mL

Normal Limit of Siravyadha

रक्तं सशेषदोषं तु कुर्यादपि विचक्षणः। न चातिनिः स्रुतं कुर्याच्छेषं संशमनैर्जयेत्। (Su.Sha.8/15)

A physician should allow a part of the vitiated Rakta to remain inside the body rather than draining it excessively. Shamana chikitsa should be adopted to remove the remaining vitiated Doshas. This is to prevent the Ati-Visravana of Rakta leading to complications.

After puncturing the vein, a wise physician should look for samyak srava lakshanas. Further, Samyak Srava can be divided into Pravara Shuddhi, Madhyama Shuddhi and Hina Shuddhi according to the symptoms obtained by proper puncturing.

Samyak Vyadha Lakshanas

सम्यक् शस्त्र निपातेन धारया या स्रवेदसृक्। मूहूर्ते रूद्धा तिष्ठेच्च सुविद्धां तां विनिर्दिशेत्॥
यथा कुसुम्भ पुष्पेभ्यः पूर्वं स्रवति पीतिका। तथा सिरासु विद्धासु दुष्टमग्रे प्रवर्तते॥ (Su.Sha.8/11-12)

When Siravyadha is done properly then the vitiated Rakta will flow in a stream and it will automatically stop without any external hindrance. Just like yellow juice oozes out of the flowers of Kusumbha initially, in the same way the vitiated blood flows out initially when the vein is punctured.

लाघवं वेदनाष्ठान्ति व्यांधेर् वेगपरिक्षयः। सम्यक् विस्राविते लिङ्गं प्रसादो मनसस्तथा॥

Samyak Vyadha Lakshanas are:
Laghava - lightness of the body or at the site of puncture
Vedhana Shanthi - mitigation of pain
Vyadhirvega Kshaya - subsidence of the severity of disease
Mana Prasadha - optimism or cheerfulness of mind

Hina Srava

तत्र, दुर्दिने दुर्विद्धे शीत वातयोर् अस्विन्ने भुक्तमात्रे स्कन्दत्वा शोणितं न स्रवत्य अल्पं वा स्रवति॥
मद मूर्च्छा श्रमार्तानां वात विण्मूत्र सङ्गिनाम्। निद्रा अभिभूत भीतानां नृणां नासृक् प्रवर्तते॥
(Su.Su. 14/27-28)

If Siravyadha, is done on a clody day, if the puncturing is improper, if affected with cold and breeze, if sudation is not done earlier and if done after meals then the vitiated Rakta does not flow out as much as required or flows out in a little quantity. In persons suffering from intoxication, fainting and exertion, who have suppressed the urges of flatus, faeces and urine and those who are in the grip of sleep and fear, blood does not flow out.

मूर्च्छितस्यातिभीतस्य श्रान्तस्य तृषितस्य च। न वहन्ति सिरा विद्धास्तथा अनुत्थित यन्त्रिता:॥ (Su.Sha. 8/13)

In Patients who have fainted, who are greatly afraid, exhausted or thirsty, vitiated Rakta does not flow out when the vein is punctured.

Treatment of Hina Srava

If the vitiated Rakta does not flow out (due to any reason) then Ela (*Elletaria cardamomum*), Kushtha (*Saussurea lappa*), Tagara (*Valeriana wallichi*), Patha (*Cissampelos pareira*), Bhadradaru (*Cearus deodara*), Vidanga (*Embelia ribes*), Chitraka (*Plumbago zeylanica*), Trikatu, Aagaradhuma, Haridra (*Curcuma longa*), Arkankura (leaf buds of *Calotropis procera*) either three, four or as many as available of these drugs should be powdered, mixed with a large quantity of salt and oil, should be rubbed on the mouth of the wound; in this way vitiated Rakta flows out properly.

Atisrava

अतिप्रवृत्तं श्चिरो अभितापमान्ध्यम् अधिमन्थ तिमिर प्रादुर्भावं धातुक्षयम् आक्षेपकं दाहं पक्षाघातम् एकाङ्ग विकारं हिक्कां श्ववास कासौ पाण्डुरोगं मरणं चापादयति॥ (Su.Su. 14/30)

Causes of Ati pravritti: Atiushna, Atisvinna and Atividdha.

Excessive Srava gives complications like:

Shiroroga – Headache
Andhata – Blindness
Adhimantha – Glaucoma
Timira – Cataract
Dhatu Kshaya – Depletion of dhatu
Aksepaka – Convulsions
Pakshaghata – Paralysis
Ekangaghata – Hemiparalysis
Trishna – Thrist
Daha – Burning sensation
Hikka – Hiccough
Swasa – Breathlessness
Kasa – Cough
Pandu – Anameia
Marana – At last in extreme cases Death may occur

Treatment of Ati Srava

चतुर्विधं यदेतद्धि रुधिरस्यनिवारणम्। संधानं स्कन्दनं चैव पाचनं दहनं तथा॥
व्रणं कषाय: संधत्ते रक्तं स्कन्दयते हिमम्। तथा संपाचयेद्भस्म दाह: संकोचयेत् सिरा:॥ (Su.Su. 14/39-40)

In Raktasrava, sthambhana is achieved by four methods, i.e. sandhana, skandhana, pachana and dahana.

a. Skandana

The above said Rakta Skandhana drugs like Lodhra etc, are sprinkled over the site of Vyadhana. It does Skandhana by binding to the site of Vyadhana.

b. Sandhana

If the above measures fails, then the above said Kakolyadi Gana Kashayas are poured over the Bandhita site of Vyadhana. It helps in coagulation of Rakta.

c. Pachana

If the above measure fails then the Kshouma Vastra Bhasma is sprinkled over the site of Vyadhana.

d. Dahana

If the above measures fails then Dahana of the Vyadhita site is carried with the help of Guda, Sneha or honey.

Other than the above said measures, the following general measures can also be carried out:

When the blood flows out greatly, the powder of Rodhra (Symplocos racemosa), Madhuka (*Madhuca indica*), Priyangu (*Callicarpa macrophylla*), Garirika, Sarjarasa (Extract of *Shorea robusta*), Shalmali Pushpa (flowers of *Salmalia malabarica)*, Shankha, Sukti and Godhuma should be sprinkled and pressed with the tip of the finger on the wound; or Churna of bark of Shala (*Shorea robusta*), Sarja (*Vateria indica*), Arjuna (*Terminalia arjuna*), Meshashringi (*Gymnema sylvestre*) and Dhava (*Anogeissus latifolia*); or ash of Kshauma; or powder of Samudraphena and Laksha may be sprinkled; then a bandage is tied tightly using any bandaging material mentioned; the patient should be covered with a moist cloth, put in a cold room, treated with application of poultices and pouring liquids or the area may be cauterized either with Kshara or Agnikarma as described (Su. Su. 14/36).

A decoction of drugs of Kakolyadi Gana added with sugar and honey and made sweet should be given to drink; or the blood of deer, antelope, camel, rabbit, or buffalo may be given to drink; he should take his meals along with milk, soup of grains or meat, added with more fats (Ghee or oil); complications or secondary diseases may be treated appropriately.

Durvidda Lakshanas

दुर्दिने दुर्विद्धे शीतवातयोर् अस्विन्ने भुक्तमात्रे स्कन्दत्वाच्छोणितं न स्रवत्यल्पं वा स्रवति।
मद मूर्च्छा श्रमार्तानं वात विण्मूत्र संगिनाम्। निद्रा अभिभूत भीतानां नृणां नासृक् प्रवर्तते।। (Su.Su. 14/28)

Causes of Apravruti: Durdina, Sheetavata, Asvinna, Buktamatre, Mada, Murccha, Shramantha, Vatavinmootra Sangi, Nidrabhibuta, Bheeta etc.

तत् दुष्टं शोणितमनिह्रियमाणं शोफदाहरागपाकवेदना जनयेत्। (Su.Su. 14/29)

Inadequate flow of vitiated blood causes accumulation of Doshas and gives rise to complications like:

Shopha – Swelling
Daha – Burning sensation
Paka – Suppuration
Vedana – Pain

Chikitsa

The above said Rakta Pravartaka drugs are to be sprinkled over the site of Vyadhana for the attainment of Samyak Vyadha Lakshanas.

Defective Siravedha

There are 20 types of defects relating to an opened vein (Dushta-Vyadhana). They are as follows: Durviddha, Atividdha, Kunchita, Pichchita, Kuttita, Aprasruta, Atyudirna, Kunita, Vepita, Anuthita Viddha, Shastra Hata, Tiryaka Viddha, Avyadha, Vidhruta, Dhenuka, Punahpunahviddha and Sira-Snayu-Asthi-Sandhi Marma Viddha.

Management of Murccha During Siravyadha

One of the major complications which lead to sudden death is Murccha (unconsciousness) due to vaso-vagal shock/excess bloodletting.
If the patient becomes unconscious while performing Siravedha, the following points should be considered:

1. Immediate removal of the instrument from the wound.
2. Cold sponging.
3. Proper ventilation and aeration.
4. Consolation and assurance to the patient.
5. Further Siravedha immediately after the management of unconsciousness is avoided.
6. If the unconsciousness disappears, then the procedure of Siravyadha can be repeated after 2–3 days.

3. Pashchat Karma

Proper Attention to Regimen

Proper Massage and Dressing : Whenever blood flows stops automatically (Yantra should be removed and the instrument should be withdrawn), Tight dressing should be applied on the wound and massage is done around the wound using any oil preparation suitable for Abhyanga, so that ecchymosis (Antah Twak Rakta Srava) will not be produced.

After Siravedha, Vata gets aggravated by bathing (the area) with cold liquids etc. (methods of controlling bleeding) and gives rise to swelling and pricking pain. This should be treated by bathing the area with lukewarm Ghee.

Diet after Siravyadha

धातुक्षयात् स्रुते रक्ते मन्दः संजायतेऽनलः। पवनश्च परं कोपं याति तस्मात् प्रयत्नतः।
तं नातिशीतैर्लघुभिः स्निग्धैः शोणितवर्धनैः। ईषदम्लैरनम्लैर्वा भोजनैः समुपाचरेत्। (Su.Su.14/37-38)

After Raktamokshana Agni (digestive power) becomes weak due to the depletion of tissues and Vata becomes aggravated due to dhatu kshaya; hence the patient should be treated with foods which are not very cold, which are light (easily digestible), unctuous, which promote blood formation and are either slightly sour or devoid of sour taste.

Food, which consists of buttermilk with Yusha, Yavagu or Peya must be given to the patient. One has to protect his Agni; the diet which promotes the formation of blood must be advised. The following are to be avoided at least for one month.

क्रोध आयास मैथुन दिवास्वप्न वाग्व्यायाम यानाध्ययन स्थानासन चङ्क्रमण।
शीतवा आतप विरुद्ध असात्म्य अजीर्णान्याबल लाभात्, मासमेके मन्यते। (Su.Sha.8/24)
शेषदोषे यतो रक्ते न व्याधिरतिवर्तते। सावशेष ततः स्थेयं न तु कुर्यादतिक्रमम्।। (Su.Su. 14/43)

If a small residue of vitiated Rakta remains inside, diseases do not get aggravated and so they can be allowed to stay, but excess flow of Rakta should not be allowed.

KNOWLEDGE OF EMERGENCY MANAGEMENT OF COMPLICATION

Water and Electrolyte Imbalance

Electrolytes play a vital role in maintaining homeostasis within the body. They help to regulate myocardial and neurological functions, fluid balance, oxygen delivery, acid-base balance and much more. Electrolyte imbalances can develop by the following mechanisms : excessive ingestion, diminished elimination of an electrolyte; less drinking or excessive elimination of an electrolyte.

Total body water is distributed in two major compartments : 55–75% is intracellular [intracellular fluid (ICF)], and 25–45% is extracellular [extracellular fluid (ECF)]. The ECF is further subdivided into intravascular (plasma water) and extravascular (interstitial) spaces in a ratio of 1:3.

Extracellular fluid volume deficit is a common fluid disorder in surgical patients. The fluid deficit is not water only, but water and electrolytes in approximately the same percentage as they exist in normal extracellular fluid.

Management: Water deficit and excess management.

Water Deficit

- Intake of water
- IV 5% dextrose or dextrose saline or normal saline
- Intake output chart should always be maintained to properly adjust the fluid administration and to prevent water intoxication.

Water Excess

- Fluid intake should be stopped, particularly the IV fluid.
- IV 200 mL hypotonic (5.85%) saline solution should be given.
- This may be added with a diuretic (patient remain in stupor with renal insufficiency).

Electrolyte Imbalance

Sodium

Hyponatraemia

Clinical Features

Sunken eyes, anxious, tongue is dry, hard and reddish brown, skin is dry, wrinkled and subcutaneous tissue feel laxed, BP reduced, pulse will be fast, urine becomes dark and scanty with high specific gravity.

Management

- IV normal saline (0.9%)
- Ringer's solution may be administered in case normal saline is not available.
- Renal function should be monitored
- When there is severe loss of plasma volume, infusion of plasma or plasma subsitutes should be considered.

Hypernatraemia

Clinical Features

Puffiness of the face, pitting edema in the sacral region and ankle region, increased weight and polyuria, in infants increased tension in anterior fontanelle.

Management

- Stopage of infusion
- Diuretics if edema present
- Treatment of apparent hypernatraemia should be according to the merit of the individual cases.

Potassium

Hypokalaemia

Clinical Features

Gradual onset of drowsiness, speech becomes slow and slurred, muscular hypotonia and weakness, incontinence of urine, peripheral BP is lowered and pulse rate becomes slow, skin remains warm and dry, reddish flush of face, severe thirst.

Management

- Oral administration of potassium is always chosen first.
- Potassium salt should be administered orally or potassium chlorides in the form of effervescent tablets 2 g 6 hourly.
- When patient is comatose or nauseous and has difficulty in swallowing, IV administration is unavoidable.
- If potassium deficit is due to excessive vomiting—potassium chloride is administered.
- If urine volume is adequate—2 g of potassium chloride may be administered IV over a period of 4 hours.

- If potassium deficit is due to diarrhoea—Orally potassium citrate 2 g is administered every 6 hourly. The IV solution should contain sodium acetate in addition to potassium chloride.

Hyperkalaemia

Clinical Features

Nausea, vomiting, intermittent, intestinal colic and diarrhoea, low BP, low heart rate, poor peripheral circulation and cyanosed skin.

Management

- Exogenous administration of potassium should be stopped.
- Temporary lowering of serum potassium and suppression of myocardial effect of hyperkalemia can be acomplished by IV administration of 10% solution of calcium gluconate.

Magnesium

Magnesium Deficiency

Clinical Features

Hyperactive tendon reflexes, muscles, tremors, tetany, irritable, aggressive and restlessness.

Management

- Magnesium deficiency is best treated by parenteral administeration of magnesium chloride oro sulphate solution about 2 mEq of magnesium per kg body weight administered daily when the renal function is good.
- Excess of Mg leads to lethargy, weakness, and progressive loss of deep reflexes.
- Acute symptoms may be controlled by slow IV administration of 5 to 10 mEq of calcium chloride or gluconate.
- Persistence of symptoms, peritoneal dialysis or Haemodialysis should be done.

Calcium

Hypocalcaemia

Clinical Features

like numbness,tingling sensation in the circumoral region and the tip of fingers and toes, hyper tendon jerk, muscle cramp with carpopedal spasms and tetany. The Chvostek's sign will be positive.

Management

- IV administration of calcium gluconate or chloride.
- Calcium lactate may be given orally with supplement of vitamin D.

Hypercalcaemia

Clinical Features

Early stage symptoms : Anorexia, nausea, vomiting, fatigue, lassitude and weakness.

Later stage symptoms: Headache, pain in the back and extremities, thirst polyuria, polydipsia, stupor and coma.

Management

- Intravenous phosphate should be given slowly over a period of 12 hours once daily for more than 2 to 3 days.
- Corticosteroids

Shock and its Management

Definition

Shock is defined as a condition where the circulatory system fails to provide the nutritional needs of the cells and also fails to remove the metabolic waste products. The main cause of shock being low blood flow to vital organs.

Types

1. Hypovolaemic Shock

a. May be due to loss of blood, e.g. Haemorrhagic shock.
b. Due to loss of plasma or water and electrolytes, e.g. Shock in burns, dehydration, etc.

2. Neurogenic Shock

Trauma to spinal cord of spinal anaesthesia, etc. cause blockage of the sympathetic nervous system resulting in loss of arterial and venous tone causing pooling of blood in the peripheral circultory system. Thus cardiac output fails.

3. Vasovagal Shock

Dilatation of peripheral vessels in the limb muscles and splanchnic system, causes reduced blood flow to the cardia and brain. This results in decreased cardiac output, bradycardia, cerebral hypoxia, loss of consciousness etc.

4. Cardiogenic Shock

In various diseases like myocardial infarction, CCF, pericardinal effusion, the heart fails to pump blood.

5. Septic Shock

Gram negative septicaemia is the cause of such a condition. e.g. Cholangitis, meningitis, peritonitis etc may lead to septic shock.

6. Anaphylactic Shock

Administration of various drugs namely Penicillin, etc., causes sudden bronchospasm, laryngeal oedema, and respiratory distress leading to total hypoxia. This is caused due to increase of histamines.

Management

1. Maintenance of airway and breathing: The trachea of the patient who is unconscious or whose airwayis obstructed has to be intubated.
2. Blood pressure: Should be kept above 90 mm Hg. In case of hypovolemic shock, adequate quantities of fluids/blood should be infused.
3. The bladder should be catheterized to measure the volume of urine output.
4. Continuous monitoring of heart rate and rhythm, blood pressure, oxygen saturation and urine output, arterial blood gases etc. is important.
5. In case of septic shock, apart from otherr general measures, the septic source needs to be identified and removed, empirical antibiotic therapy needs to be initiated; various septic sources vizpus in an abscess, necrotic or gangrenous tissue needs to be drained or excised.
6. In anaphylactic shock, apart from otherr measures, injection adrenaline 0.3–0.5 mg SC/IM/IV is administered. Injection hydrocortiosone 1.5 mg/kg and Injection Aminophylline 5 mg/kg over 20 minutes (in case of broncho-spasm) is administered.

Bleeding Per Rectum

It is the condition in which blood is lost through rectum. Blood in the stool can be bright red or maroon in color. There are chances that patient may complain of pain per rectum and anus and abdominal pain or cramping. The bleeding may arise from any part of the GI-Tract including rectum.

Management

1. Diagnostic procedures, such as endoscopy, colonoscopy or angiography, may be done to pin point the source of bleeding.
2. Blood transfusions to combat blood loss in severe rectal bleeding.
3. Drainage of stomach contents.
4. Intravenous fluid replacement.
5. Surgery may be required in severe cases.

Hematemesis

Hematemesis is the vomiting of blood. The vomited blood volume in excess of 5.5 litres could be life threatening.

Management

Minimal blood loss – Kept NPO (nil per oral)
Proton pump inhibitor (e.g. omeprazole)
Blood transfusion (if Hb% <8.0gdl)
Significant blood loss – Resuscitation
Flud/Blood is administered preferably by central venous catheter. Patient is prepared for emergency endoscopy.

Epistaxis

Epistaxis is defined as an acute hemorrhage from the nostril, nasal cavity or nasopharynx. It is one of the common problem which can rarely be life threatening. There are many different etiologies, more common one being trauma.

Management

- ❑ Direct pressure is applied by pinching the soft fleshy part of nose (Little's area) for 5–10 min.
- ❑ Tilting the head forward helps to decrease the chance of nausea and airway obstruction.
- ❑ The local application of a vasoconstrictive agent (e.g. oxymetazoline).
- ❑ Silver ntirate to cauterize bleeding blood vessels.

In severe case of epistaxis, the posterior nasal pack is necessary. In this type of pack, a Foley's catheter is inserted through the nose into the nasopharynx and the balloon is inflated with saline. Gentle forward traction is applied to stop the bleeding. Careful observation of patient is needed in this pack. Usually it is applied for 2–3 days.

CHAPTER 9

Physiotherapy

DEFINITION

Physiotherapy is a system of medicine for complete health care of all age groups in modern age. "Physiotherapy is a treatment measure of physical and electrical means to accelerate the patient's recovery from injuries and diseases that hazards the normal lifestyle. It is a form of treatment carried through the medium of physical forces such as heat, electricity, water, massage and exercise with or without resistance".

Synonyms

Physical therapy and Rehabilitation therapy.
According to WHO, Physiotherapists are one who can assess, plan and implement rehabilitative programs that improve or restore human motor functions, maximize movement ability, relieve pain syndromes, and treat or prevent physical challenges associated with injuries, diseases and other impairments.

Aims of Physiotherapy

1. To treat the disability and deformity of the patient.
2. To correct the disability and deformity of the patient.
3. To prevent the disability and deformity of the patient.
4. To prepare the patient to live with their disability and deformity.
5. Promote health and physical well being by maximizing mobility and functional ability throughout all life stages.

Utility

Physiotherapy is important for Rehabilitation in Medicine, Orthopedics, Surgery, Neurology, Gynaecology and Dermatology.

Physiotherapists use their knowledge and skills to improve a range of conditions associated with different systems of the body, such as:

- Neurological (stroke, multiple sclerosis, Parkinson's)
- Neuromusculo-skeletal (back pain, whiplash associated disorder, sports injuries, arthritis)
- Cardiovascular (chronic heart disease, rehabilitation after heart attack)
- Respiratory (asthma, chronic obstructive pulmonary disease, cystic fibrosis).

Importance of Physiotherapy

- Physiotherapy has been a very effective tool against pains and injuries ranging from minor to major
- To get rid of muscle tenderness or immobility
- Respiratory disease treatments are also carried out by physiotherapeutic techniques e.g. coughing; vibration, cupped hand technique, clapping etc involve the use of physiotherapeutic techniques frequently proving the importance of physiotherapy.
- Whiplash injury is a condition due to vehicle accidents which may result in dizziness, numbness, pain in shoulder and neck muscles, ringing of bell in ear and such others.
- Orthopedics treat sports injuries, fractures, joint disorders; amputation, back and neck pain, arthritis and post-operative conditions. Orthopedic physiotherapy takes place in a private practice, depending on the stage of the condition.
- Neurological disorders such as strokes, multiple sclerosis, Parkinson's disease, cerebral palsy and spinal cord injury make up a great percentage of a physiotherapist's caseload.
- For children suffering with cerebral palsy, physiotherapy is essential in helping to reduce spasticity and deformity, improve postural control, trains the child to use assistive devices and do all that is necessary to maximize the child's functional independence.

Modes of Physiotherapy

The employment of physical measure in building of physique, correcting deformities and restoring function after disease or injury is carried out by physiotherapist by using following modes of physiotherapy :

1. Massage

Treatment of a disease or injury by skillful manual manipulation of the body tissue. This helps in relieving pain and spasm, induces relaxation, helps in promoting absorption of exudates, and helps in stretching adhesions and increase metabolism.

2. Electrotherapy

Treatment by electrophysical modalities which include low frequency, medium and high frequency currents. This includes actinotherapy and heliotherapy .

- **Actinotherapy:** The word "actis" is a Greek word meaning "a ray". Treatment by using rays (using lamp as the source) is known as Actinotherapy .
- **Heliotherapy:** The treatment by sun radiation is known as Heliotherapy.

3. Exercise therapy

Accelerating patients recovery from injuries and diseases which have altered his normal way of living by repeated muscular activity in range, strength and duration. Mainly of 2 types—Active and Passive.

BASIC KNOWLEDGE OF STATIC EXERCISE

Exercise

Performance of physical exertion for improvement of health or correction of physical deformity. Exercise therapy is a means of accelerating the patient's recovery from a stage of disease which alters his/ her normal way of living.

Aims of Exercise Therapy

1. Promotion of activity wherever possible to minimize the effects of inactivity.
2. Correction of inefficiency of a specific or a group of muscles and regain normal range of motion in a joint.
3. To accelerate the rehabilitation process of a patient and encourage them to use the ability regained to perform normal function.

Techniques of Exercise Therapy

<table>
<tr><th>S. No.</th><th>Type of movement</th><th colspan="2">Classification</th></tr>
<tr><td rowspan="5">1</td><td rowspan="5">Active</td><td rowspan="4">Voluntary</td><td>Assisted</td></tr>
<tr><td>Free</td></tr>
<tr><td>Assisted resisted</td></tr>
<tr><td>Resisted</td></tr>
<tr><td>Involuntary</td><td>Reflex</td></tr>
<tr><td rowspan="2">2</td><td rowspan="2">Passive</td><td colspan="2">Passive manual mobilization</td></tr>
<tr><td colspan="2">Relaxed passive movements</td></tr>
</table>

Static or Muscle-setting Exercise (Isometrics) (Fig. 9.1)

Static exercises, also known as Isometrics are voluntary contraction and relaxation of skeletal muscles without changing the muscle length or moving the associated part of the body. It includes method of maintaining muscle strength and tone by alternately contracting and relaxing a skeletal muscle or group of skeletal muscles without moving the associated body part. This kind of activity is very useful in preventing atrophy of the muscles, especially in patients with conditions involving the joints. It is also beneficial in increasing the endurance, strength and tone of the muscle.

Static stretching is used to stretch muscle while the body is at rest. It is composed of various techniques that gradually lengthen a muscle to an elongated position (to the point of discomfort) and hold that position for 30 seconds to two minutes. 30 seconds is the minimum duration to get the benefits of stretching, whereas two minutes is the maximum (if a position can be held for more than two minutes, a further stretch should be performed). During this holding period or directly afterwards, participants may feel a mild discomfort or warm sensation in the muscles.

Advantages

Static stretching exercises involve specialized tension receptors in our muscles. When done properly, static stretching slightly lessens the sensitivity of tension receptors, which allows the muscle to relax and to be stretched to greater length.

Stretching helps keep you flexible and counteracts the repetitive movements of exercise. When performed correctly and at the right time, static stretches help you lengthen tight muscles and improve your balance and overall fitness. A good stretch session also helps relieve stress and tension.

Contraindication for Stretching Exercise

- Joint instability
- Disease affecting the tissue being stretched e.g RA
- Acute injury
- Vascular injury e.g. thromboembolism
- Infection
- High blood pressure

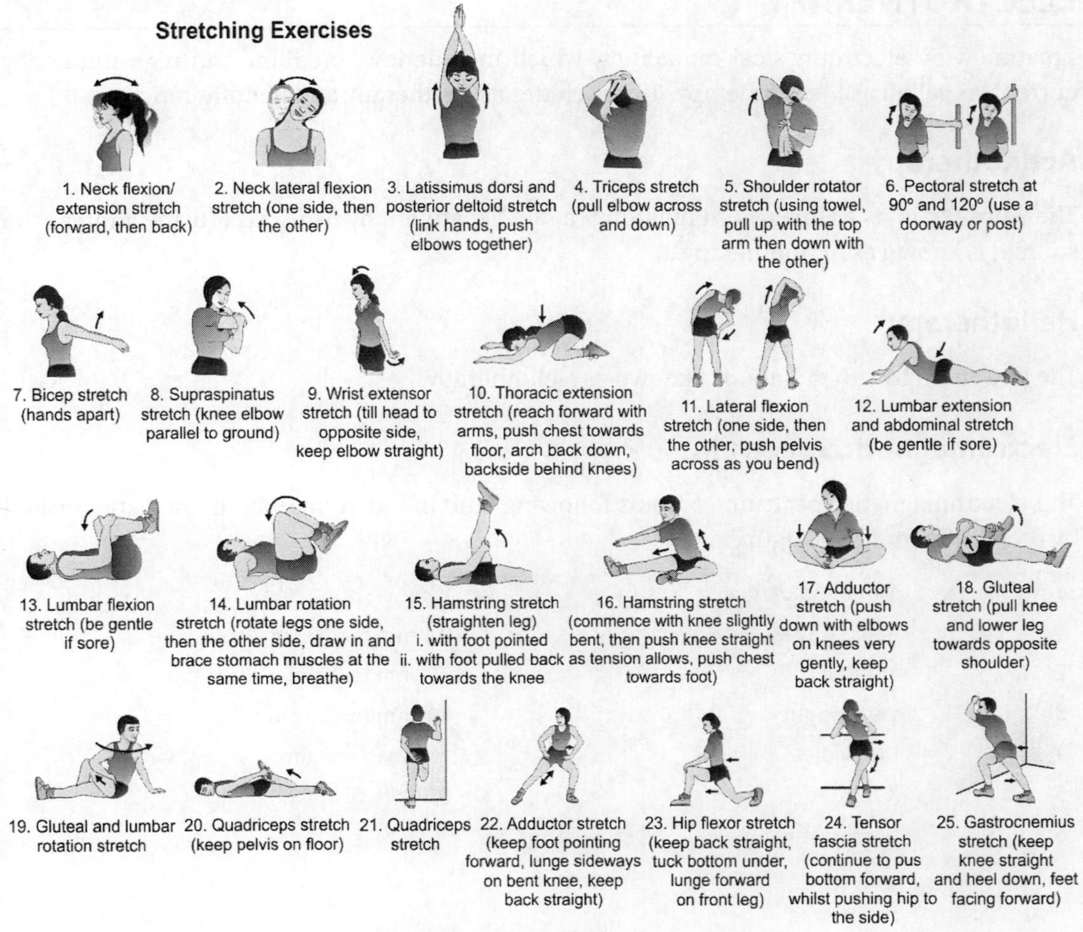

Stretching Exercises

1. Neck flexion/ extension stretch (forward, then back)
2. Neck lateral flexion stretch (one side, then the other)
3. Latissimus dorsi and posterior deltoid stretch (link hands, push elbows together)
4. Triceps stretch (pull elbow across and down)
5. Shoulder rotator stretch (using towel, pull up with the top arm then down with the other)
6. Pectoral stretch at 90° and 120° (use a doorway or post)
7. Bicep stretch (hands apart)
8. Supraspinatus stretch (knee elbow parallel to ground)
9. Wrist extensor stretch (till head to opposite side, keep elbow straight)
10. Thoracic extension stretch (reach forward with arms, push chest towards floor, arch back down, backside behind knees)
11. Lateral flexion stretch (one side, then the other, push pelvis across as you bend)
12. Lumbar extension and abdominal stretch (be gentle if sore)
13. Lumbar flexion stretch (be gentle if sore)
14. Lumbar rotation stretch (rotate legs one side, then the other side, draw in and brace stomach muscles at the same time, breathe)
15. Hamstring stretch (straighten leg) i. with foot pointed ii. with foot pulled back towards the knee
16. Hamstring stretch (commence with knee slightly bent, then push knee straight as tension allows, push chest towards foot)
17. Adductor stretch (push down with elbows on knees very gently, keep back straight)
18. Gluteal stretch (pull knee and lower leg towards opposite shoulder)
19. Gluteal and lumbar rotation stretch
20. Quadriceps stretch (keep pelvis on floor)
21. Quadriceps stretch
22. Adductor stretch (keep foot pointing forward, lunge sideways on bent knee, keep back straight)
23. Hip flexor stretch (keep back straight, tuck bottom under, lunge forward on front leg)
24. Tensor fascia stretch (continue to pus bottom forward, whilst pushing hip to the side)
25. Gastrocnemius stretch (keep knee straight and heel down, feet facing forward)

Fig. 9.1: Some static exercises

Precautions

- Static exercises tend to drive up blood pressure in an instant. Thus the people with circulation problems and high blood pressure should avoid over-exerting pressure without muscle movements.
- One should not hold the breath while performing these exercises as this would lead to increase in blood pressure.
- Professional advice is always highly recommended.
- Not recommended for children and adolescents whose bones are still growing. There are higher chances of damage to tendons and connective tissues.
- Don't force a joint beyond its normal range of motion, this can lead to instability of the joint.
- Not recommended in patients suffering from osteoporosis or taking steroids. The risk of fracture is elevated.
- Avoid aggressive stretching of muscle that have been immobilized in a splint or cast.
- Avoid stretching swollen and edematous tissue as they are more susceptible to damage.

ELECTROTHERAPY

Treatment by electrophysical modalities, which include low, medium and high frequency currents is called as Electrotherapy. This includes actinotherapy and heliotherapy.

Actinotherapy

The word "actis" is a Greek word meaning "a ray". Treatment by using rays (using lamp as the source) is known as Actinotherapy .

Heliotherapy

The treatment by sun radiation is known as Heliotherapy.

Electromagnetic Spectrum

The electromagnetic spectrum contains following kind of radiations which are distinguished by their different wavelength:

S. No.	*Name of radiation*	*Wavelength*
1	Radio waves	0.1 mm to 100 km
2	Infrared	750 nm to 0.4 mm
3	Visible light	400 nm to 750 nm
4	Ultraviolet	10 nm to 400 nm
5	X-rays	0.01 pm to 100 nm
6	Gamma rays	

INFRARED THERAPY

Infrared rays were discovered by a German scientist named Sir William Hershell in year 1800. The infrared rays are electromagnetic waves with the wavelengths of 750 nm to 40,000 nm and frequency 4 × 104 and 7.5 × 101 Hz. It lies beyond the red boundary of visible spectrum. Any hot body can produce infrared rays like the sun, electric bulb, coal fire and gas fire, etc. Sun is the natural source of infrared radiations.

IR rays are of 3 categories:

1. Near IR rays (0.76–1.56 microns)
2. Mid IR rays (1.5–4 microns)
3. Far IR rays (4–1000 microns)

According to biological research Far IR rays are absorbed very easily by the human body. It helps in all aspects of bodily growth and development. These Far IR rays are also called light of life. When its intensity is high in the body we feel healthy and will be able to overcome ailments. However, when it begins to decline, body will be subjected to ailments.

In physiotherapy infrared rays are produced by 2 types of generators:

1. Non-luminous generators produce only Infrared rays.
2. Luminous generators produce Infrared rays, UV and Visible rays.

Non-luminous Generator

1. Consists of coil wound on a cylinder of insulating material like porcelain.
2. An electric current is passed through the wire which results in the production of heat.
3. This heat produces infrared rays which are transmitted through the porcelain.
4. The porcelain gets heated and generates the radiation including visible rays.
5. To avoid this, coil is embedded in fireclay or placed behind fireclay.
7. Now the emission of rays is from the fireclay which is commonly painted black and thus very few visible rays are produced.
8. The coil is placed at a spherical reflector.
9. The reflector is mounted on an adjustable stand.

Uses

It is useful in acute inflammation or cases of recent injury.

Luminous Generator (Fig 9.2A)

1. These generators are in the form of incandescent lamps or bulbs.
2. This is lamp in which there is tungsten filaments and filled with inert gas at low pressure.

Uses

It is useful in diseases/ lesions which are chronic in nature.

Depth of Penetration

It depends on the wavelength:

S. No.	*Type of Infrared generator*	*Wavelength*	*Part penetrated*
1	Luminous generator	350–4000 nm	Dermis and epidermis
2	Non-luminous generator	750–15000 nm	Superficial dermis

Physiological Effect

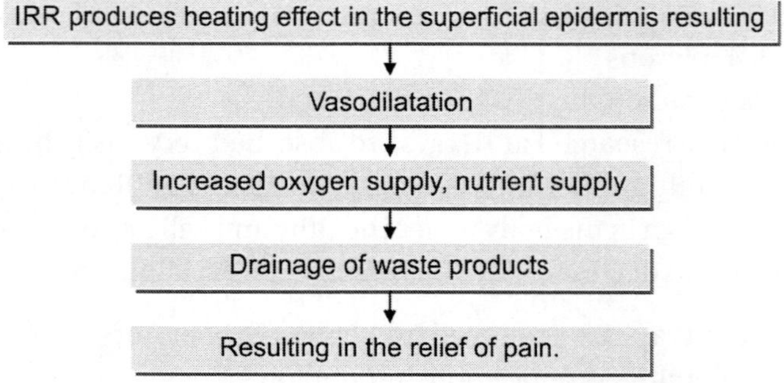

Procedure (Fig. 9.2 B)

Patient is prepared by removing the clothing from the affected part and the sensation to cold and heat is tested on the skin. Patient should be cautioned about risk of uncomfortable warmth and that it should be reported immediately to avoid burns. Undue movements during therapy should be avoided. The lamp shall be positioned about 50–25 cm away from the skin of the patient and arranged in way that the radiation falls on the skin of the patient at an angle of 90°.

Duration of the treatment is between 10–15 minutes.

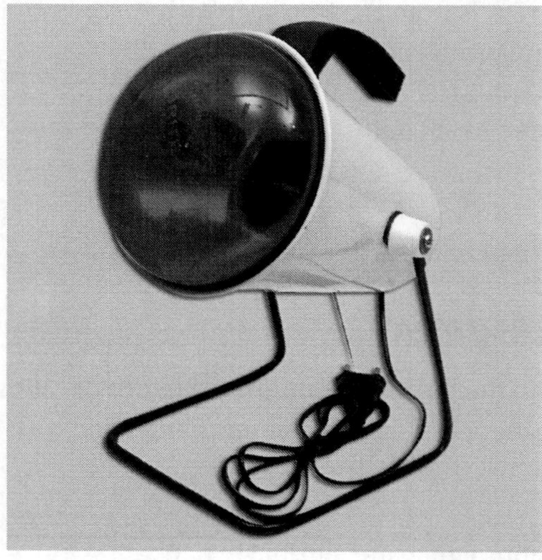

Fig. 9. 2A: Infrared bulb

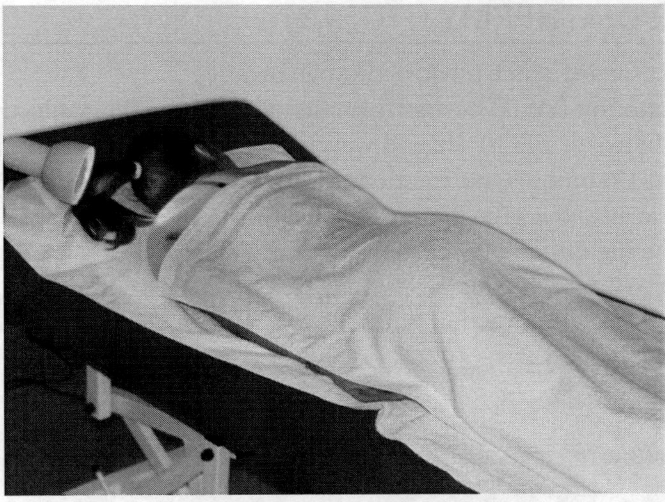

Fig. 9. 2B: Infrared therapy

Therapeutic Uses

1. Increases blood circulation
2. Wound healing
3. Decreases inflammation
4. Relieves pain
5. Improves metabolism
6. Long-term exposure improves health and immunity.
7. Induces muscle relaxation

Contraindications

1. Area of anesthesia
2. Patient of Arterial disease
3. Eczema
4. Gastric ulcer and hemorrhage

Disadvantages

1. Burns
2. Electric shock
3. Overdose headache
4. Injury to eyes
5. Faintness
6. Gangrene

SHORT WAVE DIATHERMY (FIG. 9.3)

Diathermy is a Greek word which means - through heating.

Short wave diathermy (SWD) current consists of high frequency electromagnetic waves having frequency between 10^7–10^8 Hz and wavelength between 30 and 3 m to generate heat in the body tissues. Commonly use frequency for medical use is 27.12 MHz. It provides the deepest form of heat available. The therapeutically used frequencies and wavelength are 27.12 MHz and 11 m. The high frequency current (approx 500 KHz) being used provides impulses with duration of 0.001 ms, which is beyond the range of nerve stimulation, thus, there is no discomfort and no muscle contraction is produced.

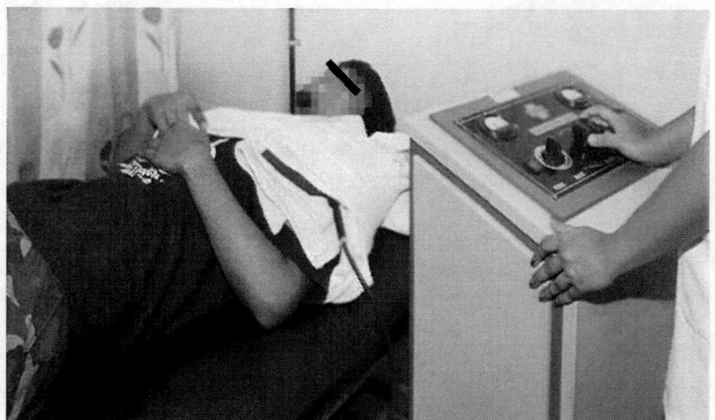

Fig. 9. 3: Short wave diathermy

Methods of Application

There are two methods of application:

1. Capacitor field method
2. Cable method

Capacitor Field Method

In this the electrodes and patient's tissue form a capacitor. The electrodes are placed on either side of the affected part, separated from the skin of patient by insulated material. The capacitance depends on:

a. The size of the electrodes
b. Distance between the electrodes
c. Tissue between the electrodes.

Cable Method

In this a thick and insulated cable is used for treatment purpose. The cable is coiled around the patient's body and is separated from patient's body by a layer of insulating material. The effect of the electric field or magnetic field or both is used in this type of diathermy. Cable method is especially useful for treating large areas which cannot be covered between the electrodes e.g. in cases of extensive RA.

Indications

1. Inflammation of joints
2. Tennis elbow
3. Degeneration of joints of neck (cervical spondylosis), knee and hip etc. (Osteoarthritis)
4. Ligament sprains and strains of muscles
5. Low back ache
6. Plantar fasciitis (heel pain)
7. Sinusitis
8. Muscle and tendon tear
9. Hematoma
10. Carbuncles

Contraindications

1. High fever
2. Fluctuating blood pressure
3. Very sensitive skin
4. Persons with untreated fits
5. Persons using cardiac pace maker
6. Severe kidney and heart problems
7. Pregnancy
8. Mentally retarded individuals
9. Tuberculosis of bone
10. Malignancy

Advantages

1. Relaxation of the muscles
2. Effective in controlling bacterial infections
3. Relieves pain
4. Reduces healing time.

Treatment Time

Initial stage—5–10 minutes
Moderate stage—10–20 minutes
Severe state—20–30 minutes.

Disadvantages

1. Burns
2. Shock
3. Electric sparking
4. Faintness
5. Scalds (boils)
6. Overdose

Precautions

The table or chair being used for patient should not contain any metal as it interferes with the electromagnetic field of SWD. Skin of the patient shall be exposed wherever possible to maximize the benefits.

ELECTROMAGNETIC THERAPY (FIG. 9.4)

Electromagnetic therapy or electromagnetic field therapy refers to therapy involving the use of electromagnets.

Substance which attracts the iron pieces and set itself in the north and south pole when it is freely suspended. This property is known as magnetism.

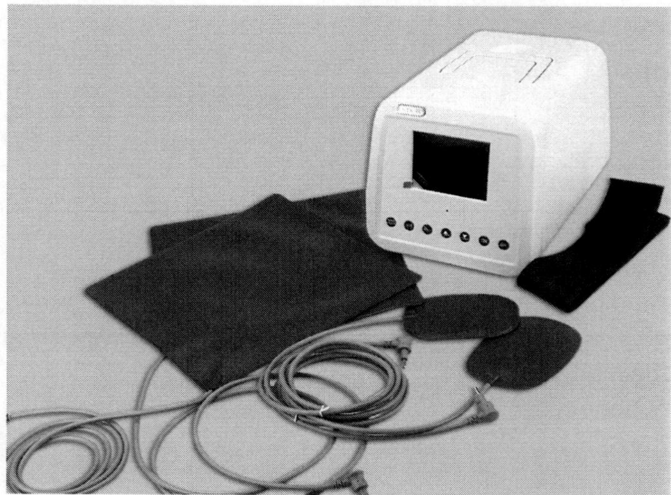

Fig. 9. 4: Electromagnetic therapy

Types of magnets: There are two types of Magnets

1. **Natural magnets:** Often irregular in shape and they are weak.
2. **Artificial magnet:** It is found that a piece of iron or steel can acquire magnetic properties, on rubbing with a magnet. Such magnets made out of iron and steel are called artificial magnets. Artificial magnets have desired shape and strength e.g. horse shoe magnet, magnetic needle etc.

Properties of the Magnet

1. A magnet attracts magnetic substances like iron, steel, cobalt, nickel towards it. The attraction appears to be maximum at the end.
2. When a magnet is suspended freely with the help of an unspun thread, it comes to rest along the North-South direction.
3. Like poles repel each other and unlike poles attract each other.
4. Hammering and heating the magnet destroys the magnetic property of the magnets.

Electromagnet

A simple electromagnet consisting of a coil of insulated wire wrapped around an iron core. The strength of magnetic field generated is proportional to the amount of current. The magnetic therapy is a type of physiotherapy as it uses electromagnetic energy and it is an effective, safe and noninvasive cure. The magneto therapy regenerates the injured cell by improving the enzyme secretion and repolarizes the cellular membrane. Furthermore, it produces an anti-stress action and promotes acceleration of all reparative phenomenon's with bio-regeneration, anti-inflammatory and analgesic action without any side effect.

Duration

It depends on the nature of disease and patient's tolerance. It can be used once a day or twice as per conditions. In the beginning it should be used for 5 min, later the duration can be increased but not more than 10 mins. In cases of joint pain, gout, arthritis it can be used up to 30 minutes. Should not take bath up to one hour after the treatment.

Benefits

- Relieves the pain, it acts as a potent analgesic
- It accelerates the healing processes
- It stimulates the cellular exchange
- It improves the flow of nutrition and the oxygenation of the tissue
- It reduce the inflammation
- It stimulates the reabsorption of edema
- Degeneration: It slows down the process of bone degeneration.

Precaution or Contraindication

- Pregnancy
- Individuals with pacemakers or similar device
- Bleeding wounds.

Complications

- Heaviness
- Headache
- Sleeping symptoms.

WAX BATH THERAPY (FIG. 9.5)

Wax bath therapy is an application of the molten paraffin wax on the body parts. The melting point of wax is 51°C–55°C. If the molten wax is poured at this temperature it may cause burn. So some impurities like paraffin or mineral oil is added to lower the melting point for safe application and the temperature of the paraffin wax is maintained at 40°C–44°C. As the wax solidifies from molten state, it conducts the heat into the tissues.

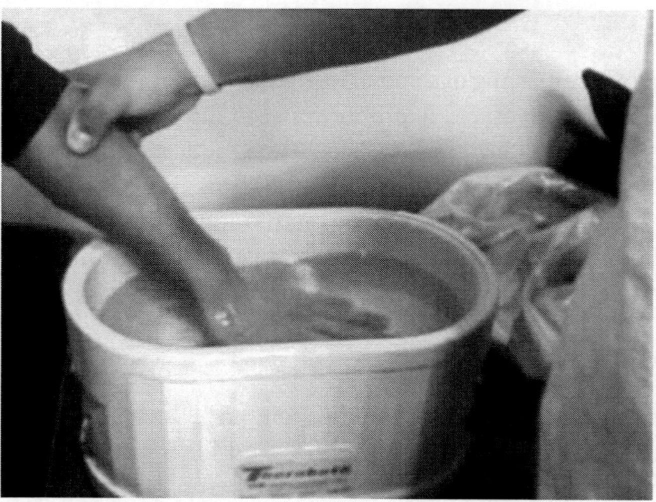

Fig 9. 5: Wax bath therapy

Methods of Application

a. Dipping and wrapping
b. Immersion
c. Direct pouring
d. Toweling or bandaging
e. Brushing method

Indication

- Edema and inflammation (sub-acute and early chronic stage)
- Swelling of hands in RA
- Degenerative joint disease
- Adhesion and scat

Treatment Time

The time duration for the treatment is about 30–45 minutes.

Contraindications

- Open wounds
- Skin rashes
- Allergic conditions
- Impaired skin sensations
- Defective arterial supply.

ULTRASONIC THERAPY (FIG. 9.6)

Ultrasound refers to mechanical vibrations which are essentially same as sound waves but of a higher frequency. Such waves are, beyond the range of human hearing and therefore also called as ultrasonic. It requires elastic medium such as air, and cannot cross a vacuum unlike electromagnetic waves

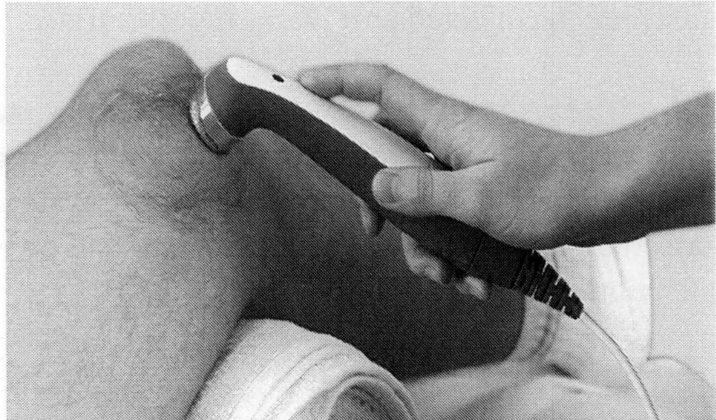

Fig 9. 6: Ultrasonic therapy

Frequency of Ultrasound

Any vibration at a frequency above the audible sound range, i.e. 20–20000 Hz. Different therapies are employed in range from 0.5–4 MHz.

At 1 MHz, frequency is most useful in individuals with a high percentage of cutaneous fat and whenever the desired effects are in the deeper structures, i.e. depth of penetration about 4 cm.

At 3 MHz, the energy is absorbed in the more superficial tissues with a depth of penetration about 2 cm. Ultrasound therapy is based on biological effects of ultrasonic oscillations which are not electric. Despite of that, this therapy is sometimes included in the list of electrotherapeutic methods (Fig. 9.7).

An ultrasound (US) therapeutic system consists of two main parts:

a. Generator of high frequency of electric current and
b. The application probes, the US source itself, which consists of a piezoelectric transducer.

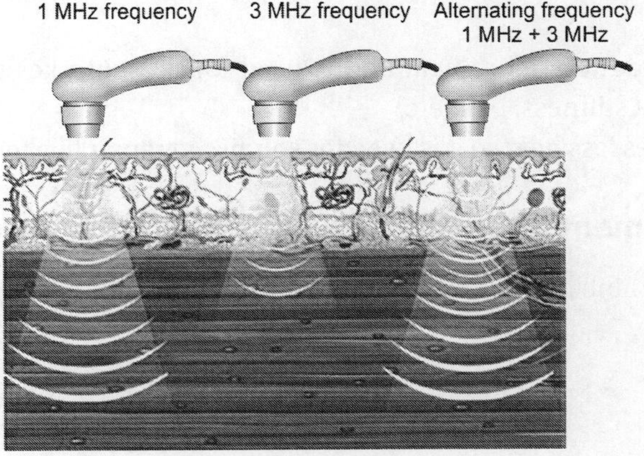

Fig. 9. 7: Different wavelengths of ultrasonic therapy

Techniques of Application

1. Direct Contact Method

In this method treatment head is applied directly over the skin of affected part and moved in small concentric circles to avoid damage by reflection and also to avoid concentration at any particular point. This technique can cover the areas up to 3 times the size of treatment head effectively. It is preferred where the affected part has a smooth surface.

2. Water Bath Method

In this technique, the treatment is given to a patient after submerging the affected part in a water bath, the distance between skin and head is kept at about 1cm. Water used for this purpose shall preferably be degassed, or if gas is present the bubbles shall be wiped of frequently to avoid any damage by reflection.

3. Water Bag Method

It is used on surfaces which are irregular. A rubber bag filled with degassed water is then placed over the skin of patient after applying a coupling medium and then the treatment head is moved over the bag as it is moved over the skin of the patient. The disadvantage of this method is that much energy is absorbed by the rubber itself.

Absorption

Ultrasound is absorbed by the tissues and converted to heat at that point. This contributes the thermal effect of ultrasound.

Dosage

Three factors determine ultrasound dosage as follows :

1. Size of the treatment area
2. Depth of the lesion from the surface
3. Nature of lesion

Mode

Continuous mode produces more heat and is used for musculoskeletal conditions such as muscular spasm, joint stiffness, pain etc.
Pulsed mode produces less heat so it is used for soft tissue repair like tendinitis etc.

Duration of Treatment

Size or the area determine the treatment time, i.e. 1-2 minute for every cm^2.
Minimum 1-2 minute.
Maximum 8 minute.
Average 5 minute.

For chronic conditions: Longer treatment time.
For acute conditions: Lesser treatment time.

Indications

- Soft tissue injuries
- Scar tissue
- Chronic indurate oedema
- Varicose ulcer
- Bone injuries
- Plantar warts.

Contraindications

- Thrombophlebitis
- Acute sepsis
- Tumours
- Pregnancy
- Cardiac disease
- Haemorrhage
- Implants (metal implants)
- Anaesthetic area.

Precaution

Care shall be taken to leave some space between the treatment head of the Ultrasonic machine and the skin of the patient to prevent damage to the head by reflection of waves.

Effects

Thermal Effects

- There is local rise in temperature of the tissues giving sedative effect and promotes healing.
- Extensibility of the collagen is increased, which helps in stretching of scars or adhesions.

Cavitation

- It is produced by the oscillation of highly compressible bodies within the tissue.
- It is a type of nonthermal effect of Ultrasound.
- When stable cavitation causes microstreaming, influencing cell permeability and the direction of movement of molecules.
- To avoid any harm due to unstable cavitation effect, the treatment head must be moved regularly.

Mechanical

- Also known as micro-massage, it is caused by compression of cells due to waves.
- It affects the movement of fluid in interstitial space.
- Reduces oedema
- Increases extensibility of scars.

Biological

It helps in healing through following methods:

Inflammatory

It increases fragility of lysome membranes, enhancing the release of enzymes in them which further helps in clearing the debris.

Proliferative

Increases the mobility of fibro and myofibroblasts to the area of repair, thus improve healing time.

Remodeling

It increases the tensile strength of the scar by affecting strength and elasticity of the fibres.

Self-Assessment

MULTIPLE CHOICE QUESTIONS

1. How many type of Sagni Sveda are there according to Charaka?
   (a) 13 (b) 15
   (c) 12 (d) 10
2. Madhyama dose of Sneha gets digested in:
   (a) 3 hours (b) 6 hours
   (c) 12 hours (d) 16 hours
3. What is the most potent treatment of Murdha taila?
   (a) Abhyanga (b) Seka
   (c) Basti (d) Pichu
4. Shirobasti is choice of treatment in:
   (a) Pratishaya (b) Kasa
   (c) Ardit (d) Badhirya
5. Sansarjana karma in Madhyam shuddhi is advised for:
   (a) 1 Day (b) 5 Days
   (c) 7 Days (d) 3 Days
6. According to Charaka Kala of Prayogika Dhumapana are:
   (a) 4 (b) 3
   (c) 8 (d) 12
7. Siravedha is indicated in:
   (a) Urdhvaga Raktapitta (b) Gridhrasi
   (c) Tamak Shvas (d) None of the above
8. What is the quantity of oil used in Matra Basti?
   (a) 30 mL (b) 40 mL
   (c) 60mL (d) 20 mL
9. How many Netra Dosha are described in case of Basti netra?
   (a) 10 (b) 12
   (c) 4 (d) 8
10. How many Basti's are administered in "Karma Basti" protocol?
    (a) 10 (b) 8
    (c) 16 (d) 30

11. Shirobasti is the choice of treatment in which of the following?
    (a) Ardita (b) Gridhrasi
    (c) Kasa (d) Shvasa
12. Frequency of changing oil in Snehadhara is:
    (a) After 2 days (b) Everyday
    (c) After 3 days (d) Never
13. Mridu sveda is indicated for which body parts:
    (a) Shira (b) Vrishana and Linga
    (c) Netra (d) All of the above
14. Jambeera pinda sveda comes under which category?
    (a) Snigdha Sankara sveda (b) Ruksha Sankara Sveda
    (c) Upnaha (d) None of the above
15. What is the height of Shirobasti Cap?
    (a) 12 Angula (b) 14 Angula
    (c) 16 Angula (d) 18 Angula
16. How many yoga of Vatsaka are described by Charaka?
    (a) 18 (b) 39
    (c) 133 (d) 545
17. Gati Vaishamya arises due to which type of Basti dosha?
    (a) Basti putaka dosha (b) Basti praneta dosha
    (c) Basti netra dosha (d) Atiyoga
18. What is the length of Vrana basti netra?
    (a) 2 angula (b) 4 angula
    (c) 6 angula (d) 8 angula
19. Which of the following is not a Nirvisha Jalauka?
    (a) Algarda (b) Indrayudha
    (c) Samudrika (d) Mushika
20. Which procedure is referred to as Ardha chikitsa in Shalya tantra?
    (a) Jalaukavcharan (b) Pracchana
    (c) Siravedha (d) None of the above
21. Snehana and Shodhana are subtypes of which kind of Nasya?
    (a) Dhuma (b) Navana
    (c) Pradhamana (d) Avapeeda
22. How many times Prayogika Dhuma is administered in a day?
    (a) 1 (b) 2
    (c) 3 (d) 4
23. According to Charaka which type of Snehapaka is advised to use for Abhyanga?
    (a) Chikkana (b) Khara
    (c) Mridu (d) Madhyama
24. Avapeedaka Sneha is given at what time?
    (a) Before meals (b) Empty stomach
    (c) Between meals (d) At bed time

25. Which of the following is not included under Ushma Sveda according to Dalhana?
    (a) Kumbhi (b) Ashmaghna
    (c) Nadi (d) Karshu
26. Who among the following has included Raktamokshana as fifth karma in Pancha karma?
    (a) Charaka (b) Chakrapani
    (c) Sushruta (d) Dalhana
27. How many Anna kala are advised for each modality under Sansarjana krama in Uttama shuddhi?
    (a) 1 Annakala (b) 2 Annakala
    (c) 3 Annakala (d) 4 Annakala
28. What is the duration of Parihara kala described after Basti Karma?
    (a) Samaguna (b) Dviguna
    (c) Triguna (d) Chaturguna
29. Navana Nasya is indicated in:
    (a) Urdhvaga Raktapitta (b) Ardita
    (c) Kasa (d) None of the above
30. What is the quantity of oil used in "Sneha" Basti?
    (a) 30 mL (b) 240 mL
    (c) 60mL (d) 120 mL
31. How many Dosha/Vyapad are described in case of Basti Praneta?
    (a) 10 (b) 12
    (c) 4 (d) 8
32. How many Basti's are administered in "Yoga Basti" protocol?
    (a) 10 (b) 8
    (c) 16 (d) 30
33. Till what level from kesha Bhumi is Sneha dravya is filled during Shirobasti procedure?
    (a) 12 Angula (b) 8 Angula
    (c) 2 Angula (d) 4 Angula
34. Frequency of changing oil in Shirodhara is:
    (a) After 2 days (b) Everyday
    (c) After 3 days (d) Never
35. Patrapinda Sveda is not done on:
    (a) Shira (b) Vrishana and Linga
    (c) Both (d) None
36. What is the frequency of changing Pottali in Shalishashtika Pinda Sveda ?
    (a) After 3 days (b) Daily
    (c) Never (d) Every second day
37. What is the height of Varti from forehead in Shirodhara ?
    (a) 2 Angula (b) 4 Angula
    (c) 6 Angula (d) 8 Angula
38. How many yoga of Madanaphala are described by Charaka?
    (a) 133 (b) 655
    (c) 233 (d) 545

39. Parihara Kala in Basti chikitsa is:
    (a) Sama (b) Dviguna
    (c) Triguna (d) None of the above
40. What is the correct sequence of mixing following in Basti Sammelan vidhi?
    1. Kvatha, 2. Kalka, 3. Sneha, 4. Madhu, 5. Saindhava
    (a) 1, 2, 3, 4, 5 (b) 4, 5, 3, 2, 1
    (c) 5, 4, 3, 2, 1 (d) 4, 5, 3, 1, 2
41. Which of the following is not a Savisha Jalauka?
    (a) Pingala (b) Karbura
    (c) Samudrika (d) Gochandana
42. What is the quantity of Rakta visravan in Madhyama Shudhi Siravedha?
    (a) 1 Prastha (b) 2 Prastha
    (c) ½ Prastha (d) 1 Kudava
43. How many types of Dushta vyadhana are described in respect to siravedha karma?
    (a) 20 (b) 40
    (c) 10 (d) 15
44. How many times is Snaihika Dhuma administered in a day?
    (a) 1 (b) 2
    (c) 3 (d) 4
45. Number of "Sadhya Snehan Yoga" mentioned in Vagbhatta are:
    (a) 5 (b) 6
    (c) 8 (d) 7
46. Treatment for Ayoga of Shirovirechana is:
    (a) Abhyang
    (b) Swedana
    (c) Repeated tikshna shirovirechana
    (d) Repeated Mridu shirovirechana
47. Treatment of Annavrit Anuvasana Basti Janita diseases are:
    (a) Phalavarti
    (b) Udavrta nashaka
    (c) Pachana and Mridu virechana
    (d) Both a and b
48. Quantity of milk in Panchprasritiki Basti is:
    (a) 2 prasrita (b) 3 prasrita
    (c) 1 prasrita (d) None of the above
49. Best vamak for Udara Rog is:
    (a) Kutaj (b) Kritwedhana
    (c) Ikshwaku (d) Dharmargava
50. According to Charak, kharapaka sneha is used for:
    (a) Nasya (b) Basti
    (c) Pana (d) Abhyanga

51. Vamana at an interval of 15 days, virechana at an interval of 1 month and Raktamoshana at an interval of 6 months is treatment of:
 (a) Udara roga (b) Rajyakshama
 (c) Visarpa (d) Kushtha
52. According to sushrut the matra for sneha in Dwadash Prasrata Niruh Basti should be:
 (a) 3 Prasrat (b) 2 Prasrat
 (c) 5 Prasrat (d) 4 Prasrat
53. Which of the following Sneha has the property Mutrabadham
 (a) Sarpi (b) Taila
 (c) Vasa (d) Majja
54. Which among following is not a Shirovirechana dravya?
 (a) Bharangi (b) Shringaber
 (c) Lashun (d) Kashmri
55. In symptom of supti which kind of Raktamokshan should be performed?
 (a) Prachan (b) Shringa
 (c) Jaluka (d) Siravedha
56. "Kuryad Adhmananam Gauravam Jwaram" is the symptom of
 (a) Bastidan at night (b) Bastidan in the day
 (c) Bastidan before meal (d) Bastidan in morning
57. According to Charaka ingredients of Kalka of taila used for abhyanga in Apsamara chikitsa are:
 (a) Goshakrit (b) Aja shakrit
 (c) Both of the above (d) None of the above
58. What are the harmful effects if Niruha Basti is not administered on empty stomach?
 (a) Daruna chhardi (b) Visuchika
 (c) Angamarda (d) A and B both
59. Anuvasan Basti is given in night in which of the following season:
 (a) Shishir, Hemanta, Vasanta.
 (b) Grishma, Sharada, Hemanta.
 (c) Sharada, Grishma, Varsha.
 (d) In any season in night Anuvasana basti can be given.
60. According to Dalhana in Abhyanga, Sneha reaches to rakta in how many matras:
 (a) 300 (b) 400
 (c) 500 (d) 600
61. Vamana is indicated in all of the following except:
 (a) Nava jwara (b) Mandagni
 (c) Atisara (d) Samvrita koshta
62. If the Bastidrava given is excessively hot, what complications may arise:
 (a) Daha and Atisara (b) Vidaha and murcha
 (c) Ayoga lakshana (d) Atiyoga lakshana
63. Vatala Dosha is present in:
 (a) Basti netra (b) Basti putak
 (c) Basti dravya (d) None of the above

64. Which of the following is a Dosha of Basti praneta:
    (a) Savata (b) Vatala
    (c) Jalika (d) Hrasava
65. No. of days required to complete a course of Panchakarma in case of Pradhana Shuddhi are:
    (a) 129 (b) 138
    (c) 130 (d) 85
66. According to Charak siddhisthan, the count of Mahadoshkar Varjya Vishaya is:
    (a) 6 (b) 8
    (c) 4 (d) 12
67. According to Charak, which kind of Snehapaka is used for Abhyantara snehapana:
    (a) Madhyama (b) Mridu
    (c) Khara (d) None of the above
68. How many types of Svedana have been described by Vagbhatta:
    (a) 6 (b) 3
    (c) 4 (d) 8
69. Pinda Sveda is a subtype of which Sveda?
    (a) Prastara (b) Nadi
    (c) Sankara (d) Bhu
70. Nasa Hi Shirso Dvaram, has been told by:
    (a) Charak (b) Sushruta
    (c) Ashtanga Hridaya (d) Sharangdhara
71. Which of the following is not amongst Ashta Mahadoshkara Varjya Vishaya
    (a) Ratha kshobha (b) Uccha bhashana
    (c) Vaidyamani (d) Atisnigdha ahara
72. Which is the right "Kala"of Virechana according to Sharangdhara
    (a) Sharad (b) Vasant
    (c) Varsha (d) Both A and B
73. What is the treatment of Vamana Atiyoga according to Shanrangdhara
    (a) Mridu Virechana (b) Tikshna Virechana
    (c) Nasya (d) None of the above
74. Vamana should be administered after a break of how many days after samyak Snehapana:
    (a) 1 (b) 2
    (c) 3 (d) 4
75. Pracchana karma can remove blood from how deep:
    (a) 1 Angula (b) 10 Angula
    (c) 2 Hasta (d) 12 Angula
76. How many Sneha Basti Vyapat are described by Charaka:
    (a) 6 (b) 8
    (c) 10 (d) 12

77. According to Sharangadhara, the minimum age after which Nasya can be administered is:
(a) 4 (b) 6
(c) 7 (d) 8

78. According to Sushruta total number of Vamana-Virechana Vyapat is:
(a) 10 (b) 12
(c) 13 (d) 15

79. The number of Virechana yoga of Tilvak is:
(a) 18 (b) 16
(c) 39 (d) 12

80. The number of Shayya dosha described under Basti dosha by Sushruta is:
(a) 11 (b) 4
(c) 7 (d) 9

81. Which of the following conditions is contraindicated for Shirovirechana
(a) Nava jvara (b) Hanugraha
(c) Apatanaka (d) Galaganda

82. Niruha Basti is contraindicated in:
(a) Shirahshula (b) Karnashula
(c) Akshepaka (d) Kushtha

83. Timir disease is an indication for which therapy:
(a) Vamana (b) Virechana
(c) Vaman and virechana (d) None of the above

84. According to kashyapa, treatment for Atisvinna condition should be similar to:
(a) Shopha (b) Atisara
(c) Visarpa (d) Vidradhi

85. According to Charaka, which of the following is contraindicated for Anuvasana
(a) Navajvara (b) Pandu
(c) KamLa (d) All of the above

86. Best form of Snehapana is:
(a) Yusha (b) Basti
(c) Accha sneha (d) Odana

87. Which of the following is best line of treatment for Tamak shvasa, Pakshaghata and Udara:
(a) Vamana (b) Virechana
(c) Basti (d) Nasya

88. Saindhavadi Anuvasana Basti is indicated in:
(a) Pakshaghata (b) Amavata
(c) Gridhrasi (d) Vatarakta

89. Which of the following Dravya is Shrestha Vamaka dravya according to Acharya Shonaka?
(a) Madanaphala (b) Katu tumbi
(c) Dhamargava (d) Jimutaka

90. What is the correct length of Basti Netra for a person aged 20 years?
    (a) 10 Angula (b) 8 Angula
    (c) 12 Angula (d) 6 Angula
91. How many karnika are there in a Basti Netra according to Charaka?
    (a) 2 (b) 4
    (c) 3 (d) 1
92. What is the correct time to administer Nasya in Hemant/Shita ritu?
    (a) Purvahna (b) Madhyahna
    (c) Aparahna (d) Ratri
93. What is the correct time to administer Nasya in Grishma Ritu?
    (a) Purvahna (b) Madhyahna
    (c) Aparahna (d) Ratri
94. What is the correct length of Basti Netra for a person aged 8 years according to Sushruta?
    (a) 10 Angula (b) 8 Angula
    (c) 12 Angula (d) 6 Angula
95. How many types of Sveda are described by Sushruta
    (a) 2 (b) 13
    (c) 4 (d) 6
96. How many yoga of Jimutaka have been described?
    (a) 39 (b) 45
    (c) 255 (d) 133
97. According to Sushruta, Anupana for Ghripana in Kaphaja disorders should be:
    (a) Saidhava lavana (b) Only ghrita
    (c) Vyosha (d) none of the above
98. Madhutailika Basti is:
    (a) Stambhana (b) Rukshana
    (c) Rasayana (d) Shamana
99. Amongst muline dravya, Shanapushpi is used for:
    (a) Shiroverechana (b) Vamana
    (c) Virechana (d) None of the above
100. In case of Pindita Rakta Dushti, choice of treatment for Raktamokshana is:
    (a) Jalauka (b) Pracchana
    (c) Alabu (d) Siravedha

SHORT ANSWER QUESTIONS

1. What are the various classifications of Snehana?
2. Write short note on contraindications of Vamana karma along with reasons.
3. Write short note on Charakokta Vamana Vyapada.
4. Write short note on Shalishashtika Pinda Sveda.
5. Write short note on importance on Purva karma in Pancha karma.
6. Describe Basti Sammelan Vidhi in short.

7. Write short note on classification of Raktamokshana.
8. Write Samyaka and Asamyaka Shuddhi symptoms of Nasya karma
9. Write short note on Short wave diathermy.
10. Write short note on Contraindications of Nasya karma.
11. Svedopaga Dravya.
12. What are the properties of Vamaka dravya.
13. Sneha yoni.
14. Svedana Atiyoga lakshana.
15. Snehana Guna.
16. Vamanopaga Gana.
17. Tarpanadi karma.
18. Properties of Ghrita.
19. Types of Upnaha Sveda according to Chakrapani.
20. Write Udvartana procedure with its indications.
21. Write Indications and Contraindications of Virechana.
22. Basti sammelan vidhi.
23. Chikitsa sutra of Raktavaha Srotasa Vikara.
24. Shirovirechanopga gana.
25. Pradhamana Nasya.
26. Types of Raktamokshana.
27. Time of administration of Nasya.
28. Differentiate between Marsha and Pratimarsha Nasya.
29. Shuddha Rakta lakshana.
30. Doses of Avapidaka Nasya
31. Write short note on Short wave diathermy.
32. Write short note on Contraindications of Raktamokshana.
33. Write short note on Basti Putaka Dosha.
34. Write short note on classification of Nasya.
35. Write Samyaka and Asamyaka shuddhi symptoms of Raktamokshana karma.
36. Write short note on Infrared treatment.
37. Write short note on Wax bath therapy.
38. Write short note on Padaghata.
39. Write short note on contraindications of Virechana karma along with reasons.
40. Write short note on Svedana Atiyoga.
41. Write short note on Shalishashtika Pinda sveda.
42. Write short note on importance on Purva karma in Pancha karma
43. Give short description of various types of Jalauka.
44. Samyak yoga of Nasya karma.
45. Shirovirechana dravya.
46. Yapana Basti.
47. Basti Netra vayapada.
48. Give schedule of Karma basti.

49. Give doses of various types of Nasya.
50. Classification of Dhumpana.
51. Avapeedaka nasya.
52. Write short note on Pracchana karma.
53. Write Kati basti procedure with its indications.
54. Define virechana and give its classification according to Sharangdhara.
55. Vamanopaga dravya.
56. Give Panchbhautikatva and properties of Virechana dravya.
57. Samyaka Snehana lakshana.
58. Ashta Mahadoshkara Varjya Vishaya.
59. Virechanopaga Gana.
60. Uttama Shuddhi Sansarjana karma.
61. Classification of Svedana according to Sushruta.
62. Mahasneha.
63. How many types of tables are used for Panchakarma therapy with its uses?
64. Differentiate amang (a) Matra basti (b) Anuvasan basti (c) Sneha basti.
65. What are the different dimensions of Basti Netra according to different ages?
66. Write about Matra of Niruha Basti according different age groups?
67. Write about indications, benefits and quantity of Matra basti.
68. Why Niruha Basti is given before meals?
69. What are the adharabhuta siddhanta of Pancha karma chikitsa?
70. Why is it advised to undertake Vamana karma before virechana in cases of Sanshodhana?
71. Role of Nasya in Ardita.
72. What are the benefits of using tail as a snehpana?
73. What are the Anupana of different types of sneha dravya?
74. What are Ashta Mahadoshakara bhava?
75. How many types of Sagni Sveda are described? Give their names.
76. Explain Niragni Sveda.
77. Explain Nadi Sveda in detail.
78. What is the correct sequence of mixing dravyas in Niruha basti?
79. What is the Pratyagaman kala for Niruha and Anuvasan Basti?
80. What is the treatment of Snehvyapad?
81. Explain procedure of Upnaha.
82. Differentiate between Gandusha and kavala.
83. Write about Mukha lepa.
84. Write heena, ati and samyag yog lakshana of Gandusha.
85. Write Vamnopaga mahakashya.
86. Write dravyas of Asthapanopaga and Anuvasanopaga Mahakashaya.
87. Write dravyas of Snehopaga Mahakashaya.
88. Describe Dhoomnetra.
89. Define Physitherapy.
90. Define Isometrics.

91. Write indications and contra indications of Static excercises.
92. Write importance of Raktamokshana in chikitsa.
93. Write description of Ksheera Basti.
94. Write names of Sneha Basti vyapat.
95. Write about Shaman Sneha.
96. Differentiate between Kavala and Gandusha.
97. Write definition of Snehana.
98. Write about Panchaprasrutikasneha Peya.
99. Write short note on Mardana and Unmardana.
100. Write about Electromagnetic therapy.

LONG ANSWER QUESTIONS

1. Describe the procedure of Shirodhara along with its mode of action.
2. Describe Purva, Pradhana and Pashchata karma of Virechana karma in details.
3. Give classification of Basti and describe Uttara basti procedure in detail.
4. Give classification of Nasya karma and describe doses and time of administration of various types of Nasya karma
5. What is the role of Virechana in Pakshaghata.
6. Define Basti and describe the procedure of Anuvasana Basti in detail.
7. Write in detail about various types of Basti vyapada along with their chikitsa.
8. Describe Purva pradhana and Pashchat karma of Jalaukavcharana in details.
9. Describe the specifications of Panchakarma speciality center along with manpower and equipments required.
10. Describe Purva, Pradhana and Pashchata karma of Abhyantara snehana in details.
11. Give classification of Basti and describe the procedure of Niruha basti in detail.
12. Write mode of action of Vamaka dravyas.
13. Write mode of action of Virechana dravyas.
14. Write mode of action of Shirodhara.
15. How Panchakarma is beneficial for a healthy person?
16. Explain vamana karma with its indications and contraindications?
17. What are the indications and contra indications of vamana karma along with their reasons?
18. What are the doshas of (a) Basti Netra, (b) Basti Putaka and (c) Basti Data
19. Explain Vaitrana basti in detail.
20. Explain Kshara basti in detail.
21. What are the Samyak, Heena and Atiyog lakshan of basti (both Anuvasan and Niruha).
22. Explain Lekhan Basti in detail and how it is beneficial for obesity?
23. What is the Nirukti of Basti? Give its importance and mode of action.
24. What are the Niruha Basti vyapad?
25. What are the Anuvasan Basti vyapad?
26. What is Yapana Basti? Explain raj Yapana basti in detail.

27. Why Niruha Basti is given on empty stomach? What are the complications if niruha is given after meals?
28. Explain Pravicharna for Snehpana along with types.
29. What are the Ayoga, Atiyog and Samyag yoga Lakshan of Snehpana?
30. What are the indications and contraindications of Snehpana?
31. What are Ashta Mahadoshakara Bhava? Write complications and treatment of each.
32. What are the indication and contraindication of svedana?
33. What is Sagni Sveda. Explain the types in details?
34. Explain Jentak Sveda in detail.
35. Explain Snehadhara in detail.
36. What are the indication and procedure of Shirodhara?
37. Explain indication and contraindication of Patrapinda sveda along with its procedure in detail.
38. Write the procedure of Shashtik Shali Pind Sveda including its Purva Pradhana and Pashchat karma
39. Explain the sizes of different types of Uttara Basti Netra and write indications of Uttara Basti in males.
40. Explain Murdha taila in detail with its indications.
41. What is Kala basti and what are its indication and mode of administration according to Kashyap?
42. Write the method of preparation of Anu Taila with its Matra in healthy individual.
43. Write mode of action of Nasya.
44. Write Pradhana karma of Vamana karma in details.
45. Write Siravedha Procedure in details.
46. Define Physiotherapy and give its importance in treatment in modern era.
47. What kind of Panchakarma procedures can be used in Nirama Sandhigata Vata. Give their mode of action on the disease.
48. Explain the Panchakarma procedures useful in Aamvata disease.
49. Why is Basti called as Ardha Chikitsa?
50. What is the importance of Panchakamra in modern era?

ABBREVIATIONS

Ch.	=	Charaka Samhita
Ch. Su.	=	Charak Samhita Sutrasthana
Ch. Si.	=	Charak Samhita Siddhisthana
Ch. Ka.	=	Charak Samhita Kalpasthana
Ch. Chi.	=	Charak Samhita Chikitsasthana
Ch. Vi.	=	Charak Samhita Vimanasthana
Su.	=	Sushruta Samhita
Su. Su.	=	Sushruta Samhita Sutrasthana
Su. Chi.	=	Sushruta Samhita Chikitsasthana
Su. Ut.	=	Sushruta Samhita Uttarastantra
Su. Sha.	=	Sushruta Samhita Sharirasthana
A.H.	=	Ashtanga Hridaya
A.H. Su.	=	Ashtanga Hridaya Sutrasthana
A.H. Ni.	=	Ashtanga Hridaya Nidanasthana
A.H. Ut.	=	Ashtanga Hridaya Uttarasthana
A. H. Chi.	=	Ashtanga Hridaya Chikitsasthana
A. H. Ka.	=	Ashtanga Hridaya Kalpasthana
A.S.	=	Ashtanga Sangraha
A. S. Su.	=	Ashtanga Sangraha Sutrasthana
A. S. Ut.	=	Ashtanga Sangraha Uttarasthana
A. S. Chi.	=	Ashtanga Sangraha Chikitsasthana
A. S. Ka.	=	Ashtanga Sangraha Kalpasthana
Ka. S.	=	Kashyapa Samhita
Ka. S. Khi.	=	Kashyapa Samhita Khilasthana
Bhe. S.	=	Bhela Samhita
Bhe. Su.	=	Bhela Samhita Sutrasthana
Bhe. Sa. Si.	=	Bhela Samhita Siddhisthana
Sha. S.	=	Sharangdhara Samhita
Sha. Pu.	=	Sharangdhara Samhita Purvakhanda
Sha. Ut.	=	Sharangdhara Samhita Uttarakhanda
C. D.	=	Chakradatta
Kai. Di. Ni.	=	Kaidev Nighantu
Dra. Gu. Vi.	=	Dravya Guna Vigyan
Ch. P.	=	Chakrapandi
SKD	=	Shabdakalpadruma
Pan. Sam.	=	Pancha karma Samhita
Bh. P.	=	Bhavaprakash

Index

Page numbers followed by, *f* refer to figure

R

T

W

Y

Z